The Trauma of Terrorism: Sharing Knowledge and Shared Care, An International Handbook

The Trauma of Terrorism: Sharing Knowledge and Shared Care, An International Handbook has been co-published simultaneously as *Journal of Aggression, Maltreatment & Trauma*, Volume 9, Numbers 1/2 and 3/4 2004 and Volume 10, Numbers 1/2 and 3/4 2005.

The Trauma of Terrorism: Sharing Knowledge and Shared Care, An International Handbook

Yael Danieli, PhD
Danny Brom, PhD
Joe Sills, MA
Editors

The Trauma of Terrorism: Sharing Knowledge and Shared Care, An International Handbook has been co-published simultaneously as *Journal of Aggression, Maltreatment & Trauma*, Volume 9, Numbers 1/2 and 3/4 2004 and Volume 10, Numbers 1/2 and 3/4 2005.

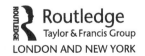

Routledge
Taylor & Francis Group
LONDON AND NEW YORK

First published 2005 by The Haworth Press, Inc
10 Alice Street, Binghamton, NY 13904-1580

This edition published in 2012 by Routledge
2 Park Square, Milton Park, Abingdon, Oxon OX14 4RN
711 Third Avenue, New York, NY 10017, USA
Routledge is an imprint of the Taylor & Francis Group, an informa business

The Trauma of Terrorism: Sharing Knowledge and Shared Care, An International Handbook has been co-published simultaneously as *Journal of Aggression, Maltreatment & Trauma*, Volume 9, Numbers 1/2 and 3/4 2004 and Volume 10, Numbers 1/2 and 3/4 2005.

The development, preparation, and publication of this work has been undertaken with great care. However, the publisher, employees, editors, and agents of The Haworth Press and all imprints of The Haworth Press, Inc., including The Haworth Medical Press® and The Pharmaceutical Products Press®, are not responsible for any errors contained herein or for consequences that may ensue from use of materials or information contained in this work. Opinions expressed by the author(s) are not necessarily those of The Haworth Press, Inc.

Cover design by Kerry E. Mack
Cover design concept by Clemens Weiss

Library of Congress Cataloging-in-Publication Data

The trauma of terrorism: sharing knowledge and shared care, an international handbook /Yael Danieli, Danny Brom and Joe Sills, editors.
    p. cm.
    "The Trauma of Terrorism: Sharing Knowledge and Shared Care, An International Handbook has been co-published simultaneously as Journal of Aggression, Maltreatment & Trauma, Volume 9, Numbers 1/2, 3/4 2004 and Volume 10, Numbers 1/2, 3/4 2005."
Includes bibliographical references and index.
    1. Terrorism–Psychological aspects. 2. Victims of terrorism–Psychology. I. Danieli, Yael II. Brom, D. III. Sills, Joe IV. Journal of aggression, maltreatment & trauma.
HV6431.T723. 2004
362.196'8521–dc22   2004023989
ISBN - 978 0 7890 2773 3

This Volume Is Dedicated
to the Victims/Survivors of Terrorism,
Their Families,
and to Those Who Care for Them.

The Trauma of Terrorism: Sharing Knowledge and Shared Care, An International Handbook

The Trauma of Terrorism: Sharing Knowledge and Shared Care, An International Handbook has been co-published simultaneously as *Journal of Aggression, Maltreatment & Trauma*, Volume 9, Numbers 1/2 and 3/4 2004 and Volume 10, Numbers 1/2 and 3/4 2005.

The Trauma of Terrorism: Sharing Knowledge and Shared Care, An International Handbook

CONTENTS

SECTION IV: PSYCHOLOGICAL FIRST AID, ACUTE
    AND LONG-TERM TREATMENT
    FOLLOWING TERRORIST ATTACKS

ABOUT THE EDITORS

Yael Danieli, PhD, is a Clinical Psychologist in private practice, a victimologist, traumatologist, and the Director of the Group Project for Holocaust Survivors and their Children, which she co-founded in 1975 in the New York City area. Dr. Danieli is also Founding President of the International Network of Holocaust and Genocide Survivors and their Friends. She has done extensive psychotherapeutic work with survivors and children of survivors. She has studied in depth post-war responses and attitudes toward them, and the impact these and the Holocaust had on their lives. She has lectured and published worldwide in numerous books and journals, translated into at least 11 languages, on optimal care and training for this and other massively traumatized victim/survivor populations, and has received several awards for her work, the most recent of which is the Lifetime Achievement Award of the International Society for Traumatic Stress Studies (ISTSS). Most recently, she has been appointed consultant to the International Criminal Court on issues related to victims and staff care. She has served as consultant to South Africa's Truth and Reconciliation Commission and the Rwanda government on reparations for victims, and has led *Promoting a Dialogue: Democracy Cannot Be Built with the Hands of Broken Souls* in Bosnia and Herzegovina. Her books are: *International Responses to Traumatic Stress . . .*; *The Universal Declaration of Human Rights: Fifty Years and Beyond*; *Sharing the Front Line and the Back Hills*; and *International Handbook of Multigenerational Legacies of Trauma*.

A Founding Director and past President of the ISTSS, the Initial Report of her Presidential Task Force on Curriculum, Education, and Training for professionals working with victim/survivors was adopted by the United Nations. She has also co-chaired the ISTSS Task Force on International Trauma Training. Dr. Danieli has been the Senior Representative to the United Nations of the World Federation for Mental Health (WFMH) and of the ISTSS. A Founding Member of WFMH's Scientific Committee on the Mental Health Needs of Victims, and its Chair, she has been active in developing, promoting, adapting and implementing the United Nations Declaration of Basic Principles of Justice for Victims of Crime and Abuse of Power and all subsequent UN victims-related work, including their right to reparation and their role in the International Criminal

Court. She has served as Consultant to numerous UN agencies and programs and to various governments concerning trauma and victim/survivor's rights and care. In the US, she has consulted for the National Institute of Mental Health, the Federal Bureau of Investigation, and various news organizations.

She taught at Brooklyn College and at John Jay College for Criminal Justice of the City University of New York, and has been a faculty member and supervisor at the (US) National Institute for the Psychotherapies. Before arriving in the United States (for a Doctorate in Psychology at New York University earned in 1981), she served as a Sergeant in the Israeli Armed Forces, earned degrees, taught and wrote in music, philosophy and psychology.

Danny Brom, PhD, is a Clinical Psychologist and founding Director of the Temmy and Albert Latner Israel Center for the Treatment of Psychotrauma at Herzog Hospital in Jerusalem, Israel. His main interest and experience lie in the prevention, treatment, and research of the consequences of traumatic stress. Dr. Brom has worked in the field of traumatic stress since 1979, first in the Netherlands where he was the Director of the Dutch Institute of Psychotrauma from 1985 until 1988. In 1989 he was appointed Director of the Latner Institute for Research in Social Psychiatry and Psychotherapy at Herzog Hospital in Jerusalem. In addition, he was Director of Research of Amcha, the Israeli National Center for Psychosocial Support of Survivors of the Holocaust and the Second Generation. Dr. Brom has also been teaching at the Department of Clinical Psychology of Hebrew University since 1998. He has published numerous articles and chapters. His books include *Coping with Trauma: Consequences, Prevention and Treatment* (Swets & Zeitlinger). He has been active in training mental health professionals in different countries. He is chair of the Israel Trauma Coalition that he initiated together with UJA-Federation of New York; the coalition includes over 40 organizations which collaborate on the development, evaluation and dissemination of trauma-related services.

Joe Sills, MA, retired from the United Nations secretariat at the end of 1998, following a 17-year career with the world organization. He remains active in UN-related matters, serving as a consultant to the UN Compensation Commission (a subsidiary body of the Security Council, established to process claims and pay compensation for losses resulting from Iraq's invasion and occupation of Kuwait), the UN Office for Drug Control and Crime Prevention, the American Council for the UN University, the International Labour Organization, and the United Nations Foundation. He co-chaired the task force of the Corporate Council on Africa on HIV/AIDS in southern Africa and is a member of the Board of the US Council for the United Nations Population Fund. Mr. Sills joined the United Nations secretariat in 1981, following eight years as Vice President of the United Nations Association of the USA. For six years, he was associate spokesman for Secretary-General Javier Pérez de Cuéllar. Concurrently, he formulated and directed the information programs for two UN conferences: The International Conference on Drug Abuse and Illicit Trafficking (Vienna, 1987) and the UN Conference on Environment and Development (Rio de Janeiro, 1992). Mr. Sills then became Director of the Communications and Project Management Division of the UN Department of Public Information. In 1996, Mr. Sills was appointed Director of the United Nations Information Center in Washington, DC. Before assignment to Washington, he was spokesman for United Nations Secretary-General Boutros Boutros-Ghali for over three years. He received his BA degree from Vanderbilt University and his MA degree in Arab Area Studies from the American University of Beirut in Lebanon.

About the Contributors

Hirad Abtahi is Deputy Chef de Cabinet and Legal Adviser in the Immediate Office of the President of the International Criminal Court (ICC). Prior to joining the ICC, he was extensively involved in the "Milosevic trial," as Chambers' Legal Officer, at the International Criminal Tribunal for the former Yugoslavia. Hirad Abtahi was also a legal consultant with the Geneva-based International Commission of Jurists, where he advised on the issues of victims and witnesses, detention and enforcement of sentences. He has lectured and published articles in English, French, and Persian on human rights, humanitarian law, and international criminal law issues.

Rhonda Adessky, PhD, is the Co-Founder and Co-Director of the Center for the Treatment of Traumatic Stress and Anxiety Disorders, a treatment, research and training center in Cognitive Behavior Therapy at Hadassah University Hospital. Dr. Adessky received her PhD in Clinical Psychology from Concordia University in 1996. She completed a Postdoctoral Fellowship in the Department of Psychology at Yale University. Dr. Adessky worked at the Yale Psychological Services Clinic and was the interim Director from 1998-1999. She has taught courses in cognitive behavioral therapy in Israel and abroad. Dr. Adessky has lived in Israel since November 2000.

Jennifer Ahern has a MPH in Epidemiology and Biostatistics from the University of California at Berkeley, and is the Senior Research Analyst for the Center for Urban Epidemiologic Studies at The New York Academy of Medicine. Her work includes research on mental health in New York City after September 11, the effects of discrimination on the mental and physical health of drug users, and mortality rates in New York City. She also conducts research on individual and neighborhood level social determinants of health, specifically in relation to birth outcomes, mental health and causes of mortality. Her previous work includes studies of work place health and wellbeing within police departments and health care settings.

Lawrence Amsel, MD, MPH, is a Psychiatric Researcher, Clinician and Educator. He is the director of Dissemination Research for Trauma Studies and Treatment at the New York State Psychiatric Institute and Assistant Professor of Clinical Psychiatry at Columbia University. Dr. Amsel has done cutting edge research on applying Decision Science and Game Theory to clinical psychiatry. Applications have included improving dissemination of evidence-based mental health practices through the use of motivational strategies, and developing a Game Theoretic model of suicidal behavior that organizes empirical findings in novel ways that may help improve the prediction and prevention of suicide.

Tali Arad was born and has lived her entire life in Jerusalem. She recalls vividly when, as a young child, a bomb inside a refrigerator on Jaffa street in downtown Jerusalem exploded, killing and injuring several people, sparing her mother and baby brother. She served in the NAHAL (Pioneer Fighting Youth, who serve both in the army and on the kibbutz). After discharge, she graduated from the David Yellin College of Education in Jerusalem. Subsequently changing her profession, she graduated from the Koteret School of Journalism and Communication in Tel-Aviv. Since 2000 she has worked at a local Jerusalem newspaper.

Alan Atkinson is a Journalist based in Adelaide with the Australian Broadcasting Corporation. Born in England, he has worked for several major newspapers, including *The Guardian*, London. He was on holiday in Bali when two bombs killed 202 people in Kuta nightclubs on October 12, 2002, and was one of the first Western reporters on the scene. An account of his family holiday which turned into reporting on horror has been published by the ABC under the title *Three Weeks in Bali*. Published by the Singapore company, Flame of the Forest, it is available through Amazon.com as *Terror in Bali*.

Enrique Baca is Chairman of the Psychiatry Department of Autonoma University of Madrid as well as the head of the Psychiatry Department of Puerta de Hierro Hospital. He is the president of the Spanish Society of Psychiatry. He is the senior author of numerous articles and editor of more than 20 books.

Enrique Baca-García, PhD, has carried out research in severe mental illnesses since 1994. He has completed his residency with a fellowship in psychiatry research at Hospital Ramon y Cajal (Madrid) and Universidad de Alcalá (Madrid). During these years he obtained the first NARSAD (National Alliance for Research on Schizophrenia and Depression) grant for Spain. He has published some 30 articles in peer-reviewed journals. Currently, he works as attending psychiatrist at Fundacion Jimenez Diaz, where he directs the psychiatry residency program, and is Associate Professor at Autonoma University of Madrid.

Martin Barber became Director of the United Nations Mine Action Service (UNMAS) in December 2000, bringing with him extensive experience in humanitarian and emergency operations and United Nations bodies. Prior to joining UNMAS, he was Chief of the Policy Development and Advocacy Branch of the United Nations Office for the Coordination of Humanitarian Affairs in New York. He served previously as the Deputy Special Representative of the Secretary-General in Bosnia and Herzegovina, and Humanitarian Coordinator of the office for the Coordination of Humanitarian Assistance in Afghanistan. From 1981 to 1988 he was Director of the British Refugee Council in London.

Naomi L. Baum, PhD, is the Director of the National School Intervention Project at the Israel Center for the Treatment of Psychotrauma, Jerusalem. She did her graduate work at Bryn Mawr College in educational psychology. She has worked as a consulting psychologist in schools and educational frameworks in both Israel and the USA for over two decades. Dr. Baum has taught psychology to teacher trainees at colleges in Israel and the USA. She was a fellow at the Mandel School for Educational Leadership in Jerusalem from 2000-2002. She is married and the mother of seven children.

Fortu Benarroch, PhD, is a Child and Adolescent Psychiatrist and the Clinical Director of the Orion Center for Treatment of Trauma in Children and Adolescents, in the department of Child and Adolescent Psychiatry in Hadassah University Hospital. He is also the Psychiatric Consultant to the Pediatric Neurology Unit in Shaarei Tzedek Medical Center. He formerly served as the Chief Psychiatrist in the IDF (Israel Defense Force) Air Force.

Bella Ben-Gershon, MSW, is a Clinical Social Worker and Psychotherapist. She attended the Hebrew University and graduated in 1990 with a diploma in psychotherapy. She has authored many papers in journals and book chapters about the psychological consequences of terrorism, social work and counseling.

Rony Berger, PsyD, is a licensed Clinical Psychologist and a Family and Couples Therapist. He is the Director of Community Services at Natal, Israel Trauma Center for Victims of Terror and War, and a researcher at the Harry Truman Center for the Advancement of Peace, The Hebrew University of Jerusalem. Between 1997-2001 Dr. Berger was a Visiting Professor for Psychology at Al Quds University, Palestine, where he taught graduate students and co-directed the Palestinian Center for Traumatic Stress Studies. Dr. Berger has also lectured, consulted and given workshops to numerous governmental agencies and organizations in the United States.

Avi Bleich, MD, MPA, is the Director of Lev-HaSharon Mental Health Center and Chairman of Psychiatry at Tel-Aviv University Medical School. In his former military career, he was the commander (Colonel) of the Mental Health Services of the Israel Defense Forces. Throughout his career, Prof. Bleich devoted his energies to clinical issues, teaching and academic affairs, and management of medical systems. One of his main research interests is traumatic stress, with its short- and long-lasting psychological effects.

Angela S. Boudreaux, BA, is Research Associate at the Stetson Institute for Social Research and a graduate candidate in the Stetson University Department of Counselor Education Mental Health Counseling Program. Since 1996, she has been involved in studies of public safety workers who have responded to terrorism in the U.S.A.

Alain Brunet, PhD, conducts biological and psychological investigations on the etiology and treatment of Post-Traumatic Stress Disorder. He is Assistant Professor at the Department of Psychiatry, McGill University (Québec, Canada). He is also a Researcher at the Douglas Hospital Research Center, and Coordinator of the Research and Education Program at the National Center for Operational Stress of Veterans Affairs Canada, at the St.-Anne Center.

Maria Luisa Cabanas is a Psychologist. She has worked as the director of the Psychological Assistance Center of the Association of Victims of Terrorism (AVT) since 1992. Currently, she is the director of the Institute of Victimology in Madrid.

Ed Cairns, BA, PhD, FBPsS, is Professor of Psychology at the University of Ulster. He has spent the last 30 years studying the psychological aspects of political violence in relation to the conflict in Northern Ireland. He has been a visiting scholar at the Universities of Florida, Cape Town and Melbourne. He is a Fellow of the British Psychological Society and Past President of the Division of Peace Psychology of the APA. His most recent books are: Cairns, E. (1996), *Children and Political Violence*; Cairns, E., & Roe, M. (Eds.), (2003) *The Role of Memory in Ethnic Conflict*. Palgrave/Macmillan: London, New York.

Andrea Campbell, BSc, is a graduate student in Psychology at the University of Ulster at Coleraine where she is currently pursuing a PhD in Social Psychology. Her research interests include Social Identity Theory and multidimensional aspects of prejudice in relation to the conflict in Northern Ireland.

Peter S. Canellos, has been Deputy Managing Editor and Washington Bureau Chief for *The Boston Globe* since 2003. A graduate of the University of Pennsylvania and Columbia Law School, he has covered national affairs, urban issues, and politics during his 16 years at *The Boston Globe*. In Boston he oversaw the *Globe's* local coverage, including Health, Science, Education, and Ideas Sections. He dedicates this contribution to his beloved partner of 13 years, Elizabeth Neuffer, an award-winning journalist and author whose voice would have been a part of this book, who died May 9, 2003, in a car crash in Iraq.

Claude M. Chemtob, PhD, is a Clinical Psychologist and Researcher specializing in trauma in adults and children. Dr. Chemtob is Clinical Professor of psychiatry and pediatrics at the Mount Sinai School of Medicine and currently serves as the Saul Z. Cohen Chair in Child and Family Mental Health at the

Jewish Board for Family and Children's Services in New York City. He is the principal investigator of a large National Institute of Mental Health-funded collaborative between Mount Sinai and JBFCS aimed at translating evidence-based approaches to child trauma assessment and intervention to community service settings. He was a consultant to the Presidential Commission of the French Republic, to the U.S. National Advisory Committee on Children and Terrorism, and currently consults on terrorism response in Israel in the context of a U.S.-Israel bi-national initiative established by the UJA Federation.

Susan and Daniel Cohen are the parents of Theodora Cohen who was killed in the terrorist bombing of Pan Am 103 on December 21, 1988. The Cohens are longtime freelance writers with some 200 books and many articles to their credit. They are the authors of *Pan Am 103* (revised edition, Signet, 2001).

Chris Cramer is Managing Director of CNN International. This includes overseeing the editorial and programming components of CNN International and associated services, with the additional responsibility of management of the 28 international bureaus. He is also the honorary president of the International News Safety Institute, a new global organization established to work toward protecting journalists. He is a fellow of the Royal Television Society, a member of the British Association of Film and Television Arts and a member of the Board of Councilors of the Jimmy Carter Center in Atlanta.

Gerald Cromer, PhD, teaches in the Department of Criminology, Bar Ilan University. He is the author of *The Writing Was on the Wall: Constructing Political Deviance in Israel* (Bar Ilan University Press: Ramat Gan, 1988), *Narratives of Violence* (Ashgate: Aldershot, 2001) and *A War of Words: Political Violence and Political Debate in Israel* (Frank Cass: London, 2004). He is presently working on a study of the use of war as a metaphor.

Barbara Crossette, a Columnist for U.N. Wire, an independent Internet news service, was *The New York Times* United Nations Bureau Chief from 1994 to 2001. She was earlier the *Times* chief correspondent in Southeast Asia and South Asia and diplomatic reporter in Washington. She authored "So Close to Heaven: The Vanishing Buddhist Kingdoms of the Himalayas;" "The Great Hill Stations of Asia;" and "India: Old Civilization in a New World." Ms. Crossette won a George Polk award for her coverage of the assassination in 1991 of Rajiv Ghandi, and an Interaction award in 1998 for coverage of international humanitarian issues.

Rabbi Zahara Davidowitz-Farkas is engaged in the response and recovery efforts of 9/11 and founded the Institute for Disaster Spiritual Care. She is a partner member of the Critical Response Team of the American Red Cross.

Previously, Rabbi Davidowitz-Farkas directed the Weiler Chaplaincy of the New York Board of Rabbis, coordinated Jewish chaplaincy at New York Hospital-Cornell Medical Center, and was Dean of Hebrew Union College-Jewish Institute of Religion in New York. She has written and lectured on topics such as spiritual care in the context of disaster, Jewish pastoral care, death and dying, and bioethics.

Joyce M. Davis, Associate Director of Broadcasting for Radio Free Europe/Radio Liberty in Prague, was previously Journalist in Residence at the Pew International Journalism Program. She is a specialist in the Middle East and Islamic movements. Her newest book, *Martyrs: Innocence, Vengeance and Despair in the Middle East*, offers insights into Islam's teaching on martyrdom and its connection to the September 11th attacks on the United States. She has been Deputy Foreign Editor of Knight Ridder Newspapers, Senior Fellow with the United States Institute of Peace, and foreign editor and Director of News Staffing for National Public Radio.

Ellen R. DeVoe, PhD, MSW, is Assistant Professor at Columbia University School of Social Work in New York City. Dr. DeVoe's work has focused on the impact of family and community violence on young children and families and on the development and evaluation of interventions designed to mitigate these effects. Dr. DeVoe has a program of federally-funded research including a study of the impact of September 11 on very young children and their families in New York City.

Amy Dorin, MS, ACSW, is Senior Vice President, Behavioral Health Services, F.E.G.S., overseeing a $46 million outpatient behavioral health network with programs in New York City and Long Island serving approximately 18,000 people annually. A graduate of Boston University and Columbia University's School of Social Work, in her 30-year career in Human Services she worked as a clinician, administrator, and government official, in the New York City Mayor's Office of Operations, Children's Aid Society, and Montefiore Hospital. Ms. Dorin received the New York State Office of Mental Health award for "Excellence in Service" for 2001.

Julie Dunsmore is a Psychologist with 25 years experience in the area of loss, grief and trauma. She is the President of the National Association of Loss and Grief and currently provides outreach and support to survivors, the bereaved, and others involved with or witness to the Bali bombing. This has worked closely with a range of support agencies including the Coroners Court and the Australian Federal Police. She is the director of Health Promotion in Northern Sydney Health and has made a number of award-winning documentaries on loss and grief, particularly related to cancer and neonatal death.

Brian Engdahl, PhD, has been a Counseling Psychologist at the Department of Veterans Affairs Medical Center for 25 years, and is Clinical Associate Professor in the Department of Psychology at the University of Minnesota, Minneapolis, Minnesota. He provides counseling to combat veterans of all wars, and to active duty soldiers of the Iraq war who have experienced spinal cord and traumatic brain injuries. His research examines health and adjustment of former prisoners of war and other combat veterans. He has published and presented his findings to national and international audiences of trauma survivors, their families, and professionals working with them.

Gerry Fairbrother, PhD, is a Senior Scientist and Fellow at The New York Academy of Medicine and Research Director of its Child Health Forum. Dr. Fairbrother holds a faculty appointment in Epidemiology and Social Medicine at the Albert Einstein College of Medicine. Her research is policy-oriented and focuses on the ability of the health care delivery system to respond to the needs of children and families. Dr. Fairbrother has examined the effects of September 11 on New York City children and the delivery system's ability to identify and serve the mental health needs of children after a terrorist attack.

Micha Feldmann is a senior member of SELAH-Israel Crisis Management Center, a volunteer network that, since 1993, has helped more than 10,000 new immigrant families struck by tragedy. From 1982 on, he has devoted his life largely to bringing Ethiopian Jews to Israel and aiding their absorption into society. He was a chief architect of "Operation Solomon" which in one weekend brought 14,310 Ethiopian Jews out of besieged Addis Ababa. In 1994, he spent four months in Rwanda assisting over 100,000 refugees in returning home to neighboring countries. In 1998 he published his first book (in Hebrew), *The Ethiopian Exodus*.

Elisheva Flamm-Oren, BSW, MSW, is responsible for the programs in the areas of community, welfare and health of the Israel Office of the UJA-Federation of New York, and has played a pivotal role initiating and developing the Israel Trauma Coalition. She received her degrees from the Paul Berwald School of Social Work, the Hebrew University of Jerusalem, where she specialized in planning, policy and management of social welfare services, later teaching strategic planning and management in social services there. For ten years she worked with Mayor Teddy Kollek at the Jerusalem Foundation as director of community welfare and health programs.

Brian W. Flynn is a Consultant, Writer, Trainer, and Speaker specializing in preparation for, response to, and recovery from, the psychosocial aspects of large-scale emergencies and disasters. In addition, he currently serves as Associate Director of the Center for the Study of Traumatic Stress, and Professor (Adj.), Department of Psychiatry, Uniformed Services University of the

Health Sciences. He is a retired Rear Admiral/Assistant Surgeon General in the United States Public Health Service. For more than two decades he directly operated, or supervised the operation of, the Federal Government's domestic disaster mental health program (including terrorism).

Victor M. Fornari, MD, is Associate Chairman for Education and Training, Department of Psychiatry, North Shore University Hospital and directs child and general psychiatry training. He is Associate Professor of Psychiatry, NYU School of Medicine and Past President, Greater Long Island Psychiatric Society (American Psychiatric Association). He belongs to the Critical Incident Response Team and the Mental Health Disaster Task Force, Nassau County. He is a leader of peer AIDS and peer traumatic stress educational programs in regional schools. He provided consultation to Long Island school districts, addressing students' mental health needs post-9/11 and improving school disaster mental health plans.

Sara Freedman, MSc, is the Co-Founder and Co-Director of the Center for the Treatment of Traumatic Stress and Anxiety Disorders, a treatment, research and training center in Cognitive Behavior Therapy at Hadassah University Hospital. She received her MSc in Psychology at the Institute of Psychiatry in England. She is currently completing her PhD from the Hebrew University in Jerusalem. She teaches cognitive behaviour therapy at the Hebrew University School of Medicine, among other places. She moved to Israel in 1991.

Matthew J. Friedman, MD, PhD, is Executive Director of the National Center for Post-Traumatic Stress Disorder (PTSD), headquartered at the Department of Veterans' Affairs Medical Center in White River Junction, Vermont, and Professor of Psychiatry and of Pharmacology at Dartmouth Medical School, Hanover, New Hampshire. He has worked with PTSD patients as a clinician and researcher for 30 years and has published extensively on stress and PTSD. Dr. Friedman is past-president of the International Society for Traumatic Stress Studies and a Distinguished Fellow of the American Psychiatric Association. He has published over 140 scientific articles, books and chapters.

Carol S. Fullerton, PhD, is Associate Research Professor in the Department of Psychiatry and Scientific Director of the Center for the Study of Traumatic Stress at the Uniformed Services University of the Health Sciences Medical School, Bethesda, Maryland. Dr. Fullerton is widely published in individual and community responses to trauma and disasters, and psychological and public health effects of terrorism on the workplace. She has consulted on research programs following the September 11th attacks. Dr. Fullerton was awarded the Department of Defense Meritorious Service Medal (1990), and the Exceptional Service Medal (1993), for her research and consultation to disaster populations.

Sandro Galea, MD, is Associate Director of the Center for Urban Epidemiologic Studies at The New York Academy of Medicine and Assistant Professor of Clinical Epidemiology at Columbia University, Mailman School of Public Health. He has a MD from the University of Toronto, an MPH in epidemiology and biostatistics from Harvard University and a DrPH in epidemiology from Columbia University. Dr. Galea is primarily interested in the social and economic determinants of health and risk behavior in urban settings. His recent research includes mental health, drug use, and sudden cardiac arrest. He has worked as a clinician in remote rural communities in Northern Canada and in Mudug Region, Somalia.

Esti Galili-Weisstub, MD, is Director of Child and Adolescent Psychiatry at Hadassah University Hospital in Jerusalem. She established the Orion Center for Treatment of Trauma in Children and Adolescents. She is the President of the Israel Child and Adolescent Psychiatric Association and Consultant to the Israeli Knesset (parliament) on Issues of Child and Adolescent Psychiatry. She is a member of the Israel Council of Mental Health, which serves as an advisory board to the Israeli Minister of Health. Dr. Galili-Weisstub is also a Training Analyst of the Israel Society of Analytical Psychology (Jungian Psychoanalysis).

Boaz Ganor, MA, is Executive Director of The International Policy Institute for Counter-Terrorism. His Doctoral thesis is entitled *Israel's Counter Terrorism Policy–Efficacy versus Liberal-Democratic Values 1983-1999*. Dr. Ganor holds an MA in Political Science from Tel-Aviv University. His Master's thesis was entitled *The Influence of Terror on Israeli Public Opinion*. He is an expert on combating terrorism and has written many articles and publications on this subject. He also conducts courses and seminars on terrorism and counter-terrorism policies. Dr. Ganor was a member of the Israeli delegation to the trilateral (American-Palestinian-Israeli) Committee for Monitoring Incitement to Violence and Terror.

Robert Gifford, PhD, is a member of the Department of Psychiatry, Center for the Study of Traumatic Stress, Uniformed Services University in Bethesda, MD. Dr. Gifford is a research psychologist with extensive experience studying the impact of deployment and combat stress on active duty military members and their units. Before retiring from the Army in 2003, he served as the Executive Officer in charge of the Walter Reed Army Institute of Research, Washington, DC.

Virginia Gil-Rivas, PhD, is Assistant Professor in the Department of Psychology at the University of North Carolina, Charlotte. Dr. Gil-Rivas has authored several papers examining the association between trauma exposure and substance abuse disorders. Her current interests are the role of close interpersonal relationships, stress and coping as they related to psychological well-being and health among adolescents and adults, cross-cultural research, and research with diverse populations within the U.S.

Dodie Gill, LPC, LSATP, CEAP, founded the Arlington Employee Assistance Program in 1980. She has broad experience in program development and administration, management consultation, and crisis intervention, as well as family treatment and individual and group counseling. Additionally, she has extensive experience working with treatment issues related to trauma. Following the terrorist attack on the Pentagon, she developed and directed the critical incident stress management response for Arlington County public safety employees. Dodie Gill is a frequent speaker at professional seminars and is internationally known for her work in advancing the employee assistance profession.

Kimberly B. Gill, MA, is Assistant Director of Mental Health Disaster Preparedness and Response at the New York City Department of Health and Mental Hygiene. Ms. Gill received a BA in psychology from Miami University in Oxford, OH and a MA in Applied Psychology from Teachers College, Columbia University. Her previous experience includes management of clinical trials at the New York State Psychiatric Institute, evaluating treatments for individuals living with co-occurring psychiatric and substance abuse disorders. Ms. Gill currently serves to assist in establishing a comprehensive mental health disaster preparedness plan for the City of New York.

Al Goodman is CNN's Madrid Bureau Chief since 2000. For most of the preceding five years, he freelanced, concurrently, from Spain for *The New York Times* and CNN. He earlier freelanced for National Public Radio and the *International Herald Tribune*. He has made numerous trips to the Basque region. He is co-author of *The World on A String: How to Become a Freelance Foreign Correspondent* (Henry Holt and Company, New York, 1997), a primer of advice and anecdotes that has been used at American journalism schools.

Sir Jeremy Greenstock, GCMG, was a career member of the British Foreign Service (Her Majesty's Diplomatic Service) from 1969 to 2004. From September 2003, he was United Kingdom (UK) Special Representative for Iraq, working alongside the Civilian Provisional Authority Administrator, Ambassador Paul Bremmer, to bring stability and economic recovery to post-conflict Iraq. Between July 1998 and July 2003, he was UK Permanent Representative at the United Nations in New York, representing the UK on the Security Council and chairing the Council's Counter-Terrorism Committee. A specialist in Arab world affairs, he has served in Dubai, Jedda/Riyadh and

Paris, as Minister in the British Embassy in Washington, and as Political Director in the Foreign & Commonwealth Office in London. Before joining the diplomatic service, Sir Jeremy taught classics at Eton College. He was educated at Harrow and Worcester College, Oxford.

Alexander Grinshpoon, MD, is a Psychiatrist. He received his MD from Kishinev State University in 1977 and his MHA at Ben-Gurion University of Negev in 1999. He has authored papers in journals and book chapters about psychiatric epidemiology, forensic psychiatry, and psychological consequences of terrorism.

Clyde Haberman, who writes the New York City column for *The New York Times*, was a foreign correspondent for that newspaper from 1982 to 1995, based in Tokyo, Rome, and then Jerusalem. He has covered major events like the overthrow of Philippine President Marcos, pro-democracy uprisings in South Korea, Communism's collapse in Eastern Europe, the Persian Gulf War and its aftermath, the breakthrough 1993 Israeli-P.L.O. agreement, and the rise of militant Islamic terrorism. Haberman, with *The New York Times* since 1977, coming from the *New York Post*, has also been City Hall bureau chief and an editor in the "Week in Review" section.

Molly J. Hall, MD, is Associate Professor and Assistant Chair in the Department of Psychiatry, Uniformed Services University Medical School. She directs the Bioterrorism Education Project for the Center for the Study of Traumatic Stress. Dr. Hall is the psychiatry consultant to the Council of Governments Bioterrorism Task Force and Animal Services Committee for Maryland, Virginia, and the District of Columbia. She provides mental health consultation to the Veterinary Medical Assistance Teams, National Medical Defense System, responding to natural disasters and epidemic livestock loss.

Brandon Hamber was born in South Africa and trained there as a clinical psychologist. He currently works in Northern Ireland. He is Research Associate of the Belfast-based think-tank, Democratic Dialogue, and a consultant to the Office of Psychosocial Issues at the Free University in Berlin. He has been the recipient of the Tip O'Neill Fellowship (1997/1998) in Northern Ireland and Rockefeller Resident Fellowship (1996) in Brazil. He is a board member of the Khulumani Victim Support Group. Previously, he coordinated the Transition and Reconciliation Unit at the Centre for the Study of Violence and Reconciliation in South Africa.

Jessica L. Hamblen, PhD, received a PhD in Clinical Psychology from the State University of New York at Buffalo in 2000. She is Associate Director for Research and Education at the National Center for PTSD. She served as the Co-Director of a project that examined New York's mental health systems' responses to 9/11. In addition, she was principal author of a 12-session cognitive behavioral intervention for continuing postdisaster disaster that was used by Project Liberty as part of their enhanced services initiative after 9/11.

Susan E. Hamilton, PhD, is Senior Associate, Disaster Mental Health Services (DMHS) of the American Red Cross and responsible for the ongoing development and implementation of the DMHS Program on a national level. She provides technical guidance to disaster relief operations throughout the United States, and works closely with the national mental health associations, Federal and State Agencies. Dr. Hamilton received her PhD in clinical psychology from the Institute of Psychiatry, University of London, England. Her career has included private practice, research, university teaching, directing programs, and serving as a consultant to a variety of organizations.

David Handschuh is Staff Photographer at the *New York Daily News* and Adjunct Professor of Photojournalism at New York University. Past President of the National Press Photographers Association, he co-authored the National Media Guide for Emergency and Disaster Incidents. During months of recovery from serious injuries suffered while covering the attack on the World Trade Center, he implemented several programs to document and address long-term physical and mental health issues for journalists who worked at Ground Zero. For this, he was awarded "Fellow of the Society," the highest honor bestowed by Sigma Delta Chi, the National Society of Professional Journalists.

Margaret Heldring, PhD, is a Clinical Psychologist and President of America's HealthTogether, a nonprofit organization promoting health and social justice. She has been Clinical Assistant Professor of Family Medicine at the University of Washington and coordinator of Behavioral Sciences for a family practice residency program at Swedish Medical Center in Seattle. Dr. Heldring served as Director of Health Policy for Bill Bradley's 2000 presidential campaign and chief health advisor to Senators Bradley and Paul Wellstone. She is editor for Family Health Policy for *Families, Systems and Health* and is on the Editorial Advisory Board for *The American Family Physician.*

Martin Herskovitz lives in Petah Tikva, Israel. He is employed as a civilian Safety Manager in the Israel Defense Forces. Among his hobbies are writing poetry and moderating a mailgroup/list-serv for children of Holocaust survivors. His poetry has been published in Midstream, Caring for a Holocaust Survivor–A Practice Manual, and on-line in a E-Journal "If Not Now." His poem "Photographs" won an Honorable Mention in the Reuben Rose Contest in 2002. He has presented his poetry in Second Generation conferences in Chicago, 2002 and Toronto, 2003.

E. Alison Holman, PhD, FNP, is Staff Research Associate at the Health Policy and Research Unit, University of California, Irvine. A health psychologist and family nurse practitioner with clinical experience with children and their families, she has studied coping in various traumatized populations. Her research addresses interactive effects of cognitive, social, emotional, and physical responses on adaptation to traumatic stress. She is co-principal investigator of a nationwide longitudinal study addressing the mental and physical health consequences of trauma following the September 11th attacks. In 2001, she received the Chaim Danieli Young Professional Award from the International Society of Traumatic Stress Studies.

Ruth Pat-Horenczyk received her PhD in Psychology from the Hebrew University of Jerusalem. She is the director of the child and adolescent clinical services at the Israel Center for the Treatment of Psychotrauma in Jerusalem, teaches in the Department of Psychology at the Hebrew University, and works as a clinical psychologist in private practice. Dr. Pat-Horenczyk is involved in clinical research and teaching courses on trauma, sleep medicine, and eating disorders. Currently she conducts a screening project of post-traumatic distress among children and adolescents, develops school-based interventions, and leads an interest group on the treatment of traumatized children.

Shelley Horwitz, MSW, Director of Planning and Allocations, Caring Commission at UJA-Federation of New York, has spearheaded bi-national collaborations between American and Israeli professionals to develop joint strategies for clinical and community interventions in response to trauma and terrorism. Following 9/11 she was instrumental in designing programs to meet a wide range of community needs for UJA-Federation agencies serving victims and their families. Ms. Horwitz serves on the executive committee of the New York City Voluntary Organizations Active in Disaster, whose objective is to organize coordinated city-wide disaster preparedness strategies for the human services sector.

Reverend Hierodeacon John Hutchison-Hall is Executive Director of Disaster Spiritual Care Services–New York. Fr. John was a part of the American Red Cross' spiritual care team on the 9/11 disaster serving as Assistant Officer for service centers. Prior to his work with the American Red Cross, he served in various senior administrative capacities with the Missionary Society of St. Constantine's outreach and chaplaincy programs in Siberia and Romania. A native of New York City, Fr. John's first life was on Wall Street, and he has over a decade of experience in international finance and trading.

Louis Jehel, PhD, is a Psychiatrist responsible for the Emergency and Psychotraumatology University Unit (University Hospital Tenon, AP-HP, Paris France). He conducts studies on the etiology and treatment of trauma survivors with Post-traumatic Disorders. He teaches psychotraumatology to medical students at the University of Paris VI and Paris XII. Recently, he has served as an expert on the assessment of PTSD in many consensus conferences in France.

Gilah Kahn-Hoffmann is the Reporting/Information Officer for the Israel Trauma Coalition. She earned her BA from McGill University. In Israel, she has worked as a journalist, writing, editing and translating for *The Jerusalem Post* and various other publications.

Sandra J. Kaplan, MD, is Vice-Chairman of the Department of Psychiatry, North Shore University Hospital (NSUH) of the North Shore-Long Island Jewish Health System and Professor of Clinical Psychiatry, NYU School of Medicine. She serves on the Steering Committee of the National Child Traumatic Stress Network (NCTSN), US Substance Abuse and Mental Health Services Administration, is Co-Director of the NSUH NCTSN Center and Principal Investigator of the NIMH supported: "Follow-up Study: Young Adults Physically Abused as Adolescents." In 2001, she received the American Psychiatric Association Agnes McGavin Award and is a member of its Council on Children and Families.

Noureddine Khaled, PhD, a doctor of psychology and social psychology, is Professor at Algiers University where he lectures and supervises graduate and postgraduate theses. He has been a practicing psychotherapist since 1987. He directed research reports and publications about adolescents, deviant behavior, school success and failure. He was president of SARP (Algerian Society for Research in Psychology) between 1997 and 2003 where he directed a psychosocial program for victims of terrorism with an epidemiological study and many publications. He is the director of the project "Psychological and Psychosocial Help for Victims of Violence in Algeria."

J. David Kinzie, MD, is Professor of Psychiatry at Oregon Health & Science University, Portland, Oregon. The founder of the Indochinese Psychiatric Program (now Intercultural Psychiatric Program), he still treats Somali, Cambodian, and Central American refugees. He is Director of the Torture Treatment Center of Oregon and of the Child Traumatic Stress Clinic, both in the Department of Psychiatry. He is a Distinguished Life Fellow of the American Psychiatric Association.

Tovah P. Klein, PhD, is Director of the Barnard College Center for Toddler Development, a research, education, and training center located in the psychology department at Barnard College where she is on the faculty. Dr. Klein's research focuses on parental influences on children's social and emotional development, particularly in young children. This work includes a study of adaptation of children under the age of five and their parents following the September 11 World Trade Center disaster.

Harold Kudler trained at Yale and is Associate Clinical Professor at Duke. He has received teaching awards from the Duke Department of Psychiatry and the American Psychiatric Association. Dr. Kudler manages mental health services for a three-state region of the U.S. Department of Veterans Affairs (VA) and co-chairs VA's Special Committee on PTSD, which reports directly to Congress. He initiated the International Society for Traumatic Stress Studies' (ISTSS) PTSD Practice Guideline process and served on the ISTSS Board of Directors. He recently helped lead development of a joint VA/Department of Defense guideline for the management of posttraumatic stress.

Ilan Kutz, MD, is on the staff of Tel-Aviv University and Shalvatah Psychiatric Center and heads the Consultation-Liaison Services at Meir General Hospital and its Acute Stress Intervention Unit. He has developed a phase-oriented intervention model for treating Acute Stress Disorder (ASD) in victims of terrorist attacks. Currently, on behalf of the Israeli Coalition of Trauma Intervention Organizations, he directs the national workshops on *Interventions in Acute Psychic Trauma*, and *General Hospital Preparedness for Treating Mass Casualties with Acute Stress Following Terrorist Attacks*.

Mooli Lahad, PhD, is Professor of Drama Therapy at Tel Hai College, Upper Galilee, Israel and at Surrey University, Roehampton, England. He directs the Community Stress Prevention Center, which he established in 1979 with the Israeli Ministry of Education. The author of numerous books and articles on communities under stress and coping with life-threatening situations, his awards include the Israeli Psychology Association's Bonner Prize for outstanding contributions to education, and the Tel Aviv University's Adler Institute's Welfare of the Child Prize. He is a consultant to national and international ministries, UNICEF, and member of the Prime Minister's Committee on Public Resiliency.

Roy Laird, PhD, CSW, has worked, taught, consulted, and developed programs in a wide variety of settings for nearly thirty years. He is currently developing an expanded multimodal service program at a psychiatric residence for F.E.G.S.

Nathaniel Laor, MD, PhD, is Professor of Psychiatry and Philosophy at Tel-Aviv University, and Clinical Professor at Yale University Child Study Center. He is a prolific contributor in the area of trauma and disaster intervention. He has led the Tel-Aviv Trauma and Mental Health Centers in response to disasters such as the 1991 missile attacks on Tel-Aviv, the 1999 earthquake in Turkey, and the individual, school, and city response to terrorist attacks. He founded and directs the Cohen-Harris Center for Trauma and Disaster Intervention and also directs the Tel-Aviv Emergency Mental Health Headquarters and the Tel-Aviv Preparedness and Resilience Program.

Roberta Leiner, CSW, Managing Director of Caring Commission of UJA-Federation of New York, provides overall management and direction for the initiatives that enable UJA-Federation to play a central role in the provision of a Jewish response to crucial human needs, ranging from palliative care and hospice, safety-net and self-sufficiency, services for children and families, and social justice. She is responsible for developing new strategies and approaches and ensuring requisite financial and human resources support for these efforts. Previously, Ms. Leiner was Vice President of Behavioral Health Care and Community Initiatives at Hudson River HealthCare, Inc., in Peekskill, New York.

Avital Laufer, PhD, received her PhD in the sociology of health from Bar Ilan University, Israel. She is a lecturere at the College of Jedea and Samaria, and a researcher at the Alder Center for the Study of Child Welfare and Protection. She specializes in the fields of children's violence, as well as children living in adverse circumstances.

Talia Levanon, MSW, is Coordinator of the Israel Trauma Coalition. She is a clinical social worker and psychotherapist with expertise in the field of trauma and bereavement. She received her degree in clinical social work from Bar Ilan University and is a graduate of the Integrative Psychotherapy program at the Hebrew University. For eight years she provided treatment at the National Insurance Institute's Rehabilitation Unit for Widows and Widowers. Her private practice focuses on bereavement and the terminally ill.

Robert Jay Lifton, MD, is Visiting Professor of Psychiatry at the Harvard Medical School. The overall themes of his work have been holocaust and transformation. His books include *Death in Life: Survivors of Hiroshima* (which won a National Book Award); *The Nazi Doctors: Medical Killing and the Psychology of Genocide* (awarded a Los Angeles Times book prize); *Home from the War: Learning from Vietnam Veterans* (finalist for a National Book Award); *Destroying the World to Save It* (about the fanatical Japanese cult Aum Shinrikyo); and, most recently, *Superpower Syndrome: America's Apocalyptic Confrontation with the World*.

Adam Lisberg is a News Reporter for the *New York Daily News*. He has previously worked for newspapers in Chicago, Vermont, and New Jersey. He had been working for *The Record* of Bergen County, New Jersey for less than a year on Sept. 11, 2001, when he drove to the World Trade Center to cover the terrorist attack and barely escaped with his life. He lives in Brooklyn with his wife, Rachel.

Tony Maddox is currently head of CNN International's news operations in Atlanta. As senior vice president, he is responsible for overseas bureaus and staff, and runs the international desk at headquarters. Before joining CNN in 1998, he was the BBC's head of news and current affairs for Northern Ireland, based in Belfast, a job he began in 1995, after working as the BBC's head of news in southwest England. He began his career as a local radio reporter, taking on his first job as news editor in 1989.

Ruth Malkinson, PhD, School of Social Work, Tel Aviv University, specializes in bereavement, family and couple therapy. She is coordinator of the Postgraduate Family Therapy Program and past president of the Israeli Association for Family and Marital Therapy. She has published, together with Rubin and Witztum, numerous articles and the book *Loss and Bereavement in Jewish Society in Israel* (1993).

John Mallett, BSc, MSc, DPhil, teaches Psychology at the University of Ulster. His research interests relate to health and community psychology, particularly in the Northern Ireland context. He has collaborated with Professor Cairns and others on perceptions of victimhood in Northern Ireland and has researched the links between religious segregation, social support and mental health. He has also studied the impact of integrated and segregated schooling on the political attitudes of Northern Irish children.

David Malone, DPhil, became President of IPA in 1998, on leave from his Government. A career Foreign Service officer, during 1994-1998, he was Director General of the Policy, International Organizations and Global Issues Bureaus of the Canadian Foreign and Trade Ministry. From 1992 to 1994, he was Ambassador and Deputy Permanent Representative of Canada to the UN, chairing the negotiations of the Special Committee on Peacekeeping Operations. Earlier, he served in Egypt, Kuwait and Jordan. He is a graduate of l'Université de Montréal, American University in Cairo and Harvard. He holds a DPhil from Oxford. He has taught at the University of Toronto and Columbia University and currently teaches at the New York University Law School and at l'Institut des Etudes Politiques in Paris. His most recent book is The *UN Security Council from Cold War to Twenty-First Century*.

Sherri Mandell has degrees from Cornell and Colorado State Universities and has taught writing at the University of Maryland and Penn State University. She authored Writers of the Holocaust (Facts on File, 2000) and numerous articles in world newspapers and she was senior writer for Wholefamily.com, an award-winning site for family wellness. Ms. Mandell is co-president of The Koby Mandell Foundation, which creates, initiates, and funds programs promoting healing for victims of terrorism and other human rights abuses, such as

Camp Koby and Yosef for children aged 9-17, the Mother's Healing Retreat for bereaved mothers and widows, and Family Healing Retreats.

Daniel N. McIntosh, PhD, Associate Professor of Psychology at the University of Denver, is a social psychologist who studies adjustment to negative life events, emotion, and the psychology of religion. His work examines social and cognitive responses to stressful and low control situations, the role of religion in coping, and cognitive deficits emerging from situations of uncontrollability.

Bill McNeil was 27-years-old and 10 months into his first job as a doctor when, on a surfing holiday in Bali, the Sari club was blown up and he found himself dealing with injuries and deaths of many of his peers. His vivid portrayals of the horrors he encountered and his actions in the face of them reflect his bravery. It is a testament to Bill's professionalism and courage that he remained to confront the catastrophe and help in every way he could. Bill has returned to work but struggled to come to terms with his experience.

Anthony J. Marsella, PhD, DHC, is Emeritus Professor of Psychology at the University of Hawaii. He is a past Director of the University's Disaster Management and Humanitarian Assistance Program and Clinical Studies Program. He has published 10 books and more than 130 book chapters, journal articles, and technical reports in the areas of cross-cultural psychopathology and international and global issues. He is the recipient of numerous grants and was awarded an honorary doctoral degree by The University of Copenhagen for contributions to peace and international understanding.

Randall D. Marshall, MD, is Director of Trauma Studies, New York State Psychiatric Institute, and Associate Professor of Clinical Psychiatry, Columbia University College of Physicians and Surgeons. His research, related to psychological trauma and other anxiety disorders, has addressed questions of diagnosis, pharmacotherapy, cognitive-behavioral therapy, dissemination of evidence-based treatments, and the biology of anxiety. Since the 9/11 attacks, he has directed a large-scale project to provide training in evidence-based psychotherapy for persons with PTSD to the greater New York community.

Fathali M. Moghaddam, PhD, is an Iranian born, British-educated researcher, currently Professor of Psychology at Georgetown University. He has previously worked at McGill University, Canada, and at the United Nations Development Programme. His most recent books are *The Individual and Society* (2002), *The Self and Others* (2003, with Rom Harre), and *Understanding Terrorism* (2004, co-edited with A. J. Marsella).

Conny Mus has been a Correspondent for RTL4 Nieuws, The Holland Media Group, the Netherlands, since 1982. He has covered, among many events, the Gulf wars in 1991 and 2003, the Palestinian uprising and terror attacks in

Israel, the Balkan conflict (Former Yugoslavia/Kosovo), earthquakes in Turkey, war in Lebanon and revolution in Rumania.

Kathleen Nader, DSW, has worked nationally and internationally in post traumatic stress and related fields since 1974. Between 1985 and 1993, she was Director of Evaluations for the UCLA Trauma, Violence, and Sudden Bereavement Program. Her work has included the provision of consultation, training, and specialized interventions for children and adults following catastrophic events. Dr. Nader has written and co-authored various publications, screening instruments, and videotapes regarding trauma and traumatic bereavement in youth, culture, and school interventions. Her book, *Honoring Differences: Cultural Issues in the Treatment of Trauma and Loss* (co-edited with Dubrow and Stamm) was published in 1999. Her book on *Assessing Trauma in Children and Adolescents* will be published in 2004.

Yuval Neria received his Doctorate in Clinical Psychology from Haifa University, Israel. Over the last 15 years, as researcher and clinician, he has worked in trauma, loss and post-traumatic stress disorder. His research has involved, among others, prisoners of war, American and Israeli war veterans, and patients initially hospitalized for psychosis. As Associate Director of the Trauma Studies and Services at the New York State Psychiatric Institute, Dr. Neria is conducting psychosocial and epidemiological research on individuals with PTSD and grief reactions following 9/11, and editing a book on the psychological aftermath of the 9/11 attacks for Cambridge University Press.

Fran H. Norris, PhD, received a PhD in Community Psychology from the University of Louisville in 1983. She is presently a Research Professor in the Department of Psychiatry at Dartmouth Medical School and a Research Associate of the National Center for PTSD. Dr. Norris has directed several large-scale studies of disasters, including Hurricanes Hugo, Andrew, and Paulina, and floods in Appalachia and Mexico. She also directed a "lessons learned case study" of New York's mental health system's response to 9/11 that was conducted for the Center for Mental Health Services and the Office of the Director of the Substance Abuse and Mental Health Services Administration (SAMHSA).

Carol S. North, MD, MPE, is a Board Certified Psychiatrist and Professor of Psychiatry at Washington University School of Medicine in St. Louis, Missouri. She serves as Director of Consultation-Liaison Psychiatry and Director of Emergency Psychiatry at Washington University/Barnes-Jewish Hospital in St. Louis. Dr. North is a Fellow of the American Psychiatric Association and member of its disaster preparedness committee, past president of the Eastern Missouri Psychiatric Society, and a Fellow of the American Psychopathological Association.

Ann E. Norwood, MD, is Senior Advisor for Public Health Risk Communication, Office of the Assistant Secretary for Public Health Emergency Preparedness at the Department of Health and Human Services. A graduate of Vassar College, Dr. Norwood obtained her medical degree from the Uniformed Services University (USU) where she later served for 15 years as a billeted faculty member and as Associate Chair of Psychiatry at USU until April, 2003. Dr. Norwood has written and spoken extensively on the psychological, behavioral, and social effects of trauma and violence with a special focus on Weapons of Mass Destruction and risk communication.

Eleanor Pardess, MA, is a Clinical Psychologist who teaches at Tel Aviv University and chairs the Steering Committee of Psychologists at the Israel Crisis Management Center (Selah). Over the past ten years she has facilitated support groups for families coping with traumatic loss and conducted nature-based workshops that harness the power of metaphors and the expressive arts to facilitate transformative processes of grieving and the reconstruction of meaning. She leads training seminars for volunteers throughout Israel and teaches courses for mental health professionals on crisis management, psychotherapy, and post-traumatic growth.

Tamara Pearl is Danny's sister. She holds a masters degree in psychology, works as a Certified Homeopath, and serves as vice president of the Daniel Pearl Foundation which was formed to promote the ideals that inspired Daniel's life and to address the root causes of his tragic death.

David Pelcovitz, PhD, is Director of Psychology at North Shore University Hospital, Manhasset, NY and Clinical Professor of Psychology in Psychiatry at NYU School of Medicine. Dr. Pelcovitz has published and lectured extensively on a variety of topics related to child and adolescent abuse, child exposure to domestic violence and post-traumatic stress disorder in adolescents. He has served as an adviser to the Task Force on DSM-IV for Relational Disorders, as co-site coordinator of the PTSD DSM-IV Field Trials for adolescents, and as co-director of the SAMHSA adolescent trauma treatment development center.

Betty J. Pfefferbaum, MD, JD, is a General and Child Psychiatrist and Chairman of the Department of Psychiatry and Behavioral Sciences at the University of Oklahoma College of Medicine, holding the Paul and Ruth Jonas Chair. Dr. Pfefferbaum is the Director of the Terrorism and Disaster Branch of the National Center for Child Traumatic Stress. She helped plan and organize clinical services and research after the 1995 Oklahoma City bombing, assisted in mental health efforts after the 1998 United States Embassy bombings in East Africa, and provided consultation regarding clinical and research efforts associated with the September 11, 2001, terrorist attacks.

Giandomenico Picco is President and CEO of GDP Associates, a consulting company based in New York he founded in 1994. Mr. Picco was a United Nations official from 1973 until 1992. He headed the UN task force that led to a cease fire between Iraq and Iran in 1988; was a member of the team for the Geneva Agreements on Afghanistan; and was the negotiator who brought about the release of several Western hostages from Lebanon. Educated in Italy, the US and the Netherlands, Mr. Picco received awards from the US, UK, Germany, Italy and Lebanon for his work in the Middle East.

Judith Pizarro is a PhD student in the Department of Psychology and Social Behavior at the University of California, Irvine. Her primary research interests include mental and physical health outcomes after exposure to traumatic experience. She has examined the long-term health outcomes of veterans after exposure to combat experience, as well as how initial reactions to the experience of the September 11th terrorist attacks are associated with levels of distress, posttraumatic stress symptoms, and health outcomes over time.

Ilona Pivar, PhD, is a Health Science Specialist at the National Center for PTSD, Department of Veterans Affairs, Menlo Park, California. She received her PhD in Clinical Psychology from the Pacific Graduate School of Psychology in Palo Alto, California in 2000. Her dissertation measured complicated grief as a distress syndrome distinct from PTSD and depression in combat veterans. She is currently engaged in clinical work, education and research in disaster mental health and bereavement and is developing a group treatment for complicated grief in combat veterans.

Alexander M. Ponizovsky, MD, is a Psychiatrist and Senior Scientist. He received his MD at Moscow Medical Academy in 1970 and his PhD in Psychiatry in 1980. He was a Senior researcher at the Psychiatry Epidemiology Research Unit in Talbieh MHC, Jerusalem from 1991-1998 and Sha'ar Menashe MHC from 1998-2001. He has authored papers in journals and book chapters about the epidemiology of suicide behavior in adult and adolescent immigrants from USSR to Israel, psychological distress, depression, quality of life in schizophrenia, RBC membrane aberrations in schizophrenia and the psychological consequences of terrorism.

Michael Poulin is a PhD student in the Department of Psychology and Social Behavior at the University of California, Irvine. His research interests center on individuals' cognitive representations of the world, or world views. In his work on responses to the September 11th terrorist attacks and subsequent events, he has examined the ways in which individuals' world views are associated with distress following the attacks, and the ways in which world views shift over the life span.

Holly G. Prigerson, PhD, is Associate Professor of Psychiatry, Epidemiology and Public Health at Yale University School of Medicine, received Master's degrees in History and Sociology and a PhD in Sociology in 1990 from Stanford University. She completed a postdoctoral fellowship in Epidemiology at Yale School of Medicine in 1991. During her US National Institute Of Mental Health (NIMH) K01 Scientist Development Award she initiated her studies of complicated grief as a psychiatric disorder distinct from bereavement-related depression and anxiety. Dr. Prigerson's NIMH-funded research has focused on psychiatric responses to impending and recent loss, including loss from suicide, and trauma.

Beverley Raphael, MD, is Director of the Centre for Mental Health for New South Wales (NSW) and Emeritus Professor in Psychiatry, the University of Queensland. She holds professorial appointments at The University of NSW, The University of Sydney and The University of Newcastle. She authored *The Anatomy of Bereavement* (1983), *When Disaster Strikes* (1986), co-edited *International Handbook of Traumatic Stress Studies* (1993), and *Psychological Debriefing: Theory, Practice and Evidence* (2000), and wrote numerous scientific articles. She led the mental health disaster response planning for the Sydney Olympics and was integral to mental health responses following the World Trade Center bombing.

Dori B. Reissman, MD, MPH (CDR, USPHS), provides leadership and vision to address the psychosocial and behavioral health dimensions of public health emergency events and to promote resilience initiatives at the Centers for Disease Control and Prevention (CDC). Commissioned as a medical officer in the U.S. Public Health Service and a medical epidemiologist at CDC since 1997; serving in the Bioterrorism Preparedness and Response Program, the National Center for Environmental Health, and the Epidemic Intelligence Service Program. She has specialty medical training in psychiatry, and occupational and environmental medicine; and a Masters degree in Pharmacology and Toxicology.

Heidi Resnick, PhD, is Professor in the Department of Psychiatry and Behavioral Sciences at Medical University of South Carolina. Dr. Resnick received her PhD in clinical psychology from Indiana University. Her major research interest is the etiology of post-traumatic stress following civilian trauma. Recent research has included the study of rape victims' immediate post-rape biological and psychological response profiles in association with specific assault characteristics and as predictors of long term PTSD. In addition, she is studying rape victims' concerns about their physical health following rape, and development of appropriate medical care and health care counseling for rape victims, including information about HIV and risk reduction.

María Mercedes Pérez-Rodríguez has worked on various research projects, including a short collaboration at University of California at Los Angeles medical hospital. Currently working as Investigator at the Ramón y Cajal and Fundación Jiménez Díaz University Hospitals, she is doing her PhD in Psychiatry and taking part in various research projects in emergency settings focusing particularly on immigration and coping with stress.

Gina Ross, MFCT, is founding President of International Trauma-Healing Institute (USA) and co-founder of the Israeli Trauma Center in Jerusalem. Trained in cognitive behavioral and somatic approaches, she specializes in trauma therapy and cross-cultural therapy in seven languages. Ross has presented at international conferences and appeared on radio and television as a trauma expert. Currently she works with Israeli and Palestinian society and media to bring about understanding of the role of trauma in Middle Eastern politics. She has authored *Beyond the Trauma Vortex: The Media's Role in Healing Fear, Terror, and Violence* and several other scholarly articles.

Lee Ann Ross was the Deputy Mission Director for the US Agency for International Development's (USAID), Kenya program on August 7, 1998, when the US embassy in Nairobi was bombed. She managed a $37 million bomb recovery program for two years following the bombing and received USAID's Distinguished Honor Award for her work with the victims. She joined USAID in 1976 and served in Yemen, Sri Lanka, Indonesia, twice in Kenya, and finished her career in Washington as USAID's Senior Policy Advisor on Victims of Terrorism. She has an MS in Economics from Colorado State University.

Joshua F. Rubin, MPP, is Chief Administrative Officer of the Division of Mental Hygiene in the New York City Department of Health and Mental Hygiene. Previously, he was the Special Assistant to the Executive Deputy Commissioner for Mental Hygiene. Mr. Rubin began his career as a Program Associate for the Coalition of Voluntary Mental Health Agencies, a nonprofit organization representing community-based providers of outpatient mental health services in New York City. He has a Masters in Public Policy from the John F. Kennedy School of Government at Harvard University and a Bachelors degree in Religion and the Humanities from the University of Chicago.

Kelly L. Ryan, MA, MPH, Director of the Office of Mental Health Disaster Preparedness and Response at the New York City Department of Health and Mental Hygiene, has an MPH from Harvard University and is ABD in clinical psychology from Temple University. She received her Bachelor in Psychology and Public Health from the University of Rochester. Previously,

Ms. Ryan consulted to healthcare and public health organizations around project and program evaluation as well as strategic planning. She intends to focus her dissertation on the issues of burden of illness and quality of life, impacted by mood disorders, in the professional environment.

Lloyd I. Sederer, MD, Executive Deputy Commissioner for Mental Hygiene Services in the New York City Department of Health and Mental Hygiene, has had a wide-ranging career spanning clinical work, advocacy, scholarship, and leadership, including serving as Director of Clinical Services for the American Psychiatric Association and as Medical Director and Executive Vice President of McLean Hospital, a non-profit psychiatric hospital of Harvard Medical School. He is a Distinguished Fellow of the American Psychiatric Association, a Fellow of the New York Academy of Medicine and a recipient of the Exemplary Psychiatrist Award from the National Alliance for the Mentally Ill.

Simon Shimshon Rubin, PhD, Professor of Psychology at the University of Haifa, specializes in bereavement, clinical practice, psychotherapy training, and professional ethics. He has chaired his university's Clinical Psychology Program, Postgraduate Psychotherapy Program, and ethics committee.

Miriam Schiff, PhD, MSW, is a licensed School Psychologist and a lecturer at the Hebrew University School of Social Work in Jerusalem, Israel. Dr. Schiff's research focuses on the consequences of trauma and political violence on adolescent mental health and substance use. She is also studying long-term consequences of children's functioning and mental health in out-of-home placements. Dr. Schiff's clinical activity includes work with children and adolescents traumatized by the recent extensive political violence in Israel.

William E. Schlenger, PhD, Director of the Center for Risk Behavior and Mental Health Research at the Research Triangle Institute, is a psychologist with a diverse background in applied research focused on psychiatric epidemiology and mental health and substance abuse services research. He is best known for his substantive work in the epidemiology of post-traumatic stress disorder (PTSD), and for his work in evaluating mental health and substance abuse service interventions.

John K. Schorr, PhD, a member of the Stetson University sociology faculty since 1975 and Director of the Stetson Institute for Social Research since 1997, is an expert in disaster sociology as it relates to communities experiencing and responding to natural and man-made disasters. He co-authored the book *Demanding Democracy After Three Mile Island* (1991) with Raymond L. Goldsteen, and has written numerous articles.

Roxane Cohen Silver, PhD, is Professor in the Department of Psychology and Social Behavior and Department of Medicine at the University of California, Irvine. An expert in stress and coping, she is a Fellow of the American Psychological Association and the American Psychological Society. Dr. Silver is principal investigator of the only ongoing national study of psychological responses to the September 11th attacks, funded by the National Science Foundation. In December 2003, she was appointed by U.S. Department of Homeland Security Secretary Tom Ridge to the Academe and Policy Research Senior Advisory Committee of the Homeland Security Advisory Council.

Zahava Solomon, PhD, is the Director of the Adler Research Center and Professor of psychiatric epidemiology and social work at Tel Aviv University, Israel. She has published over 200 scientific articles and 6 books on man-made psychological trauma. Her work focuses on war, captivity, the Holocaust and terror. She is the recipient of numerous grants and awards, including the International Society for Traumatic Stress Studies Laufer award for outstanding scientific achievement in the field of PTSD.

Daya Somasundaram, MD, is currently Senior Professor in Psychiatry and Head of the Department of Psychiatry at the Faculty of Medicine, University of Jaffna in Sri Lanka. He is also a Consultant Psychiatrist to the General (Teaching) Hospital, Jaffna; District Hospital, Tellipallai and Base Hospital, Point Pedro. His research interest includes war trauma and consciousness. He has published his studies in international journals and books.

Shauna Spencer is a Consultant to the D.C. Department of Mental Health (DMH), directing one of the nation's 9/11 FEMA Crisis Counseling Programs offering community-based recovery services. Ms. Spencer co-authored the Project's, *Discovering Resilience*, a workshop targeted to caregivers and urban youth. She has over 22 years of senior management experience in health systems delivery and has created innovative outreach, quality improvement and operational effectiveness strategies for healthcare organizations across Metropolitan Washington. She earned her MBA and BA in Behavioral Science at Westminster College in Salt Lake City, Utah and is nationally certified as a health care quality professional.

Smadar Spirman, MSW, MA, is a Social Worker who specialized in urban planning. She directs the Emergency Treatment Services for the City of Tel-Aviv–Jaffa, which coordinates about 900 professionals in various areas of human care, and is Associate Director of the Cohen-Harris Center for Trauma and Disaster Intervention. Following the 1991 missile attacks on Tel-Aviv, she developed a comprehensive model for multi-systemic response to municipal emergencies which serves as blueprint for many other cities in the country.

Bradley D. Stein, MD, PhD, is Health Services Researcher at the RAND Corporation, Associate Director for Mental and Behavioral Health in the RAND Center for Domestic and International Health Security, and Assistant

Professor of Child Psychiatry at the Keck School of Medicine, University of Southern California. His major research interests include the emotional and behavioral effect of terrorism and other traumatic events, and quality improvement efforts for children's mental health care delivered in schools and other community settings.

Ellen Stoller, ATR, a registered Art Therapist, oversees Disaster Relief Services at F.E.G.S. She is also the Assistant Vice President of Community Services, Training and Consumer Affairs.

Nadine Strossen, PhD, Professor of Law at New York Law School, has written, lectured and practiced extensively in the areas of constitutional law, civil liberties and international human rights. In 1991, she was elected President of the American Civil Liberties Union, the first woman to head the nation's largest and oldest civil liberties organization. (Since the ACLU Presidency is non-paid, she continues in her faculty position as well.) Strossen graduated Phi Beta Kappa from Harvard College (1972) and magna cum laude from Harvard Law School (1975), where she was an editor of the *Harvard Law Review*.

Jennifer Stuber, PhD, is a Post-Doctoral Fellow at The New York Academy of Medicine. Dr. Stuber is engaged in research tracking the psychological impact of the September 11 terrorist attacks on the general population of New York City residents including children. Her work has addressed unmet mental health needs and barriers to mental health care in a post-disaster context. She is particularly interested in behavior problems in children pre- and post-September 11 attacks; the associations between parent and child well-being; and areas where parents are reliable informants of children's exposure to terrorism, their psychological responses, and service utilization.

Eun Jung Suh, PhD, is Training Coordinator of Trauma Studies and Services, New York State Psychiatric Institute, and Instructor of Clinical Psychology, Columbia University. She has completed postdoctoral fellowships in psychiatric epidemiology at Columbia University School of Public Health and in the study of ethno-political conflict at Solomon Asch Center, University of Pennsylvania. Her current research focuses on culturally-sensitive assessment of psychological trauma and the development and dissemination of contextually-relevant, evidence-based treatments of posttraumatic stress reactions. She has extensive experience in training clinicians in the treatment of PTSD and in evaluating this training, both in New York and South Africa.

Terri L. Tanielian, MA, is a Social Research Analyst at the RAND Corporation, where she also serves as Associate Director for Mental and Behavioral Health in the RAND Center for Domestic and International Health Security and Deputy Director for the Center for Military Health Policy Research. She conducts mental health services and policy research in both the civilian and military sector. Her major research areas include the mental and behavioral effects of and public response to terrorism, psychological consequence management and community preparedness, as well as mental health service delivery and system organization.

Samuel B. Thielman, MD, PhD, is Chief of Crisis Management for Mental Health Services at the Department of State in Washington, DC. He is currently involved in formulating and implementing the Department's response to mental health issues raised by diplomatic service in potential war zones around the world. From 1999-2003, he was the Department's regional psychiatrist for East and Central Africa and has worked extensively with victims of the bombings in Nairobi and Dar Es Salaam. He is Adjunct Assistant Professor in the Department of Psychiatry and Behavioral Sciences at Duke.

Robert J. Ursano, MD, is Chairman of the Department of Psychiatry and Director of the Center for the Study of Traumatic Stress at the Uniformed Services University of the Health Sciences, Bethesda, Maryland. Dr. Ursano's work is at the forefront of public health policy planning to combat bioterrorism. He was a national consultant for planning clinical care responses and research programs following the September 11th terrorist attacks and the Department of Defense Pentagon response groups. He is widely published in the areas of post-traumatic stress disorder and the psychological effects of terrorism, traumatic events and disasters, and combat.

Moshe Vardi, MD, was born in Poland in 1946. He graduated in 1974 from the Technion Medical School, Haifa, Israel and specialized in General Psychiatry and in Child and Adolescent Psychiatry in Geha Psychiatric Hospital, Israel. Since 1981, working at Loewenstein Rehabilitation Center, Tel Aviv University Medical School, Ra'anana, Israel, his main foci have been traumatic brain injury rehabilitation, neuropsychiatry, trauma and post-trauma in children and adults. Dr. Vardi is the Head of Psychiatric Services and of the Post Trauma Unit for Children victims of Accidents and Terror at Loewenstein Rehabilitation Center.

David Vlahov, PhD, is Director for the Center for Urban Epidemiologic Studies at The New York Academy of Medicine, Professor of Clinical Epidemiology at the Mailman School of Public Health at Columbia University and Adjunct Professor in Epidemiology at the Johns Hopkins School of Public Health. Dr. Vlahov has been Principal Investigator of the Natural History of HIV Infection among Injection Drug Users (the ALIVE Study). For the ALIVE study, the National Institutes of Health (NIH) recognized Dr. Vlahov with their MERIT Award. He is the Editor-in-Chief of the Journal of Urban

Health and has been appointed to the National Advisory Council on Drug Abuse within the Department of Health and Human Services.

Jonas Waizer, PhD, has been with F.E.G.S. Health and Human Services System since 1991, is its Chief Operating Officer for Behavioral & Health Related Services and is Treasurer for the New York City Coalition of Voluntary Mental Health Agencies, Inc. He served as Associate Commissioner for the New York State Office of Mental Health and as Assistant Director for the New Jersey Mental Health Department. He worked at Downstate Medical Center-SUNY and other general and public New York hospitals. He has a doctorate in Psychology, is licensed to practice in New York State, and has published and presented extensively.

Patricia J. Watson, PhD, received a PhD in Clinical Psychology from Catholic University in 1994 and completed a fellowship in Pediatric Psychology at Harvard Medical School in 1995. She is presently the Deputy of Education at the National Center for PTSD and Assistant Professor in the Department of Psychiatry at Dartmouth Medical School. She has published on early interventions for PTSD and is currently co-editing a book on interventions for trauma following disasters and mass violence.

Gabriel Weimann, MD, is Full Professor of Communication and Chair, Department of Communication at the University of Haifa, Israel. His research interests include media effects and public opinion, political communication and modern terrorism. His books include *Hate on Trial, The Theater of Terror, The Influentials: People Who Influence People*, and *Communicating Unreality*, and he has published over a hundred papers in scientific journals. A Visiting Professor at universities in North America and Europe, he is a (2003-2004) Senior Fellow at the United States Institute of Peace, Washington, DC, working on *Terror in the Internet: The New Arena, the New Challenges*.

Zeev Wiener, MD, is a Family Physician and a Psychiatrist. He is the Director of Community Interventions at the Cohen-Harris Center for Trauma and Disaster Intervention, an instructor of primary care professionals in community psychiatry, and Program Director of the School for the Study of Trauma, Preparedness and Community Resilience established by the Cohen-Harris Center.

Eliezer Witztum, MD, is Professor in the Division of Psychiatry, Faculty of Health Sciences, Ben-Gurion University of the Negev and Director of Psychotherapy Supervision, Mental Health Center, Beer Sheva. He is co-editor of *Sihot–The Israel Journal of Psychotherapy*. He has published, together with Malkinson and Rubin, numerous articles and the book *Traumatic and Non-traumatic Loss and Bereavement: Clinical Theory and Practice* (2000).

Leo Wolmer, MA, is Clinical Psychologist, Director of Research at the Tel-Aviv Community Mental Health Center, and Director of School Interventions at the Cohen-Harris Center for Trauma and Disaster Intervention. He developed a unique model for Teacher-Based School Reactivation, which was implemented and tested empirically in Israel, Turkey, and Italy. His scientific publications have emphasized trauma in children as well as adults covering domains such as developmental psychopathology, psychophysiology, psychotherapy research and the systemic aspect of disaster intervention.

Sally Wooding, PhD, is Clinical Psychologist and Senior Project Officer at the Centre for Mental Health with the NSW Health Department. She is involved with disaster response and planning for the state of New South Wales and liaises with other Australian states and territories planning for national response to terrorist incidents and disaster. She has published in the area of child and adolescent trauma and abuse, attachment, and traumatic grief and bereavement following disaster and terrorism. She has extensive clinical experience working with children, adolescents, and families who have experienced trauma.

Deena Yellin is a Reporter at *The Record* in Hackensack, New Jersey. She has also written for *The New York Times*, *Newsday*, *The Jerusalem Post* and *Parents Magazine*. She earned her Master's degree from Columbia University's Graduate School of Journalism.

Acknowledgments

First and foremost, we thank the contributors who brought to the volume broad expertise and rich experience and those who shared with candor their personal experiences, hearts, and wisdom through their voices. Their care and dedication joined in making the volume a labor of love.

We are honored that David Malone, President of the International Peace Academy, contributed the Foreword, and Sir Jeremy Greenstock, former Ambassador of the United Kingdom to the United Nations and Chairman of the Security Council Counter-Terrorism Committee, contributed the Epilogue.

Clemens Weiss generously designed the cover of this volume.

This volume was made possible by the commitment and support of F.E.G.S. in New York, with the help of Jonas Waizer and Amy Dorin.

John P. Wilson believed in the idea of the book from its inception and, with Mary Beth Williams and Jacqueline Garrick, helped create the connections to make the volume and the special issue of the *Journal of Aggression, Maltreatment & Trauma* a reality.

Chris Cramer, Betty Pfefferbaum, Brian Engdahl, Felicity Barringer, Ruth Bar-on, Joop T.V.M. de Jong, and Ziad Abdeen generously enriched all of us by suggesting and enlisting some of the contributors.

Brian Engdahl and William E. Schlenger reviewed and commented in detail on some of the articles. They and Dorathea Halpert, Roger S. Clark, and Patricia Saunders helped with the Introduction and Conclusion. So did Necla Tschirgi for the Introduction and Danilo Türk for the Conclusion. Youssef Mahmoud kindly translated the Palestinian Voices and Naomi Baum, The Terrorism Poem.

We thank Robert Geffner for taking on the dual challenge and for providing constant, supportive editorial presence, and the editorial staff of the *Journal of Aggression, Maltreatment & Trauma* for their dedicated work.

Elizabeth Neuffer had planned to contribute her voice to this volume. Tragically, on May 8, 2003, she was killed in Iraq while covering the war for the *Boston Globe*. A compassionate and courageous journalist, she held human rights, justice, and friendship paramount.

This book has been blessed with the kind of generosity that helps transcend its sometimes heart-wrenching substance and make the world freer of terror. We are thankful for that as well.

FOREWORD

Terrorism:
The United Nations
and the Search for Shared Solutions

David Malone

Terrorism is today a topic of vital importance to the lives of millions of people around the world. It occurs in both wealthy and poor countries. Terrorists operate in democracies and in authoritarian states. There is no single root cause of terrorism, or even a common set of causes. Sharing the different experiences of terrorism is therefore key to our ability to understand, deal with and eradicate terrorism and its effects. This remarkable volume provides a timely and important step in this process of building a common understanding of the horror of terrorism, a step toward shared solutions.

The importance of terrorism was well understood by global policy-makers prior to the attacks in the United States on September 11, 2001. It took those terrible events, though, to raise the profile of terrorism as an avenue of academic and clinical inquiry and to force the issue to the top of international policy-makers' agendas. The United Nations system has long provided a forum for discussion of the issue of terrorism, but the events of September 11, 2001, followed by the terrorist attack on United Nations headquarters in Baghdad on

Address correspondence: David Malone, DPhil, Ten, The Driveway, Apartment 1811, Ottawa, Ontario, Canada K2P 1C7 (Email: david.malone@international.gs.ca).

[Haworth co-indexing entry note]: "Terrorism: The United Nations and the Search for Shared Solutions." Malone, David. Co-published simultaneously in *Journal of Aggression, Maltreatment & Trauma* (The Haworth Maltreatment & Trauma Press, an imprint of The Haworth Press, Inc.) Vol. 9, No. 1/2, 2004; and: *The Trauma of Terrorism: Sharing Knowledge and Shared Care, An International Handbook* (ed: Yael Danieli, Danny Brom, and Joe Sills) The Haworth Maltreatment & Trauma Press, an imprint of The Haworth Press, Inc., 2005.

August, 19, 2003, made clear its role would be central in the worldwide fight against terrorism.

Those attacks challenged the United Nations to confront terrorism in ways it had not previously imagined. Terrorism is now much more than an abstraction for the world organization. The UN General Assembly has for too long been engaged in a debilitating debate over the definition of terrorism, unable to reach consensus on the relationships between states and terrorism and national liberation movements and terrorism. That failure even to define terrorism has hurt the organization and the fight against terror. It has weakened the entire United Nations system's credibility.

The efforts of the United Nations to deal with terrorism have accelerated in recent times. Since 1973, twelve anti-terrorism Conventions have been adopted within the framework of the General Assembly. These play an important role in providing for universal jurisdiction and a global extradition regime. Over the last decade, the United Nations Security Council (UNSC) has adopted sanctions regimes against several states involved in assisting and harboring international terrorist organizations. The Security Council responded promptly to the attacks of September 11, 2001, issuing an unequivocal condemnation of the terrorist attacks the next day (UNSC Resolution 1368). This was followed on September 28, 2001, with Resolution 1373, a landmark resolution that requires all member states, under Chapter VII of the United Nations Charter, to take specific actions to combat terrorism. UNSC Resolution 1373 created for the first time uniform obligations for all 191 member states in responding to terrorism, going beyond the twelve international treaties that bind only those that accede to them. It specifically requires all states to deny all forms of financial support for terrorist groups; to suppress the provision of safe haven, sustenance, or support for terrorists; and to share with other governments information about any groups practicing or planning terrorist attacks. It bars active and passive assistance by governments to terrorists. The resolution also established the Counter-Terrorism Committee to assist member states in developing the legal, political and operational capacity to carry out their responsibilities under this resolution.

Both the General Assembly and the Security Council have also addressed the relationship between human rights and the fight against terrorism, the former in Resolution 219 of December 18, 2002, and the latter in Resolution 1456 of January 20, 2003. However, it is broadly recognized that much more needs to be done in order to enable the United Nations to play an even stronger role in mobilizing governments and non-governmental organizations (NGOs) to deal cooperatively with the continuing threat of international terrorism. The UN–its programs, its funds and its agencies–must do more to explore how it can focus more directly on the roots of terrorism and work harder to resolve festering conflicts that can give rise to acts of terrorism.

To that end, the International Peace Academy (IPA) has worked to assist the United Nations community in responding to the complex challenges of international terrorism through its "The United Nations and International Terrorism" project. IPA actively participated in a Policy Working Group established by the UN Secretary-General and organized two workshops bringing outside experts together with members of the Policy Working Group in developing major themes of the report. The recommendations of the Group were presented to the Security Council and the General Assembly on September 10, 2002.

In addition, IPA convened on October 25-26, 2002 a conference on "Responding to Terrorism: What Role for the United Nations?" This conference was aimed at ensuring the active participation of speakers from the developing world in sharing their perspectives, often overlooked in the western policy dialogue on terrorism, with officials and diplomats based in New York (International Peace Academy, 2002). These voices are critical of the United Nations system's response to terrorism, and particularly of the role of the major powers in shaping the approach of the Security Council to the terrorism challenge. These views, however controversial, reflect a broad segment of public opinion in the developing world. They emphasize the need for exactly the kind of international sharing of experiences and understandings of terrorism that this volume seeks to provide. (For complete information on IPA programs, research studies and reports see www.ipa@ipacademy.org)

On June 9-11, 2003, IPA brought together in Oslo an international panel of leading experts on terrorism to discuss the root causes of terrorism. This expert meeting represented the contribution of the academic and research community to the high-level conference on "Fighting Terrorism for Humanity," which convened in New York on September 22, 2003.

The then High Commissioner for Human Rights, the late Sergio Vieira de Mello, suggested in the spring of 2003 that more rigorous thinking was needed concerning the different ways terrorism affected human rights and what his office and the rest of the United Nations system should do to uphold human rights while fighting terrorism. Tragically, the High Commissioner, along with 21 other UN colleagues and friends, was killed in a terrorist attack in Baghdad on August 19, 2003. Determined to do justice to the memory of these murdered colleagues and friends, IPA brought together experts on terrorism, security, human rights and international policy, along with senior officials from the United Nations and several regional inter-governmental organizations–the Organization of American States (OAS), the African Union (AU) and the Organization for Security and Cooperation in Europe (OSCE)–at a conference on November 7, 2003, in New York, entitled "Human Rights, the United Nations and the Struggle Against Terrorism."

These discussions have served to generate a body of understanding within the United Nations system, and outside, concerning the nature and effects of terrorism. It is common ground that "no political goal or cause justifies intentionally attacking civilians. Terrorism can never be justified or excused" (International Peace Academy, 2003a, p. 3). Similarly, commentators and experts agree that the causes of terrorism are difficult to pinpoint. The discussions facilitated by IPA suggest, however, that terrorism is triggered by a range of factors, including: inequalities of power creating incentives for recourse to asymmetrical warfare tactics and creating resentment of foreign intervention or repression; failures of state capacity and control; non-democratic, illegitimate or corrupt government; alienation of social groups by the state; rapid modernization or the experience of social injustice or discrimination; and a culture of violence and extremist ideology and leadership.

The discussions also suggest that, contrary to widely held belief, there is only a weak and indirect relationship between poverty and terrorism. At the individual level, terrorists are generally not drawn from the poorest segments of their societies. Typically, they are at average or above average levels in terms of education and socio-economic background. However, poverty has frequently been used as justification for social revolutionary terrorists, who may claim to represent the poor and marginalized without being poor themselves. Perceptions of marginalization and exclusion require long-term initiatives in which the UN should have a key role. Eradicating terrorism requires new policies toward non-traditional security threats, including finding solutions to economic, environmental and social problems that extremists manipulate and exploit.

Equally, these discussions indicate that terrorists are not insane or irrational actors. Symptoms of psychopathology are not common among terrorists. Neither do suicide terrorists, as individuals, possess the typical risk factors of suicide. There is no common personality profile that characterizes most terrorists, who appear to be relatively normal individuals. Alienation breeds terrorists who are isolated. The challenge is how to engage them. One way is to encourage debate within and between open societies. This volume will play an important role in improving our understanding of the psychological aspects of terrorism and in encouraging the exchange of information on this phenomenon, which open societies must engage in if they are to understand the complexities of engaging terrorists.

The exchange of information represented by this volume is, in itself, a powerful antidote to the conditions which act as crucibles for terrorism. Terrorism takes root in chaos and the absence of good governance. Democracy and proper governance, including free expression and a vibrant civil society, respect for human rights and a functioning, fair judiciary, allow dissent to be expressed in non-violent and legitimate ways.

This raises important questions for the future of the United Nations' response to terrorism. The UN must consider how best it can address the absence of the rule of law and effective governance in states that often enable terrorists to flourish. States that lack legitimacy and control over the economy and other traditional levers of power provide the space and oxygen for terrorist groups to flourish. State sponsorship of terrorism can be either active and involve acts of commission, or passive and involve acts of omission. In either case, the UN faces a dilemma: member states enjoy legitimacy in the United Nations system even though they may be hosting, tolerating and/or supporting terrorists. States also resent what they deem as interference in their internal affairs. The United Nations has lowered the barriers of sovereignty over the past few years but the fight against terrorism will require a further realignment of the fluid border between internal matters and those of universal concern.

The fight against terrorism provides further opportunity for the United Nations to redefine the boundaries between state sovereignty and issues that are legitimately the concern of the international community. The UN might, for example, reassess its relationship with religions, including the sponsorship of discussions about the role of religion in international affairs. Some have suggested that the United Nations Department of Public Information could undertake a public relations campaign promoting tolerance and understanding among all cultures and religions. Another area of particular importance–touched on by some of the contributions to this volume–is the relationship between education and terrorism. Education is of paramount importance as a tool to achieve tolerance and respect; but equally, its capacity to generate hatred and to act as a breeding-ground for terrorist sympathy means that education can no longer be regarded as a purely domestic concern. Organizations such as the United Nations Educational, Scientific and Cultural Organization (UNESCO), the United Nations Children's Fund (UNICEF) and the UN Human Rights Committee are already engaged in activities that help ensure that education promotes human rights and respect for diversity. Efforts could be made to bring this work forward through all relevant UN agencies, as well as other international, regional and national governmental and non-governmental organizations.

Terrorism challenges the fundamental principles of the United Nations. Can the United Nations forge effective policies, beyond the national interests of its most powerful member states, to deal with international terrorism? The fight against terrorism provides opportunities and challenges for creative change within the entire United Nations system. The effectiveness of the Security Council's Counter-Terrorism Committee (CTC) should be improved.

There should be more effective cooperation, enhanced networks and shared intelligence databases. At the same time, the Office of the High Commissioner for Human Rights (OHCHR) must play a greater role in ensuring the UN's counter-terrorism activities reinforce–and do not erode–human rights. The UN must make full use of all available tools. The United Nations should take the lead in promoting dialogue, diplomacy–and human rights (International Peace Academy, 2003a, p. 8).

Terrorism raises a range of complex questions for human rights discourse: are terrorist acts human rights violations? Do human rights violations cause terrorism? How should human rights limit state responses to terrorism? How can we ensure that counter-terrorism does not provide a pretext for human rights abuses? And how can human rights inform terrorism-prevention strategies? The central point is that there must be no trade-off between human rights and terrorism; human rights abuses in fact fuel terrorism, along with misery, ignorance and despair. In counter-terrorism efforts, it is crucial to uphold democratic principles and maintain moral and ethical standards while fighting terrorism. Increased repression and coercion are likely to feed terrorism, rather than reducing it. Extremist ideologies that promote hatred and terrorism should be confronted on ideological grounds by investing more effort into challenging them politically, and not only by the use of coercive force.

Equally, respect for human rights helps prevent terrorism. States that do not allow their residents freedom of expression, association or assembly, and that control power without allowing citizens a free choice in who governs them, are themselves encouraging terrorism. Such violations create legitimate grievances, which terrorists then exploit to advance their own unlawful agendas that further damage human rights. States that respect human rights and basic democratic principles, however, must not subvert these freedoms in the search for security. This is not only counter-productive but also provides justification to authoritarian states to crack down further on peaceful and legitimate opposition, in the process increasing the danger for everyone (International Peace Academy, 2003b, p. 4).

Without adequate understanding of the nature and effects of terrorist activity we cannot hope to answer adequately any of these questions–the place of human rights in our response to terrorism, the role of the United Nations, or the causes of terrorism. This volume will greatly improve that understanding. Particularly notable, from that perspective, is the inclusion of not only academic and clinical commentaries and analysis, but also the first-hand accounts of what it is like to live through terrorism. The "Voices" strategically distributed through this volume bring an immediacy and realism to this discussion that is often sorely lacking. These Voices not only inform our understanding of how terrorism operates, and its effects, but also help to build an anti-terrorist culture. They help us avoid the romanticization of terrorism, focusing on the reality and horror of terrorists' acts.

Today's terrorist threat is global. To respond adequately, we must share experiences and knowledge from around the globe to build a more complete understanding of the nature and effects of that threat. This volume is a timely and important step in this process. Through it, shared solutions to the horror of terrorism grow one step closer. The three editors of this volume, all of whom know the United Nations intimately, have done us a major favor in drawing to our attention the multiple policy challenges that terrorism raises for the United Nations and for other multilateral institutions. I am deeply grateful to them.

REFERENCES

International Peace Academy. (2002, October). *Responding to terrorism: What role for the United Nations?* New York: Chadbourne & Park.

International Peace Academy. (2003a, September). *Fighting terrorism for humanity: A conference on the roots of evil*. Conference report. Retrieved May 5, 2004 from, http://www.ipacademy.org/PDF_Reports/Terrorism_web_031218.pdf

International Peace Academy. (2003b, November). *Human rights, the United Nations, and the struggle against terrorism*. New York.

INTRODUCTION

The Trauma of Terrorism: Contextual Considerations

Yael Danieli
Danny Brom
Joe Sills

SUMMARY. This introductory article maps some of the key contextual issues for this volume. Stating the challenges posed by the "new normality" thrust upon the world by the September 11 attacks, it reviews historical trends and definitional distinctions, including non-state, state and state-sponsored terrorism, and the international institutional and legal structures for combating it. The introduction proposes a multidimensional, multidisciplinary, integrative framework conceptualizing the consequences of the trauma of terrorism and informing optimal interventions. It critically reviews formulations in existing nosologies and

Address correspondence to: Yael Danieli, PhD, Group Project for Holocaust Survivors and their Children, 345 East 80th Street (31-J), New York, NY 10021 USA (E-mail: YAELD@aol.com).

[Haworth co-indexing entry note]: "The Trauma of Terrorism: Contextual Considerations." Danieli, Yael, Danny Brom and Joe Sills. Co-published simultaneously in *Journal of Aggression, Maltreatment & Trauma* (The Haworth Maltreatment & Trauma Press, an imprint of The Haworth Press, Inc.) Vol. 9, No. 1/2, 2004; and: *The Trauma of Terrorism: Sharing Knowledge and Shared Care, An International Handbook* (ed: Yael Danieli, Danny Brom, and Joe Sills) The Haworth Maltreatment & Trauma Press, an imprint of The Haworth Press, Inc., 2005.

summarizes the volume, addressing consequences and mitigation of terrorism's effects on people, communities, societies, and nations.

KEYWORDS. Definitional issues of terrorism, PTSD, framework of trauma, United Nations, global treaties, long-term effects

The terrorist attack on September 11, 2001 is a watershed event, a defining moment in the way of being not only in the United States, but also in the world. As with other massive human-made catastrophes, it became for many a demarcating rupture that continues to map and orient other events and experiences as before or after it. After a short period, many felt that "nothing will ever be the same," that there is no "back to normal." Thus, the individual and collective challenge is to create a new normality: follow new rules of behavior; search for new ways of being safe and secure; relate in new ways to oneself, others, and the world; and reassess and find meaning and values on personal, interpersonal, societal, national, and international levels. Subsequent terrorist attacks in places such as Bali, Madrid, and Istanbul, including the increasing number of suicide bombings in Israel and elsewhere, make it hard to envision a world without terrorism.

The central question for the "new normality," for which there is neither a single nor a simple answer, is: *How do we live with growing levels of threat, anxiety, fear, uncertainty, and loss?* The post-September 11 demoralization has been compounded not only by the economic downturn, but also by the crises of civil liberties and of trust in governments' ability to protect their citizens, by the lingering threats of other forms of terrorism, and ongoing and imminent wars. Whom can we trust? On whose judgment can we rely? Do our governments have a meaningful direction? Do we have a meaningful direction? Do our values still hold?

Many survivors of previous trauma living in the United States were particularly shaken by September 11 because, until then, they had viewed America as their "last place of safety." For some, specific aspects of the terrorist attacks served as triggers as well as aspects symbolic of past trauma, and reactivated past symptoms (e.g., incineration for Holocaust survivors and their offspring; absence of remains for relatives of the "disappeared" from some Latin American countries; see also, e.g., Kinzie, Boehnlein, Riley, & Sparr, 2002). American former prisoners of war (POWs), having lived through the attack on Pearl Harbor, combat, and imprisonment, and who were already well aware of life's unpredictability and fragility, were also affected by 9/11. Rodman and Engdahl (2002) found a small but significant increase in PTSD-related distress among 117 World War II and Korean War POWs surveyed in July 2002.

September 11 has created an unprecedented surge of interest in trauma (and self-proclaimed expertise thereof). Many existing groups committed themselves to volunteer their service to those in need following the terrorist attacks. Others, particularly around New York City, were created specifically for this purpose. Many professions responded overwhelmingly on all levels. Various societies, institutions, and organizations generated feature publications from their unique perspectives. Providers who had attempted to meet the psychosocial needs of victims of massive trauma worldwide applied approaches based on their experience and training (Danieli, Rodley, & Weisaeth, 1996; Green et al., 2002; Weine, Danieli, Silove, Van Ommeren, Fairbank, & Saul, 2002).

TERROR AND TERRORISM

The word "terror" comes from the Latin word *"terrere"* which means "to frighten" or "to scare." Terrorism has entailed a mass psychological aspect from its inception. The first use of large-scale terrorism was during the "popular" phase of the French Revolution: in September 1793, the "regime de la terreur" (reign of terror) was officially declared and implemented, causing the execution of 17,000 people. Executions were conducted before large audiences and were accompanied by sensational publicity, thereby spreading the intended fear.

Terrorism has mushroomed in scope and intensity over the past few years. Targets, traditionally military and political, have shifted and now include civilian, public, and communal settings. A single act of terrorism can thus claim more victims and affect many more people than before. Even when terrorism is directed at an individual, it is directed at the community. Its randomness amplifies the whole community's fear. As such, terrorism is indeed psychological warfare. Modern terrorists have also become aware of new opportunities for exerting a mass psychological impact as a result of technological advances in communications.

Terrorism has a profound, multidimensional impact on society and has become a pivotal factor in the policies of governments around the world. Elie Wiesel (2002) noted that the 21st century has seen a marked shift in the very nature of terrorism. Driven by hate, it does not care about innocent victims.

This parallels the shift in war casualties: at the dawn of the 20th century, 10% were civilians; the 21st century began with 90%. No society is immune to the current wave of terrorism or to the sense of vulnerability that it engenders. Security, safety, conflict, and war have all assumed a different meaning.

ISSUES OF DEFINITION

The editors and contributors of this volume have generally approached terrorism from the perspective that "we know it when we see it." This is consistent with the approach taken by the United Nations Security Council in its remarkable, unanimously adopted Resolution 1373 (UNSC Res. 1373, 28 September, 2001), which imposes heavy counter-terrorism responsibilities on States, especially regarding the financing of terrorism, as elaborated in the Foreword and Epilogue of this volume. That Resolution also created a Counter-Terrorism Committee that closely monitors what States do to control terror. But efforts to devise a comprehensive definition of terrorism, and thus to further its prevention, suppression, and control by treaty, have not yet been crowned with success at the United Nations. A draft Comprehensive Convention on International Terrorism is agonizingly close to fruition as we write. Nevertheless, it is possible to obtain agreement that certain of those activities we think of as terrorist are utterly unacceptable to the international community and that there is a global obligation to bring to justice those who engage in such acts.

The most recently adopted treaty, the 1999 International Convention for the Suppression of the Financing of Terrorism (U.N.Doc.A/Res.54/109 [1999]), is also consistent with our approach. The intellectual source of much that is in Security Council Resolution 1373, it proscribes "acts of terrorism" fitting into two categories. In the first are those types of terrorism that have been specifically banned by treaty: hijacking of aircraft, unlawful acts against the safety of civil aviation, crimes against internationally protected persons, hostage-taking, unlawful acts involving nuclear material, unlawful acts against airports serving international aviation, unlawful acts against the safety of maritime navigation, unlawful acts against the safety of fixed platforms on the continental shelf, and terrorist bombings. The second, residual category is "Any other acts intended to cause death or serious bodily injury to a civilian, or to any other person not taking an active part in the hostilities in a situation of armed conflict, when the purpose of such act, by its nature or context, is to intimidate a population, or to compel a government or an international organization to do or abstain from doing any act" [Article 2(1)(b)]. The residual category or "generic terrorism" in fact subsumes the kind of actions specifically proscribed by treaty and also captures the essence of the phenomenon with which we are concerned in this volume. While it provides a useful working definition, we should note that, in terms of legal definitions (and legal strategies for dealing with the phenomenon), many of the atrocities that we discuss fit alternatively (and sometimes more appropriately) into such categories as war crimes and crimes against humanity. We would have no problem, for example, in characterizing the 9/11 attacks as crimes against humanity.

For the most part, the terrorist activities focused on in this volume are carried out by non-state actors. Sometimes, however, the actor will in fact be operating (clandestinely) on behalf of or assisted in some way by a State. We are mindful of the Security Council's reaffirmation in one of the preambular paragraphs to Resolution 1373, of the principle established by the General Assembly in its Friendly Relations Declaration of October 1970 (resolution 2625 [XXV]) and reiterated by the Security Council in its resolution 1189 (1998) of 13 August 1998, namely, that every State has the duty to refrain from organizing, instigating, assisting, or participating in terrorist acts in another State or acquiescing in organized activities within its territory directed toward the commission of such acts.

The United States Department of State defines terrorism narrowly as: "... premeditated, politically motivated violence perpetrated against non-combatant targets by sub-national groups or clandestine agents, usually intended to influence an audience" (Title 22, United States Government, Section 2656(d)). Many would argue that so narrow a definition is inadequate, primarily because it excludes the role of states, specifically, state-sponsored terrorism and state terrorism.

The concept of state-sponsored terrorism is the clearer of the two. It entails adding to the definition above a role for a sovereign state in planning and financing the activity and providing the terrorists with needed logistical and other supports. The destruction of Pan Am 103 over Lockerbie by terrorists acting as agents of the Libyan government is an example of what is widely accepted as state-sponsored terrorism.

Things become less clear when the discussion turns to state terrorism. Increasingly, the term terrorism is used for a broad range of state actions deemed evil. Indeed, some find it tempting to characterize as state terrorism any actions of states with which they take issue, however far these diverge from more conventional views of terrorism.

An earlier volume by the senior editor, *International Handbook of Multigenerational Legacies of Trauma* (Danieli, 1998), concentrated on massive human-made atrocities, including state terrorism, and their long-term and multigenerational effects. A second, *The Universal Declaration of Human Rights: Fifty Years and Beyond* (Danieli, Stamatopoulou, & Dias, 1999), critically evaluated the degree to which the international human rights system has reached the people by protecting individual human beings or averting their victimization. This volume, then, does not focus on the particular problems that arise when a Government engages in depredations against its own population, such as disappearances and other crimes against humanity. In at least one respect, the search for solutions in those cases is even more difficult than in the case of depredations by non-State actors. The Government, empowered to be a protector, has become a persecutor. The victim must cope not only with individual and other loss but also with the fundamental loss of trust in those in power.

TRAUMA AND THE CONTINUITY OF SELF: A MULTIDIMENSIONAL, MULTIDISCIPLINARY INTEGRATIVE (TCMI) FRAMEWORK

A most relevant model to conceptualize the consequences of terrorism is the multidimensional, multidisciplinary integrative framework proposed by Danieli (1998) and Danieli, Engdahl, and Schlenger (2003). An individual's identity involves a complex interplay of multiple systems, including: biological and intrapsychic; interpersonal, including the familial, social, and communal; ethnic, cultural, ethical, religious, spiritual, and natural; educational/occupational; material/economic, legal, environmental, political, national, and international. These systems coexist along the time dimension, creating a sense of life continuous from past through present to the future. Ideally, one should have free psychological access to and movement within all these identity systems. Each system is the focus of one or more disciplines that may overlap and interact, such as biology, psychology, sociology, economics, law, anthropology, religious studies, and philosophy. Each discipline has its own views of human nature and it is those that inform what the professional thinks and does.

TRAUMA EXPOSURE AND "FIXITY"

Trauma exposure can cause a rupture, a possible regression, and a state of being "stuck" in this free flow, which Danieli (1998) has called "fixity." The intent, place, time, frequency, duration, intensity, extent, and meaning of the trauma for the individual, and the survival strategies used to adapt to it, will determine the degree of rupture and the severity of the fixity.

Fixity can be intensified in particular by the *conspiracy of silence* (Danieli, 1982, 1998), the survivors' reaction to the societal (including healthcare and other professionals) indifference, avoidance, repression, and denial of the survivors' trauma experiences (see also Symonds, 1980). Society's initial emotional outburst yet its demand for rapid return to apparent normality is an important example. This *conspiracy of silence* is detrimental to the survivors' familial and sociocultural (re)integration by intensifying their already profound sense of isolation and mistrust of society. It further impedes the possibility of their intrapsychic integration and healing, and makes the task of mourning their losses impossible. Fixity may increase vulnerability to further trauma. It also may render *chronic* the immediate reactions to trauma (e.g., acute stress disorder), and, in the extreme, become life-long (Danieli, 1997) *post-trauma/victimization adaptational styles* (Danieli, 1985). This occurs when survival strategies generalize to a way of life and become an integral part of one's personality, repertoire of defense, or character armor.

Recognition of the possible long-term impact of trauma on one's personality and adaptation and the *intergenerational* transmission of victimization-related pathology still await explicit inclusion in future editions of the diagnostic nomenclature. Until they are included, the behavior of some survivors, and some children of survivors, may be misdiagnosed, its etiology misunderstood, and its treatment, at best, incomplete. This framework allows evaluation of each system's degree of rupture or resilience, and thus informs the choice and development of optimal multilevel intervention. Repairing the rupture and thereby freeing the flow rarely means, "going back to normal." Clinging to the possibility of "returning to normal" may indicate denial of the survivors' experiences and thereby fixity.

Immediately after September 11, Danieli (2001) suggested that, more than ever, issues related to the time dimension emerged as paramount. *First* was the imperative to resist the culturally prevalent (American) impulse to do something, to find a quick fix, to focus on outcome rather than process, to look all too swiftly for closure, and to flee "back to normal." *Second*, knowing that there will be long-term effects not only of the disaster itself but also of the immediate interventions, we must recognize the necessity for and importance of long-term commitment, and systematically examine every short-term decision from a long-term perspective. Since the urge to act and help others and oneself in the immediate aftermath is near universal, it should be harnessed and incorporated into long-term planning. Danieli (2001) also noted the necessity of considering *at-risk times* (e.g., family holidays, anniversaries) as well as the *at-risk groups*.

Integration of the trauma must take place in *all* of life's relevant (ruptured) systems and cannot be accomplished by the individual alone. Systems can change and recover independently of other systems. Rupture repair may be needed in all systems of the survivor, in his or her community and nation, and in their place in the international community. To fulfill the reparative and preventive goals of trauma recovery, perspective and integration through awareness and containment must be established so that one's sense of continuity and belongingness is restored. To be healing and even self-actualizing, the integration of traumatic experiences must be examined from the perspective of the *totality* of the trauma survivors' and family and community members' lives.

REACTIONS AND RESPONSES TO TERRORISM

The process of coping with terrorism often takes victims through oscillating between re-experiencing the event or parts of it in multiple experiential modalities, and avoiding the memories or sensations, places, people, or activities that trigger those memories (Kleber & Brom, 1992). In the course of this flow and the lessening of the swing of the pendulum, people look for meaning and revisit their experience by talking or thinking about it and, as this process advances, the symptoms subside. Periods of difficulty in, or lack of, concentration and sleeping are common during the coping process, as are bodily tensions and symptoms that also tend to subside with the progress of healing the rupture. Much of the trauma literature for the past 20 years has often limited itself to the psychological consequences of such events. Approaches that concentrate on healthy coping patterns or more complex adaptational styles (Danieli, 1985; Felsen, 1998) do exist, but have not yet received adequate attention. The shock and sense of powerlessness that many people experience in the face of terrorism may be buffered and processed differently by different cultures (Danieli, 1998).

Exposure to trauma may also prompt review and reevaluation of one's self-perception, beliefs about the world, and values. Although changes in self-perception, beliefs, and values can be negative, at least some of those exposed to trauma report what they perceive to be positive changes as a result of coping with the aftermath of trauma ("posttraumatic growth"; Tedeschi & Calhoun, 1996). Survivors have described an increased appreciation for life, a reorganization of their priorities, and a realization that they are stronger than they had thought. This is related to Danieli's (1994) recognition of competence vs. helplessness in coping with the aftermath of trauma. Competence (through one's own strength and/or the support of others), coupled with an awareness of options, can provide the basis of hope in recovery from traumatization.

Within the same context, Peterson (2002) assessed the values, strengths, and virtues before and after 9/11 in convenience samples of Americans, using a cross-sectional, Internet-based survey approach. Among the 24 strengths assessed, six were higher after 9/11 than before: love, gratitude, hope, kindness, spirituality, and teamwork. This finding is consistent with the predictions of the "terror management theory," which holds that people "manage" the terror of confronting their mortality by increasing their identification with culturally salient values. By six months post-9/11, however, gratitude, hope, and love scores were lower, although only gratitude had returned to its pre-9/11 level.

Kindness, spirituality, and teamwork, however, were higher at six months post-9/11.

Children exposed to large-scale traumatic events may experience significant worries and fears, concerns about personal safety and security, nightmares (either resembling or seemingly unrelated to the traumatic events), separation anxiety, and somatic complaints. In addition, children may experience changes in sleep and appetite, and school performance may be adversely impacted due to difficulties with attention, concentration, and increased activity levels. Other reactions common in children include an increased sensitivity to sounds such as sirens, increased startle response, and a decreased interest in once pleasurable activities. As they attempt to cope with and process traumatic events, younger children may engage in post-traumatic play and ask questions or talk about the event repeatedly. Among older children, concerns about safety and security may extend to a sense of a foreshortened future. In addition, adolescents may exhibit withdrawal, substance abuse, and risk-taking behaviors, as well as a fascination with death and suicide. Finally, extensive viewing of media coverage appears to negatively affect children of all ages. Interventions with children must consider the distinct differences between adult and child responses (Gurwitch, Sullivan, & Long, 1998).

The psychological effects of the trauma of terrorism in the most seriously affected individuals are defined narrowly in both of the world's primary nosologies: the ICD-10 (World Health Organization [WHO], 1992) and DSM-IV (American Psychiatric Association [APA], 1994). The most directly relevant syndromes include acute stress disorder (ASD) in the short term, and posttraumatic stress disorder (PTSD) in the longer term. Additional disorders that frequently occur after exposure to trauma include depression, other anxiety disorders, and substance abuse. Conversion and somatization disorders may also occur, and are more likely to be observed in non-Western cultures (Engdahl, Jaranson, Kastrup, & Danieli, 1999). Complicated bereavement (Horowitz, 1976) and traumatic grief (Prigerson & Jacobs, 2001) have been noted as additional potential effects.

Shear and colleagues (2001) define "traumatic grief" as a constellation of symptoms, including preoccupation with the deceased, longing, yearning, disbelief, and inability to accept the death, bitterness or anger about the death, and avoidance of reminders of the loss. Research shows that traumatic events that are human-made and intentional, unexpected, sudden, and violent have a greater adverse impact than natural disasters (Norris, 2002).

The proposed diagnoses of "complex PTSD" (Herman, 1992) and "disorder of extreme stress not otherwise specified" (DESNOS; Roth, Newman, Pelcovitz, van der Kolk, & Mandel, 1997) that were considered for but not included in the DSM-IV (APA, 1994) represent attempts to go beyond the basic

17 symptoms of PTSD and associated features. Although several of the DESNOS descriptions, such as survivor's guilt, are included as associated features of PTSD, many believe that it is a construct in its own right. Similarly to Danieli (see the TCMI Framework above), the descriptions of complex PTSD and DESNOS emphasize profound personality changes following repeated exposure to human-made traumata. These recognize alterations in the survivor's world assumptions and values but allowed in the *current* DSM only as associated features and not as a distinct diagnosis.

In each of these instances, however, the entity represents a hybrid that mixes aspects typically conceptualized as belonging to Axis I (clinical syndromes defined by the presence of specific symptom constellations) and Axis II (personality disorders, "enduring pattern of inner experience and behavior that . . . is pervasive and inflexible . . . is stable over time, and leads to distress or impairment" [APA, 1994, p. 629]). The ICD-10 (WHO, 1992) category of *"enduring personality change after catastrophic experience"* is more consistent with Danieli's notion of *post-trauma/victimization adaptational styles,* but the ICD-10 description focuses on *adjustment* rather than *adaptation*, and is far narrower than Danieli's. Adaptation may include both healthy and pathological styles and is not constrained by a given diagnostic system.

THE TRAUMA OF TERRORISM:
SHARING KNOWLEDGE AND SHARED CARE

Our primary motivation for publishing this volume is to make sense of the reality of living with terrorism. We barely experienced a sense of choice about this undertaking. We felt an urgent need to learn as much as possible from everywhere in the world that has experienced the terrifying and tragic reality of terrorism. The volume focuses on some of the critical questions that must be answered: how do we address the human consequences of terrorism, and mitigate its effects on people, communities, societies, and nations?

The reader will find that many of the articles in this volume focus on the United States and Israel. There are two reasons for this. First, the aftermath of the events of 9/11 in the U.S. and the continuing attacks against Israeli targets by suicide bombers are at the forefront of attention to terrorism today. Second, the current research in the United States and Israel on the effects of terrorism is more comprehensive than elsewhere. However, we have made every possible effort to include studies from around the world, as indicated by articles on Japan, Northern Ireland, France, Kenya, Sri Lanka, Spain, Algeria, and Indonesia. We hope that this volume will spur further worldwide scientific research into the effects of terrorism and methods for addressing them.

Section I consists of five articles that explore the origins of terrorism in modern society. Marsella and Moghaddam trace the origins of terrorism from ancient times to the present day, and review important efforts to conceptualize the phenomenon. Ganor focuses on the ability of a small group of individuals, utilizing modern technology, to manipulate public opinion to force decision makers to meet their demands. Cromer details the history and nature of Lehi (Lohamei Herut Yisrael/Fighters for the Freedom of Israel) and relates its justification of violence to four kinds of narratives: contemporary, historical, metaphysical, and biographical. Lifton discusses the worldwide impact of the use of sarin gas in a Tokyo subway in 1999 by the Aum Shinrikyo cult, whose apocalyptic vision crossed the crucial threshold from dreaming about Armageddon to attempting to bring it about. Picco distinguishes between "tactical terrorism," whose political objectives are well-known, precise, and negotiable; and "strategic terrorism," based on non-negotiable, perpetual confrontation with the enemy: anyone who is different.

Section II consists of 18 articles comprising an extensive and varied examination of the psychological consequences of terrorism. The first four are on adults in the United States. Schlenger reviews the initial, preliminary studies post-9/11 and, while noting their value, especially due to their immediacy, calls for more comprehensive studies to confirm these initial findings. Ahern, Galea, Resnick, and Vlahov discuss the finding of a post-9/11 random digit-dial telephone survey of New York City residents that, among those directly affected by the attacks or who had prior traumatic experience, watching television was associated with a higher probability of PTSD. Cohen Silver, Poulin, Holman, McIntosh, Gil-Rivas and Pizarro analyze a nationwide longitudinal investigation of psychological responses to 9/11 that focused on the relationship between exposure/proximity to the attacks and levels of acute and posttraumatic stress syndromes. North summarizes the field of somatization and applies its principles to recommendations for disaster and terrorism research and post-disaster interventions.

The next 10 articles cover findings from around the world. Baca, Baca-Garcia, Pérez-Rodríguez, and Luisa Cabanas analyze the short- and long-term effects revealed by a study of 3,000 victims of terrorism in Spain between 1997 and 2001. Campbell, Cairns, and Mallett review the effects of the "Troubles" in Northern Ireland both on individuals and, more significantly and longer-term, on intergroup relations. Jehel and Brunett discuss the development and functioning of a French medico-psychological network to deal with the aftermath of terrorist attacks, augmenting traditional rescue teams. Khaled presents the results of epidemiological surveys conducted between 1999 and 2001 on the effects of terrorism-induced trauma in two representative areas in Algiers. Somasundaram reports on epidemiological surveys in Sri Lanka, primarily

among the Tamil population, which show widespread traumatization and consequent psychosocial problems, and on the need for community-based interventions to reverse these effects. Thielman, utilizing case histories and written
narratives, comments on the effects of the 1998 bombing of the U.S. embassy in
Nairobi, the response from the Kenyan mental health community, and the collaboration between Kenyan and American responders. Raphael, Dunsmore, and
Wooding describe the acute, intermediate, and ongoing mental health responses
to the 2002 bombing of a night club in Bali, Indonesia, and include a number of
survivors' narratives. Engdahl reviews findings on the impact of terrorism outside of the United States, including the wide cultural variations that characterize
the responses. Pivar and Prigerson examine studies addressing traumatic loss after terrorist-related and other violent deaths, and stress the importance of including specific assessments of grief in studies of terrorism within a cultural and
community context. Hall, Norwood, Fullerton, Gifford, and Ursano focus on
planning for the public's psychological and behavioral reactions to a bioterrorist
attack, including individual and community preparedness, response, recovery,
and early public health interventions.

The last four articles in Section II focus on the psychological impact of terrorism on children. Pfefferbaum et al. review the literature on the psychological impact of terrorism on children across the developmental span, and on the
relationship between the reactions of parent and child following the 1995
Oklahoma City bombing and the 9/11 attacks. Galili-Weisstub and Benarroch describe 260 young terror victims treated in the emergency room of two Israeli hospitals for acute clinical reactions and intrapsychic difficulties. Pat-Horenczyk
reports on the Jerusalem Screening Project, which examined the effects of direct
and indirect exposure to terrorism on PTSD and functional impairment among adolescents living in Jerusalem and in a settlement in the West Bank. Solomon and
Laufer examine the effects of terror on world assumptions in Israeli youth, sampling 2,999 adolescents aged 13-16.

Section III consists of five articles on the impact of terrorism on individuals, groups and society. Strossen calls attention to the dangers to civil liberties
that may accompany measures taken in the name of national security in reaction to terrorist attacks, specifically in the United States post-9/11. Weimann
discusses the use and manipulation of modern communications by terrorist organizations that have led governments and media organizations to evaluate
critically their responses. Nader and Danieli analyze cultural differences as
important elements in the prevention, assessment, and treatment of post-terrorism psychological sequelae. Kinzie reviews the results of clinical studies of
the effects of television coverage of the events of 9/11 on refugees from five
ethnic groups currently residing in Oregon (U.S.), and of the negative effects
on these refugees of countermeasures aimed at combating terrorism.

Section IV consists of four articles on psychological first aid and acute and long-term treatment following terrorist attacks. Kutz and Bleich, based on an analysis of clinical syndromes following terrorist attacks in Israel, outline the organizational principles and state of preparedness that hospitals should maintain to respond effectively. Adessky and Freedman use case material to illustrate the challenges faced when conducting treatment of PTSD during prolonged adversity. Kaplan, Pelcovitz, and Fornari, utilizing vignettes at various developmental levels of children and adolescents, analyze experiences in the treatment of children and families who were traumatized by, and lost relatives in, the attack on the World Trade Center. Malkinson, Rubin, and Witztum use two case vignettes to posit that trauma (including terror attacks) and bereavement co-occur and overlap and are thus best treated as mixed rather than separate or independent phenomena.

Section V consists of three articles devoted to school- and community-based interventions in the face of terrorist attacks. Baum presents the Israeli National School Intervention Project, begun in 2000 in response to the outbreak of attacks on civilians, and focused on the ongoing and long-term effects on children and adolescents of exposure to these attacks. Waizer, Dorin, Stoller, and Laird review the post-9/11 Project Liberty in New York City, the largest disaster counseling effort to date, which included substantial outreach to the city's large foreign-born community. Berger analyses a case study of a terrorist attack on a kibbutz in Israel, and an approach toward building community resilience in the aftermath of such a traumatic event.

Section VI consists of 10 articles that present a multicomponent model of preparing providers in communities affected by terrorism. Friedman sets forth a public mental health approach for survivors of terrorist attacks, stressing the need to develop early prevention programs for the minority of victims of such attacks who will develop clinically significant disorders. Heldring and Kudler stress the importance of integrating mental health services within the primary health care system, and advocate strongly for a national strategy to direct these efforts. Vardi analyzes emotional and behavioral symptoms in Israeli children following terrorist attacks and presents a program to train primary care providers to carry out long-term follow-up of these children. Davidowitz-Farkas and Hutchinson-Hall describe the different roles clergy played in providing spiritual care following 9/11 and the requirements for training clergy to enable adequate response to trauma and grief following a terrorist attack. Schorr and Boudreaux report firefighters' accounts of on-site terrorism experiences and their emotional aftermath, including reflections five years after the bombing in Oklahoma City. Solomon and Berger assess the psychological consequences of body handling in the aftermath of terrorist attacks through a survey of volunteers of ZAKA, the primary Israeli organization that removes bodies and body parts following terrorist attacks. Pardess offers guidelines for screening, assigning, and ongoing training and support of volunteers, based on the experience of SELAH, the Israel Crisis Center's countrywide volunteer network. Hamilton details the reexamination by the American Red Cross of national security and disaster response following terrorist acts beginning with the Oklahoma City bombing in 1995, whose strategic basis is increased collaboration among federal, state, and local agencies and voluntary organizations. Amsel, Neria, Marshall, and Suh describe the development, delivery, and initial evaluation of an attempt to address the fact that most clinicians have little training in evidence-based assessment and treatment of the psychological consequences of terrorism. Norris, Watson, Hamblen, and Pfefferbaum, utilizing a systems perspective, explored in Oklahoma City seven years after the 1995 bombing the views of local people who had developed, implemented or provided disaster mental health services, with a goal of learning the lessons from their experiences.

Section VII consists of seven articles addressing individual and community preparedness and new methods of mental health services for the 21st century. Lahad examines the effects of terrorism on communities from the standpoint of resiliency rather than psychopathology, and describes the work of the Community Stress Prevention Center, Kiryat Shmona, Israel. Laor, Wiener, Spirman, and Wolmer explore the Tel Aviv, Israel model for meeting the challenge of mass disasters, in which responsible planning is based on a broad system of mediators and activities maintained in normal times, supplemented by intervention personnel and techniques set in motion during emergencies. Sederer, Ryan, Gill, and Rubin concentrate on the particular challenges facing mental health disaster planning in an urban setting (e.g., New York City), where factors such as population density, reliance on mass transportation, and varied ethnic demography come into play. Reissman, Spencer, Tanielian, and Stein discuss the need for public and private mental and behavioral health networks to participate in joint planning and response exercises with other response system components, including public health, emergency management, and law enforcement. Chemtob argues that, facing terrorism, a nation has a choice of becoming more resilient or merely more vigilant, and presents the outline of a plan to increase resilience through a national strategy for psychosocial security. Levanon, Flamm-Oren, and Kahn-Hoffman describe the work of the Israel Trauma Coalition, which embodies the evolving concept of the Continuum of Trauma Services to address the needs of victims of terrorist attacks. Ben-Gershon, Grinshpoon, and Ponizovsky discuss the comprehensive emergency response system in general hospitals and communities in Israel to meet, at both the individual and the population levels, the psychological needs resulting from terrorism. Flynn reviews the organization and delivery within the United States of psychological services to victims of terrorism, which he regards as a relatively young science, rapidly growing, but with much knowledge, wisdom, and maturity yet to be gained.

Both the Foreword and the Epilogue review and analyze international standards and measures against terrorism. The "voices" among the articles are of individuals whose stories add the personal dimension to the understanding of the origins and impact of terrorism. The "guides" present brief statements of principles.

REFERENCES

American Psychiatric Association. (1994). *Diagnostic and statistical manual of mental disorders* (4th ed.). Washington, DC: Author.

Danieli, Y. (1982). *Therapists' difficulties in treating survivors of the Nazi Holocaust and their children.* Dissertation Abstracts International, 42(12-B, Pt 1), 4927. (UMI No. 949-904).

Danieli, Y. (1985). The treatment and prevention of long-term effects and intergenerational transmission of victimization: A lesson from Holocaust survivors and their children. In C. R. Figley (Ed.), *Trauma and its wake* (pp. 295-313). New York: Brunner/Mazel.

Danieli, Y. (1994). Resilience and hope. In G. Lejeune (Ed.), *Children worldwide* (pp. 47-49). Geneva: International Catholic Child Bureau.

Danieli, Y. (1997). As survivors age: An overview. *Journal of Geriatric Psychiatry, 30*(1), 9-26.

Danieli, Y. (Ed.). (1998). *International handbook of multigenerational legacies of trauma.* New York: Kluwer Academic/Plenum Publishing Corporation.

Danieli, Y. (2001). ISTSS members participate in recovery efforts in New York and Washington, DC. *Traumatic Stress Points, 15*(4), 4.

Danieli, Y., Engdahl, B., & Schlenger, W. E. (2003). The psychological aftermath of terrorism. In F. M. Moghaddam & A. J. Marsella (Eds.), *Understanding terrorism: Psychological roots, consequences, and interventions* (pp. 223-246). Washington, DC: American Psychological Association.

Danieli, Y., Rodley, N. S., & Weisaeth, L. (Eds.). (1996). *International responses to traumatic stress: Humanitarian, human rights, justice, peace and development contributions, collaborative actions and future initiatives.* Amityville, NY: Baywood Publishing Company, Inc. Published for and on behalf of the United Nations.

Danieli, Y., Stamatopoulou, E., & Dias, C. J. (Eds.). (1999). *The universal declaration of human rights: Fifty years and beyond.* Amityville, NY: Baywood Publishing Company, Inc. Published for and on behalf of the United Nations.

Engdahl, B., Jaranson, J., Kastrup, M., & Danieli, Y. (1999). Traumatic human rights violations: Their psychological impact and treatment. In Y. Danieli, E. C. Stamatopoulou, & J. Dias, (Eds.), *The universal declaration of human rights: Fifty years and beyond* (pp. 337-356). Amityville, NY: Baywood Publishing Company, Inc.

Felsen, I. (1998). Transgenerational transmission of effects of the Holocaust: the North American research perspective. In Y. Danieli (Ed.), *International handbook of multigenerational legacies of trauma* (pp. 43-68). New York: Kluwer Academic/Plenum Publishing Corporation.

Green, B., Friedman, M., de Jong, J., Solomon, S., Keane, T., Fairbank, J. et al. (Eds.). (2003). *Trauma in war and peace: Prevention, practice, and policy.* New York: Kluwer Academic/Plenum Publishers.

Gurwitch, R. H., Sullivan, M. A., & Long, P. J. (1998). The impact of trauma and disaster on young children. *Child & Adolescent Psychiatric Clinics of North America, 7,* 1932.

Herman, J. L. (1992). *Trauma and recovery.* New York: Basic Books.

Horowitz, M. J. (1976). *Stress response syndrome.* New York: Aronson, Inc.

Kinzie, J. D., Boehnlein, J., Riley, C., & Sparr, L. (2002). The effects of September 11 on traumatized refugees: Reactivation of posttraumatic stress disorder. *Journal of Nervous and Mental Disease, 190*(7), 437-441.

Kleber, R. J., & Brom, D. (1992). *Coping with trauma: Consequences, prevention and treatment.* Lisse, The Netherlands: Swets.

Norris, F. H. (2002). Psychological consequences of disasters. *PTSD Research Quarterly, 13*(2), 1-7.

Peterson, C. (2002, August). Character strengths before and after September 11. In R. G. Tedeschi (Chair), *Posttraumatic growth in the aftermath of terrorism.* Symposium conducted at the meeting of the American Psychological Association, Chicago, IL, USA.

Prigerson, H., & Jacobs, S. C. (2001). Traumatic grief as a distinct disorder: A rationale, consensus criteria, and a preliminary empirical test. In M. S. Stroebe, R. O. Hansson, W. Stroebe & H. A. W. Schut (Eds.), *Handbook of bereavement research: Consequences, coping, and care* (pp. 613-645). Washington, DC: American Psychological Association.

Rodman, J., & Engdahl, B. (2002, August). Posttraumatic growth and PTSD in WWII and Korean War veterans. In R. G. Tedeschi (Chair), *Posttraumatic growth in the aftermath of terrorism.* Symposium conducted at the meeting of the American Psychological Association, Chicago, IL, USA.

Roth, S., Newman, E., Pelcovitz, D., van der Kolk, B., & Mandel, F. (1997). Complex PTSD in victims exposed to sexual and physical abuse: Results from the DSM-IV Field Trial for Posttraumatic Stress Disorder. *Journal of Traumatic Stress, 10,* 539-555.

Shear, K. M., Frank, E., Foa, E., Cherry, C., Reynolds, C. F., Vader Bilt, J. et al. (2001). Traumatic grief treatment: A pilot study. *American Journal of Psychiatry, 158,* 1506-1508.

Symonds, M. (1980). The "second injury" to victims. [Special issue]. *Evaluation and Change,* 36-38.

Tedeschi, R. G., & Calhoun, L. G. (1996). The posttraumatic growth inventory: Measuring the positive legacy of trauma. *Journal of Traumatic Stress, 9,* 455-471.

Weine, S., Danieli, Y., Silove, D., Van Ommeren, M., Fairbank, J. A., & Saul, J. (2002). Guidelines for international training in mental health and psychosocial interventions for trauma exposed populations in clinical and community settings. *Psychiatry, 65*(2),156-164.

Wiesel, E. (2002, January 17). A conversation with Elie Wiesel [Television series episode]. In Y. Vega (Execute Producer), *The Charlie Rose Show*. New York: WNET.

World Health Organization. (1992). *International classification of diseases* (10th rev.). Geneva: Author.

SECTION I
THE ORIGINS OF TERRORISM
IN MODERN SOCIETY

The Origins and Nature of Terrorism:
Foundations and Issues

Anthony J. Marsella
Fathali M. Moghaddam

SUMMARY. Terrorism has been present for centuries in a myriad of forms and locations. However, the events of September 11, 2001 gave terrorism a new meaning in the United States and many other nations. Following a brief historical review of terrorism, we examine the background of *Al Qaeda*. We then look at definitions of terrorism and review factors that contribute to its development. In the conclusion, we note the challenge that faces the world in combating terrorism, not only with mil-

Address correspondence to: Anthony J. Marsella, PhD, DHC, Department of Psychology, University of Hawaii, Honolulu, HI 96822 USA.

[Haworth co-indexing entry note]: "The Origins and Nature of Terrorism: Foundations and Issues." Marsella, Anthony J., and Fathali M. Moghaddam. Co-published simultaneously in *Journal of Aggression, Maltreatment & Trauma* (The Haworth Maltreatment & Trauma Press, an imprint of The Haworth Press, Inc.) Vol. 9, No. 1/2, 2004; and: *The Trauma of Terrorism: Sharing Knowledge and Shared Care, An International Handbook* (ed: Yael Danieli, Danny Brom, and Joe Sills) The Haworth Maltreatment & Trauma Press, an imprint of The Haworth Press, Inc., 2005.

19

itary means, but also by acknowledging and treating its diverse origins, expressions, and consequences.

KEYWORDS. Terrorism, definition, *Al Qaeda*

HISTORY

There are a number of useful scholarly sources that trace the origins of terrorism across time (e.g., Center for Defense Information [CDI], 2003; Nash, 1998; Rapoport, 2001; Reich, 1998). Many consider the earliest acts of terrorism to have started in ancient Palestine during the first century CE, when Jewish citizens sought freedom from Roman occupation by engaging in assassinations of Romans and suspected Jewish collaborators. One group was called the *Sicari* because of their favored use of the *sica* or short dagger to murder Jewish collaborators. Another group, led by Simon Ben Koseba, exhibited intense fanaticism by killing mainly Romans and Greeks, often in open displays of violence similar to those seen today. This group was called the *Zealots*, and it is from them that we derive the present meaning of the word for individuals who are fanatics (CDI, 2003).

By the early middle ages, a radical Muslim group in the Middle East began to kill those who failed to follow fundamentalist versions of Islam. It was rumored that these killers used hashish prior to their killings and it is from the term "hashish" that the modern word "assassin" is derived (CDI, 2003). Another group in India that functioned between the 7th and the 19th centuries, the *Thugees* (it is from them that we derive the word "thug"), strangled their victims as an offering to the Hindu goddess of terror and violence (CDI, 2003).

It is widely held that the beginnings of modern terrorism occurred in Russia around 1880 when a radical ideological group, *Narodnaya Volya* (The People's Will), used terrorism to attempt to overthrow the Czarist state. In the years that followed, anarchists, political ideologues, and demented individuals used assassination and bombings (e.g., United States President William McKinley in 1901; Ferdinand, Archduke of Austria, in 1914).

The English word "terrorism" comes from the French term "regime de la terreur" that swept across the country between 1793-1794 in the course of the French Revolution. Always value-laden, terrorism was viewed as legitimate and positive by the revolutionaries because it was deemed vital for the revolutionary government to gain power over the royalty and survive the forces seeking to destroy it in its infancy. As Maximilien Robespierre proclaimed in 1794, "Terror is nothing other than justice, prompt, severe, inflexible; it is therefore an emanation of virtue; it is not so much a special principle as it is a consequence of the general principle of democracy applied to our country's most urgent needs" (cited in CDI, 2003, p. 8). Governments, especially those led by despots, have long used harsh methods to control their citizens. The best example of state-sponsored terrorism is Stalinist Russia. Josef Stalin used brutal methods to control the Russians during his reign of terror.

ATTACKS ON AMERICA

The September 11, 2001, bombing was not the first terrorist attack on American soil, nor was it the first attack on American international interests and possessions (see Nash, 1998 for a detailed listing). There was the 1993 attack on the World Trade Center (WTC) led by Ramzi Ahmed Yousef, in which six people were killed and hundreds injured. This attack failed to bring down the WTC but it did signal American vulnerability on its own soil as well as overseas as evidenced by the attacks on the Khobar Towers in Saudi Arabia, the American Embassies in Kenya and Tanzania, and the USS Cole in Yemen. The message of these attacks was clear: America and Americans would no longer be safe. They would join a world that had been at war for decades in more than 60 low-intensity conflicts in which civilians, not soldiers, were now the primary victims.

In time, it became known that the September 11 attacks, as well as the others around the globe, were part of a larger master plan guided by an international terrorist group known as *Al Qaeda*, a well organized and richly-funded Muslim fundamentalist group headed by an educated and wealthy Saudi Arabian citizen, Osama Bin Laden (Bodansky, 2001; Williams, 2002). In the words of Osama Bin Laden, he and *Al Qaeda* [translation: The Source or Base] were seeking revenge for what they viewed as America's many economic, political, and cultural exploitations of Islamic people and cultural traditions. In an interview conducted in 1998, long before the September 11 attacks, Osama Bin Laden had already registered his contempt for America:

> . . . The people of Islam had suffered from aggression, iniquity, and injustice imposed on them by the Zionist-Crusaders' alliance . . . the latest of these aggressions incurred by the Muslims since the death of the Prophet is the occupation of the land of the two Holy Places . . . by the armies of the American Crusaders and their allies. . . . For over seven years

the United States has been occupying the lands of Islam in the holiest of places, the Arabian Peninsula, plundering its riches, dictating to its rulers, humiliating its people, terrorizing its neighbors, and turning its bases in the Peninsula into a spearhead through which to fight the neighboring Muslim people. (Osama Bin Laden, 1998; Source: Strategic Studies Institute, www.army.mil.usassi)

In subsequent remarks aired on October 8, 2001, and published by the Associated Press, Osama Bin Laden commented on the attack of September 11, 2001:

What America is tasting now is something insignificant compared to what we have tasted for scores of years. Our nation [the Islamic World] has been tasting this humiliation and this degradation for more than 80 years, its sons are killed, its blood is shed, its sanctuaries are attacked, and no one hears and no one heeds. (Osama Bin Laden, October 8, 2001; Source: Associated Press)

The intent and purpose of Osama Bin Laden and the *Al Qaeda* network was clear. America was to be punished for its many offenses against the Muslim people and Islam. Revenge would be had and it would be meted out in destructive scenarios designed to bring the *Al Qaeda* cause to people around the world. Osama Bin Laden knew very well that his destructive acts would bring cheers from many who shared his views of America's perceived role as "Satan," and not all among them would be Muslims. Others who perceive America to be the source of their problems would use this opportunity to condemn America's foreign and economic policies. For example, Arundhati Roy, a popular English journalist with the *Manchester Guardian*, likened Osama Bin Laden to America itself. He wrote:

What is Osama bin Laden? He's America's family secret. He is the American President's dark "doppelganger." The savage twin of all that purports to be beautiful and civilized. He has been sculpted from the spare rib of a world laid to waste by America's foreign policy: its gunboat diplomacy, its nuclear arsenal, its vulgarly stated policy of "full-spectrum dominance," its chilling disregard for non-American lives, its barbarous military interventions, its support for despotic and dictatorial regimes, its merciless economic agenda that has munched through the economies of poor countries like a cloud of locusts. Its marauding multinationals who are taking over the air we breathe, the ground we stand on, the water we drink. The thoughts we think. Now the family secret has been spilled, the twins are blurring into one another and gradually becoming interchangeable. (Roy, 2001, p. 1)

Roy's comments were cheered by many who saw the events of September 11, 2001, as a declaration of war against American political and economic policies. While this is offensive to many Americans who accurately see themselves as good and caring citizens of a great nation that has done much to advance human civilization through intellectual, cultural, and humanitarian means, it is necessary for American society to open its eyes to the dynamics and consequences of life in a global community. Above all, there is a need to evaluate the complexities of today's globalized world within the historical and situational contexts that shape the meaning and perception of the many frightening events unfolding before us.

THE CONUNDRUMS OF DEFINITION

The stinging words of Osama Bin Laden (a terrorist) and Arundhati Roy (a popular journalist) communicate some of the many controversial issues surrounding the nature and meaning of international terrorism today. First, let it be said clearly and without doubt that the actions of *Al Qaeda* on September 11, 2001 constitute a crime of mass murder and destruction and demand punishment and retribution. The acts meet the criteria needed to define terrorism and as such are subject to international legal action. Murder of innocent civilians to promote political, economic, or social aims is a horrendous crime, and cannot be justified by cries of oppression or abuse. Efforts to alter political, economic, or social conditions by sub-national groups are not crimes in themselves, but the efforts must be conducted within the constraints of law and morality as codified in local, national, and international systems. Nevertheless, it is now obvious that in an age of easy access to weapons of mass destruction, even a few individuals can wreak havoc on nations. There is an urgent need to refine conceptualizations and definitions of "terrorism."

Although there are many definitions of terrorism (see Burgess, 2003; Hallett, 2003; Moghaddam & Marsella, 2003), an obvious sign of its controversial and confusing nature, many legal and scholarly experts accept the definition used by the United States Department of State in Title 22 of the United States Code, Section 2656f(d): " . . . premeditated, politically-motivated violence perpetrated against non-combatant targets by sub-national groups or clandestine agents, usually intended to influence an audience" (quoted in Reich, 1998, p. 262). The essential elements of terrorism are thus: (a) The use of force or violence; (b) by individuals or groups; (c) directed toward innocent civilians; (d) intended to influence or coerce changes in political or social decisions and policies; (e) by instilling fear and terror. This definition is, however, a narrow one. As discussed below, others advocate a broader definition, which would include state-sponsored terrorism and state terrorism.

The fact of the matter is that the non-State terrorist position of powerlessness *vis-à-vis* a given government or State may encourage secretly planned acts of violence designed to give a "media" or "theatrical" portrayal to the act; the greater the damage, the greater the value of the act in the eyes of the terrorists and their supporters. However, this cannot condone nor rationalize the violence disguised as a guerrilla liberation movement or anti-colonial act by people seeking freedom from oppression. To right the wrongs of centuries or moments is best accomplished through patient diplomacy and constructive peaceful actions rather than violence, a fact the United States is learning in Iraq.

ADDITIONAL ISSUES REGARDING THE DEFINITION AND CONCEPTUALIZATION OF TERRORISM

As this article is being written, there have been numerous bombings in Russian cities, resulting in the murder of hundreds of innocent victims by Chechen groups seeking freedom from Russian Federation domination and rule. Chechnya was not granted its independence as the former Soviet Union collapsed. Indeed, its struggle for freedom from Russia and the Soviet Union has been going on for more than 150 years. Finally, in 1994 Russian troops invaded Chechnya. The resulting war has left more than 40,000 dead and hundreds of thousands as refugees. In response to the Chechen rebel bombings in Russian cities, which are clearly acts of terrorism, Russian troops then destroy and kill Chechen fighters and innocent civilians caught in the crossfire, especially in Grozny, its capital. The cycle of hate and violence continues unabated. It is noteworthy that Chechnya has extensive oil and mineral reserves. Obviously, this encourages Russia to maintain control in spite of the violence.

In this struggle, many of the dilemmas surrounding the origin, definition, and prevention of terrorism can be found. Which side is the victim? Which side is the terrorist? Research and professional psychologists have responded to the new threat, as evident by the broad variety of critical assessments already available (e.g., Atran, 2003; Chomsky, 2001; Moghaddam & Marsella, 2003; Stout, 2002). At the heart of the challenge are questions central to all of psychology. Such questions concern the role of unique and contextual factors: To what extent does terrorism arise because of the particular personality characteristics of terrorists? To what extent is terrorism a result of broader cultural conditions? The first question leads to explorations of the supposedly "abnormal" characteristics of individual terrorists. An alternative approach has been to dig deeper into the cultural characteristics of the contexts that give rise to terrorism, in the tradition of experimentalists who explored the conditions in which individuals selected to represent the 'normal' population obey an authority figure and do extreme harm to others (Moghaddam, 2003).

While the contextual or 'sociocultural' (Moghaddam & Marsella, 2003) approach to understanding terrorism seems to be the most promising, it is also in many ways the most challenging, particularly given the traditional reductionist leanings of mainstream psychology. After all, the sociocultural and contextual approaches require us to consider individual behavior in the larger historical, political, economic, and social context, an approach still only found in the more recent and innovative (and still less influential) areas of psychological research (e.g., social constructivist, cultural, and post-modernist psychologies). These approaches require us to conduct deeper and more serious assessments of such questions as hatred toward the U.S., as well as the long-term foreign policies of the U.S. on lower-income and impoverished societies.

There are numerous other struggles between governments and disaffected minority groups who seek independence. Consider the situations between the Israelis and the Palestinians, Spain and the Basques, England and the IRA in Northern Ireland, China and the Tibetans, and, of course, the Shiite and Kurdish efforts against the former government of Saddam Hussein in Iraq. But what is it that justifies the use of violence and the label guerilla, insurgent, or freedom fighter rather than terrorist? Many unresolved issues remain surrounding the nature, definition, meaning, and legal implications of terrorist acts (e.g., Burgess, 2003). Do any of the following conditions warrant consideration in reaching legal and/or moral definitions of terrorism:

1. If the government is oppressive and not duly constituted by the vote of all the people (e.g., Saddam Hussein's former government in Iraq, Chinese occupation of Tibet)?
2. If the act is directed beyond military targets and personnel and involves the intentional murder and harming of innocent civilians (e.g., the events of September 11, 2001 in New York, Washington, DC, and the airline crash in Shanksville, PA)
3. If the government is corrupt and exploits the people it is intended to represent, as often occurs in Sub-Saharan nations in Africa (e.g., Sierra Leone, Liberia, Rwanda, Zimbabwe)?
4. If the government is dominated by foreign interests to the exclusion of the perceived interests of its people (e.g., Cuba under Fulgencio Batista prior to his overthrow by Castro; the Russian presence in Afghanistan between the 1970s and 1990s)?
5. If a subgroup of ethnic and cultural minorities desire and wish for separation because of their desire to pursue cultural identification and preservation and/or economic well-being (e.g., Chechnya and Russia)?

6. If the government is a colonial power (e.g., Great Britain in Palestine/ Israel, Kenya, or India; France in Tahiti; China in Tibet)?
7. Can religion be used as a source of peace rather than the source of war and conflict? Consider the fact that in the majority of conflicts in the world today, intolerance for religious variation constitutes a major reason for anger and hatred (e.g., Philippines, Bosnia, Sri Lanka, Northern Ireland, Russia, Indonesia, East Timor, Israel/Palestine).

These questions are not intended to justify the murder, kidnapping, and arson by any individuals or groups or by any government, but rather to point out that the historical and situational context must be considered in arriving at judgments. The questions are provided to provoke discussion and thought among the readers, compelling them to weigh their conclusions against certain criteria that may or may not be shared by others. It is the relativity, the problem of alternative perspectives, that poses a serious problem for courts and even for individual moral judgments.

Ultimately, the best example of a moral and ethical effort in pursuit of a group or peoples' interests against oppression and colonization is Gandhi's non-violent approach in India. Non-violence can be an effective means for change (e.g., Bondurant, 1969; Paige, 2002) but the people seeking change must be willing to endure the often punishing consequences of their actions in favor of a sense of ethical and moral righteousness. One can only wonder if non-violent protests would result in any progress in the current situations in Russia, China, Northern Ireland, or Israel. We are compelled to argue that non-violence must be considered as the legal, moral, and ethical approach rather than acts of "terroristic" violence.

CONCEPTUALIZING AND CLASSIFYING TERRORISM PATTERNS

Even as we call attention to the conundrums of defining terrorism, it is useful to discuss the patterns or types of terrorist groups. This too has been the source of considerable debate, but what is emerging in recent years is an increased clarity regarding categories and classifications of terrorism and terrorist acts.

Early efforts to classify terrorism relied on analyses of (a) motives (e.g., political, economic, psychosocial, religious), (b) methods (e.g., bombs, kidnappings, chemicals), and (c) goals (e.g., instilling fear, collapse of governments, altering policies, establishing a power base). More recent efforts have recognized the complex patterns and variations in terrorism related to sponsorship and support. For example, Post (2002a) proposes that terrorism be separated into (a) sub-state terrorism (e.g., groups not affiliated with a national government); (b) state-supported terrorism (e.g., Libya, North Korea, Sudan); and (c) state or regime terrorism (e.g., use of state resources to terrorize citizens or neighboring states). Post noted that sub-state terrorism was the most diverse and included revolutionary leftist groups (e.g., *Sendero Luminoso* in Peru), rightist groups (e.g., Nazi/Fascist groups), national separatist groups (e.g., *ETA* in Spain, IRA in Northern Ireland), religious extremists (e.g., *Aum Shinryko*), and single-issue groups (e.g., anti-abortion). He also divided the religious extremists into two groups: fundamentalists (e.g., *Al Qaeda*) and new religions (e.g., *Aum Shinryko*).

Post's classification illuminates the spectrum of terrorist groups, orientations, and purposes. In this respect, it is a welcome addition to the research literature. Others have been critical of his classifications because, they argue, it is ethnocentric. For example, Montiel and Anuwar (2002) argue that there are other forms of "terrorism," including "global structural violence," economic exploitation, and U.S. legitimated acts of terrorism. They contend that U.S. economic, political, and military hegemony fosters inequities around the world and cultural domination. They also propose that the United States belongs in the category of state-sponsored terrorism because it has supported rightist regimes in Central and South America and in the Middle East.

ENABLING TERRORISM

The causes of terrorism are complex and reside within formative, precipative, exacerbative, and maintenance causes (Marsella, 2003). That is to say, some of the causes have historical roots (formative) reflecting antagonisms that may have origins in past struggles against a government (e.g., Northern Ireland) or group of people (e.g., Palestinian-Israeli conflicts). These causes often are brought forward in recent conditions of oppression and punishment (precipative and exacerbative) by the dominant groups, leading to an endless cycle of violence in which each new action is considered yet another provocation (consider the Israeli-Palestinian conflict).

The simple fact of the matter is that military action against terrorism will never be sufficient unto itself. It must be combined with diplomatic, political, economic, psychological, and humanitarian efforts. Oppression, exploitation, abuse, marginalization, poverty, indignity, and cultural destruction are root causes of most terrorism, albeit some terrorist acts obviously emerged from the demented psyches of some individuals (e.g., Unabomber, Oklahoma City bombing).

As long as military actions remain the primary response to terrorism, then the precipitating, exacerbating, and maintenance causes of terrorism will remain and terrorism will continue. Even if *Al Qaeda* is defeated, history indicates that other terrorist groups and other leaders will arise. The response to terrorism must be multidimensional. It must be part of a long-term commitment to global peace and cooperation, not of suppression or oppression (e.g., Marsella, 2003). This means that governments must be prepared to negotiate and engage in creative diplomatic dialogues and interactions with terrorist groups. The doors must be kept open for discussion and resolution through international conflict mediation. This does not require yielding or surrendering national security. Pride and hubris must be set aside as the sole arbiters of governmental action. This is not an endorsement of terrorist actions but rather a realistic consideration of the origins, consequences, and complexities of contemporary terrorism.

For example, it is fashionable among many government officials to say that, contrary to the claims of academic scholars, poverty does not cause terrorism. They point to the fact that the 9/11 terrorists came from middle-class backgrounds and were educated. What this contention fails to recognize is that revolutions are often led by the wealthy speaking on behalf of the poor because the former are better educated and have more access to the power needed for action. It is the perceived injustice that often leads the educated to take action against the powerful as witnessed in the formation of unions.

Poverty is fertile ground for recruiting terrorists because of the hopelessness and helplessness it breeds. When there is poverty, there is also social injustice, prejudice, deprivation, and shame. When there is poverty, social cohesion breaks down, and the result of the disintegration is often crime, illness, social deviancy, identity confusion and loss, and cries for massive structural changes. Poverty, in the opinion of the authors of this article, is a major enabling condition for terrorism (e.g., Marsella, 2003; Moghaddam, 2003). When a country has 50% unemployment, cries for revolutionary change emboldened by terrorism often emerge as the preferred choice for discharging anger and for stimulating social and political change.

It must be recognized that the enabling conditions for terrorism still require the presence of actual persons whose individual beliefs, motives, goals, and leadership skills and talents can respond to the conditions with terrorist actions. Marsella (2003) reviews some of the psychological characteristics and qualities that may interact with certain contexts to promote the risk of terrorism (e.g., aggression, anger, authoritarian personality qualities, "true believer" qualities). Thus, the origins of terrorism reside in a spectrum of factors including individual personality predispositions and acquired behavior patterns, historical and situational contexts of oppression and punishment, and some interactions of the two. Each terrorist act is unique in its determinants, and yet it also reflects certain commonalities with other terrorist acts.

SUICIDE BOMBERS

Among the many acts of terrorism that have emerged through the centuries, one of the most terrifying and deadly has been suicide bombings in which the perpetrators willfully destroy themselves as they detonate deadly bombs in crowded civilian settings (i.e., buildings, restaurants, bars, supermarkets, buses). For many counter-terrorist agencies, suicide bombers have been a source of bewilderment. While courage in carrying out a terrorist mission might be understood, the willingness of suicide bombers to die for their cause has led to the incorrect assumption that these individuals are deranged or mentally ill. Nothing could be more inaccurate.

The rewards for suicide bombers are numerous and varied, including the promise of an eternal afterlife; financial support for families; a post-death status of prestige and honor in their community; a felt sense of righteousness and justification; and revenge for indignity, abuses, and perhaps the deaths of family members. The Israeli-Palestinian situation is the best example of the suicide bombing. While no one can condone the deaths of innocent non-combatants (i.e., civilians), the hatred and anger that has built up against the Israelis among the Palestinian communities and terrorist groups is so strong that it readily justifies the bombings in the minds of the Palestinians. The fact remains that men, women, and children who commit these bombings find rewards for doing so in religious martyrdom, heroic revenge, implacable anger, and fiscal awards to their family.

CONCLUSION

The number of terrorist acts and terrorist organizations is growing. In a global community, this growth poses a critical challenge to everyone's security and safety. While the reflexive response to the increased tide of terrorism may be increased military actions, it is obvious that root causes are not being addressed. The result is that the history of terrorism is being written each day in headlines and television images. The struggle for recognition and for retribution will continue through bombings, assassinations, kidnappings, cyberwars, and agroterrorism. The low intensity wars and conflicts, now considered to be in excess of 60, will continue as groups turn to terrorism as a way of achieving their political and social aims. World leaders have shown little imagination, vision, or creativity in addressing terrorism beyond increased military responses. The result will be continued global unrest and insecurity. Terrorism, an ancient tactic and strategy rooted in hate, anger, and revenge, viable because of its low risk and cost, increasingly deadly because of access to weapons of mass destruction, will continue until it is re-construed by nations, governments, and people everywhere as a response that is part of the closely-woven tapestry of other challenges present in our world. Isolating terrorism from the problems of poverty, injustice, indignity, prejudice, hate, fundamentalism, oppression, helplessness, and hopelessness that is spurred on by political, economic, and religious abuse assures its continuation and empowerment. Until such time as this spectrum of problems is also addressed, terrorism will remain a daily threat across the globe.

REFERENCES

Atran, S. (2003). Genesis of suicide terrorism. *Science, 299,* 1534-1539.

Bodansky, Y. (2001). *Bin Laden: The man who declared war on America.* New York: Random House.

Bondurant, J. (1969). *Conquest of violence: The Gandhian philosophy of conflict.* Berkeley, CA: University of California Press.

Burgess, M. (2003). *Terrorism: Problems of definition.* Available from www.cdi.org/program/ issue/index.cfm?

Center for Defense Information. (2003). *Terrorism. A brief history of terrorism.* Retrieved August 18, 2003 from www.cdi.org/friendlyversion/printversion.cfm?document ID = 1502.

Chomsky, N. (2001). *9-11.* New York: Seven Stories Press.

Hallett, B. (2003). Dishonest crimes, dishonest language: An argument about terrorism. In F. Moghaddam & A. J. Marsella (Eds.), *Understanding terrorism: Psychosocial roots, consequences, and interventions* (pp. 49-67). Washington, DC: American Psychological Association.

Marsella, A. J. (2003). Reflections on international terrorism: Issues, concepts, directions. In F. Moghaddam & A. J. Marsella (Eds.), *Understanding terrorism: Psychosocial roots, consequences, and interventions* (pp. 11-48). Washington, DC: American Psychological Association.

Moghaddam, F. (2003). Cultural pre-conditions for potential terrorist groups: Terrorism and societal change. In F. Moghaddam & A. J. Marsella (Eds.), *Understanding terrorism: Psychosocial roots, consequences, and interventions* (pp. 103-118). Washington, DC: American Psychological Association.

Moghaddam, A., & Marsella, A. J. (Eds.) (2003). *Understanding terrorism. Psychosocial roots, consequences, and interventions.* Washington, DC: American Psychological Association.

Montiel, C., & Anuwar, M. (2002). Other terrorisms, psychology, and media. *Peace and Conflict: Journal of Peace Psychology, 8,* 201-206.

Nash, J. (1998). *Terrorism in the 20th century: A narrative encyclopedia from anarchists through the Weathermen, to the Unabomber.* New York: Evans.

Paige, G. (2002). *Non-killing global political science.* Honolulu, HI: Exlibris Corporation.

Post, J. (2002a). Differentiating the threat of chemical and biological terrorism: Motivations and constraints. *Peace and Conflict: Journal of Peace Psychology, 8,* 187-200.

Post, J. (2002b). Response. *Peace and Conflict: Journal of Peace Psychology*, *8*, 223-227.

Rapoport, D. (Ed.) (2001). *Inside terrorist organizations*. Portland, OR: Frank Cass Publishers.

Reich, W. (Ed.) (1998). *Origins of terrorism: Psychologies, ideologies, theologies, states of mind.* Washington, DC: Woodrow Wilson Center Press.

Roy, A. (2001, September 29). The algebra of infinite justice. *Manchester Guardian*, p. 1.

Stout, C. E. (Ed). (2002). *The psychology of terrorism: Four volumes.* Westport, CT: Praeger.

Williams, P. (2002). *Al Qaeda: Brotherhood of terror.* New York: Alpha Press.

Terrorism as a Strategy
of Psychological Warfare

Boaz Ganor

SUMMARY. The ability of a few individuals to manipulate public opinion, thus influencing the highest policies of the land, makes terrorism a strategic threat to democratic societies. Terrorism undermines the sense of security and disrupts everyday life, harming the target country's ability to function. This strategy seeks to drive public opinion to pressure decision-makers to surrender to the terrorists' demands. The population becomes a tool in advancing the political agenda in the name of which terrorism is perpetrated. Only by understanding how terrorism manipulates the target population can we learn how to avoid falling into the trap of such psychological warfare.

KEYWORDS. Terror strategy, psychological warfare, anxiety, media

---

Address correspondence to: Boaz Ganor, PhD, The International Policy Institute for Counter-Terrorism, The Interdisciplinary Center Herzliya, P.O. Box 167, Herzliya 46150, Israel (E-mail: ganor@idc.ac.il; Website: http://www.ict.org.il).

[Haworth co-indexing entry note]: "Terrorism as a Strategy of Psychological Warfare." Ganor, Boaz. Co-published simultaneously in *Journal of Aggression, Maltreatment & Trauma* (The Haworth Maltreatment & Trauma Press, an imprint of The Haworth Press, Inc.) Vol. 9, No. 1/2, 2004; and: *The Trauma of Terrorism: Sharing Knowledge and Shared Care, An International Handbook* (ed: Yael Danieli, Danny Brom, and Joe Sills) The Haworth Maltreatment & Trauma Press, an imprint of The Haworth Press, Inc., 2005.

CLASSICAL TERRORISM AND MODERN TERRORISM

Academics researching the phenomenon of terrorism disagree as to when, exactly, terrorism first appeared in the history of mankind. Some historians believe that it started with the Sicariis in the Judean kingdom during the 1st Century; others cite the Assassins of the 11th Century, the Jacobin rule in France in the 18th Century, or the operations of individual groups in the 19th Century. Of course, identifying terrorism in any particular historical period depends on the definition of terrorism chosen.

One of the classic tools for changing policy and gaining power has been political aggression, or, in other words, "classical terrorism." It focused on rulers, symbolic figures close to the center of power, or other "elite" targets, in order to bring about regime change or intimidate those in power so they would alter their policies to suit the attackers. Sometimes the terrorist's goal was more modest: simply to take revenge on rulers or their functionaries for felt grievances.

Modern terrorism is essentially indiscriminate. The identities of the victims are irrelevant to the perpetrators, so long as they belong to a group singled out for attack, and the attack conveys the intended message to the target population. However, in contrast to classical terrorism, modern terrorism aims to inflict the greatest possible number of casualties and damage. The goal is to undermine the government, to spread panic and anxiety among the targeted population and demoralize the public.

Technological developments, mainly in the second half of the 20th century, provided the soil in which modern terrorism was able to root and grow, giving birth to a new type of terrorist organization. Technological inventions include small arms that are lethal, mobile, and difficult to trace, as well as soft targets such as public transportation. The most obvious example of how modern terrorism has evolved in parallel with modern technology is commercial air transportation, which furnishes the terrorist with both target and escape route. The development of modern mass communications, particularly television, has enabled information to be broadcast in real time to every corner of the globe. Satellites, targeted TV, the multiplicity of communication channels, and the competition for ratings have all provided modern terrorists with unprecedented tools to get their message straight into the living rooms of their intended audience. An attack on one thus becomes an attack on all.

At the same time, developments in the international political scene have also played a significant role in the development of modern terrorism. As the costs of conventional warfare have risen, and the danger of using non-conventional weapons becomes more and more concrete, terrorism and guerilla warfare have become a convenient means for achieving political goals. Terrorism has become a weapon of convenience for a number of countries who see terrorist organizations and guerilla groups as deniable tools for advancing their interests.

The growth of modern liberal democratic values (e.g., freedom to organize, the right to self-determination, the emphasis on the value of human life) have also influenced the development of terrorist organizations and the evolution of their tactics. Consider, for example, the explanations offered by Abu Iyad, Yasser Arafat's deputy, who was in charge of the Fatah "United Security" and responsible for the perpetration of many terrorist attacks against Israelis. Referring to the kidnapping of a British aircraft to Tunisia, Abu Iyad contended that he was asked by the Egyptian Foreign Minister, Ismail Fahmi, to persuade the hostage-takers to release the hostages unharmed. Abu Iyad (1983) states that he requested them to do their utmost to persuade the kidnappers to agree to his plan, mostly to convince them that there was no chance that their blackmailing would succeed, as most of the hostages were not Europeans or Americans. "Who cares what happens to Pakistanis, Indians or other Asians? It . . . is a fact: the West cares only for their own nationals, while people from the third world are second-class citizens, and very often are treated accordingly. Therefore, it would be best if the kidnappers were to satisfy themselves with a compromise which would enable them to retreat with dignity, in other words, my offer meant that they would be allowed to leave unharmed and would not be punished" (pp. 7-8).

THE STRATEGY OF TERRORISM

Modern terrorist attacks are perpetrated to achieve a resounding media echo in order to reach public opinion. The attack usually causes limited physical damage in international terms (e.g., in comparison to the physical and property damage caused in traffic accidents). Yet, its explosive echo grows in volume as it is amplified by the media; the message conveyed by the attack is sharpened and magnified. A terrorist attack is intended to influence public opinion. Its message is really a combination of three different messages aimed at three different audiences: the people whom the terrorists claim to represent, the targeted population, and lastly, the international community.

Terrorist operations are intended to advance the interests of a particular population external to the terrorist organization itself (i.e., a nation, an elite, a social stratum, or a group of sympathizers). The message sent to this population is one of empowerment and heightened morale, which is meant to strengthen its support of the terrorist organization and encourage enlistment into its ranks. Merari (1987) contends that almost every organization seeks to grow: "With the exception of a small number of elitist anarchist organizations which do not want to expand their ranks, the large majority strive to sweep into their ranks as many supporters and members as possible, and this they manage to do via the media" (p. 1).

The message sent to the targeted population is the exact opposite of that sent to the terrorists' supporters; the attack is meant to undermine morale, lessen confidence and sense of personal security, and spread panic, anxiety, and the conviction that only concessions and the realization of the terrorists' political ambitions will restore peace and security. Last, but not least, the terrorist attack is intended to draw the attention of the international community to the plight of those the terrorist organization claims to represent. George Habash, head of the Popular Front for the Liberation of Palestine, states that, "by perpetrating terrorist attacks, we remind the world that a Holocaust has occurred here and justice must be done . . . " (Merari & Elad, 1986, p. 27).

The question of the gains achieved in perpetrating terrorist attacks are, therefore, a function of time and place and depend on the terrorist organization's ideology, internal structure, and international circumstances, as well as the stage of the organization's development. The dichotomy between the need to draw the world's attention to a specific problem and the wish not to suffer the consequences of their actions means that terrorist organizations will sometimes either avoid claiming responsibility for their attacks, or do so under a fictitious name.

THE 9/11 ATTACKS AND MODERN TERRORISM STRATEGY

The events of 11 September 2001 awakened the world to a new danger. The kind of terrorism confronting the world today is totally different from that which existed before the attacks on the United States. This is not merely due to the scale of the 9/11 atrocities, but also because they took place on American soil. After 9/11, no place is safe; not even a superpower can consider itself immune. This is the message of modern terrorism. Osama bin Laden was not just a trigger-happy maniac out to kill as many Americans as possible. Rather, he had a cynical political goal that he sought to achieve through the use of horrific terrorist atrocities, a goal that could be attained only by spreading fear and anxiety throughout American society. (See other articles in this volume for analyses of other instances of contemporary terrorism.)

Bin Laden and other al-Qaida spokesmen have declared their ultimate goal countless times. Put simply, they want to conquer the world, to spread their version of radical Islam to every part of the globe by violent means so that there will be no place outside the sway of Islamic religious law. This ambition is based on the distinction in fundamentalist Islam between "Dar el-Harb" and "Dar el-Islam." The Realm of Islam (i.e., that part of the world ruled by Islamic law) stands forever opposed to the War Zone (i.e., those regions not yet under Islamic control. In this war there is no gray area: either you are a fellow Islamic radical or you are an enemy.

It is important to differentiate between *Islamism*, or Islamic radicalism, and Islam as a generality. The Islamic religion as a whole is not necessarily any more (or less) violent than any other religion. The radicalism of Islamism is an outgrowth of one particular and idiosyncratic interpretation of Islam, and does not follow perforce from the basic tenets of the faith. This emerging perversion of Islam, which presents itself as the only "true Islam," poses a major challenge to moderate Muslims. Islamist radicals see violent Jihad (holy war) as the supreme religious duty, above all other values of traditional Islam. In fact, the Islamists view moderate Muslims as infidels, and thus as enemies no less than Jews, Christians, and Hindus. Islamists may feel even more hostility toward moderate Muslims than they do toward members of other religions, since the moderates are seen as heretics and traitors rather than as mere enemy infidels.

Islamic radicals see their first task as the conquest of the moderate Muslim countries, and the establishment there of fundamentalist Muslim regimes. In order to achieve their ultimate goal of world conquest, Al-Qaida has adopted a three-staged global strategy. The first stage is to spread their version of Islam to Muslim countries in central Asia and the Middle East. These states are already home to Islamic radical organizations, some of which have many supporters. Among the countries with strong Islamist movements that could serve as agents for destabilization and eventual Islamist takeover are Afghanistan, Pakistan, Saudi Arabia, Yemen, other Persian Gulf countries, Egypt, Israel, and Jordan. Once this first stage is achieved, these "Islamized" countries would serve as the staging ground for the second stage: the spread of radical Islam to countries with large Muslim communities, such as Kosovo, Bosnia, Germany, the former Islamic republics of the USSR, China (especially Xinjiang), the Philippines, Indonesia, Malaysia, and finally the nations of northern Africa. Only after the completion of this stage will Islamic radicalism be ready for the final stage: the ultimate battle to spread their rule to the non-Muslim world.

Given this phased strategy, why did Bin Laden attack the United States in 2001? The United States, after all, is a target for the third stage of the campaign, not the first. The reason appears to be that bin Laden believed that America needed to be induced to stop meddling in the Muslim world, and to cease supporting moderate Muslim regimes. Only with America out of the picture could the Islamists complete the first stage of their strategy. Bin Laden felt that he must force Americans to withdraw their military forces, financial support, and influence from Arab soil, especially from Saudi Arabia and Kuwait. In effect, the spread of radical Islam to these states could not be accomplished unless the United States could be forced into isolationism.

Bin Laden planned to accomplish this American withdrawal by using the tactic of modern terrorism: a campaign directed against American interests, combined with a propaganda blitz designed to reinforce his message. The terrorist campaign was epitomized by the horrific attacks in New York and Washington and the plane crash in Shanksville, PA in September 2001. But these attacks in themselves would not be sufficient to make the Americans isolationists; they must be accompanied by the appropriate propaganda. Thus, Al-Qaida launched a campaign to sell their message to the American audience, via videotapes and speeches designed to reinforce the message: withdraw from Arab lands, stop trying to spread your values in our region, stop supporting Israel and the moderate Muslim regimes, and you will be safe. But the American media did not fall for this campaign. They refused to broadcast or transmit these tapes in full in America. So bin Laden's media campaign failed. Moreover, Americans were not terrorized by the 9/11 attacks. They were afraid, but their reaction was a wave of patriotism, the very opposite of what Bin Laden wanted to achieve.

TERRORISM AND PSYCHOLOGICAL WARFARE

The modern terrorist's strategy differs from that of the common criminal in that the terrorist is motivated by a political agenda. His actions (e.g., murder, sabotage, blackmail) may be identical to those of the common criminal. However, for the terrorist, these are all means to achieve wider goals, whether ideological, religious, social, or economic. The way to the terrorist's ultimate political goal runs through a vital interim objective: the creation of an unremitting paralyzing sensation of fear in the target community. Thus, modern terrorism is a means of instilling in every individual the feeling that the next attack may have his or her name on it. Terrorism works to undermine the sense of security and to disrupt everyday life so as to harm the target country's ability to function. The goal of this strategy is to drive public opinion to pressure decision-makers to surrender to the terrorists' demands. Thus, the target population becomes a tool in the hands of the terrorist in advancing the political agenda in the name of which the terrorism is perpetrated.

Terrorists are not necessarily interested in the deaths of three, thirty, or even three thousand people. Rather, they allow the imagination of the target population to do their work for them. In fact, it is conceivable that the terrorists could attain their aims without carrying out a single attack. The desired panic could be produced by the continuous broadcast of threats and declarations, on radio, TV, videos, and all the familiar methods of psychological warfare.

Modern terrorism, in defiance of the norms and laws of combat, focuses its attacks on civilians, thus turning the home front into the frontline. The civilian population is not only an easy target for the terrorist, but also an effective one; the randomness of the attack contributes to the general anxiety. The message is that anyone, anywhere, at any time, may be the target of the next attack. This threat undermines the ability of the civilian population to live a normal life. When every action must involve planning how to survive a potential terrorist attack at a random time and place, the daily routine becomes fraught with anxiety.

A "conventional" terrorist attack usually has a fairly limited physical effect. Its effectiveness lies in its ability to get the terrorists' message across. These messages are intended for three different audiences. To the terrorist organization's supporters, and the population it purports to serve, the message is: "We have succeeded. We have neutralized the power of the enemy and hit them at their most sensitive point." The attack thus serves to strengthen this public's support of the terrorist organization, to encourage enlistment to their ranks and, in general, to raise the morale of this community.

To the community and government targeted by the terrorist attack, the opposite message is sent: "Despite all your defenses–your army, your police force, your military hardware–you are never safe from us." Once civilians feel unsafe in their own homes and workplaces, daily life is disrupted, causing considerable harm to personal and national morale. The message is: "until you accede to our demands, you will not be safe."

At the same time, the terrorist attacks send still a third message to international public opinion. To the rest of the world, the terrorists present the attacks as examples of their determination to achieve their political aims by any means and at any cost. The terrorist attacks are intended to draw the attention of international public opinion to the conflict and the terrorists' demands. A more sinister message is concealed in this show of determination: "You, the countries uninvolved in the conflict, must put pressure on our enemies to give us what we want. Otherwise you might be next."

The terrorists' primary aim is to create fear within the target population, with the intention that this fear is translated into pressure on the government to accede to the terrorists' demands in order to stave off further terrorist attacks. The success of this strategy is dependent on the degree to which the fear of attack can be magnified out of proportion to the actual danger. The fear engendered in a population living in the shadow of terrorism has two components, one rational and one irrational. The rational fear is simply a product of the possibility of meeting a violent death or sustaining an injury as a result of a terrorist attack, with the degree of anxiety being proportional to the actual likelihood of the event occurring. In a society experiencing a large number of attacks, such anxiety is natural. However, there is also a more insidious element, an "irrational" anxiety, a fear that bears no relation to the actual statistical probability of being killed or injured in a terrorist attack, or even of a terrorist attack taking place at all (Ganor, 2003).

It is this irrational anxiety that is the interim goal of the terrorist organization, and the means by which it exerts pressure on the target population. By magnifying the threat, by making it seem that violent death lies around every corner, the terrorists hope to amplify the victim's anxiety to the point where she or he loses a sense of proportion. Modern terrorism is psychological warfare pure and simple. It aims at isolating the individual from the group, to break up a society into so many frightened individuals, hiding in their homes and unable to go about their daily lives as citizens, employees, and family members. Further, the terrorist aims to undermine the individual's belief in the collective values of society by amplifying the potential threat to the extent that security appears to outweigh all other political concerns (see Strossen, this volume). Terrorism uses the victim's own imagination against him or her.

Modern terrorist organizations invest much time and effort, as well as extensive resources, in psychological warfare. They carefully observe their target population to find weaknesses and cracks in the society that can be widened or exploited. The terrorists study the target country's media to learn how best to get their threats across and how to magnify the fears of the population and stimulate or amplify criticism of the government and its policies. Dissenting views in the society are carefully collected and used to undermine the population's beliefs in the rightness of its own ways. The terrorist organization knows from the outset that it will not achieve its goals purely by means of attacks. It must enlist the help of its victims themselves in gaining its objectives. A victory that would be impossible by military means is thus brought within reach through a protracted, gnawing campaign of psychological warfare, a war of attrition that gradually erodes the target population's will to fight and turns the tables against the stronger power.

PERSONALIZATION OF TERRORISM

One of the most telling examples of such a policy in action is the effect that a terrorist attack has on members of the target population not directly hit by the attack. This influence, the "personalization of the attack," can be seen immediately after a terrorist attack on a busy street or crowded shopping center. The immediate reaction of most people upon hearing of the attack is: "I was there only last week!" or "my wife works on the next block," or "my aunt lives just down the street." People have a natural tendency to seek a personal connection to events, a tendency of which the terrorist organization is well aware. By such "personalizing" of terrorist attacks, the effect on the target population is made to extend beyond the immediate victims to include people who were not even in the area at the time of the attack. The message conveyed, even though totally unfounded, is nevertheless highly dangerous. Members of the target population come to believe that only by a coincidence were they, or someone dear to them, saved from harm, and that such a coincidence cannot be counted upon next time.

Governments and policies have floundered under the influence of terrorism. The ability of a small group of individuals to manipulate public opinion, and thus the highest policies of the land, is what makes terrorism a strategic threat to Israel and other democratic societies.

CONCLUSIONS

Decision-makers and security personnel in countries affected by terrorism, not to mention members of the media, often appear to be woefully ignorant of the psychological manipulations used by terrorist organizations. These people all too often play into the hands of the terrorists, helping to increase the effectiveness of the terrorists' psychological campaign. The media often grant the terrorists a platform to publicize their views and psychological manipulations, not only through the coverage of the attack itself, but also in airing interviews with terrorists and videotapes made by them. Decision-makers publicly make reference to baseless threats made by the terrorists, thus granting them a credibility that they would not otherwise have. All of this naturally increases the public's anxiety. In addition, security personnel sometimes choose to publish vague intelligence warnings of impending attacks, even where such publicity does not add to public security. This increases the level of anxiety and contributes to a feeling of insecurity and confusion among the public, who have no idea how to act in the light of these warnings.

In their public statements, military and police spokesmen must take into consideration the psychological effect of terrorism. Otherwise, they risk winning the battle (i.e., succeeding in detecting and foiling a specific attack) while losing the war. When terrorism succeeds in creating such anxiety within a society that daily life becomes impossible, then that society has lost the war against terrorism. Some of the "irrational" anxiety stems, therefore, from a lack of knowledge. People tend to be afraid of the unknown.

It is the responsibility of the State to provide its citizens with the tools and information necessary to counter the terrorist's psychological manipulation. This should be done through education, arming the population with knowledge in order to prevent the strategic damage inflicted by modern terrorism. Terrorism can be fought using the knowledge of the actual risk of terrorism to the citizen, in contrast to the perceived risk, as well as information on the terrorists' psychological campaign and on the misuse of the media by them. This must be based on comprehensive research into how the terrorists use psychological manipulations to achieve their goals. On the basis of this information, tools can be developed to neutralize these manipulations.

The target community must be taught to view media coverage of terrorist attacks with a critical eye, in order to avoid falling for terrorist manipulation. Individuals must be taught to recognize the moment when the manner in which they relate to terrorism changed, the instant when "rational" fear became "irrational" anxiety. At this stage, the instruction should give individuals psychological tools to enable them to lower the level of personal "irrational" anxiety on their own. As a rule, members of a targeted population must constantly ask themselves: how do the terrorists expect me to behave in the light of their attacks? Am I willing to play the part that they have assigned to me in their terrorism strategy? (Numerous articles in this volume provide additional preventive measures on individual, family, community, and national levels.)

The media need not be a tool in the hands of the terrorist organization. On the contrary, they can play a crucial role in neutralizing the psychological damage of terrorism (see G. Ross, this volume). In a democratic society, the media's role is to provide reliable information in real time. However, reporters must be wary of their natural tendency to amplify the horror of a terrorist attack, and thus serve as a platform for the terrorists. The media should avoid taking close-ups while a terrorist attack is underway and should downplay expressions of extreme fear and panic in the heat of the moment. Above all, they should avoid broadcasting tapes made by terrorist organizations and interviews with individual terrorists.

In a democratic society there is no place for censorship, even on such a problematic and sensitive issue. However, journalists must be aware of their responsibility as members of society. and avoid being used as a tool by the terrorists to attain their political aims.

Psychological victory and the ensuing changes in public policy are the primary strategic goals of terrorist groups. This manipulation of governments through public opinion is especially dangerous to democracies. Thus, the decision-makers and politicians have a responsibility to their constituencies to help neutralize the effects of terrorist manipulation. Among other things, decision-makers can help by allocating the necessary funds for educational and instructional activities within their community. In addition, they must be careful not to intensify the fear of terrorist attacks by using the attacks as a tool in inter-party political struggles.

In conclusion, a terrorist attack is not an end in itself, but only a means to an end. Those faced with countering terrorism must have as thorough an understanding of the terrorists and their methods as the terrorist has of his target society. Often, the knowledge that one is being manipulated and how this is being done is itself a powerful weapon for countering such manipulation.

REFERENCES

Ganor, B. (2003). *The counter-terrorism puzzle, a guide for decision makers* (Hebrew). Hertzliya, Israel: Mifalot The Interdisciplinary Center.

Iyad, A. (1983). *Without a country: Conversations with Erik Rolo*. Mifras 3 Publishers, pp. 7-8.

Merari, A. (1987, July 22). Interview in *Bamahane* (an Israel Defense Forces weekly magazine) (Hebrew), pp. 1-3.

Merari, A. & Elad, S. (1986). *Hostile terrorist activities abroad*. Tel Aviv: Hakibbutz Hameuhad Publishing House. (Hebrew)

Ross, G. (2004). Media guidelines: From the "trauma vortex" to the "healing vortex." *Journal of Aggression, Maltreatment & Trauma, 9*(1/2/3/4), 391-394.

Strossen, N. (2004). Terrorism's toll on civil liberties. *Journal of Aggression, Maltreatment & Trauma, 9*(1/2/3/4), 365-377.

Tales from the Underground

Gerald Cromer

SUMMARY. This study of the propaganda of Lehi (Lohamei Herut Yisrael/Fighters for the Freedom of Israel) shows how it is best analyzed as a series of stories. Movement leaders tried to justify their resort to violence by telling four kinds of narratives: contemporary, historical, metahistorical, and biographical. After providing a description of these terrorist tales, the article draws attention to their internal structure, the interaction among them, and the way in which they were in dialogue with the prior religious discourse.

KEYWORDS. Terrorism, narrative, terrorist propaganda, freedom fighters

Studies of the propaganda of nationalist and separatist movements draw attention to the widespread tendency among academics to politicize terrorism. While this approach may be suitable for the analysis of ideologically oriented

---

Address correspondence to: Gerald Cromer, PhD, Department of Criminology, Bar Ilan University, Ramat Gan, Israel (E-mail: cromeg@mail.biu.ac.il).

This article is a highly abridged version of a chapter that appeared in Cromer (2001, pp. 1-44).

[Haworth co-indexing entry note]: "Tales from the Underground." Cromer, Gerald. Co-published simultaneously in *Journal of Aggression, Maltreatment & Trauma* (The Haworth Maltreatment & Trauma Press, an imprint of The Haworth Press, Inc.) Vol. 9, No. 1/2, 2004; and: *The Trauma of Terrorism: Sharing Knowledge and Shared Care, An International Handbook* (ed: Yael Danieli, Danny Brom, and Joe Sills) The Haworth Maltreatment & Trauma Press, an imprint of The Haworth Press, Inc., 2005.

groups, it is thought to be totally inappropriate for the study of nationalist ones. Tololyan (1988) and others have argued that political reductionism fails to take into account the extent to which the latter are an integral part of the wider cultural context. Terrorist propaganda is intertextual, and it is therefore imperative to consider the different ways in which it is in dialogue with mainstream national discourse and the master narratives of the culture in question.

The cultural specificity of each nationalistic group makes it difficult to generalize about terrorist propaganda. Nevertheless, a review of the few studies that have been carried out suggests that it is possible to delineate certain similarities in the way in which different movements try to justify their resort to violence. For the purposes of analysis, they are best considered under two broad headings: the construction of histories and life histories and the appropriation of religion.

The propaganda of all nationalist and separatist movements is replete with historical references. The terrorists and their enemies, both external and internal, are compared to famous and infamous figures from bygone days. Consequently, the analogies always take the form of narratives about earlier examples of resistance to oppression.

Clearly, the resort to history is meant not only to help understand old facts of heroism but also to engender new ones. Terrorist propaganda hails past acts of bravery and resistance in order to encourage similar ones in the present. It therefore consists of a series of projective narratives that are both descriptive and prescriptive. "They not only tell a story of the past, but also map out future actions that can imbue the time of individual lives with collective values . . . [and] tell individuals how they would ideally have to live and die in order to contribute properly to the collectivity and its future" (Tololyan, 1988, p. 218).

Projective narratives of the ideal life and death are backed up by a martyrology (Zameret, 1974, pp. 85-88) or regulative biographies (Tololyan, 1988, p. 230) of those who personified them. Thus, the life histories of those who fell in the struggle for independence are constructed in such a way that they can be portrayed as examples of the national ideal. Those who are engaged in violence are depicted not as outcasts from society but as paradigmatic figures of its deepest values. They are to be praised rather than punished for their actions.

This particular reading of history and life histories is, of course, very different from earlier ones, especially that of the religious authorities. Their concentration on divine intervention, for instance, is replaced by an emphasis on human action or what Schatzberger (1985, p. 57) aptly referred to as "the motif of the active deed." Notwithstanding this and other disagreements, the terrorists find it difficult to attack the defenders of the faith head on. If and when they do, their criticism is often couched in religious terms. Nationalist and separatist propaganda is replete with symbols made effective by centuries of ecclesiastic rhetoric and practice.

As a result of this tendency to appropriate religious language and rituals, traditional models are rarely discarded. They are rather transformed and infused with new meanings (Aretxaga, 1993, p. 240; Arthur, 1996, p. 272). Although the concepts of sacrifice and martyrdom are as central to the propaganda of both the Armenian Secret Liberation Army (ASALA) and the Irish Republican Army (IRA) as they are to church sermons and other forms of religious discourse, the message conveyed is exactly the opposite. Sacrifice is redefined as heroic death and hailed as the harbinger of national renewal. Consequently, resignation to suffering in this world is derided. Active resistance to oppression and the creation of a better world is the order of the day (Aretxaga, 1993, p. 244; Tololyan, 1987, p. 100).

By attacking religion in this way, nationalist and separatist groups clearly damage the authority of the church and synagogue. However, this is only half the story. Paradoxically perhaps, the terrorists' offensive against the spiritual authorities endows their violent actions with a religious aura of their own. By using the vocabulary and imagery of the church, they secularize religious myths and sacralize their own cause at one and the same time (Arthur, 1996, pp. 276-277; Tololyan, 1987, 95).

A FIGHTER'S MORALITY

An acronym for Lohamei Herut Yisrael (Fighters for the Freedom of Israel), Lehi was an underground organization that fought against the British presence in Palestine and for the establishment of an independent Jewish state.[1] Movement leaders pointed to the failure of both political and practical Zionism in achieving these ends. Neither of them, they argued, had succeeded in bringing the British mandate to an end. It was therefore both necessary and justifiable to use force against the "foreign ruler." That was the only way to achieve freedom and independence.

However, Lehi's use of violence was not only defended as a strategy of last resort. Movement leaders and rank and file members alike tended to vindicate themselves on moral as well as pragmatic grounds. They appealed to "the sphere of eternal ideas such as freedom, liberty and equality." Thus Lehi members swore allegiance to "the law of the movement of Hebrew freedom fighters" and adhered to "the supreme command, the command of life for our people." Its authority, they argued, derived from the natural law concerning "the right of each nation to freedom in its homeland, and to fight against the oppressor and the exploiter." This supreme law took precedence over all others.

Lehi propaganda, in common with that of other terrorist movements, devoted more space to negative portrayals of internal and external enemies than it did to positive self-depictions. Time and again, the British laws regarding Palestine were attacked not only for being contrary to the stipulations of the mandate but also as unjust and immoral. Movement activists who were brought to trial therefore rejected the jurisdiction of the courts. They neither denied their actions nor offered excuses for having committed them. Without exception, they insisted on being recognized as a belligerent party and being tried as prisoners of war, or totally rejected the right of the British to sit in judgment.

This "accusation of the accusers" was by no means limited to British actions against the *yishuv* (the pre-state Jewish settlement in Palestine). Lehi propaganda often emphasized the fact that the movement was fighting against the very existence of a foreign ruler, "not against a bad commissioner but against the commission, not against the implementation of the mandate but against the fact that it was not given to the Hebrew people." It was the mere presence of the British in the Promised Land rather than the way they behaved there that constituted the core of the problem. The mandatory authorities were thus an "a priori enemy" and, in turn, a justifiable target of the Freedom Fighters of Israel.

Lehi leaders were confident that they would prove victorious in the struggle against the British. They insisted that "there is hope because brute physical force, the force of violence and malice, cannot stand up against the force of those who fight with firearms and for an ideal." According to this view of things, the movement's spiritual strength gave it "an extra weapon that cannot be measured in material terms." When taken into account though, Lehi had a distinct advantage over the physically superior empire. It was, therefore, just a matter of time until victory was achieved.

IN THE MIRROR OF THE PAST

This ultimately optimistic reading of the ongoing struggle against the British mandate was backed up by "the lessons of history." Lehi propaganda was replete with comparisons between contemporary events and those of yesteryear. Of course, this interpretive process was not conceived of as an intellectual exercise. It was meant to be both a guide and a goad to action. "The past demands. History is binding."

Each and every protagonist was compared to figures from bygone days. Heroes and villains alike were portrayed as being essentially similar, or even as better or worse than those that preceded them. Thus, the British were compared to all the arch enemies of the Jewish people from Pharaoh until modern times. Significantly, however, Lehi propaganda most frequently likened them to Amalek, the apogee of evil in Jewish tradition and the only nation that the Jews were commanded to destroy completely.

Lehi propaganda also included comparisons between the British mandate and Nazi Germany. The latter was not regarded as an ahistorical phenomenon or even as *sui generis*. Hitler was essentially the same as other enemies of the Jewish people: "the Hitlers of yesterday, the Hitlers of today and the Hitlers of tomorrow." In fact, some, including the British, were worse. Not only did they fail to prevent German atrocities and commit many of their own; they also occupied the Hebrew homeland. And that, according to Lehi, is the most hideous crime of all, "the absolute evil that everything else stems from."

Lehi leaders also used historical analogies to attack their enemies within the yishuv. The leaders of the Jewish settlement in Palestine were likened to the Judenrat in the lands occupied by Nazi Germany and to the Hellenists at the time of the destruction of the First Temple. Lehi, in contrast, was compared to a long list of heroes who had fought for national liberation from biblical to modern times. It was the latest link in "the chain of heroes of the Jewish people, a people who had fought for its freedom with more force, more strength, more sacrifice, and more determination than any other nation in the world."

Lehi propaganda invariably emphasized the resolve of Jewish freedom fighters rather than the extent to which they were successful. The fact that they fought, not that they won, was regarded as the crucial factor. However, this dichotomy is somewhat misleading because all those involved in the struggle for Jewish independence are victorious in the end. Even if they lose a battle, they transmit the love for freedom to their contemporaries and to future generations. The struggle therefore continues unabated and will eventually be crowned with success. Victory is assured.

THE IRON LAW OF LIBERATION

The "Jewish liberation struggle" like that of other nations, Lehi leaders argued, is in certain ways unique. Each one depends on "the people, geography, and historical circumstances" concerned. However, these differences are of relatively minor importance. They relate to form and not to content. Consequently, it is important to understand and explain not only the lessons of Jewish history, but also those of other nations who fought or are still fighting for their freedom.

Lehi propaganda invariably portrayed British imperialism as more despotic than any other kind of foreign rule, and even as "the most perfect regime of oppression." Nevertheless, frequent reference was also made to the cruelty and fate of other colonial powers. The collapse of the Austro-Hungarian and Ottoman empires, for instance, as often cited as proof of the fact that the mightiest rulers could be brought down by determined action on the part of subjugated nations. Leaders of the yishuv should therefore follow the example of foreign heroes as well as those of the Jewish people. Garibaldi, de Gaulle, and others were also appropriate models for the struggle against the British presence in Palestine.

In order to drive this message home, Lehi took the argument a step further. The fact that the stories were taken from "throughout the ages and all around the world" suggested that they were not just examples of a longstanding and worldwide phenomenon, but proof of a universal law, the iron law of liberation: "any subjugated nation that is not contaminated by a spirit of degeneration and has a desire to live will fight for its freedom. Any nation that fights for its freedom will in the end be victorious."

This law is explained, in part at least, by the fact that national liberation movements do not need to achieve an outright military victory in order to gain independence. It is enough to create "a permanent state of war that demands constant preparedness of large forces and causes an ongoing feeling of unrest." This forces the oppressor to ask the question whether "the gains are not outweighed by the losses" and, in turn, to decide that it is in his best interest to concede defeat and grant independence to the fledgling nation.

Even this limited victory though cannot be explained in terms of the physical power of the liberation movement. It is due rather to "the force of justice that guides the hand holding the weapon." Previous struggles for national independence indicate that looks can be deceiving. "Not everything that appears weak is in fact weak, and not everything that gives the impression of being strong is in fact strong." Spiritual superiority has to be included in the balance of forces. When it is taken into account, the final result is clear. In the end, right always overcomes might.

BODY AND SOUL

Even though Lehi's projective narratives were filled with references to those who throughout the ages had fought and died in the struggle for national independence, the movement understandably took special pride in the feats of its own members. Regulative biographies of Lehi heroes hailed the physical bravery and spiritual courage of those who met their death in combat or on the scaffold. However, this was by no means the whole story. Portrayals of the fallen were not limited to the period during which they fought in the underground. The life histories also related to their formative years and posthumous influence.

Lehi propaganda drew attention to critical events in the lives of the fallen that had led them to join the movement. For Eliahu Hakim, one of Lord Moyne's assassins, the sight of Arab rioters was "the first spark." In the case of his partner, Beit Zuri, it was the presence of British police in the Hebrew homeland that convinced him that "the only way to fight the British rule that is based on violence is to use force . . . and to attack their representatives that are responsible for our troubles."

Those who took up arms against the British portrayed themselves and were portrayed by others as the continuation or renewal of "the tradition of bravery in Israel." However, the need to ensure complete secrecy prevented Lehi from describing the exploits of its members in any detail. Attention was concentrated instead on how they met their death in the underground. The movement's propaganda was replete with references to the physical bravery of those killed and injured by the British. Stories were told about how they fought against seemingly insurmountable odds and to the bitter end. Frequent mention was also made of the fighters' willingness to endanger themselves to save their colleagues and their refusal to reveal the secrets of the underground even when subjected to the infamous British methods of torture. Despite undergoing "superhuman pain," Lehi's members went to their death with "the purity of the silent."

Time and again, Lehi propaganda was at pains to point out that the British only killed the bodies and not the souls or the spirit of the Fighters of the Freedom of Israel. They sacrificed their ephemeral life, but in doing so they gained an eternal one "in the memory of the free nation in an independent homeland." Obituaries for those who died at the hands of the British declared that "the blood of earlier heroes flowed in their veins and now their blood flows in ours," or in more traditional Jewish terms, that "their souls are bound in the bond of our lives, and our lives are bound in the bond of their magnanimous deep souls."

The relationship between the fallen and those who follow in their footsteps was often portrayed as a reciprocal one. According to this view of things, each side helps the other. Those killed by the British provide a role model for future generations. However, it was the knowledge that their sacrifice will be emulated by others that enabled them to take up arms and risk being killed in the first place. Thus, when recruits swore allegiance to the movement, they promised they would go to the gallows with pride and peace of mind in the belief that their death "will educate thousands of other fighters who will continue to struggle and ensure the victory of our mission."

PRAYING WITH A RIFLE

All the terrorist tales described so far were directed against the narratives of the British government and the leaders of the Jewish yishuv. Lehi's major external and internal enemies were criticized for their presence in the Promised Land and their failure to take the appropriate actions against it respectively. However, in addition to these two targets, the propaganda was also directed against traditional Judaism and those who lived according to its dictates. Religious Jews were lambasted repeatedly for believing in divine help rather than human action and their consequent failure to take part in the struggle for national liberation.

Significantly, Lehi's attack on "the official representatives of the Torah" was invariably couched in religious terms. The movement's propaganda was replete with citations of those religious commandments that were viewed as endorsing the movement's resort to violence. They included both biblical precepts (e.g., an eye for an eye, a tooth for a tooth) and talmudic injunctions (e.g., if anyone comes to kill you, kill him first). Lehi's understanding of these and other texts was often very different from the traditional interpretations. The law of retaliation, for instance, was only applied in cases of personal damages and has long been abandoned in favor of monetary compensation for the injured party. This departure from tradition was even more marked with regard to mourning customs and the Jewish festivals. However, despite or maybe because of their criticism of these rituals, Lehi leaders felt the need to appropriate them in support of their resort to violence.

Significantly, this tendency was particularly marked with regard to Passover and Hanukah, the festivals that, respectively, commemorate the liberation of the Jewish people from Egyptian bondage and Greek dominion. Thus, in contrast to the traditional idea that the lights of the menorah are holy and must therefore only be used for the purpose of "publicizing the miracle" of the rededication of the Temple, Lehi leaders declared, "Let our bodies turn into burning candles. Let our blood be the holy blood of Hanukah. This blood and these candles are sacred, and it is a religious obligation to use them." Only "redemptive actions" of this kind, it was argued, can fulfill the ultimate aim of the Jewish festivals, "not just a recollection of a past event, but its transformation into a living Torah in the present and the future."

For Lehi, the struggle for national liberation was "the Torah" or "the holiest idea" of the Jewish people. Alluding to the Shema, a prayer that traditional

Jews recite three times a day and on their deathbed, those who had taken up arms against the British were called upon to carry out each mission "with all your heart, with all your soul, and with all your might." Freedom, like God, is holy. It also demands unlimited and endless love.

The sacred nature of Lehi's ends led to a deification of those who fought to achieve them. Alluding to God's deliverance of the Children of Israel from Eygpt, they were hailed as "the outstretched arm of the Hebrew people." An announcement of the death of one of Lehi's members concluded with the opening words of the Kaddish, the traditional prayer in memory of the dead. However, the emphasis was completely different. The fallen hero rather than the eternal God was being sanctified. The nature of the argument is clear: Lehi's aim of liberating the Hebrew homeland was holy. So were all those who fought for it, and any means by which they did so.

CONCLUSION

The propaganda of nationalist and separatist groups differs from that of ideological ones in two ways: in form and in content. It is based on narratives rather than accounts (Scott & Lyman, 1968) and presents the contemporary situation as a repetition of the past rather than as an entity in its own right. Before concluding, the major characteristics of these narratives will be delineated by describing their internal structure, the interaction between them, and the way in which they are in dialogue with the prior religious one.

All the terrorist tales meet the essential requirement for a narrative: an evaluative framework in which good or bad character helps produce unfortunate or happy outcomes (MacIntyre, 1981, p. 456). Each story pitted the forces of light against the forces of darkness and showed how the former had prevailed or would eventually do so. Drawing attention to the fact that the few were confronting the many, the narratives contended that their numerical inferiority was more than compensated by enormous spiritual strength that derives from the rightness of their cause. It is these virtues that enable freedom fighters to expel the foreign ruler and achieve national independence. The struggle may be a long and arduous one, and may involve heavy losses and much bloodshed, but right is might and it will, therefore, prevail in the end.

Since all the stories took the form of a morality play between the forces of good and evil, they comprise an intricate network of nested narratives (Gergen & Gergen, 1983, p. 263). The life histories invariably related to how the fallen first learned, then lived, and finally became an integral part of the movement's projective narrative. In doing so, they provide a classic example of the way in which biographies are embedded in the story of the group within which those concerned find their identity (Connerton, 1989, p. 21). In addition, the contemporary tale is conceived of as a repetition of earlier episodes in the struggle for national independence and these, in turn, are portrayed as the enactment of broader meta-historical narratives. Together these terrorist tales transmit the "timeless truths" about the relationship between the oppressor and the oppressed and the inevitable result of the conflict between them.

"Any given telling," Bruner and Gorfain (1984, p. 60) have argued, "takes account of previous and anticipated tellings, and responds to alternative and to challenging stories." In the case of nationalist groups, this dialogic narration assumes a particularly interesting form. The frontal attack on the religious reading of history goes hand in hand with the widespread appropriation of religious language, texts, and rituals. While the content of the rhetoric emphasizes discontinuity, its style points to a certain continuity with the past. Together they are meant to show how terrorism is both anchored in and a radical alternative to traditional religion.

The ongoing dialogue with the prior religious narrative is by no means the only one that national terrorists engage in. They are also involved in a war of words with the external enemy (the foreign narrative) and the more moderate leaders of the nascent nation (the dominant narrative). Future research should therefore analyze the nature of these dialogues. Doing so is a necessary prerequisite for a deeper understanding of the content and form of terrorist tales.

NOTE

1. The different kinds of Lehi propaganda (e.g., event–related communiqués, newspapers, doctrinal texts, and radio broadcasts) have been published in Fighters for the Freedom of Israel (1982). All quotations are taken from this collection. Exact citations can be found in Cromer (2001).

REFERENCES

Aretxaga, B. (1993). Striking with hunger: Cultural meaning of political violence in Northern Ireland. In K. Warren (Ed.), *The violence within: Cultural and political opposition in divided nations* (pp. 219-253). Boulder, CO: Westview Press.

Arthur, P. (1996). Reading violence: Ireland. In D. E. Apter (Ed.), *The legitimization of violence* (pp. 234-291). New York: New York University Press.

Bruner, E. M., & Gorfain, P. (1984). Dialogic narration and the paradoxes of Massada. In E. M. Bruner (Ed.), *Text, play and story: The construction and reconstruction of self and society* (pp. 56-79). Washington, DC: American Ethnological Society.

Connerton, P. (1989). *How societies remember.* Cambridge: Cambridge University Press.

Cromer, G. (2001). *Narratives of violence.* Aldershot: Ashgate.

Fighters for the Freedom of Israel. (1982). *Collected works, 2 volumes.* Tel Aviv: Yair Publications (Hebrew).

Gergen, K. J., & Gergen, M. M. (1983). Narratives of the self. In T. R. Sarbin & K. E. Scheibe (Eds.), *Studies in social identity* (pp. 254-273). New York: Praeger.

MacIntyre, A. (1981). *After virtue: A study in moral theory.* South Bend, IN: University of Notre Dame Press.

Schatzberger, H. (1985). *Resistance and tradition in mandatory Palestine.* Ramat Gan: Bar Ilan University Press. (Hebrew)

Scott, M. B., & Lyman, S. M. (1968). Accounts. *American Sociological Review, 33*(1), 48-62.

Tololyan, K. (1987). Martyrdom as legitimacy: Terrorism, religion and symbolic appropriation in the Armenian diaspora. In P. Wilkinson & A. M. Stewart (Eds.), *Contemporary research on terrorism* (pp. 89-103). Aberdeen: Aberdeen University Press.

Tololyan, K. (1988). Cultural narrative and the motivation of the terrorist. In D. C. Rapoport (Ed.), *Inside terrorist organizations* (pp. 217-233). London: Frank Cass.

Zameret, Z. (1974). *The educational activities of Lehi.* Unpublished Masters Thesis, Hebrew University of Jerusalem.

Aum Shinrikyo:
The Threshold Crossed

Robert Jay Lifton

SUMMARY. Aum Shinrikyo and its guru, Shoko Asahara, burst into world consciousness in 1995 when the cult released sarin, a highly lethal nerve gas, into the Tokyo subway. Aum Shinrikyo emerged from the apocalyptic underbelly of Japanese society, but there is little that is uniquely Japanese about it. It epitomizes a category of cult led by a megalomanic guru who guided his disciples into induced mystical experiences in pursuit of his apocalyptic vision of renewing the world spiritually by initiating World War III and bringing about a biblical Armageddon.

KEYWORDS. Aum Shinrikyo, sarin, guru, apocalyptic, mystical experiences, Armageddon

---

Address correspondence to: Robert Jay Lifton, MD, 19A Berkeley Street, Cambridge, MA 02138 USA (E-mail: rlifton@challiance.org).

[Haworth co-indexing entry note]: "Aum Shinrikyo: The Threshold Crossed." Lifton, Robert Jay. Co-published simultaneously in *Journal of Aggression, Maltreatment & Trauma* (The Haworth Maltreatment & Trauma Press, an imprint of The Haworth Press, Inc.) Vol. 9, No. 1/2, 2004; and: *The Trauma of Terrorism: Sharing Knowledge and Shared Care, An International Handbook* (ed: Yael Danieli, Danny Brom, and Joe Sills) The Haworth Maltreatment & Trauma Press, an imprint of The Haworth Press, Inc., 2005.

Aum Shinrikyo, the fanatical Japanese cult, crossed a threshold of violence with five years still remaining in the twentieth century. Though a relatively small group, it acted upon a vision of cosmic purification that included the murder of just about everyone on earth.

Aum Shinrikyo and its guru, Shoko Asahara, burst into world consciousness when the cult released sarin gas on a number of Tokyo subway trains in March 1995. Though tens of thousands of passengers might have been threatened with death, the attack was hurried and inefficient, killing just twelve people, because the group had received word that the police were closing in. Its plan had been to release enormous amounts of sarin later that year in order to create a major disaster and set in motion a series of catastrophic events and so fulfill its guru's world-ending vision. According to the plan, Japanese authorities would believe that America had released the sarin. The Americans would, in turn, assume that the Japanese had done it and a war would break out between the two countries. Other great powers would join in, leading to World War III which would then bring about a biblical Armageddon.

ULTIMATE WEAPONS AND ULTIMATE ZEALOTRY

Of course that was wild fantasy, but it was a fantasy combined with all-too-real weapons of mass destruction. Aum had produced considerable amounts of sarin, a highly lethal nerve gas (though the guru ordered much of the cult's stockpile destroyed when he became fearful of discovery), and had released various amounts of it on several occasions prior to the Tokyo subway attack. It had also produced biological weapons, notably botulinus and anthrax, and made several attempts to create disasters in major urban areas by spraying them, but was unsuccessful because of problems with their release.

Aum pursued any avenues it could find for obtaining nuclear weapons. It looked into uranium deposits (even acquiring a ranch in an area of Australia thought to be rich in such deposits) and sought contacts with disaffected Russian nuclear scientists. Particularly active in Russia, Aum made use of its huge financial resources to purchase various kinds of weapons and to bribe officials with access to more weapons. Hence the provocative question found in the Russian diary of Aum's leading weapons procurer: "How much does a nuclear warhead cost?"

Aum could not in the end acquire those warheads, and instead made sarin gas its signature weapon. Asahara was fascinated by weapons of mass destruction in general, but sarin might have had a deeper attraction for him as he greatly admired Hitler and expressed delight when told that the Fuhrer's horoscope closely resembled his own. The gas was first produced (though not used) by Hitler's scientists. The guru was thought to have instructed Aum scientists to look into the specific Nazi method of producing sarin.

But whether or not the Hitler connection influenced Aum's use of sarin, Asahara's greatest passion was with nuclear weapons. Those were what he really craved. He was obsessed with them as a potential victim of a nuclear attack to come, as a survivor (of the atomic bombings of Japan), and as a fierce nuclearist who yearned to possess and use them.

His obsession with nuclear weapons began with Hiroshima. On a number of occasions he declared that Japan would experience "a hundred Hiroshimas," and many of his visions and "meditations" involved that city. In one of these he described traveling to Hiroshima on the "astral plane" and finding there grotesque evidence of a World War III nuclear holocaust that had already occurred. Always drawn to the most apocalyptic means of destruction, Asahara viewed chemical agents like sarin and biological agents like botulinus not only as "the poor man's nuclear weapons" (as many have) but also as "energy-saving nuclear weapons" (highly effective without requiring the enormous explosive capacity of nuclear weapons or their elaborate production methods). Asahara also spoke with great enthusiasm about "laser weapons" and "plasma weapons," which he came to believe already existed and were even more powerful than the nuclear variety. But it was nuclear weapons that remained his measure and his passion.

Asahara and Aum represent an extreme case of what I call "trickle-down nuclearism" in which ever smaller nations, cults, or transnational groups seek to obtain ever less expensive and easier to produce nuclear weapons. Trickle-down nuclearism is partly technological, having to do with the miniaturization of the weapons, the spread of knowledge about how to make them, and the improved technical skills of groups seeking them. But it is also a state of mind as the weapons, an ever longer-standing presence in our world, sink yet deeper into us; that of an intense yearning for and embrace of them as sources of ultimate power, especially on the part of those who imagine world-ending or world-purifying events. Over the course of the Cold War, most cults on the order of Aum Shinrikyo would not have imagined the possibility of acquiring nuclear weapons. But the above developments have combined with a failure on the part of prominent nuclear powers to rid themselves of their own stockpiles. The result has been an expanding sense of nuclear entitlement and an impetus toward proliferation, as nations and militant movements increasingly equate possession of the weapons with international respect.

One must recognize a remarkable trickle-down effect when such intense nuclear desire extends to a cult like Aum, consisting of no more than 10,000 Japanese members and only 1,400 full-time "monks." It seems that "living with nuclear weapons" can have its hidden dangers, because increasingly smaller groups can develop strong impulses to live with them too, and, in cases like Aum, to seek to use them to end life. It used to be that the United States and the Soviet Union had something of a monopoly, not just on the weapons market, but on the dangerous passions associated with them. Aum suggests that there is no limit to how far these passions can "trickle down."

With Aum, we may speak of a marriage between ultimate zealotry and ultimate weaponry, or between an ideology of violent apocalypse and weapons with an apocalyptic essence. Each fed malignantly on the other: Aum's apocalyptic zealotry pushing it to seek the weapons, whose apocalyptic essence further intensified the zealotry.

APOCALYPTIC JAPAN

The society that gave rise to Aum had experienced an extraordinary degree of psychological and historical dislocation, dating back to Japan's traumatic emergence from feudalism in the late nineteenth century. That dislocation culminated in devastating defeat in World War II, which included an element of something close to physical annihilation as well as psychic collapse in the breakdown of the emperor-centered religion that had so dominated the society. Indeed, the devastating bombing of all of Japan's major cities, followed by the atomic bombings of Hiroshima and Nagasaki, created a uniquely apocalyptic wartime experience.

The behavior of the Japanese themselves during the war had its own apocalyptic dimensions. The extent of their wartime atrocities, never officially acknowledged in the post-war years, rivaled those of the Nazis. They included policies in China we would now call "ethnic cleansing"; the massacre and systematic rape of Chinese, notably in Nanking; slave labor on an unprecedented scale; extensive use of biological warfare; grotesque medical experiments on prisoners; the forcing of more than 100,000 women, mostly Korean, into prostitution to serve Japanese military personnel; and the systematic bombing of civilians in Chinese cities that some have viewed as a forerunner of allied strategic bombing. The Japanese were apocalyptic perpetrators as well as victims.

The reverberations of that double experience have been evident throughout the post-World War II era. Underneath the seemingly stable Japanese society, there has been a powerful apocalyptic undercurrent, visible in novels, in highly popular cartoon narratives (or graphic novels), in films for television and movie theaters (the Godzilla films are the best known in America), and in wildly successful television series. There are endless stories of the destruction or threatened destruction of the world and of post-apocalyptic nuclear wastelands.

Nothing better indicates the apocalyptic explosion in Japanese popular culture than its strange embrace of the writings of the sixteenth-century French astrologer and physician Nostradamus, who loosely predicted (on the basis of the Book of Revelation) that the end of the world would come with the year 2000. Even looser Japanese translations of his work, some of which suggested that a savior would arrive from the East, have undergone more than 400 printings since 1973 and sold in the millions, making the Japanese the world's greatest consumers of his murky message. Young Japanese were especially responsive to the extremity of that message because post-war society, though democratic in form, was perceived as authoritarian in its lockstep requirements, and profoundly corrupt in its political and economic behavior. Many young and well-educated Japanese were primed and ready to respond to the apocalyptic extremity of Shoko Asahara's message.

Also feeding Asahara's and Aum's extremity, and public appeal, was the nuclear drumbeat of the Cold War, and various threats by the United States and the Soviet Union to initiate something close to world destruction. After the end of the Cold War, Asahara found himself fascinated by the Gulf War of 1990-1991. He identified with the Iraqi dictator Saddam Hussein, whom he saw as a non-white target of American aggression, but at the same time he was excited by America's high-tech, laser-guided weapons systems because they seemed a harbinger of the Armageddon he so craved. As a late-twentieth-century apocalyptic figure, Asahara associated Armageddon with the most advanced weapons technology; and as a paranoid and megalomanic guru close to madness, he was thrilled by the mass killing such technology could bring about. The ultimate lure, for him, of course, was nuclear weapons, which conveyed to him the image that he alone–or with a few disciples–could achieve his ultimate goal of destroying the world.

AUM AND THE WORLD

Aum Shinrikyo was a cult that emerged from the apocalyptic underbelly of its own society. But I would emphasize that there was little that was uniquely Japanese about it. Certainly its impulse toward forcing the end, its fascination with Armageddon, and its attraction toward ultimate weaponry are increasingly common denominators in the global apocalyptic mindset and can take shape in any culture. Aum's Japanese circumstances probably caused it to go further in these areas than other groups previously had (since then Islamist and American extremists have more than caught up). Rather than being unique, Aum epitomizes a category of cultic movement bent on world-ending violence (for definitions of strategic terrorism, see Picco, this volume).

Despite its totalistic, one-sided sense of mission, Aum's doctrine and practice were almost desperately eclectic and many-sided, contributing to what could be called apocalyptic multiculturalism. The cult was primarily Buddhist, but focused on elements of early Tibetan Buddhism closely tied to Hinduism. Asahara chose the world-destroying and restoring Hindu deity Shiva as his personal god and embraced the Christian Armageddon narrative as the basis for his apocalyptic vision. He referred as well to apocalyptic ideas in Hinduism and Buddhism, but these tended to be less precise and schematic than the Christian version, less of a road map to the end of time and more gradualistic depictions of spiritual and moral decline (though there is in Hinduism powerful imagery of Shiva dancing the cosmos to nonexistence in order to renew it).

In addition to its Tibetan roots, the Buddhism he practiced and taught had lively New Age components, including an emphasis on high states or "mystical experiences." Disciples whom I interviewed after he was arrested stressed how appealing this was, in contrast to the "deadness" of ordinary Japanese Buddhism, which had little to do with their life experience. The yoga Asahara quite skillfully taught had a similar combination of the very old and very new. He also was influenced at least to some extent by a violently apocalyptic fringe of the American right, through translations of their writings distributed in Tokyo, though the virulent anti-Semitism he often expressed probably derived mainly from strong Japanese roots.

Such eclecticism has been common in "new religions" and cultic movements in Japan and elsewhere. Aum's version of eclecticism enabled it to be ancient and current, as well as vastly inclusive in its claimed connection (however superficial or distorted) to much of the world's varied religious and cultural fare. This eclecticism contributed to an aura of universality, of being beyond any single religion or culture in its mission of cosmic purification.

Aum was eclectic in its finances as well. It was focused intensely on acquiring wealth, and made enormous amounts of money by aggressively merchandising its religion, including the sale of ritual objects and literature, exorbitant charges for initiations and practices, and a requirement (sometimes enforced through coercion and threat) that converts donate their total assets or those of their families–as well as through a great variety of businesses, such as computer companies, noodle shops and restaurants, bookstores, dating bureaus, and real estate agencies. Such commercial enterprises, ordinarily considered by Asahara part of Japan's cultural "pollution," in Aum's hands became a sacred form of service.

Everything was subsumed to the guru's murderous apocalyptic project (even if many followers were unclear about its exact nature or the violence it was to involve), and such projects can generate extraordinary amounts of energy. The 1,400 or so full-time Aum religionists seemed to be everywhere, doing everything–conducting strenuous religious practices, manipulating other members, running profitable businesses, scouring Russia for ordinary and exotic weaponry, bribing officials, manufacturing and stockpiling and releasing chemical and biological weapons, threatening and sometimes killing people.

THE GURU AND HIS VISIONS

Megalomanic gurus tend to go through life with a sense of grievance or resentment, which in Asahara's case involved lifelong bitterness over having been sent to a school for the blind. He was indeed without vision in one eye and his vision was impaired in the other, but he was not legally blind and was sent to the school by his impoverished parents for reasons of convenience (i.e., it provided free tuition and board) and because his completely sightless older brother had already been enrolled there. While the childhood of a guru can never completely explain his remarkable adult behavior, we can say that, as a boy, Asahara lived out, quite literally, Erasmus's dictum that "in the country of the blind the one-eyed man is king." In the school, he proved to be a manipulative and bullying force, though he could be tender to his completely blind followers. Even then he was extremely interested in accumulating money, intensely involved in drama (writing and acting in plays), and had grandiose ambitions including becoming prime minister of Japan or at least a great doctor–all characteristics that were present in him as an adult.

He had some brushes with the law, one soon after leaving the school, for causing bodily injury to another person, and one in Tokyo a bit later for selling fake medicines in a Chinese herbal pharmacy he had started. He entered the wide-open world of Japanese new religions in the early 1980s, joining a relatively established one before striking out on his own as a religious teacher and guru. He later described "achievements" of a kind generally required to create a guru's myth. These involved overcoming personal failures and psychological difficulties by spiritual means and, above all, experiencing cosmic visions, two of which were to become the basis for his guruism. At age thirty, he imagined himself leading an army of the gods to a victory of the forces of light over the forces of darkness, and the following year achieved "final enlightenment" while meditating in the Himalayas.

In living out his impulse toward extremity, Asahara not only embraced the principle of "forcing the end," but developed an ideology of killing to heal, even of altruistic murder and altruistic world destruction. This was accomplished by "attack guruism" and "action prophecy," which combined lethal prediction with lethal action. An ancient Buddhist principle called *poa* means that the killing of a person of inferior spiritual status by a person of high spiritual attainment was beneficial to the victim, enhancing his next rebirth and thereby his immortality. The more general principle here is that killing on a vast scale, whether by Aum, Islamist zealots, or superpower visionaries, is only possible when accompanied by a claim to virtue.

Asahara's one talent in life was being a guru, and he demonstrated a great ability for attracting and holding disciples through intense and innovative forms of religious practice and mind manipulation. He revealed the complexities and contradictions that make up the mind of a guru (and the human mind in general): a man of superficial brilliance, he could be dignified and empathic, spiritually genuine, childish and inconsistent, fraudulent and manipulative, grandiose and schizoid, paranoid and delusional, megalomanic and murderous.

THE EXPERIENCE OF TRANSCENDENCE

The "mystical experiences" into which he guided disciples were generally induced by rapid-breathing exercises, which deoxygenated the brain and readily brought about altered states of consciousness, sometimes in combination with drugs and states of sleeplessness. This form of the *experience of transcendence*, with or without drugs, is extremely important to apocalyptic groups, secular as well as religious. In the case of a cult like Aum, its apocalyptic component brings strong psychic energy to bear on whatever physiological state is created. Aum disciples embraced these high states to the point of addiction. When interviewed, they told me of ignoring or numbing themselves to evidence of duplicity and violence in the cult because they did not want to see or hear anything that might cause them to be denied access to their mystical experiences. Months or even years after leaving the cult, toward which they felt much disillusionment, they still longed for those lost mystical states, which, they repeatedly insisted, provided the most intensely satisfying spiritual moments they had ever known. The exact state of the brain at such moments is not scientifically understood, nor can one be certain about the specific influence of an apocalyptic vision in rendering the oxygen-deprived "high state" still more intense (as compared, for instance, to the classical experiences of transcendence described by mystics). What one can say is that the mind/brain experience combined extreme euphoria with an impulse to struggle, even violently, on behalf of the world (and the guru) promoting such euphoria.

The content of such an experience of transcendence is determined by the immediate environment, which, in Aum, meant images of the guru and of the expected apocalyptic event. Hence, there were frequent visions in which disciples achieved one of Aum's ultimate aims and had a sense of merging completely with the guru. Another typical vision was that of a world in ruins with fires raging everywhere, a landscape without people except for a small group of Aum disciples, sometimes with the guru at its center, all of whom were quietly meditating.

THE SOLE SURVIVOR TO RENEW MANKIND

A post-apocalyptic vision was key to the cult's overall project because in it Aum members become the *only survivors*, a tiny remnant of gentle but steadfast purity, ready to re-spiritualize a cleansed and vacant world–the kind of survivor remnant described in the Book of Revelation. There was in this a parallel to Pierce's vision in *The Turner Diaries* of the induced nuclear devastation of most of the world, leaving a remnant of white patriots, also sharing in a steadfast and gentle purity and ready to repopulate the earth.

That post-apocalyptic vision is reminiscent of a famous figure in the psychiatric literature who envisioned himself as the "sole survivor to renew mankind." That impulse, if acted upon, can become a form of addiction to continuous survival, and such addicts "need corpses," as the writer Elias Canetti put it (1962, p. 443). The great majority of Aum disciples did not, of course, know that the cult was stockpiling biological and chemical weapons or seeking nuclear devices (for a more complete study, see Lifton, 1999). But they were expecting an apocalyptic event and imagined themselves taking part in an "Armageddon-like battle" against evil forces. Only a few top disciples were privy to the guru's violent plans, though many others had a mindset that is sometimes referred to as "middle knowledge" (both knowing and not knowing) about it.

The murderous side of Aum could thus be called its mystical secret, something on the order of the Germans' knowledge of Nazi mass murder. Certainly everyone in Aum had a sense, however amorphous, that remaining loyal to the group was the only way to survive a cataclysm sure to come. For such a group, the only means of survival becomes killing everyone else. That turned out to be a task beyond Aum's capacities. But the cult's combination of ultimate zealotry and ultimate weapons made it imaginable, and in acting on these imaginings Aum crossed a crucial threshold, from dreaming of or praying for Armageddon to attempting vigorously to bring it about.

REFERENCES

Canetti, E. (1962). *Crowds and power.* New York: Viking.

Picco, G. (2004). Tactical and strategic terrorism. *Journal of Aggression, Maltreatment & Trauma, 9*(1/2/3/4), 71-78.

Lifton, R.J. (1999). *Destroying the world to save it: Aum Shinrikyo, apocalyptic violence, and the new global terrorism.* New York: Metropolitan Books.

Lifton, R. J. (2003). *Super power syndrome: America's apocalyptic confrontation with the world.* New York: Thunder's Mouth Press/Nation Books.

Voice:
Murdered Twin Buddhas
and Annihilated Twin Towers:
Traumatized Civilization

Hirad Abtahi

The United Nations' 2001 Year of Dialogue Among Civilizations witnessed the destruction of the Buddhas of Bamiyan and the Twin Towers. Manifestations of civilizations were hit by a trans-continental violence spread out by a ruling faction, the Taliban, and a nebulous organization, Al Qaeda.

While the Dialogue Among Civilizations attracted little attention, September 11 stimulated debates on the clash of civilizations between the "Muslim world" and the West. This partial reading of events reflected the fact that the post-September 11 advocates of the "clash of civilizations" forgot, or did not see as fitting their intellectual construction, that before attacking the United States, the Taliban/Al Qaeda nexus had inflicted severe pain on Muslim civilization, in the name of which they claimed to have attacked the West. Because

Address correspondence to: Hirad Abtahi, LLB, LLM, Deputy Chef de Cabinet, Immediate Office of the President. International Criminal Court, Maanweg 17425 16 AB, The Hague, The Netherlands (E-mail: hirad.abtahi@icc-cpi.int).

This Voice is an abstract of an legal essay entitled: *From the destruction of the Twin Buddhas to the destruction of the Twin Towers: Crimes against civilizations under the ICC Statute,* published in the *International Criminal Law Review,* 4(1), 2004.

[Haworth co-indexing entry note]: "Voice: Murdered Twin Buddhas and Annihilated Twin Towers: Traumatized Civilization." Abtahi, Hirad. Co-published simultaneously in *Journal of Aggression, Maltreatment & Trauma* (The Haworth Maltreatment & Trauma Press, an imprint of The Haworth Press, Inc.) Vol. 9, No. 1/2, 2004; and: *The Trauma of Terrorism: Sharing Knowledge and Shared Care, An International Handbook* (ed: Yael Danieli, Danny Brom, and Joe Sills) The Haworth Maltreatment & Trauma Press, an imprint of The Haworth Press, Inc., 2005.

of a hazy cultural perception of Muslim civilization, most of them did not conceive of anything occurring in Afghanistan. But war and warlordism are perceived as an almost anthropological specificity of Afghans, a "tribal habit" of living through and for war, and being accustomed to accompanying pains.

In truth, following the cynical principle "the enemy of my enemy is my friend," throughout the 1990s, Muslim fundamentalists were left alone in Afghanistan to combat the "enemies," turning that country into a black hole into which foreign powers surged. Hence, the lack of reprimand, let alone impunity, *vis-à-vis* the 1998-2001 crimes against humanity committed in the "Islamic Emirate of Afghanistan." This subjection to "banality" of those crimes, which fell within the realm of impunity, provided them with enough space to expand. Hence, the September 11 crimes that, far from being a "banal" crime against humanity, attracted worldwide attention, particularly from one of the supposedly least expected countries, Iran, where people held candlelight vigils for the victims. September 11 was certainly not a clash of civilizations.

September 11 was part of a joint criminal enterprise led by a nexus of fundamentalists who rejected any projection of the world other than their own. Initially, the Taliban's introverted attack on civilization consisted of purifying their Islam in territories under their control. Noting the world's lack of reprimand for the 1998 "Afghan Srebrenica," these Muslims, who massacred thousands of Muslims, acquired space to mature. Through continuous intercourse with Al Qaeda, their introverted approach evolved towards an extroverted one, defying the world with the demolition of the Twin Buddhas. Noting the international community's helplessness before this most visible act, this criminal enterprise reached its critical mass; its expansion outside Afghanistan could continue unimpeded.

In fact, occurring in a temporal continuum, these two crimes against humanity constituted a wider crime against humanity designed to annihilate civilization. What matters is not so much the extent to which each of the entities was involved in this multifaceted criminal enterprise, but the fact that the Taliban provided safe haven to Al Qaeda, protecting it from external pressure, and enabling it to acquire sufficient space to refine its criminal plans. Although the Taliban repeatedly heard the allegations concerning Al Qaeda masterminding criminal acts outside Afghanistan, they refused to withdraw their protection from Al Qaeda, knowingly taking at least the risk of facilitating Al Qaeda's crimes. The Taliban were willing to be attacked by the United States' overwhelming might to the point of losing their own power, following their refusal to hand over Osama Ben Laden and his accomplices. Their taking of such fatal risk provides more than a hint as to the morphism of the Taliban/Al Qaeda nexus.

While initially each might have had different objectives, their interaction led to an anti-civilization criminal pattern designed to shape the world around their perception of the dawn of Islam by destroying what had polluted its purity: culture. In Afghanistan, this encompassed cultural heritage, physical representations, such as the Persian manuscripts or the pre-Islamic Twin Buddhas, but also human life, when the vehicle of that pollution was human thought, such as Shi'a Islam, or the pre-Islamic Iranian Nowrooz. To kill humans was to destroy their polluting thought responsible for propagating culture. Similarly, Al Qaeda sought to destroy "Western imperialism," through both its human life and cultural heritage, as illustrated by the events of September 11. Furthermore, the Bamiyan Buddhas initially caught the Western scholars' attention as evidence of the influence of Classicism on eastern Iranian art, and it was upon Classicism that the universalizing values of the Enlightenment have been shaping Western democracies. In this context, Al Qaeda's involvement in the destruction of the Twin Buddhas may be viewed as a reaction to the Enlightenment's hegemonic cultural, economic, and political power.

Viewed together, the Taliban/Al Qaeda nexus' joint criminal enterprise equated to a wider crime against humanity intended to annihilate civilization. It was a widespread, systematic attack, requiring a multi-continental sophisticated level of organization, but also a repetition of criminal acts, the destruction of the Twin Buddhas and the targeting of American monuments being its most visible aspects. This attack, directed on discriminatory grounds against both humans and their cultural heritage, was the crime against humanity of persecution. The aim of the perpetrators' joint criminal enterprise was to attack every manifestation of culture with which they disagreed. To attack culture was to disfigure civilization.

Although opaque, the border is, regrettably, not static. Since September 11, sites such as Westminster Abbey, the Statue of Liberty, or the Eiffel Tower have been cited as potential targets. Regardless of the validity of those fears, what remains is that all these sites pertain to cultural heritage. Whether or not consciously, it has been realized that the attack was directed against civilizations. With the passing of time, future generations will wonder what was the United States before September 11, or Afghanistan before the Taliban/Al Qaeda nexus. While little trace of their victims will remain, the images of the destruction of the World Trade Center and the Bamiyan Buddhas will be available. These scars, the lost cultural heritage, will be the testimony of deep wounds: the victims' suffering.

Tactical and Strategic Terrorism

Giandomenico Picco

SUMMARY. Terrorism may well be one word, but its forms are multiple and accordingly the ways to combat it differ. In recent history, we have been exposed to "tactical terrorism," whose political objectives were well known and unchangeable and were pursued by groups with a place and a stake in their own countries. By contrast, Al Qaeda has introduced strategic terrorism, perpetual confrontation with the enemy being anyone who is "different." Furthermore, the political objectives change frequently, since they are not what matters; for strategic terrorism, the perpetual confrontation is more important than any political objective per se.

KEYWORDS. Tactical terrorism, strategic terrorism, negotiations, enemy

Memory is often faulty, at times partial and at times selective. It cannot be otherwise; we all view reality from where we stand. In time of war, it is well

Address correspondence to: Giandomenico Picco, GDP Associates, Inc., 150 East 58th Street, 23rd Floor, New York, NY 10155 USA (E-mail: gdpassociates@worldnet.att.net).

[Haworth co-indexing entry note]: "Tactical and Strategic Terrorism." Picco, Giandomenico. Co-published simultaneously in *Journal of Aggression, Maltreatment & Trauma* (The Haworth Maltreatment & Trauma Press, an imprint of The Haworth Press, Inc.) Vol. 9, No. 1/2, 2004; and: *The Trauma of Terrorism: Sharing Knowledge and Shared Care, An International Handbook* (ed: Yael Danieli, Danny Brom, and Joe Sills) The Haworth Maltreatment & Trauma Press, an imprint of The Haworth Press, Inc., 2005.

known that truth is the first victim. Many of the today's states were born out of acts that would be and were called, by some, acts of terrorism. Throughout history, rebels became leaders and revolutionaries became members of the establishment, and they re-wrote history, for better or for worse. Yet the killing of civilians in declared or undeclared wars in relation to military casualties has increased dramatically: from a 10/90 ratio between civilians and military to the very opposite at the end of the 1900s. It seems that civilians have become the target of choice: whatever definition of terrorism we choose, the killing of civilians as bystanders is surely a part of it. We tend to be kinder in labeling some as terrorist, and less kind toward others. The difference is not just a stark one, such as between those who call one person a terrorist and others who call the same person a freedom fighter; there are also those who feel uneasy with both definitions.

But then Al Qaeda came onto the scene, adding some clarity to defining terrorism. There is a profound difference between Al Qaeda terrorism and the types of terrorism in which other groups engage. Al Qaeda is engaged in "strategic terrorism" rather than in "tactical terrorism."

TACTICAL TERRORISM

The Iran Contra Affair was a scheme devised by some political figures in Washington to deliver weapons to Iran indirectly for the purpose of securing Iran's help in the liberation of U.S. hostages held in Lebanon. The scheme worked only partially, since three hostages gained their freedom through it. A few years later, direct negotiations with the hostage takers led to the release of the remaining captives (Picco, 1999). An even more famous example transpired in the 1990s, when the U.S. administration engaged in negotiations with the political wing of the Irish Republican Army (IRA). In 1998, the Friday Agreement was reached for peace in Northern Ireland.

There is no question that these groups had used terrorism in order to achieve a political end that was not only well known and declared but remained constant. Their actions were focused on the direction of the proclaimed political objective. The terrorists' actions sought the attention of the victim's sympathizers for the injustice that they felt. The actions were therefore instrumental in the pursuit of a political goal that was well known and politically achievable.

Such tactical use of terror was confirmed by the very fact that these groups did not shy away from negotiations with officialdom. Negotiations and clarity of political objectives are key elements of tactical terrorism.

The structure of both Hezbollah, a terrorist group operating primarily in Southern Lebanon, and the IRA consists of a political as well as a military wing. They are supported by and responsible for a civilian constituency that is much larger than the number of its operatives and militants. Indeed, a network of welfare arrangements is in place to provide jobs, salaries, medical care, schooling, and so forth to a fixed-based civilian society that does not have the luxury of moving around and hiding, since it is part of the population of a given area.

Both the IRA and Hezbollah have had, for a long time, political representation in Parliament and represent an important voice of the political spectrums in their respective national scenes. The political and the military side of the two organizations is key to their modus operandi and may well be to their destiny. The modus operandi is clearly affected by the fact that they have a constituency of civilians for which they carry a degree of responsibility. They are not leading just an army, or even groups of armed militants, who have no tomorrow.

No matter what the slogans, it is the social network of that civilian constituency which provides the base. That constituency cannot be destroyed on the altar of a slogan or political rhetoric as could groups of militarily trained individuals. In other words, the civilian base of these organizations represents the stake in the future but also the stake in the existing reality of the nation of which they are a part.

Both the IRA and Hezbollah have been involved in negotiations: while the Irish group was involved in the negotiation with the United States for the achievement of some of their political objectives in exchange for relinquishing the tactic of terrorism, Hezbollah has been so far engaged only in spot negotiations with some Western countries over time and with Israel–indirectly but openly–as well as with the United Nations. This in itself is very telling. Involvement in negotiations with a party that objects to the tactic that the group uses and, to a large extent, also objects to its most radical declared political goals, indicates some ability to compromise.

Negotiations are an integral part of tactical terrorism; in fact, they are proof that we are facing tactical terrorism. If negotiations are undertaken, by definition the methodology is sacrificed to the idea of securing some goal. Further, in negotiations by definition the goal can only partially be achieved, as that is the very nature of negotiations: no side gets 100% of what it wishes.

The very use of negotiations for a terrorist group implies readiness to dispose of the terrorist method on one hand and to compromise on the goals on the other. It is indeed tactical terrorism that we have seen so far when dealing with groups like the IRA and Hezbollah. Here people matter more than the ultimate objective.

How otherwise would the US-led negotiations in Northern Ireland have succeeded? How would the negotiations in Lebanon have brought about the liberation of the Western hostages? While governments officially maintain that negotiations with terrorists are out of the question, they have almost consistently agreed to engage when terrorist groups have shown willingness to do so. In this sense, the key decision is taken by the groups themselves rather than by the official institutions. The door is usually opened at first by the groups that have engaged in terrorist activities. Then, the methodology for pursuing the negotiations may vary, but the record seems to prove that in a variety of ways, despite obstacles, governments have found ways to take advantage of such openings.

Negotiations can only be entered into with groups involved in tactical terrorism. The agreement by governments to deal with them de facto is proof that such groups are prepared to be involved in the process of negotiations as they accept, consciously or not, that the mechanism of direct negotiations requires that each side concedes some to the other. The reason why this is possible is because for these groups terrorism is a tool to achieve a specific clear and identifiable political objective, not an end in itself.

As societies afflicted by terrorism over the last few decades, we have been witness to attacks where the terrorist groups tried to attract the attention of the victims and their sympathizers rather than attracting the sympathies of the perpetrator's sympathizers. The media were used for this purpose throughout the saga of the hostages who were taken in Lebanon. Tapes, photographs, and messages were directed at the world of the victims. These were geared to raise the awareness of the "outside world" of the issues dear to the terrorist groups.

Furthermore, the practitioners of tactical terrorism do not define their enemies in ideological terms but in operational terms; that is why they do not rule out possible contacts and negotiations. For Hezbollah or the IRA, the world is not divided into "us and them"; there is also the "in between," the irrelevant, and those who are not part of their fight either in favor or against. Tactical terrorism is rather specific about who the enemy is and does not commit the error of creating more enemies than is necessary. The enemy is usually specifically defined as a government or two, not a people, not a civilization, not a religion.

For instance, Hezbollah believes that the American "people" are not the enemy. Indeed, they accepted communication with them over time. The U.S. government was, at different times, identified as an enemy, but even in this case communication with that government was seen as a sign of power. No later than 2002, the leader of Hezbollah, Sheik Nasrallah, was quoted as saying that he had some quasi-constant communication with the U.S. Government. Whether this statement is true or not, the fact remains that he must never declare war on the world but has been very specific about who his enemies are and indeed he has maintained some kind of contact even with them. The IRA, for instance, found it possible to deal with the U.S. government, a clear and well-known ally of the British government, which was regarded by the IRA as the enemy.

Tactical terrorism needs to focus its actions; otherwise, the "cause" would not be helped. Thus, by way of example, Hezbollah and the IRA did not hit Chinese targets or Indian targets or, for that matter, Italian targets. To be sure, tactical terrorism is no less lethal than strategic terrorism as far as its victims are concerned. The victims are still innocent civilians.

AL QAEDA AND STRATEGIC TERRORISM

By 1994, Afghanistan had been experiencing a civil war among the various factions that had claimed victory over the Soviets and their local allies. The decision in the spring of 1992 by the United Nations Secretary General to allow his Representative in Afghanistan and Pakistan to engineer the physical removal from Kabul of the Communist leader Najibullah was a bad one. The result was to leave the country with a power vacuum which developed into a civil war until the Taliban came into the picture.

Indeed, Afghanistan had become a failed state by 1994, a perfect target for a criminal or terrorist organization to seize. The Taliban were not an indigenous movement of Afghanistan; actually, they were born and organized within the borders of Pakistan. Like a parasite grows within the body of another creature so did Al Qaeda in the Taliban structure. Al Qaeda offered the Taliban a backbone or support structure from which to branch. Within a very few years, Al Qaeda had identified and conducted operations first against Afghans themselves (most notably Shiite Afghans) then moved on to mount attacks against Iranians along the borders and inside Afghanistan, Chinese within the western provinces of China, Indians in Kashmir, and Russians in Chechnya.

The "all" concept of the enemy was an expanding one. It became a concept that was coming to mean "everybody who is not us." In reality, Al Qaeda had begun to consider as an enemy "the different," "the other," and, accordingly, everybody else. The list was topped off, of course, on September 11th. By that time, Al Qaeda was in fact targeting everybody except its very own people.

By 2001, the U.S., Russia, China, and India felt themselves to be the targets of choice of Al Qaeda's new kind of terrorism. They were very likely correct.

The foundation of strategic terrorism is to perceive diversity as a threat. The political objectives of Al Qaeda have been as fleeting as the wind. It took until 1998 for the propaganda of the group to even mention the Palestinian issue. As of late, the Al Qaeda media machine had made clear that Morocco, Saudi Arabia, and Pakistan would be targeted. This happened.

The variety of issues and targets that Al Qaeda trumpets at different times demonstrates that they are just excuses and indeed cover for the real objective. The real objective of the ideology behind the Al Qaeda type of terrorism is simply to fight "the other." In theory, Al Qaeda needs an enemy to exist; it needs perpetual war.

In October of 2002, in a tape attributed to Bin Laden, the voice calls on the "infidels" to convert to Islam or to face dire consequences. The stage for the clash of civilizations, the real objective of Al Qaeda and of strategic terrorism, was explicitly set. Ultimately, the groups engaged in tactical terrorism can "survive" without an enemy; those involved in strategic terrorism cannot.

A major difference between these two types of terrorism is that there is no social constituency to take care of as a strategic terrorist group. There are no job opportunities to be created nor hospitals and farms to be run, and no elections to Parliament to be won. Furthermore, we have never heard of negotiations with Al Qaeda either being offered or sought. Strategic terrorism cannot afford negotiations because there is nothing to negotiate; it is confrontation to the death of one side or the other. Almost any other terrorist group has been involved in some negotiations, but not Al Qaeda.

The virtual cells, the sleeper cells, the seizing of political causes a la carte according to the moment in time, are a far cry from the consistent political objectives of tactical terrorism. Furthermore, the acts of terrorism perpetrated by the Al Qaeda type of groups are aimed at creating sympathy for the perpetrators in order to obtain more recruits; the attacks of tactical terrorism are aimed at gaining the attention of the sympathizers of the victims.

The "home base" of tactical terrorism does not change. Lebanon or Northern Ireland, Palestine or Peru, have remained the "home base" for the most famous groups. Al Qaeda has no home base. It does not need one because it has no social constituency to serve. The search for a failed or quasi-failed state as a trampoline for further action is thus only tactical and surely replaceable. Can we imagine the IRA home base being moved from Ireland or Hezbollah from Lebanon?

Is the IRA or Sendero Luminoso, the rebel movement in Peru, interested in a clash of civilizations? I doubt it. But as the alleged tape of October 2002 spells out, Al Qaeda is indeed. In fact, that is its real objective.

THE UN AND STRATEGIC TERRORISM

At the moment of this writing, at the beginning of 2004, we do not know who actually perpetrated the heinous attack against the UN building in Baghdad. But for those who acted surprised at the event, since the UN was in Iraq in a humanitarian mode to help the Iraqi people, it may perhaps be helpful to recall that strategic terrorism had already threatened the UN and that there is a very clear logic for the Al Qaeda-type groups to attack the UN.

As stated above, by definition, strategic terrorism feeds on the existence of an enemy. Al Qaeda is a sectarian based organization with the arrogance to believe that they are in the sole possession of the truth and that those who disagree with them are wrong and should be restrained or suppressed. These are the exact opposites of the philosophy of the UN Charter. Al Qaeda is exclusion; the UN is inclusion. For the UN, every human being counts while for Al Qaeda, only its own count. Diversity is the core of the UN's mission; it is the seed of betterment and growth. Reconciliation is pursued by the UN in respect of each unique identity. Al Qaeda recognizes no other identity as a positive value. The UN is based on the use of force as a last resort; strategic terrorism uses force as the first and only resort. The UN claims no sole, undisputed knowledge of the truth, nor tries to convert people from their religious belief. The UN is the nemesis of Al Qaeda, for the two visions of the world are diametrically opposed.

WHAT NEXT?

Strategic terrorism's ultimate objective appears to be a clash of civilizations, a clash between the West and the Islamic world, or a perpetual war between the Arab world and the U.S. The difficulty in combating this type of terrorism is that the terrorists involved apparently have nothing to lose. By contrast, those involved in tactical terrorism have much to lose: the well-being of the people for whom they are directly responsible on a daily basis.

Lumping together these two types of terrorism may increase the likelihood that they will collaborate with each other when the opposite would be in the interest of those combating terrorism. The lack of a geographical or national basis and its totally sectarian, almost racist, view, makes strategic terrorism quite literally the enemy of our era.

Above and beyond the ignominy of the attack, the culture of strategic terrorism should be of major concern to us all. The battle they are fighting is not just to achieve a clash of civilizations but also to conquer the hearts and minds of new generations of individuals in various parts of the world. The culture of exclusion and of the arrogance of claiming to be the sole possessor of the truth may well be the seed for a very long-term confrontation and much suffering. Terrorism of this kind may well have to be confronted not only with the tools of war, law, and regulations, but those of culture (Picco, 2001). Any sectarianism and arrogance, of being the only one who is right, even when practiced by those who do not resort to terrorist acts, may eventually feed into the culture of terrorism. The policies and people who seem to indulge and build political careers on the hatred of groups of people based on differences, on the arrogance of group supremacy, be it at a political, religious, or cultural level, and whose lives are dominated by the perception that diversity is a threat, are all helping the culture of strategic terrorism, rather than fighting it.

There are fundamentalists who wear a beard and a turban, and there are others who with their words and their behaviors disseminate poison and, though dressed in jackets and ties, are also fundamentalists. They will all be held accountable.

Christian extremists, Muslim extremists, Jewish extremists, Hindu extremists are responsible for feeding the culture of strategic terrorism, best described by the words of Isaiah Berlin (1981):

> Few things have done more harm than the belief on the part of individuals or groups that he or she or they are in the sole possession of the truth: especially about how to live, what to be and do, and that those who differ from them are not merely mistaken but wicked or mad, and need restraining or suppressing. It is a terrible and dangerous arrogance to believe that you alone are right; have a magical eye which sees the truth and that others cannot be right if they disagree. (p. 12)

To be met successfully, such major challenges require more than just weapons and theories. They require heroes, such as those, UN and NGO workers on humanitarian and human rights missions who fight strategic terrorism not with arms but with the courage and the dignity of a life in the service of others, not only of their family, but also of those unknown to them. Our heroes believe in inclusion and in diversity, but most of all in the value of each human being irrespective of his or her faith. Many were struck down by the cowardly hand of a strategic terrorist. Their names have to become known, their lives have to be told. We shall thus provide inspiration to a new generation to believe in the essential decency and dignity of the human being. We need to exalt those heroes, for without them how can we win the battle for the hearts and minds of the next generation?

REFERENCES

Berlin, I. (2001). Notes on prejudice. *The New York Review of Books, 48*(16), p. 12.

Picco, G. (1999). *Man without a gun: One diplomat's secret struggle to free the hostages, fight terrorism, and end a war.* New York: Times Books/Random House.

Picco, G. (2001). *Crossing the divide: Dialogue among civilizations.* South Orange, New Jersey: Seton Hall University.

Voice:
Do They Kill for Their Mothers?

Joyce M. Davis

"Nobody has to force Palestinian boys to become martyrs," say the men who send them out to die and to kill. More often than not, they have to force them not to. "They beg us to pick them for an operation. They beg us to teach them how to fire an M-18. They beg us for the grenades. They make pests of themselves until we give in and say, ok, it is your time. Of course, we all know that death is with us, always, but for the istishhadi, the ones you call suicide bombers, they yearn for death. And do you know why they do it? You think we force them, don't you? You think we trick them? You think we brainwash them? No, we are not so smart as that. These boys do it for one reason, for their mothers. They do it for the women who they see crying every time an Israeli tank destroys a home. For the women, black shawls wrapped around their creased faces, who collapse as the bloodied bodies of their sons are wrapped in the white shrouds for burial. They do not do it for us. No, the martyrs kill for their mothers. You don't believe me? You find this unbelievable? Have you spoken to a Palestinian mother? Do you know that they are filled with rage at the memories of their dead sons, and now their dead daughters? Go talk to a Palestinian mother, then you will understand."

Address correspondence to: Joyce M. Davis, Radio Free Europe/Radio Liberty, Vinohradska 1, 110 00 Prague 1, Czech Republic, or Radio Free Europe Washington Office, 1201 Connecticut Avenue, Suite 400, Washington, DC 20036 USA (E-mail: jdavis11007@msn.com).

[Haworth co-indexing entry note]: "Voice: Do They Kill for Their Mothers?." Davis, Joyce M. Co-published simultaneously in *Journal of Aggression, Maltreatment & Trauma* (The Haworth Maltreatment & Trauma Press, an imprint of The Haworth Press, Inc.) Vol. 9, No. 1/2, 2004; and: *The Trauma of Terrorism: Sharing Knowledge and Shared Care, An International Handbook* (ed: Yael Danieli, Danny Brom, and Joe Sills) The Haworth Maltreatment & Trauma Press, an imprint of The Haworth Press, Inc., 2005.

"My son was only 13 years old when the Israelis shot him down in the street, not far from here," said Munabrahim Daoud, seated on a plush sofa in the living room of her home in Ramallah. "He was a good boy. A smart boy and a Boy Scout. He was the best in his class at English. He was very affectionate and he would come and help me in the morning. He had that innocence of a child and just at that age when he was coming closer to me, he left us. I will not let them forget Mohammed. I will never let them forget him, or the other boys they killed. I will not let them forget the land we lost . . . it is our land. It is not theirs. What if someone took your land? They took our land, our wealth and even our children. This Intifada is not over yet. We have been suffering since 1948. Every time it calms down, we make sure the fire comes again because we insist on results."

Mothers such a Munabrahim, whose sons have been killed in battles with Israeli soldiers, are powerful voices inside Palestinian communities. They can either work for peace or for war. Munabrahim had chosen to do the latter, but not all Palestinian mothers had done so. Some took a different view of the mayhem that had gripped the West Bank and Gaza. Some were ready for the long nightmare to be over.

"Do you think I would have let him go if I knew what he was going to do?" asked Um Iyad with barely disguised disgust. "I would never have allowed him to go. I would have tied him down. I would have locked the house up. I would have chained him to the bed and bolted every door and locked every window. We did not train Izzidene to hate." Yet Izzidene al Masri, 22, walked into the Sbarro Pizzeria in downtown Jerusalem, past baby carriages and laughing children, and blew himself up. "We did not teach him that kind of hate," Um Iyad said. "We had Israeli friends. We had even served Israeli soldiers in our restaurant here in Jenin before this madness broke out, this stupidity. He was very religious, he was obsessed with the afterlife. He wanted to meet God in heaven, but what can I tell you? It was not a good thing that he did, there were many innocents there, and so many children! We do not support it when the Israelis kill our people, so we cannot support it when their innocent people are killed. We just cannot condone that kind of martyrdom."

Yet as much as mothers such as Um Iyad pain over the continued bloodshed between Israelis and Palestinians, the number of istishhadi, those who sacrifice themselves, continues to rise, including an increasing number of women. "From Mary's womb issued a child who eliminated oppression, while the body of Wafa became shrapnel that eliminated despair and aroused hope," wrote Dr. Abdel Sadeq, head of the Department of Psychiatry at Cairo University, speaking of Wafa Idris, a divorcee who was unable to have children, who is believed to be the first Palestinian female suicide bomber (Al-Arabi, 2002). She was 28 years old when she blew herself up on Jaffa road in downtown Jerusalem in January 2002, killing an 81-year-old man and wounding more than 100 others. According to Davis (2003), Idris probably took her cue from Loula Abboud, one of the first female suicide bombers, who reportedly said:

> I couldn't stay in Beirut, dancing and singing about our glorious land on the quai every night, when the Israelis were pillaging my home. I had to go back. I had to fight for Aoun. It was hard lying to my mother, but I knew she would understand, eventually, when it was all over. She had been a rebel in her day, a Communist when that was far from a popular thing to be. She had a cause and she had thrown herself into it. She was out in the streets when she was young, marching, protesting. I'm doing the same, but with a gun.

> I'm only 19 but I believe in something greater than that. I believe in God, in Jesus Christ, my country, in my family. Why shouldn't I fight? My friends from the village are ready to go with me. If I die, I'll be ready for it. And when it's all done, she'll be proud, even though she'll wish I were with her, that I had not gone back. Won't it be wonderful to fight with the resistance? To fight the Israelis. To defend our home. I won't be afraid, and I won't let the others be afraid, either.

> Whatever comes, we know God is with us. One thing is sure, I'll never let them take me alive. I'll fix it so that when the end comes, when I'm surrounded, I'll be ready. I'll keep a few grenades in reserve just in case the Israelis come for me, and when I go, I'll make sure to take a few of them with me. The one thing I feel bad about, though, is lying to mummy. But when it's all done, she, above all, will understand. I can't bear to see her crying and do nothing. If it happens, she'll know that I died, and killed, for her.

REFERENCES

Davis, J. M. (2003). *Martyrs: Innocence, vengeance, and despair in the Middle East.* New York: Palgrave Macmillan.

Sadeq, A. (2002). *Al-Quds Al-Arabi (Arab Jerusalem).* Retrieved February 4, 2002 from http://moise.sefarad.org/print.php?id=374.

Voice:
Palestinian Voices

THE FIRST STORY: AASIM YUSIF MOHAMED RIHANE

The name is Aasim Yusif Mohamed Rihane, born July 2, 1980, a male bachelor from the town of Tel in Nablus. He is in his third year at the university studies majoring in economics. He comes from a family of 12, eight males and four females. One brother was killed in a martyrdom operation and two are in prison. The first was serving a ten year sentence, the other, a five year sentence. Aasim conducted his own martyrdom operation in Qalqaliya. Ten people were killed and 40 were injured as a result of this operation. His political affiliation is Hamas.

Further Details on the Life of a Martyr

He was a studious, intelligent and athletic young man. He distinguished himself in Karate, in chanting the Koran by heart, and in calligraphy. He was known to be a quiet but a kind and caring person. He was also known to hold fanatical views on issues relating to religion, honor, and land. The following events motivated his action. The first event was when he witnessed the forceful and public removal of a scarf off of a woman's face by Israeli forces. The second event was the martyrdom (killing) of his older brother after a prolonged and violent fire exchange with Israeli forces during which he killed a number of soldiers.

Address correspondence to: The senior editor of this volume, Yael Danieli, PhD, Group Project for Holocaust Survivors and Their Children, 345 East 80th Street (31-J), New York, NY 10021 USA (E-mail: yaeld@aol.com).

[Haworth co-indexing entry note]: "Voice: Palestinian Voices." Co-published simultaneously in *Journal of Aggression, Maltreatment & Trauma* (The Haworth Maltreatment & Trauma Press, an imprint of The Haworth Press, Inc.) Vol. 9, No. 1/2, 2004; and: *The Trauma of Terrorism: Sharing Knowledge and Shared Care, An International Handbook* (ed: Yael Danieli, Danny Bron, and Joe Sillis) The Haworth Maltreatment & Trauma Press, an imprint of The Haworth Press, Inc., 2005.

How Was the Operation Carried Out?

He and a group of friends stationed themselves under an olive tree, not far from the crossroads where the operation took place. Moments before executing the operation he called his mother and father and asked for their blessing. Soon after a bus came by, carrying (Israeli) settlers. He stopped the bus. The bus stopped because he was wearing the uniform of an Israeli soldier. He got on with his weapon and after asking two children to get off the bus and run home, he started shooting, indiscriminately, the remaining passengers. After ascertaining that all the travelers were either killed or injured, he returned to his hiding place under the tree where his friends were waiting for him. He told his friends to leave without him. He needed to stay because his mission was not completed. A jeep carrying soldiers appeared. He ran to it and started shooting. A violent fight ensued. He continued to shoot until the Jeep managed to drive over his body and kill him. His friends filmed this operation before they fled.

THE STORY OF MOHAMED RIHANE: AS TOLD BY HIS WIFE

Mohamed Rihane was born on February 11, 1980 in the village of Tell to a conservative, religious family. He started learning the Koran at an early age and completed his primary and secondary education. He went on to marry his cousin. A year after his marriage (in 1998) he was imprisoned by the Israeli authorities, but managed to escape. Two days after his escape, he was arrested by the Palestinian authorities and was jailed for two and a half years. During a brief furlough, his wife got pregnant and they had a son. He was released from jail in April 2001.

In his life, he was a good natured-man, kind to his siblings and old people in his village. He was considerate towards all those who came in contact with him, particularly families who had members that were martyred or imprisoned. He felt that he and his family were lucky to have a roof over their heads and not refugees like others who did not know where their next meal was coming from. He was particularly pained by the killing of innocent children and old people, by the uprooting of trees and the destruction of houses. One day, he was deeply outraged when he heard of an incident during which the Israeli army physically and verbally attacked a woman at one of the roadblocks. He wished he could catch the soldier who perpetrated that act. He was a jealous man and wanted his wife to protect her face from the stares of other men, particularly when she paid him visits at the prison.

On November 11, 2001, after the evening prayer and dinner with his family, he chatted with his relatives until midnight. After playing with his son and sipping tea, he heard a horn of a car in front of the house. It was 1:30 in the morning but he went out to inquire. He did not return immediately and I fell asleep while he was out.

While I was asleep, he returned to see his mother around 2:00 am and inquired about the planes that were hovering overhead. His mother then heard voices outside the house. After looking outside she saw Jews surrounding the house and she called out to him to find out what was going on. He went out with his gun and started shooting from a distance of two meters while saying "God is great." He was killed. I do not know what woke me up, his invocations to Allah, or the sound of the bullets flying off the wall of the house.

We soon saw a man lying on the ground and we did not know his identity because it was dark. It turned out to be Mohamed. In her grief, his mother thanked God for giving him what he wanted, namely to be a martyr. The wife felt the same way and also thanked God. His mother approached the body and kissed it. The Israelis did not want us to move the body inside. It remained outside the house from 3:00 in the morning until 11 am. His parents and I watched the body from inside the house until it was transported to the morgue.

After his burial the boys in the hospital gave the family the clothes he was wearing. A few days later, it was discovered that some of his flesh got stuck to the pants. A hundred days after his martyrdom, the family went to build his grave. His brothers then decided to open the grave and bury his clothes with him.

Voice:
Remembrance Day/Independence Day

Martin Herskovitz

Lately I've had a jumble of emotions
On the one hand I know it could have been worse
A different angle, a change in position
And the shrapnel . . . (certain things are better left unsaid).
In any case I am thankful that we gained a life.
On the other hand I mourn for the child that was,
Smiling and serene,
Whose biggest worry was the upcoming matriculation test,
To whose load fate has now added a few more parcels.
And along comes Remembrance Day
And my private mourning
Is confronted by the bereavement of thousands,
Dwarfed by it.
As I hear the suffering of the parents,
I make room for them within my own pain to cry.
So I feel today
that our personal mixture of gratitude and mourning
Is not unlike the prevailing feeling on this day,
A day of mourning on Independence eve–

Address correspondence to: Martin Herskovitz, 143 Rothschild Street, Petah Tikva, 49370, Israel (E-mail: hmartin@bezeqint.net or E-mail: hemartin@zahav.net.il).

[Haworth co-indexing entry note]: "Voice: Remembrance Day/Independence Day." Herskovitz, Martin. Co-published simultaneously in *Journal of Aggression, Maltreatment & Trauma* (The Haworth Maltreatment & Trauma Press, an imprint of The Haworth Press, Inc.) Vol. 9, No. 1/2, 2004; and: *The Trauma of Terrorism: Sharing Knowledge and Shared Care, An International Handbook* (ed: Yael Danieli, Danny Brom, and Joe Sills) The Haworth Maltreatment & Trauma Press, an imprint of The Haworth Press, Inc., 2005.

Grieving amidst expectation,
Sadness and thanksgiving,
One eye cries while the other tries to heal itself,
Determined to continue.

On March 28, 2001 my son, Netanel (Tani), then aged 16, was injured in a terrorist suicide bombing in Israel near Kfar Saba in a gas station adjacent to the Kalkilya border crossing as he waited for a bus to take him to his High School, Bnei Chayil, in Kedumim. His right eye was badly injured and the prognosis for restoring sight was pessimistic. He has indeed lost sight in the eye, but this poem was written before all hope was lost.

As a child of a Holocaust survivor in a family that did not discuss the Holocaust, I learned to cope with problems by denying them and putting them behind me as quickly as possible. I was raised in the shadow of one war and now am living in the heart of another. That year, on Israel's Remembrance Day (April 25), commemorated on the eve of our Independence Day, I, together with the entire country, mourned our fallen soldiers. In that setting I was also able to connect with my emotions regarding my son's injury and this poem was the result.

Voice:
Terrorism Poem

While you were showering
A mortar fell
And three people died.
While you were sleeping
Shots were fired
And eight soldiers were wounded.
While you were eating
Terrorists infiltrated
A house where children were sleeping.
And while you were saying the grace after meals
All that remained of the children
Were pieces.
While you were playing
A terrorist entered
A hall full of people.
And while you were losing
Their souls left their bodies
The guests, the bride and the groom.
So let's hurry, let's run, let's get organized, let's finish, let's do as much as we can
For who knows what will happen,
The next time someone sits down to eat.

Irit
14 years

Address correspondence to: Yael Danieli, PhD, Group Project for Holocaust Survivors and Their Children, 345 East 80th Street (31-J), New York, NY 10021 USA. (E-mail: yaeld@aol.com).

Poem translated by Naomi Baum.

[Haworth co-indexing entry note]: "Voice: Terrorism Poem." Co-published simultaneously in *Journal of Aggression, Maltreatment & Trauma* (The Haworth Maltreatment & Trauma Press, an imprint of The Haworth Press, Inc.) Vol. 9, No. 1/2, 2004; and: *The Trauma of Terrorism: Sharing Knowledge and Shared Care, An International Handbook* (ed: Yael Danieli, Danny Brom, and Joe Sills) The Haworth Maltreatment & Trauma Press, an imprint of The Haworth Press, Inc., 2005.

SECTION II
THE PSYCHOLOGICAL
CONSEQUENCES OF TERRORISM

Adults in the United States:
Voice:
Grounded on Sept. 11

David Handschuh

If the desire to flee in life-threatening situations is strong, the desire to stay and document them is often stronger. It's not a feeling of being invincible. It's just a need to keep recording the truth. It's something I've been doing for more than 20 years as a newspaper photographer in New York City, using my camera to bring reality to the readers.

Sept. 11 was a bit different from the start. I was scheduled to work Election Day returns, starting at 5 p.m. I remember waking up that morning and looking out the window and noting what a beautiful day it was. It was the first day of a graduate level photojournalism class I was scheduled to teach at New York University. Class was to begin at 9:30 a.m. and I wanted to be in my classroom, ready, by 9 a.m.

Address correspondence to: David Handschuh, *New York Daily News*, 450 West 33rd Street, 3rd Floor Photo, New York, NY 10001 USA (E-mail: David@FocusOnMentoring.org).

[Haworth co-indexing entry note]: "Adults in the United States Grounded on Sept. 11." Handschuh, David. Co-published simultaneously in *Journal of Aggression, Maltreatment & Trauma* (The Haworth Maltreatment & Trauma Press, an imprint of The Haworth Press, Inc.) Vol. 9, No. 1/2, 2004; and: *The Trauma of Terrorism: Sharing Knowledge and Shared Care, An International Handbook* (ed: Yael Danieli, Danny Brom, and Joe Sills) The Haworth Maltreatment & Trauma Press, an imprint of The Haworth Press, Inc., 2005.

Driving across the George Washington Bridge, I sat in traffic and gazed out at the beautiful skyline. The Empire State building clearly stood out in Midtown. The Twin Towers of the World Trade Center held up the southern end of the panoramic view. I had no idea that in a few hours the city skyline would be dramatically changed and that thousands of families would be ripped apart.

I was fiddling with the FM radio, the police scanner, and tucking receipts and papers under rubber bands on the sun visor in my car while sitting in bumper-to-bumper traffic. Then I looked up. There was a massive column of smoke coming from lower Manhattan. The voices from the Manhattan Fire Department on the police scanner in my car were yelling to send every piece of apparatus available to the World Trade Center. My first thought was that some knucklehead had accidentally flown his Cessna or Piper into the building.

I called the office of the New York Daily News, told them I was on 14th street and the West Side Highway, and asked if they wanted me to go. They said to go. I called NYU and left a message to place a note on my classroom door stating, "Professor Handschuh will be late today due to a news emergency." I didn't realize I would be an entire semester late. My next phone call was to my home. "A plane hit the World Trade Center. I'm going," was the message I left on the answering machine.

As Fire Department Rescue One rushed southbound in the northbound lane of the West Side Highway, I swerved across the traffic island and followed it on its rear bumper. Their rear door was open and I could see the firefighters as they strapped on their air packs and pulled tools from compartments, getting ready to do battle with the flames and smoke. Several firefighters waved to me out the back door, recognizing me as a friendly face who had covered their heroics for more than 20 years. Less than two hours later, all 11 of the firefighters on Rescue One would be dead.

I arrived at the World Trade Center at 8:53 a.m. I remember looking at the clock on my dashboard and praying that many would be spared. I hoped that a few people were delayed by voting, or just took a few extra minutes outside to enjoy the crisp, clear morning.

I had no inkling of danger and no concern for my personal safety. I just thought I would be recording the largest challenge that the paramedics, firefighters, and police officers of the City of New York would ever face. No one standing in the street or arriving soon after had a clue that the beautiful morning would soon turn into a field trip to hell. I had no idea that I would be covering one of the biggest stories in the history of the modern world.

There was massive destruction looming 90 floors up, but it was eerie and quiet on the street. In a city in which the curses of cab drivers and banging of garbage cans often serve as a wakeup alarm, it was like someone had hit the mute button. People were coming to work with their coffee and breakfast in a bag, silently standing and watching. You could hear the flames crackling and the glass breaking. You could see debris falling.

As I turned my camera lens on the flaming North tower, I realized that not all the debris falling to the street was glass and metal. I can't begin to describe what it looked like as some jumped to their deaths rather than be burned alive.

Many photographers recorded images that morning worse than the most horrible nightmares anyone could have. West Street was littered with debris: office papers, broken glass, and body parts. These were sights I never want to see again. I took photographs that I will never show anyone.

I walked south to the corner of Liberty Street, hoping to take pictures of people leaving the towers. There were few, yet the smoke and flames continued to spread. People were fleeing the Marriott Hotel. Women ran carrying their high heels so they could run faster. A few were covering their heads with serving trays as they fled across West Street. People were helping others run to avoid the blizzard of debris. Medics were starting to arrive to care for the many who needed medical attention.

And then came this noise, a loud, high-pitched roar that seemed to come from everywhere, but nowhere. The second tower exploded. In just seconds, it became obvious that what at first appeared to be a horrible accident was really an act of terrorism. I didn't see the second plane, though I was looking at the tower at the time it hit. I have no recollection of making the picture that appeared on page two of the Daily News the next day, a photograph taken milliseconds after the plane hit the South tower. Taken from street level looking up at the World Trade Center, the photograph is framed by an achingly beautiful blue sky as an ominous black cloud of smoke billows out of the North tower. A brilliant orange fireball spews glass, concrete, aircraft parts, and melting steel.

Time stood still as I documented the horror. But all too soon, it seemed, another loud terrifying noise shook the ground. I looked up as the South tower began to crumble and disintegrate in slow motion. By instinct, I grabbed my camera and brought it up to my eye, but in the back of my mind I heard a voice that said, "Run! Run! Run!" I've been doing this for more than 20 years, and I've never run from anything. Listening to that voice that morning saved my life.

I managed to get about 40 or 50 feet and had just rounded the corner of Liberty Street when I was picked up by a tornado of night. It was like getting hit in the back by a wave at the beach. Instead of salt water, this wave was made of hot gravel, glass, cement, and metal. Suddenly, I was flying, with no control of my feet or legs. I had no choice as to which direction I was heading. I was literally flying.

The noise was overwhelming. There was cracking and creaking and things flying. The debris and the choking cloud kept coming. The locomotive-like noise lasted forever and was followed by silence. I don't think I lost conscious-ness, despite being picked up and thrown almost a full city block, landing under a vehicle, and becoming trapped by debris. I couldn't breathe, but eventually cleared my nose and mouth of debris.

I thought I was going to die, scared and alone, face down in the gutter of a lower Manhattan street. I reached for my cell phone to call home and tell ev-eryone that I loved them, but it was gone. My pager was gone. My glasses were gone. But somehow I had held onto my cameras. In them were two disks, with a total of 180 images recorded on them. Those two small disks held mil-lions of pixels of history.

I started calling for help and was soon answered by words that I will never forget. "Don't worry, brother. We'll get you out." Firefighters call each other brother. The moment I heard those words, I knew I would be okay. The men and women I've photographed saving lives in New York City for 20 years were there to save my life this time. My guardian angels, I later found out, were a team of firefighters from Engine 217 and Ladder 131, Brooklyn. They dug me out of my tomb and went off in search of others more severely injured. I later learned that two firefighters from Engine 217 lost their lives that day, most likely after saving mine.

Another team of firefighters picked me up minutes later and carried me a block to a delicatessen in Battery Park City. Shortly after leaving me on the floor of what they believed to be a safe place, the second tower collapsed, causing the façade of the deli to collapse. We were trapped again. There were 15 men inside: medics, cops, and firefighters who were holding onto each other for their lives. Some were calm. Others were crying or screaming, with just the desire to live. And there was my co-worker, fellow Daily News pho-tographer Todd Maisel, who ran after a team of rescuers carrying an injured victim to safety. Todd was in shock, realizing that the victim he had photo-graphed was me. I gave Todd my cameras and equipment to take into the of-fice. He then photographed me lying on the floor of a deli, injured but alive.

I don't know how long it was until the dust cloud from the second collapse subsided. "We're getting you out of here," my guardian angels said. Using small hand tools, sheer strength, and the will to survive, they broke through the debris that was trapping us. Three rescuers carried me to a New York Police Department harbor boat. I was strapped onto a backboard and placed at the front of a boat heading across the Hudson River toward Ellis Island with an in-jured police lieutenant, a firefighter, and a few walking wounded.

It was an amazing boat ride with a beautiful blue sky and bright sun shining on my face. Under different circumstances it was the perfect weather for a Hudson boat cruise. Every wave we hit sent shocks of pain through my body and brought me back to reality. We were in the shadow of the Statue of Liberty, upon which is written the words, "Give me your tired, your poor, your huddled masses yearning to breathe free."

And I'll always remember the image before me as I squinted to see without my glasses, smoke rising from the World Trade Center, a symbol of New York, a symbol of the United States, a symbol of the American economic system in ruins.

And I didn't have a camera.

Psychological Impact
of the September 11, 2001 Terrorist Attacks:
Summary of Empirical Findings in Adults

William E. Schlenger

SUMMARY. The terrorist attacks in the US on September 11, 2001 stimulated an unprecedented rapid response by the social and health research communities into the aftermath. This article summarizes the findings of the major studies that assessed various types of "psychological distress," and identifies some of the important gaps that remain in our understanding of the nature and etiology of human distress following purposeful, unpredictable mass violence.

KEYWORDS. Terrorism, posttraumatic stress disorder, adults, epidemiology, September 11, psychological distress

Address correspondence to: William E. Schlenger, PhD, Research Triangle Institute, P. O. Box 12194, Research Triangle Park, NC 27709 USA (E-mail: BS@RTI.org).

[Haworth co-indexing entry note]: "Psychological Impact of the September 11, 2001 Terrorist Attacks: Summary of Empirical Findings in Adults." Schlenger, William E. Co-published simultaneously in *Journal of Aggression, Maltreatment & Trauma* (The Haworth Maltreatment & Trauma Press, an imprint of The Haworth Press, Inc.) Vol. 9, No. 1/2, 2004; and: *The Trauma of Terrorism: Sharing Knowledge and Shared Care, An International Handbook* (ed: Yael Danieli, Danny Brom, and Joe Sills) The Haworth Maltreatment & Trauma Press, an imprint of The Haworth Press, Inc., 2005.

This article reviews what has been learned since the attacks on the World Trade Center (WTC) and the Pentagon about the psychosocial consequences of such acts of terrorism for adults. It summarizes the main findings from the empirical literature, critiques the methods, and identifies some of the important gaps in our knowledge.

SUMMARY OF EMPIRICAL STUDIES OF PSYCHOSOCIAL IMPACT OF SEPTEMBER 11

Initial Population-Based Surveys of Adults

Initial empirical information about the psychological effects of the September 11 attacks, based on epidemiological surveys of the nation and/or of the areas most affected, became available relatively quickly. The following presents the studies in chronological order but begins with those for which the clinical significance (e.g., treatment implications) of the findings is unknown, because the psychological symptoms were assessed with instruments whose relationship to clinical diagnosis has not been established (i.e., no evidence is presented linking endorsement of the symptoms with clinically-diagnosed disorder).

A poll of 1,200 U.S. adults (PEW Research Center, 2001) found that the percentage of Americans who reported "feelings of depression" as a result of the attacks peaked at 71% in mid-September and declined steadily to 24% by November 8. At about the same time, Schuster et al. (2001) conducted a national, random-digit dialing (RDD) survey of 560 U.S. adults conducted in the three to five days following September 11. Findings indicated that 44% of Americans were bothered "quite a bit" or "extremely" by at least one of five selected PTSD symptoms. Results varied by gender, race/ethnicity, and distance from the WTC, and 35% of the adults surveyed said that their children had one or more of such symptoms. In a subsequent follow-up of this sample, Stein et al. (in press) reported a substantial reduction two months later in the prevalence of the five selected PTSD symptoms, from 44% to 16%.

Similarly, Smith, Rasinski, and Toce (2001) conducted telephone interviews with a national probability sample of 2,126 U.S. adults between September 13 and September 27, asking about physical and emotional responses to the September 11 attacks. More than half of the respondents reported having cried, having felt nervous and tense, or having had trouble getting to sleep, which were the most commonly reported symptoms. Investigators noted, however, that although levels of reported "negative affect" were somewhat elevated in New York City, levels for the U.S. population as a whole were close to normal levels.

The American Psychological Association commissioned a RDD survey of 1,900 Americans nationwide, including oversamples in New York and Washington, in the fourth month after the attacks (Bossolo, Bergantino, Lichtenstein, & Gutman, 2002). Findings indicated that about one quarter of Americans reported "feeling more depressed than at any other times" in their lives, and that levels of PTSD symptoms were much higher in New York than elsewhere in the country. Additionally, people who reported exposure to other traumatic events prior to the September 11 attacks were significantly more likely than those who had not to report higher levels of symptoms of depression, anxiety, and PTSD.

These initial studies share several strengths, including assessment in the immediate aftermath of the attacks and nationally representative samples. Some of their common problems include the use of mental health symptom measures whose relationship to clinical diagnosis is unknown, incomplete coverage of the sites that were directly attacked, and lack of quasi-experimental comparisons that would enhance our ability to make inferences about causality.

Community Epidemiologic Studies of Adults

The next wave of studies is best described as community epidemiologic studies, because the interviews included instruments whose relationship with comprehensive clinical assessment had been established. They thus provide an empirical basis for population estimates of the prevalence of specific disorders or conditions, including both mental health and substance use outcomes.

Mental Health Outcomes. Galea et al. (2002a) studied the prevalence of PTSD and depression among adults living south of 110th Street in Manhattan. Using RDD techniques, they conducted telephone interviews with a sample of more than 1,000 adults in the second month after the attacks, focusing on September 11 exposures and the symptoms of PTSD and major depression, using mental health and substance use screening measures adapted from the Diagnostic Interview Schedule (Robins, Helzer, Croughan, & Ratliff, 1981). Findings indicated that 7.5% of the adults living in Manhattan south of 110th Street were probable cases of PTSD, and 9.7% were probable cases of major depression. Additionally, those living south of Canal Street (i.e., closest to the WTC site) were nearly three times as likely to be probable cases of PTSD as those living further away, and those who reported two or more life stressors (from a checklist of eight) in the year before the attacks were more than five times as likely to be probable cases of PTSD as those who reported having experienced none of the listed stressors.

Galea and his colleagues (2002b) subsequently conducted a second, independent cross-sectional survey of New York in the fourth month following the attacks, to provide information about the course of symptomatic responses over time. Using the same probability sampling methods applied to the earlier survey but expanding the sampling frame to cover all of New York City, they found the current prevalence of probable, September 11-related PTSD in the area of Manhattan south of 110th St. (to be comparable with the prevalence estimate from the first study) to be 2.9% in the fourth month after the attacks. Thus, the prevalence of probable PTSD in the fourth month after the attacks was about one-third the size of the prevalence in the second month after the attacks.

Galea et al. (2003) subsequently assessed a third cross-section that sampled the full New York metropolitan area in months 6-9 after the attacks. The prevalence estimate for probable PTSD at this time point was 0.9%, indicating a further drop from earlier estimates. That the prevalence of probable September 11-related PTSD 6-9 months following the attacks was about one-eighth of the prevalence in the second month suggests a substantial "recovery" rate.

Schlenger et al. (2002) surveyed a probability sample of 2,273 adults across the country, including oversamples of the New York City and Washington, DC metropolitan areas, in the second month after the attacks. The sample was selected from the Knowledge Networks (KN) Web-enabled Panel, a standing research panel that, at the time the study was conducted, had recruited nearly 60,000 households nationwide using multistage probability sample methods that began with RDD (see Schlenger et al. [2002] for full details of KN's sampling methods). The survey focused on specific exposures to the September 11 attacks and on mental health symptoms, assessed using well validated measures of PTSD symptoms (the PTSD Checklist; Weathers, Litz, Herman, Huska, & Keane, 1993) and of clinically significant psychological distress (the Brief Symptom Inventory-18's [BSI-18] global symptom index; Derogatis, 2001). Findings indicated that the prevalence of probable PTSD in the New York metropolitan area (11.2%) was significantly higher than the prevalence in the Washington, DC metropolitan area (2.7%), in other major metropolitan areas of the U.S. that were not attacked (3.6%), and in the rest of the country (4.0%). In addition, they found that the prevalence rates for Washington, DC, other major metropolitan areas, and the rest of the U.S. did not differ significantly from each other or from the overall prevalence estimate for the nation (4.3%). No significant differences were found among these geographic areas in the prevalence of clinically significant but nonspecific distress, which was found to be generally within normal limits in New York (16.6%), Washington (14.9%), other major metropolitan areas (12.3%), and the rest of the country (11.1%; overall U.S. prevalence 11.6%).

Further, Schlenger et al. (2002) reported the findings from multivariate analyses of their New York sample that included both detailed exposure measures and sociodemographic characteristics as predictors. These indicated that age, gender, direct exposure to the attacks, and number of hours of television coverage of the attacks watched were independently associated with PTSD symptom levels, but that only gender, hours of television watched, and a television content index (number of different horrifying aspects of the attacks that the person saw on television) were independently associated with nonspecific distress. Schlenger et al. interpreted these findings as indicating that direct exposure to the attacks was closely related to PTSD symptomatology but not to nonspecific distress, and that extended watching of television coverage of the attacks was better interpreted as a coping mechanism for people who were already distressed than as an exposure that caused distress.

Using the depression scale of the BSI-18 (Derogatis, 2001), a brief, well-validated screening instrument that identifies likely cases of depressive disorders, including major depression, dysthymic disorder, and others, Schlenger, Federman, Ebert, and Caddell (in press) found that 14.2% of adults in the New York metropolitan area were likely cases of depressive disorders, compared with 11.9% in Washington and 11.2% in the rest of the U.S. Although the rate in New York was numerically higher, the differences between New York and elsewhere were not statistically significant, and all of the rates fell in the normative range.

Subsequently, Silver, Holman, McIntosh, Poulin, and Gil-Rivas (2002) reported findings from a three-wave, longitudinal study that began with a national sample of more than 2,700 adults that was also drawn from the KN Web-enabled panel. Assessment included direct and indirect exposures, psychological symptoms, and coping mechanisms. Descriptive findings indicated that acute stress and PTSD symptom levels decreased over time, and longitudinal models indicated that exposure and losses associated with the attacks, pre-attack mental health status, exposure to other traumas, and six specific coping styles were independently associated with PTSD symptom levels. Only active coping was associated with symptom reduction; the five other coping styles assessed (behavioral disengagement, denial, support-seeking, self-blame, and self-distraction) were associated with increased symptom levels.

Grieger, Fullerton, and Ursano (2003) reported findings from a study that focused on a specific high-exposure group: military and civilian staff who worked at the Pentagon. The study involved an internet-based, anonymous survey of 685 staff of a specific, Pentagon-based command, 77 of whom replied. Findings indicated that about 14% of respondents had probable PTSD, and about 13% reported increased alcohol use subsequent to the attacks. Also, PTSD symptom levels, increased alcohol use, and female gender were all independently associated with lower levels of perceived safety, based on scores on a three-item index that covered safety at home, at work, and in usual daily activities and travel.

Substance Use Outcomes. In addition to studying PTSD and other psychiatric disorders, some of the studies also reported on substance use following the attacks. For example, Vlahov et al. (2002) described alcohol, tobacco, and marijuana use reported in the cross-sectional study of the sample of residents of Manhattan south of 110th Street described above (Galea et al., 2002a). Significant percentages of study participants reported higher levels of use of each of these substances after September 11 relative to before (assessed retrospectively). Vlahov and colleagues also found that the prevalence of probable PTSD was significantly higher among those whose use of cigarettes and marijuana increased, and the prevalence of depression was significantly higher for those who increased use of all three of the substances.

Because Vlahov et al.'s (2002) study has a post-only design, however, the findings depend on retrospective assessment of pre-September 11 use levels to identify changes in use, which is subject to a variety of biases. The Office of Applied Studies (OAS) at the federal Substance Abuse and Mental Health Services Administration (SAMHSA), however, was able to study substance use in New York and elsewhere following September 11 (OAS, 2002) using data from the National Survey of Drug Use and Health (NSDUH, formerly known as the National Household Survey on Drug Abuse). NSDUH is a large, annual, cross-sectional, community-based survey of substance use in the U.S. based on national probability samples of adults (and adolescents aged 12-17). Because the of the scope, large sample sizes, and repeated surveying (annual, independent cross-sectional samples), secondary analyses of NSDUH data can provide a more definitive assessment of the impact of events like September 11 on substance use.

Investigators at OAS and at SAMHSA's National Analysis Center used data from NSDUH for a quasi-experimental study of the impact of the terrorist attacks on substance use that does not depend on retrospective recall of use. The design included comparisons that control both for retrospective recall bias and for potential seasonal factors in substance use.

For a variety of reasons, the sample for each annual NSDUH is fielded in quarterly replicates, such that each quarterly sample is itself a probability sample of the nation. Also, one of the primary measures of substance use is use "in the past 30 days." Since September 11 is near the end of the third quarter of the year (the fourth quarter begins on October 1), virtually all of the participants interviewed in the fourth quarter of 2001 reported on substance use after the attacks, and virtually all of those interviewed in the first three quarters reported on substance use before the attacks. Therefore, comparison of use levels reported by the fourth quarter sample to use levels reported by the first three quarter samples provides a relatively clean pre-post assessment.

It could be the case, however, that seasonal factors influence substance use and, as a result, substance use levels in the fourth quarter might be consistently different from use in the first three quarters (e.g., the presence of major holidays in November and December could create higher or lower substance use in the fourth quarter). Therefore, the study included a comparison of quarters 1-3 vs. quarter 4 estimates of substance use from the prior year's (2000) NSDUH. It also included estimates for a sample of residents of other major metropolitan areas to assess whether any changes in use levels that might be observed in New York could be understood as a "big city" phenomenon.

The pattern of findings that emerged from multiple comparisons across multiple outcomes and population subgroups was clear. Although many comparisons were made and some were statistically significant, the overall pattern of results suggested that there was not a meaningful change in substance use or in substance abuse treatment participation in New York (or elsewhere in the U.S.) in the three months following the terrorist attacks.

CRITIQUE

Empirical information about reactions to the events of September 11 based on probability samples of the U.S. population became available quickly following the attacks. Initial cross-sectional findings showed that many adults in the U.S. were deeply disturbed by the attacks, but subsequent longitudinal findings suggested that much of the distress documented in the initial assessments was self-limiting (i.e., resolved over time without professional treatment). Later, studies focusing on clinically significant symptoms and probable disorder prevalence generally showed that probable PTSD prevalence was strongly associated with direct exposure (or "connection") to the attacks, and that the PTSD problem following the attacks was concentrated in the New York metropolitan area. Additionally, the studies that (retrospectively) assessed pre-September 11 exposure to traumatic events found such exposure to be an important risk factor for the development of PTSD following the attacks.

The strengths of this body of literature include the speed with which preliminary information about reactions to the attacks was made available (i.e., reports from four major studies published in first-tier, peer-reviewed journals within 12 months of the attacks), the use of probability samples, documentation of both direct and indirect exposures, and inclusion in some studies of well validated screening measures of clinically significant symptomatology. As a result, policy makers and others have a much clearer early picture of the aftermath of the September 11 attacks than has previously been possible following large-scale traumatic events.

Nevertheless, it is important that these initial findings be confirmed as extensively as possible with more comprehensive studies that have longitudinal designs. Such studies provide a stronger basis for causal inference with respect to exposure (i.e., to what extent did the events of September 11 cause the symptoms observed at follow-up?) because they include both between-subjects and within-subjects comparisons that allow more comprehensive ruling out of alternative hypotheses.

Additionally, studies that use comprehensive clinical assessments rather than screening instruments are needed. Community epidemiologic studies of large-scope events rely on screening instruments primarily for logistical reasons, and the use of screeners with established correspondence to clinical diagnosis in community-based studies is a critical component of the study's internal validity. Because of the resources required and other logistic issues associated with comprehensive clinical assessment, however, its use in studies of large-scope events has typically been limited to studies targeted at high exposure groups, and such studies of high exposure samples are underway in New York and Washington. These studies should add substantially to our understanding of the impact of the attacks on those most directly affected.

It is also important that the next round of studies employ methods that maximize sample member participation (i.e., minimize nonresponse) and include components aimed at clarifying the specific impact of nonresponse on study findings. All of the studies described above depended at least in part on RDD to develop their probability samples. Given the proliferation of telephone answering machines and other privacy-management devices, response rates to RDD surveys are low by historical survey standards. The thinking about nonresponse bias has evolved substantially over recent years, however, based on better conceptualizations of the problem (e.g., Little & Rubin, 1987; Schafer, 1997) and on both direct empirical evidence and evidence from simulation studies (e.g., Schafer & Graham, 2002). Schafer and Graham summarize findings indicating that nonresponse in probability samples of the general population is less likely to introduce bias in the outcomes studied than nonresponse in studies whose samples are selected based on specific inclusion criteria (e.g., clinical trials studying interventions for a specific disorder). Though these developments are reassuring, more work is needed in these areas.

North and Pfefferbaum (2002) provided comprehensive methodological comments on the initial set of epidemiologic studies of the September terrorist attacks. They noted the importance of the timing of post-exposure assessment; the need for longitudinal follow-up; the importance of comparison groups;

and the need for careful interpretation of findings from observational studies. These authors also raise the important question of indirect exposure, given the massive (and repetitive) media coverage of the events. They point out that the DSM-IV criteria mention "witnessing" as an exposure, but also note that "No provision is made, however, for classification of indirect witnessing through viewing media images of the event" (p. 635).

It seems unlikely that the committees that have deliberated over detailed specification of the PTSD syndrome for the three versions of the DSM that have been published since PTSD was included in 1980 thought about events like September 11, where large numbers of people who were thousands of miles away from the danger and physical damage could view on television (live, on tape, or both) buildings where they could reasonably expect their loved ones to be located purposefully attacked and completely destroyed. Although not emphasized in the main-findings paper, Schlenger et al. (2002) found that more than 10 million adults in the U.S. reported that they had a family member, friend, or coworker killed or injured in the attacks, including about 7.5 million outside of the New York and Washington, DC metropolitan areas. This is an issue that should receive much more attention, both conceptually and empirically. North and Pfefferbaum (2002) also make the distinction between symptoms and distress, on the one hand, and diagnosable psychiatric illness on the other. Although they prefer structured, survey interview-based assessments that mimic the DSM criteria, it remains that the gold standard for case identification (diagnosis) is comprehensive, multisource-multimethod clinical assessment conducted by well-trained, experienced clinicians. All assessments that fall short of this standard should be considered to be "screening instruments," which are subject to increased but under many circumstances "acceptable," levels of diagnostic error. Therefore, the critical issue in selecting among candidate screeners is empirical documentation of their correspondence with comprehensive clinical diagnosis in community-based samples, not the content of the assessments themselves.

Relatedly, Neria and his colleagues (Neria, Bromet, & Marshall, 2002) point out an important limitation of standard community epidemiologic assessment methods. Those methods ask respondents to make a link only between traumatic exposures and PTSD symptoms but not the symptoms of other psychiatric disorders or of other adverse outcomes. As a result, these methods may mask the relationship of other outcomes (e.g., depression) with trauma. If so, the current body of epidemiologic research may underestimate substantially the full impact of trauma on the lives of those exposed. Given the emphasis in recent (and presumably future) versions of the DSM on empirical bases for diagnostic criteria, this masking may have produced distortions or biases in the diagnostic nomenclature as well. These issues should be high on the agenda for researchers and clinicians interested in documenting and treating the symptomatic responses of people exposed to terrorism and related events.

CONCLUSION

Empirical documentation of psychosocial distress based on acceptable research methods became available quickly following the terrorist attacks of September 11. The findings of these studies as a group demonstrated that although a majority of Americans were "distressed" in one or more ways by the attacks, much of the distress was not clinically significant and proved to be self-limiting (i.e., subsided relatively quickly, without formal intervention). Additionally, a much smaller proportion experienced clinically significant symptomatology, including symptoms of PTSD and depression. These clinically significant reactions were concentrated in the New York area, where the damage and direct exposure was greatest, and the evidence suggests that much of it was also self limiting.

Although those whose clinically significant symptoms do not resolve relatively quickly (e.g., within 3-6 months following exposure) typically represent a relatively small proportion of all of those exposed: (a) even a small proportion of a large population represents a large number of cases (e.g., because there are more than 10 million adults living in the New York metropolitan area, a condition whose prevalence there is only 1% means that more than 100,000 New York area adults have that condition), and (b) their PTSD and other symptoms are likely to be chronic. Danieli, Engdahl, and Schlenger (2003) provide an overview of issues related to this subgroup, whose lives are forever changed by the event. Briefly, the focus of interventions with this subgroup should be on "adapting to the new reality" rather than "returning to normal."

Finally, although the September 11 studies represent a valuable resource to policy makers and others with responsibility for dealing with large-scale traumatic events, the findings of the initial studies must be considered preliminary. Additional studies that include comprehensive clinical assessment and more complete participation by those selected via probability sampling techniques are required to confirm the validity of this important work.

REFERENCES

Bossolo, L., Bergantino, D., Lichtenstein, B., & Gutman, M. (2002). *Many Americans still feeling effects of September 11th; are reexamining their priorities in life.* Retrieved February 22, 2002, from APA Online: http://www.apa.org/practice/poll_911.html

Danieli, Y., Engdahl, B., & Schlenger, W. (2003). The psychological consequences of terrorism. In F. Moghaddam, & A. Marsella (Eds.), *Understanding terrorism* (pp. 223-246). Washington, DC: American Psychological Association.

Derogatis, L. (2001). *Brief Symptom Inventory 18: Administration, Scoring, and Procedures Manual*. Minneapolis, MN: NCS Pearson, Inc.

Galea, S., Ahern, J., Resnick, H., Kilpatrick, D., Bucuvalas, M., Gold, J. et al. (2002a). Psychological sequelae of the September 11 terrorist attacks in New York City. *New England Journal of Medicine, 346*, 982-987.

Galea, S., Resnick, H., Ahern, J., Gold, J., Bucuvalas, M., Kilpatrick, D. et al. (2002b). Posttraumatic stress disorder in Manhattan, New York City, after the September 11th terrorist attacks. *Journal of Urban Health, 79*(3), 340-353.

Galea, S., Vlahov, D., Resnick, H., Ahern, J., Susser, E., Gold, J. et al. (2003). Trends in probable posttraumatic stress disorder among adults in New York City after the September 11 terrorist attacks. *American Journal of Epidemiology, 158*(6), 514-524.

Grieger, T, Fullerton, C, & Ursano, R. (2003). Posttraumatic stress disorder, alcohol use, and perceived safety after the terrorist attack on the Pentagon. *Psychiatric Services, 54*(10), 1380-1382.

Little, L., & Rubin, D. (1987). *Statistical analysis with missing data*. New York: Wiley.

Neria, Y., Bromet, E., & Marshall, R. (2002). The relationship between trauma exposure, post-traumatic stress disorder (PTSD) and depression. *Psychological Medicine, 32*, 1479-1480.

North, C., & Pfefferbaum, B. (2002). Research on the mental health effects of terrorism. *Journal of the American Medical Association, 288*, 633-636.

Office of Applied Studies. (2002). *Impact of September 11, 2001 events on substance use and mental health* (Analytic Series: A-18, DHHS Publication No. SMA 02-3729). Rockville, MD: Substance Abuse and Mental Health Services Administration.

PEW Research Center. (2002, January 11). *Worries about terrorism subside in Mid-America*. [PEW Research Center website]. Retrieved November 8, 2001 from, www.people-press.org/110801rpt.htm

Robins, L, Helzer, J, Croughan, J, & Ratliff, K. (1981). National Institute of Mental Health Diagnostic Interview Schedule: Its history, characteristics, and validity. *Archives of General Psychiatry, 45*, 977-986.

Schafer, J. (1997). *Analysis of incomplete multivariate data*. London: Chapman & Hall.

Schafer, J., & Graham, J. (2002). Missing data: Our view of the state of the art. *Psychological Methods, 7*(2), 147-177.

Schlenger, W., Caddell, J., Ebert, L., Jordan, B., Rourke, K., Wilson, D. et al. (2002). Psychological reactions to terrorist attacks: Findings from the national study of Americans' reactions to September 11. *Journal of the American Medical Association, 288*, 581-588.

Schlenger, W. E., Federman, E. B., Ebert, L., & Caddell, J. M. (in press). Probable PTSD and depression following the terrorist attacks of September 11, 2001: Evidence from the national study of Americans' reactions to September 11. In T. Smith (Ed.), *Social, psychological, and political impact on the American public of the September 11th terrorist attacks*. New York: Russell Sage Foundation.

Schuster, M. A., Stein, B. D., Jaycox, L. H., Collins, R. L., Marshall, G. N., Elliott, M., et al. (2001). A national survey of stress reactions after the September 11, 2001, terrorist attacks. *New England Journal of Medicine, 345,* 1507-1512.

Silver, R. C., Holman, E. A., McIntosh, D. N., Poulin, M., & Gil-Rivas, V. (2002). Nationwide longitudinal study of psychological responses to September 11. *Journal of the American Medical Association, 288*(10), 1235-1244.

Smith T. W., Rasinski K. A., & Toce, M. (2001). *America rebounds: A national study of public response to the September 11th terrorist attacks: Preliminary findings.* Chicago: National Opinion Research Center, University of Chicago.

Stein, B. D., Elliott, M. N., Jaycox, L. H., Collins, R. L., Berry, S. H., Klein, D. J. et al. (in press). A national longitudinal study of the psychological consequences of the September 11, 2001, terrorist attacks. *Psychiatry.*

Vlahov, D., Galea, S., Resnick, H., Ahern, J., Boscarino, J., Bucuvalas, M. et al. (2002). Increased use of cigarettes, alcohol, and marijuana among Manhattan, New York, residents after the September 11th terrorist attacks. *American Journal of Epidemiology, 155,* 988–996.

Weathers, F, Litz, B, Herman, D, Huska, J, & Keane, T. (1993, October). *The PTSD Checklist [PCL]: Reliability, validity, and diagnostic utility.* Paper presented at annual conference of the International Society for Traumatic Stress Studies, San Antonio, TX.

Television Watching and Mental Health in the General Population of New York City After September 11

Jennifer Ahern
Sandro Galea
Heidi Resnick
David Vlahov

SUMMARY. The September 11, 2001 terrorist attacks were watched on television by millions. Using data from a telephone survey of New York City residents in January 2002 ($N = 2001$), we examined the relations between television watching and probable posttraumatic stress disorder (PTSD) after the attacks. Among those who were directly affected by the attacks or had prior traumatic experiences, watching television was associated with probable PTSD. Experiencing a peri-event panic reaction accounted for some of the association between television watching and probable PTSD. Future research directions are suggested for better understanding the mechanisms behind observed associations between television watching and PTSD.

Address correspondence to: Sandro Galea, MD, MPH, DrPH, Center for Urban Epidemiologic Studies, Room 556, New York Academy of Medicine, 1216 Fifth Avenue, New York, NY 10029-5283 USA (E-mail: sgalea@nyam.org).

[Haworth co-indexing entry note]: "Television Watching and Mental Health in the General Population of New York City after September 11." Ahern, Jennifer et al. Co-published simultaneously in *Journal of Aggression, Maltreatment & Trauma* (The Haworth Maltreatment & Trauma Press, an imprint of The Haworth Press, Inc.) Vol. 9, No. 1/2, 2004; and: *The Trauma of Terrorism: Sharing Knowledge and Shared Care, An International Handbook* (ed: Yael Danieli, Danny Brom, and Joe Sills) The Haworth Maltreatment & Trauma Press, an imprint of The Haworth Press, Inc., 2005.

KEYWORDS. PTSD, television, panic, trauma, September 11, World Trade Center

The September 11, 2001 terrorist attacks were broadcast live on television and watched by millions as they unfolded. Many networks repeatedly broadcast vivid images of the September 11 attacks, including the collision of the airplanes with the World Trade Center (WTC) towers, people falling from the towers, the towers collapsing, and people running for their lives. One survey conducted soon after the attacks found that 98% of people in the U.S. watched at least an hour of television coverage on September 11 (Schuster et al., 2001). Considering the wide reach of television into homes across the country, it is important to examine the role television watching may play in shaping psychopathology in the aftermath of a disaster.

Media coverage plays an essential role of communication in disaster situations and also has the potential to affect powerfully those watching (Holloway, Norwood, Fullerton, Engel, & Ursano, 1997). The relation between television watching and psychopathology in the context of major traumatic events is controversial, with most extant research conducted among children and adolescents (Nader, Pynoos, Fairbanks, Al-Ajeel, & Al-Asfour, 1993; Pfefferbaum, 2001; Pfefferbaum, Gurwitch et al., 2000; Pfefferbaum, Moore et al., 1999; Pfefferbaum, Nixon et al., 1999; Pfefferbaum, Nixon, Tivis et al., 2001; Pfefferbaum, Nixon, Tucker et al., 1999; Pfefferbaum, Seale et al., 2000).

After September 11, four studies that assessed mental health in the general population of adults demonstrated associations between watching television coverage of the attacks and symptoms of PTSD (Ahern et al., 2002; Schlenger et al., 2002; Schuster et al., 2001; Silver, Holman, McIntosh, Poulin, & Gil-Rivas, 2002). Our research team conducted a telephone survey of Manhattan residents one month after the September 11 attacks and found associations between watching the image of people falling or jumping from the World Trade Center and probable PTSD (Ahern et al., 2002). This effect was strongest in persons who were directly affected by the attacks (Ahern et al., 2002). Other research found associations between several measures of television watching and symptoms of PTSD in the days and months following the September 11 attacks (Schlenger et al., 2002; Schuster et al., 2001; Silver et al., 2002).

Current research suggests that the prior experiences of adults watching television may be important factors that shape the association between watching television and psychological distress after a disaster. First, it has been suggested that among those who have been directly affected by a disaster (e.g., those who were injured or lost a close family member in the attacks), watching repeated television images of that disaster may be associated with more substantial negative psychological consequences. This may be due to a personal connection with the event among those who are directly affected and suggests that television watching may exacerbate the effects of a traumatizing experience (Ahern et al., 2002). Second, among people who have experienced other traumatic events in the past, posttraumatic stress symptoms may be exacerbated by watching violent television images (Elliott, 1997; Kinzie, Boehnlein, Riley, & Sparr, 2002; Kinzie et al., 1998; Long, Chamberlain, & Vincent, 1994; Moyers, 1996; Pittman, Orr, Forgue, deJong, & Claiborn, 1987), suggesting that those with prior traumatic experiences may be more affected by television images of a disaster. Third, we have recently shown that those who watch more television after a disaster are more likely to also have experienced a panic attack in the immediate aftermath of the disaster (Ahern, Galea, Resnick, & Vlahov, in press). Other work has shown that there is a strong relation between experiencing a panic attack soon after a traumatic experience and subsequent posttraumatic stress symptoms (Bryant & Panasetis, 2001; Deering, Glover, Ready, Eddleman, & Alarcon, 1996; Falsetti & Resnick, 1997; Galea et al., 2002), suggesting the possibility that peri-event emotional reactions may play an important role in the relation between television watching and posttraumatic stress symptoms.

Building on this previous research we explore the relations between television watching and probable PTSD in New York City (NYC) after the September 11 terrorist attacks. This exploratory analysis was aimed at generating hypotheses and directions for future research about television watching and its potential relation with posttraumatic stress symptoms among adults after disasters.

METHODS

Participants

We conducted a random digit dial telephone survey of NYC residents in January and February of 2002. All persons at least 18 years of age and living in NYC on September 11, 2001 were eligible to participate. We called each telephone number up to 10 times in an effort to contact the residents and interviewed one person in each household contacted, using a most recent birthday selection method. The interview was approximately 35 minutes in length. All five boroughs of NYC were included in the survey, with an oversample in Manhattan south of 110th Street for comparison with a prior survey. All participants gave informed consent, and the cooperation rate was 63.5%. The cooperation rate is the proportion of persons who were contacted who agreed to participate in the survey, calculated as the completed interviews and screen-outs as a percentage of completed interviews, screen-outs, refusals, and premature terminations. The study protocol was approved by the institutional review board of the New York Academy of Medicine.

Measures

Television Watching. We assessed television watching by asking how many times respondents had seen the images of "An airplane hitting the World Trade Center," "Buildings collapsing," "People running away from a cloud of smoke or debris," and "People falling or jumping from the towers of the World Trade Center" in the seven days following the attacks. The specific television images and a combined sum of all images were divided into thirds of the number of times people saw them (33.3% of the population in each group), creating low, medium, and high categories of frequency of watching.

Probable PTSD. We used the National Women's Study (NWS) PTSD module to measure PTSD symptoms. The NWS PTSD module was validated in a field trial against the PTSD module of the Structured Clinical Interview for DSM-III-R (SCID; Spitzer, Williams, Gibbon, & First, 1992) administered by mental health professionals (Kilpatrick et al., 1998). In the field trial, inter-rater kappa coefficients were 0.85 for the diagnosis of lifetime PTSD and 0.86 for the diagnosis of current PTSD. Comparing the NWS PTSD module to the SCID, the kappa coefficient of the NWS PTSD module with SCID diagnosis of PTSD was 0.77 for lifetime PTSD and 0.71 for current PTSD (Kilpatrick et al., 1998). Instrument sensitivity was 99% and specificity was 79% when compared to SCID diagnosis (Kilpatrick et al., 1998; Resnick, Kilpatrick, Dansky, Saunders, & Best, 1993). The NWS PTSD module assesses the presence of criteria B, C, and D symptoms and determines content for content-specific PTSD symptoms (e.g., content of dreams or nightmares). We assessed probable PTSD since September 11 based on the presence of necessary PTSD criteria B, C, and D symptoms during that time period. To measure probable PTSD that was related to the September 11 attacks, all re-experiencing symptoms (criterion B) and all content-specific (e.g., avoidance of thoughts or feelings) avoidance symptoms (criterion C) were required to be related to the September 11 attacks. A subset of avoidance symptoms and all the arousal symptoms (criterion D; e.g., being easily startled or jumpy) were linked to the attacks by time frame (occurrence since September 11). We use the term "probable PTSD" to reflect the fact that interviews were conducted by lay interviewers using a standard instrument.

We were interested in the role of three factors in shaping the relation between television watching and PTSD.

Being Directly Affected by the Attacks. We assessed whether respondents to our survey were directly affected by the attacks by creating a composite variable of several different potential exposures. We asked respondents about their experiences related to the attacks on September 11, including seeing the WTC attacks in person, being in the WTC complex, being injured in the attacks, having relatives or friends who were killed in the attacks, having possessions lost or damaged in the attacks, being involved in the rescue efforts, and losing a job following the WTC attacks. A respondent experiencing any of the above September 11 experiences was considered "directly affected" by the attacks.

Lifetime Traumatic Events. We assessed lifetime traumatic event experiences by asking if respondents had previously experienced any of the following: a major natural disaster, a serious accident, being attacked with a weapon, being attacked without a weapon but with the intent to seriously injure or kill, forced sexual contact, other serious injury, other situation with potential to seriously injure or kill, seeing someone seriously injured or killed, or any other extraordinarily stressful situation. In this analysis, people who had experienced any of these events were classified as having experienced a previous traumatic event.

Experiencing a Peri-Event Panic Attack. We measured a peri-event panic attack after September 11 by using a modified version of the Diagnostic Interview Schedule measure for panic attack (Centers for Disease Control and Prevention, 1989). Those who reported having four or more symptoms occurring in the "first few hours after" the events of September 11 were considered to have experienced a peri-event panic attack.

Statistical Analyses

All analyses were conducted in SUDAAN, a statistical software package designed for analysis of cluster-correlated and weighted data (Shah, Barnwell, & Bieler, 1997), with weighting to account for the probability of selection for interview based on the number of persons and telephone lines in the household as well as the Manhattan oversample.

Relations between the categories of television watching and probable PTSD were assessed in cross-tabulations with two-tailed chi-square tests, and relations between continuous measures of television watching and probable PTSD were assessed in bivariate logistic regression models. As the findings revealed the same associations, results for categories of television viewing are presented for ease of interpretation.

We assessed the bivariate associations of the number of times the four television images and a sum of images were viewed with probable PTSD. Next, we assessed these same relations, stratified by whether respondents were directly affected by the attacks. Finally, we assessed the relations between television watching (sum of images) and probable PTSD among combined strata of directly affected and prior traumatic events, and among strata of directly affected with peri-event panic.

RESULTS

Among survey respondents ($N = 2001$), mean age was 41 years, 53.3% were female, and the racial/ethnic composition was 40.5% White, 5.4% Asian, 25.7% African American, 25.0% Hispanic, and 3.3% of other race/ethnicity. Event exposures were common: 24.6% saw the attacks on the WTC in person, 12.1% had a friend or relative killed, 8.8% were involved in the rescue efforts, and 5.9% lost a job following the attacks. Overall, 41.2% were directly affected by the attacks, 69.7% had a previous traumatic event experience, and 16.7% experienced a peri-event panic attack.

The image of an airplane hitting the WTC was watched relatively frequently in the 7 days following September 11 ($M = 41.1, Mdn = 30, SD = 35.8$) as were the images of the buildings collapsing ($M = 36.9, Mdn = 20, SD = 34.8$) and people running from a cloud of smoke ($M = 36.7, Mdn = 21, SD = 34.2$). The image of people falling or jumping was watched less frequently ($M = 11.9, Mdn = 2, SD = 23.8$). For all images, the range was 0 to 97 times, with 97 representing 97 or more times in the past 7 days. The sum of all images had a mean of 111.9 times, a median of 70 times and a standard deviation of 111.2.

Respondents who reported watching television images of the attacks on the WTC more frequently in the seven days following September 11 had higher prevalences of probable PTSD, as depicted in Figure 1. Among those who saw an airplane hitting the WTC most frequently, 10.3% had probable PTSD, while among those who saw it least frequently 4.5% had probable PTSD ($p = 0.003$). Similar associations were present for the images of buildings collapsing and people running. For the image of people falling or jumping, there was more probable PTSD among those who saw the image most frequently, but the difference was not statistically significant ($p = 0.27$). As all four images had similar patterns of association with probable PTSD, we created a measure of

FIGURE 1. Associations between watching television images related to the September 11, 2001 terrorist attacks and probable PTSD, New York City 2002 (N = 2001)

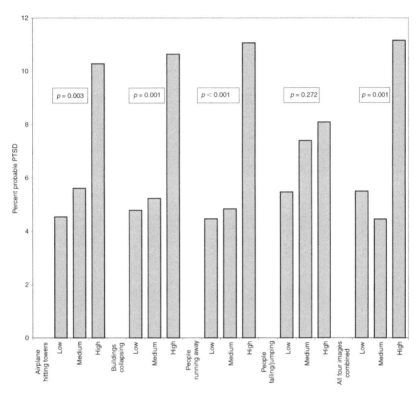

Note: Low, medium and high categories of watching television images correspond to thirds of the number of times respondents reported seeing each image in the seven days following the September 11 terrorist attacks

combined images. For those who saw the most combined images, the prevalence of probable PTSD was 11.2%, and among those who were in the middle and lowest thirds of combined images, the prevalences of probable PTSD were 4.5% and 5.5%, respectively ($p < 0.001$; see Table 1).

The associations between television image watching and probable PTSD, stratified by whether respondents were directly affected, are presented in Table 1. Among those who were directly affected by the attacks, by low, medium, and high thirds of watching the image of an airplane hitting the WTC, the prevalences of probable PTSD were 7.3%, 9.0%, and 14.6%, respectively ($p = 0.07$). The corresponding prevalences for the image of the buildings collapsing were 7.3%, 8.3%, and 15.3% ($p = 0.03$); for the image of people run-

TABLE 1. Associations Between Watching Television Images of September 11 and Probable PTSD, Stratified by Directly Affected, New York City 2002 (N = 2001)

	Total NYC					Directly affected*					Not directly affected*				
	n	%	n PTSD	% PTSD	p-value	n	%	n PTSD	% PTSD	p-value	n	%	n PTSD	% PTSD	p-value
Thirds															
Airplane hitting towers															
Low	545	33.98	23	4.54	0.003	211	28.12	15	7.34	0.07	334	38.14	8	3.08	0.12
Medium	441	26.12	31	5.61		194	26.51	22	8.96		247	25.84	9	3.17	
High	665	39.9	70	10.28		327	45.37	45	14.56		338	36.02	25	6.46	
Buildings collapsing															
Low	556	34.31	23	4.79	0.001	216	29.32	14	7.31	0.03	340	37.95	9	3.36	0.21
Medium	527	30.89	34	5.23		226	29.72	24	8.34		301	31.74	10	3.1	
High	609	34.81	67	10.64		313	40.96	45	15.33		296	30.31	22	6.01	
People running															
Low	557	33.46	22	4.47	0.0002	205	27.26	12	6.4	0.005	352	37.76	10	3.5	0.10
Medium	555	32.46	32	4.84		252	33.61	23	7.54		303	31.66	9	2.85	
High	597	34.09	70	11.06		294	39.13	46	16.13		303	30.58	24	6.55	
People falling/jumping															
Low	708	36.6	37	5.47	0.27	280	31.74	24	7.84	0.24	428	40.04	13	4.13	0.90
Medium	593	32.19	47	7.4		274	34.35	33	12		319	30.65	14	3.75	
High	543	31.21	52	8.09		251	33.91	34	12.46		292	29.31	18	4.51	
Four television images combined															
Low	640	33.58	33	5.5	0.0001	239	28.27	21	9.59	0.004	401	37.28	12	3.33	0.06
Medium	641	33.14	37	4.46		287	33.81	26	6.79		354	32.68	11	2.77	
High	643	33.28	74	11.16		314	37.92	49	16.3		329	30.04	25	6.63	

*Directly affected includes seeing the WTC attacks in person, being in the WTC complex, being injured in the attacks, having relatives or friends who were killed in the attacks, having possessions lost or damaged in the attacks, being involved in the rescue efforts, and losing a job following the WTC attacks ning, they were 6.4%, 7.5%, and 16.1% ($p = 0.005$); and for the image of people falling or jumping, they were 7.8%, 12.0%, and 12.5% ($p = 0.24$). For the sum of all images combined, the prevalence of probable PTSD was 9.6%, 6.8%, and 16.3% ($p = 0.004$) for low, medium, and high thirds of watching, respectively.

Among those not directly affected by the attacks, there were no significant associations between television images viewed and probable PTSD, although there was a borderline association with the sum of all images. The prevalence of probable PTSD in the highest category of watching combined images was 6.6%, while it was 2.8% and 3.3% in the medium and low categories, respectively ($p = 0.06$; see Table 1).

Examining the association between television watching and probable PTSD in combined groups of directly affected and past traumatic experiences revealed that associations were not consistent across strata (see Table 2). Among those who were both directly affected and experienced a prior potentially traumatic event, there was an association between television watching and probable PTSD: the prevalences for increasing thirds of watching were 12.1%, 7.9%, and 15.6% ($p = 0.05$). There were also associations between television watching and probable PTSD in those directly affected but with no past trauma, and in those with past trauma who were not directly affected ($p = 0.02$, $p = 0.01$, respectively). However, among those who were not directly affected and had no past trauma there was no association between television watching and probable PTSD; the prevalences from low to high frequency of watching were 3.6%, 1.9%, and 0.9% ($p = 0.37$).

By combined categories of directly affected and peri-event panic, the association between watching television images and probable PTSD was not consistent across strata (see Table 3). Among those who experienced peri-event panic and were directly affected, the prevalence of probable PTSD was high (20-40%) but did not differ by frequency of watching television images ($p = 0.37$). Among those who experienced peri-event panic but were not directly affected, the prevalence of probable PTSD was high as well, but with no relation to television watching ($p = 0.29$). Among those who did not experience peri-event panic, the directly affected and not directly affected groups both had borderline associations between television watching and probable PTSD ($p = 0.06$, $p = 0.07$, respectively).

DISCUSSION

In this analysis, we showed an association between watching television related to September 11 and probable PTSD both for a range of different images

TABLE 2. Association Between Television Images and Probable PTSD, Stratified by Directly Affected and Past Traumatic Experience, New York City 2002 (N = 2001)

Four television images combined		Directly affected*					Not directly affected*				
		n	%	n PTSD	% PTSD	p-value	n	%	n PTSD	% PTSD	p-value
Past traumatic events	Low	167	25.83	17	12.14	0.05	241	33.73	9	3.16	0.01
	Medium	228	34.77	25	7.87		249	33.56	9	3.19	
	High	247	39.39	40	15.61		244	32.71	23	8.94	
No past traumatic events	Low	72	35.94	4	3.84	0.02	160	44.03	3	3.58	0.37
	Medium	59	30.78	1	2.97		105	31.01	2	1.92	
	High	67	33.27	9	18.85		85	24.96	2	0.89	

* Directly affected includes seeing the WTC attacks in person, being in the WTC complex, being injured in the attacks, having relatives or friends who were killed in the attacks, having possessions lost or damaged in the attacks, being involved in the rescue efforts, and losing a job following the WTC attacks

TABLE 3. Association Between Television Images and Probable PTSD, Stratified by Directly Affected and Peri-Event Panic, New York City 2002 (N = 2001)

Four television images combined			Directly affected*					Not directly affected*				
	n	%	n PTSD	% PTSD	p-value	n	%	n PTSD	% PTSD	p-value
Peri-event panic	Low	33	20.72	11	37.23	0.37	43	29.97	9	20.56	0.29
	Medium	46	27.75	13	23.12		37	28.31	4	8.25	
	High	88	51.54	31	35.03		63	41.72	11	12.85	
No peri-event panic	Low	206	30.28	10	4.57	0.06	358	38.42	3	1.23	0.07
	Medium	241	35.42	13	3.39		317	33.36	7	2.05	
	High	226	34.3	18	8.82		266	28.22	14	5.2	

* Directly affected includes seeing the WTC attacks in person, being in the WTC complex, being injured in the attacks, having relatives or friends who were killed in the attacks, having possessions lost or damaged in the attacks, being involved in the rescue efforts, and losing a job following the WTC attacks

and for a combined measure of frequency of television watching. The majority of this association was present among those directly affected by the September 11 attacks. Consistent with previous research (Ahern et al., 2002), these results suggest the importance of a personal connection (e.g., knowing someone who was killed, being in the WTC towers, being injured in the attacks) to the images watched. Those who have a personal connection to the images may be more traumatized by watching those images, or conversely, those with a personal connection who begin to develop psychopathology may be more inclined to watch television related to the precipitating incident.

When we examined the combined contribution of being directly affected by the attacks and having had prior traumatic experiences, we found that among those who were not directly affected by the attacks and who had experienced no prior traumatic events there was no relation between television watching and probable PTSD. However, among those who were directly affected by the attacks, who experienced a prior traumatic event, or both, watching television about the attacks was associated with symptoms of probable PTSD. If future research demonstrates that watching television images of a disaster increases the risk of posttraumatic stress symptoms among those directly affected by the attacks or with a prior traumatic experience, then a reduction in television viewing for this population would be an effective public health intervention to decrease post-disaster psychopathology. The relation between watching images of traumatic events and psychological symptoms among those with previous traumatic experiences has been demonstrated in experimental settings and also in relation to September 11 television watching (Kinzie et al., 1998, 2002); however, these findings have mainly been among those with preexisting PTSD or depression. Similarly, among the respondents to our survey who had posttraumatic stress symptoms as a result of prior traumatic experiences, television viewing related to September 11 may have reactivated symptoms. Our findings in a general population sample raise the question of whether prior traumatic experience in combination with current television watching of an unfolding disaster are sufficient to explain the observed association with probable PTSD, or whether pre-existing psychopathology related to a prior traumatic event is a necessary factor that may explain this relation. Research suggests that media may be a trigger of suppressed traumatic memories (Elliott, 1997) and thus may have the ability to affect those with prior traumatic experiences who have not developed PTSD. More research in this area would enrich our understanding of these associations.

Examining the relation between being directly affected by the September 11 attacks and peri-event panic, we found that among those who experienced peri-event panic, the prevalence of probable PTSD was very high but unrelated to the September 11 television images, regardless of whether respondents were directly affected. The strong association between panic and posttraumatic stress symptoms is consistent with research that demonstrates strong associations between panic and PTSD (Bryant & Panasetis, 2001; Deering et al., 1996; Falsetti & Resnick, 1997; Galea et al., 2002), but the association between television watching and panic has not been much explored (Ahern et al., in press). Among those who did not experience peri-event panic, there were borderline associations between television watching and probable PTSD for the directly affected and those not directly affected. In particular, the relation for those who were directly affected but did not panic was much reduced from the overall association between television watching and probable PTSD among the directly affected. These findings suggest the importance of experiencing peri-event panic reactions as a key part of the relation between television watching and posttraumatic stress symptoms.

There are some limitations that should be considered when interpreting this analysis. The cooperation rate of 65.3% suggests we were unable to interview a substantial proportion of the households we attempted to contact. However, the demographic similarity between the achieved sample and Census figures suggests our sample is representative. The associations observed between television and probable PTSD do not demonstrate causality. Extensive television viewing may be a marker of early psychopathology, or the viewing may contribute to symptoms of psychopathology. Longitudinal assessment that determined the timing of the development of symptoms in relation to television viewing would help address the question of causality.

Future Directions

The findings in this analysis generate some questions to be addressed in future research. The relation between television watching and probable PTSD among those with prior traumatic experiences raises the question about what types of prior traumatic events may be more important in this context. Research among refugees suggests that images with similarity to the original traumatic event are more likely to elicit a response (Kinzie et al., 1998), and the recency of the prior traumatic experience and the proximity of the current traumatic event geographically and culturally to the individual (Kinzie et al., 2002) may be important predictors of the response to televised images of the current event. Exploration of these issues in general population samples may help us understand the relation between television and probable PTSD in a group with prior traumatic experiences who were only exposed to the current potentially traumatic event through television.

The finding that a large portion of the relation between television watching and probable PTSD can be removed by accounting for the experience of a peri-event panic attack raises important questions about the nature of the relation between television watching and peri-event panic. Primarily, it would be interesting to explore whether watching more television images of a disaster can contribute to precipitating a panic attack, or whether those who experience a peri-event panic attack later watch more television because of the panic attack. Experimental research among patients with PTSD suggests that watching television images of distressing events can cause physiological arousal, suggesting that television images might contribute to the development of a panic attack (Kinzie et al., 1998). This is a question that merits further exploration.

In the current era of constant television news coverage of events across the globe, the potential impact of watching disasters, wars, terrorism, and other traumatic events on television will only grow as a concern. A greater understanding of the mechanisms behind the observed associations between television watching and posttraumatic stress may help us understand and better prepare for the effects of future disasters.

REFERENCES

Ahern, J., Galea, S., Resnick, H., Kilpatrick, D., Bucuvalas, M., Gold, J. et al. (2002). Television images and psychological symptoms after the September 11 terrorist attacks. *Psychiatry, 65*(4), 289-300.

Ahern, J., Galea, S., Resnick, H., & Vlahov, D. (in press). Television images and probable PTSD after September 11: The role of background characteristics, event exposures and peri-event panic. *The Journal of Nervous and Mental Disease.*

Bryant, R., & Panasetis, P. (2001). Panic symptoms during trauma and acute stress disorder. *Behavior Research and Therapy, 39*(8), 961-966.

Centers for Disease Control and Prevention. (1989). Diagnostic Interview Schedule (DIS). *Health Status of Vietnam Veterans. Supplement C: Medical and Psychological Procedure Manuals and Forms* (pp. 405-499). Atlanta, GA: Author.

Deering, C. G., Glover, S. G., Ready, D., Eddleman, H. C., & Alarcon, R. D. (1996). Unique patterns of comorbidity in posttraumatic stress disorder from different sources of trauma. *Comprehensive Psychiatry, 37*(5), 336-346.

Elliott, D. M. (1997). Traumatic events: Prevalence and delayed recall in the general population. *Journal of Consulting and Clinical Psychology, 65*(5), 811-820.

Falsetti, S. A., & Resnick, H. (1997). Frequency and severity of panic attack symptoms in a treatment seeking sample of trauma victims. *Journal of Traumatic Stress, 10*(4), 683-689.

Galea, S., Ahern, J., Resnick, H., Kilpatrick, D., Bucuvalas, M., Gold, J. et al. (2002). Psychological sequelae of the September 11 terrorist attacks in Manhattan, New York City. *The New England Journal of Medicine, 346*(13), 982-987.

Holloway, H. C., Norwood, A. E., Fullerton, C. S., Engel, C. C., & Ursano, R. J. (1997). The threat of biological weapons, prophylaxis and mitigation of psychological and social consequences. *The Journal of the American Medical Association, 278*(5), 425-427.

Kilpatrick, D., Resnick, H., Freedy, J., Pelcovitz, D., Resnick, P., Roth, S. et al. (1998). The posttraumatic stress disorder field trial: Evaluation of the PTSD construct–Criteria A through E. In T. A. Widiger, A. J. Frances, H. A. Pincus, R. Ross, M. B. First, W. Davis, & M. Kline (Eds.), *DSM-IV Sourcebook* (Vol. 4, pp. 803-844). Washington DC: American Psychiatric Association Press.

Kinzie, J. D., Boehnlein, J., Riley, C., & Sparr, L. (2002). The effects of September 11 on traumatized refugees: Reactivation of posttraumatic stress disorder. *The Journal of Nervous and Mental Disease, 190*(7), 437-441.

Kinzie, J. D., Denney, D., Riley, C., Boehnlein, J., McFarland, B., & Leung, P. (1998). A cross-cultural study of reactivation of posttraumatic stress disorder symptoms. *The Journal of Nervous and Mental Disease, 186*, 670-676.

Long, N., Chamberlain, K., & Vincent, C. (1994). Effect of the Gulf War on reactivation of adverse combat-related memories in Vietnam veterans. *Journal of Clinical Psychology, 50*(2), 138-144.

Moyers, F. (1996). Oklahoma City bombing: Exacerbation of symptoms in veterans with PTSD. *Archives of Psychiatric Nursing, 10*(1), 55-59.

Nader, K. O., Pynoos, R. S., Fairbanks, L. A., Al-Ajeel, M., & Al-Asfour, A. (1993). A preliminary study of PTSD and grief among the children of Kuwait following the gulf crisis. *British Journal of Clinical Psychology, 32*, 407-416.

Pfefferbaum, B. (2001). The impact of the Oklahoma City bombing on children in the community. *Military Medicine, 166*(suppl. 2), 49-50.

Pfefferbaum, B., Gurwitch, R. H., McDonald, N. B., Leftwich, M. J. T., Sconzo, G. M., Messenbaugh, A. K. et al. (2000). Posttraumatic stress among young children after the death of a friend or acquaintance in a terrorist bombing. *Psychiatric Services, 52*(3), 386-388.

Pfefferbaum, B., Moore, V. L., McDonald, N. B., Maynard, B. T., Gurwitch, R. H., & Nixon, S. J. (1999). The role of exposure in posttraumatic stress in youths following the 1995 bombing. *Journal of the Oklahoma State Medical Association, 92*(4), 164-167.

Pfefferbaum, B., Nixon, S. J., Krug, R. S., Tivis, R. D., Moore, V. L., Brown, J. M. et al. (1999). Clinical needs assessment of middle and high school students following the 1995 Oklahoma City bombing. *American Journal of Psychiatry, 156*(7), 1069-1074.

Pfefferbaum, B., Nixon, S. J., Tivis, R. D., Doughty, D. E., Pynoos, R. S., Gurwitch, R. H. et al. (2001). Television exposure in children after a terrorist incident. *Psychiatry, 64*(3), 202-211.

Pfefferbaum, B., Nixon, S. J., Tucker, P. M., Tivis, R. D., Moore, V. L., Gurwitch, R. H. et al. (1999). Posttraumatic stress responses in bereaved children after the Oklahoma City bombing. *Journal of the American Academy of Child and Adolescent Psychiatry, 38*(11), 1372-1379.

Pfefferbaum, B., Seale, T. W., McDonald, N. B., Brandt, E. N., Rainwater, S. M., Maynard, B. T. et al. (2000). Posttraumatic stress two years after the Oklahoma City bombing in youths geographically distant from the explosion. *Psychiatry, 63*(4), 358-370.

Pittman, R. K., Orr, S. P., Forgue, D. F., deJong, J., & Claiborn, J. M. (1987). Psychophysiologic assessment of posttraumatic stress disorder imagery in Vietnam combat veterans. *Archives of General Psychiatry, 44*, 970-975.

Resnick, H. S., Kilpatrick, D. G., Dansky, B. S., Saunders, B. E., & Best, C. (1993). Prevalence of civilian trauma and posttraumatic stress disorder in a representative national survey of women. *Journal of Consulting and Clinical Psychology, 61*, 984-991.

Schlenger, W. E., Caddell, J. M., Ebert, L., Jordan, B. K., Rourke, K. M., Wilson, D. et al. (2002). Psychological reactions to terrorist attacks. Findings from the national study of Americans' reactions to September 11. *The Journal of the American Medical Association, 288*(5), 581-588.

Schuster, M. A., Stein, B. D., Jaycox, L. H., Collins, R. L., Marshall, G. N., Elliott, M. N. et al. (2001). A national survey of stress reactions after the September 11, 2001, terrorist attacks. *The New England Journal of Medicine, 345*(20), 1507-1512.

Shah, B., Barnwell, B., & Bieler, G. (1997). *SUDAAN user's manual, release 7.5*. Research Triangle Park, NC: Research Triangle Institute.

Silver, R. C., Holman, E. A., McIntosh, D. N., Poulin, M., & Gil-Rivas, V. (2002). Nationwide longitudinal study of psychological responses to September 11. *The Journal of the American Medical Association, 288*(10), 1235-1244.

Spitzer, R., Williams, J., Gibbon, M., & First, M. (1992). The structural clinical interview for DSM-III-R (SCID) I: History, rationale, and description. *Archives of General Psychiatry, 49*, 624-629.

Voice:
Too Close to Ever Forget

Adam Lisberg

I feel much better now, two years later, but I still try to avoid the site. It looks nothing like it did then. It looks like any other big construction site with cranes, dump trucks, and union guys in hard hats. The edges of the job are smooth and clean, all fresh-poured concrete and angular scaffolds. No dust. No disorder. The tourists still come, but instead of the fires and smoke and crumpled buildings they saw on TV, all they can see is men building things behind sturdy steel fencing.

To look at the site now is to see nothing. There are cars, stores, a rebuilt bike path, men in suits, and women in dresses. This is as it should be; the city needs to rebuild and recover. But I fight an intense urge to shake these people and ask, "Don't you know what happened here?"

West Street. All six lanes were buried under piles of steel beams 10 feet high. I walked along them gingerly, like a giant jungle gym, hopping from one beam to the next above the crushed ambulances and the people buried in gray muck. For months it was shut down for a mile; crews picked up the steel and the ambulances and the people, laid new pavement, and made it whole again. It's a major artery. But every time I cruise down it, I can only compare it to what I saw then.

I watched trucks rumble in and out of the lots where command posts, feeding tents, and transfer stations were carved out of parking lots. They operated for months, 24 hours a day, endless grim work. I spent a Christmas morning there,

---

Address correspondence to: The senior editor of this volume, Yael Danieli, Group Project for Holocaust Survivors and Their Children, 345 East 80th Street (31-J), New York, NY 10021.

[Haworth co-indexing entry note]: "Voice: Too Close to Ever Forget." Lisberg, Adam. Co-published simultaneously in *Journal of Aggression, Maltreatment & Trauma* (The Haworth Maltreatment & Trauma Press, an imprint of The Haworth Press, Inc.) Vol. 9, No. 1/2, 2004; and: *The Trauma of Terrorism: Sharing Knowledge and Shared Care, An International Handbook* (ed: Yael Danieli, Danny Brom, and Joe Sills) The Haworth Maltreatment & Trauma Press, an imprint of The Haworth Press, Inc., 2005.

and it was as gray and featureless as any other day. Now the lots are bright, cheery, and unnervingly green; they are a place for children and softball teams. But I can't watch them play without wondering how they can be happy on that ground.

Liberty Street. Husbands sit in cars on summer evenings, waiting to pick up their wives. Joggers and bikers buzz past on the new path. Thousands of people work in the office towers there, and thousands more live nearby. I envy them, for what they've been able to put behind them, or maybe for what they don't know. They can move through their lives normally where I dodged chunks of falling metal, where I walked past cops and firefighters living their final minutes. They can walk without memory along the street where I literally ran for my life, past the patch of sidewalk where I expected to suffocate, through the spot where I first heard a man say, "I found two more dead guys."

I avoid the site because of what it makes me remember, but really, I can't avoid the memories. There's always something to remind me, crawling into my mind, unbidden, for no obvious reason, in the shower, in line at the grocery store, I guess just because it's always there.

I had been a news reporter for nine years on that morning. I felt a little too old to cover a fire. On the radio, the guy in the traffic helicopter said he saw smoke pouring from one of the towers; I figured it was a blown transformer. But I called my office, and they told me to check it out.

I used up a lifetime of luck that morning. In the time it took the south tower to fall 110 stories, I was able to make it around a corner and wedge myself against a building. I spent a long time trying to reconcile the end of the world with my everyday life, trying to find some reason why I survived when people died all around me.

In the days that followed, I panicked at the rumble of freight elevators and low-flying planes; I dreamed about running for my life. There was no way to escape. Every day I went to work and sat at my desk, distracted and numb, while I wrote about terrorism, anthrax, and memorials. Every night I went home where the air smelled of smoke, the missing stared from fliers on every corner, and my wife never wanted to let me out of her sight again.

My editors offered to let me off the story, but I threw myself into it. I spent months writing about firefighters, bagpipers, and funerals, about bottomless grief and what the dead left behind. At every funeral I covered, I couldn't help wondering what my own would have been like.

Writing those stories was gut wrenching. I realize now, that by spending so much time talking about death, talking to cops, firefighters, and the next of kin, I was trying to find some way to talk about what I saw, heard, and tasted, some way to articulate the emptiness that crawled beneath my skin. I immersed myself in pain in order to bring out some of my own.

I had to stop writing about it. I started writing the stories I used to scoff at, softer stories, feature stories, and articles that celebrated good things that usually get overlooked in the newspaper. I had once thrived on adrenaline and deadlines, but I learned that my priorities have changed. Getting right up close to the big story isn't so important to me anymore; I'd rather make it home in one piece, in time to have dinner with my wife.

Exploring the Myths of Coping with a National Trauma: A Longitudinal Study of Responses to the September 11th Terrorist Attacks

Roxane Cohen Silver
Michael Poulin
E. Alison Holman
Daniel N. McIntosh
Virginia Gil-Rivas
Judith Pizarro

SUMMARY. A longitudinal investigation of psychological responses to the September 11, 2001 terrorist attacks was conducted on a U.S. national probability sample. Using an anonymous Web-based survey methodology, data were collected among over 1,900 adults at 2 weeks and 12 months post-9/11 to consider whether direct and proximal exposure were

Address correspondence to: Roxane Cohen Silver, PhD, Department of Psychology and Social Behavior, 3340 Social Ecology II, University of California, Irvine, CA 92697-7085 USA (E-mail: rsilver@uci.edu).

Project funding was provided by the National Science Foundation grants BCS-9910223, BCS-0211039, and BCS-0215937.

[Haworth co-indexing entry note]: "Exploring the Myths of Coping with a National Trauma: A Longitudinal Study of Responses to the September 11th Terrorist Attacks." Silver, Roxane Cohen et al. Co-published simultaneously in *Journal of Aggression, Maltreatment & Trauma* (The Haworth Maltreatment & Trauma Press, an imprint of The Haworth Press, Inc.) Vol. 9, No. 1/2, 2004; and: *The Trauma of Terrorism: Sharing Knowledge and Shared Care, An International Handbook* (ed: Yael Danieli, Danny Brom, and Joe Sills) The Haworth Maltreatment & Trauma Press, an imprint of The Haworth Press, Inc., 2005.

necessary preconditions for high levels of acute and posttraumatic stress symptoms, and whether greater exposure/proximity led to greater traumatic stress symptoms. Results suggest that the requirement of direct and proximal exposure to the attacks and the expectation of a dose-response relationship between exposure and traumatic stress response are myths.

KEYWORDS. Terrorism, September 11th, acute stress response, posttraumatic stress response, exposure

On September 11th, 2001, the worst terrorist attack against the U.S. in modern history was perpetrated on its soil. Americans have had limited opportunities to study the psychological effects of domestic terrorism, but a useful starting point for understanding these phenomena is an examination of the literature on the psychological impact of traumatic life events in general. Many traumas are random, unpredictable and uncontrollable (Silver & Wortman, 1980). When such events are community disasters, the experience is shared by many. But in several ways, terrorism is unique. To the aforementioned characteristics one must add a faceless enemy with political undertones whose specific goal is to create ongoing anxiety in the populace.

A great deal has been written about how individuals will respond to traumatic life events and disasters (Norris, Byrne, & Diaz, 2001). In fact, theory and clinical lore paint a rather clear and consistent picture of responses to trauma–one that shapes societal expectations about responses to tragedy. However, many of these assumptions appear to be myths; these expectations concerning responses to trauma have not fared well when scrutinized against data addressing their validity (see Silver & Wortman, 1980; Wortman & Silver, 1989, 2001). One myth is that psychological responses to traumatic events are predictable; that is, that there are universal reactions to traumatic events. A second myth is that psychological response to traumatic events will follow a pattern, or orderly sequence of stages. A third myth is that psychological response to trauma requires direct, proximal exposure to the stressor, and that traumatic stress response is proportional to the degree of exposure, amount of loss, or proximity to the trauma (i.e., as "objective" loss increases, so will its impact). This third and final set of expectations is addressed directly in this article.

There are many possible psychological and behavioral consequences of traumatic events, including generalized distress, intrusive ruminations, physical symptoms, increased health care utilization, disruptions in functioning, decreased subjective well-being, meaning-making, construal of personal benefits, and positive community effects. One of the most widely researched domains is the extent to which trauma results in a psychopathological stress response, such as Acute Stress Disorder (ASD) or Posttraumatic Stress Disorder (PTSD). Such outcomes have been the focus of many research agendas and interventions, and have been the dominant concern following direct exposure to a trauma (Yehuda, 2002).

According to the *Diagnostic and Statistical Manual of Mental Disorders* (DSM-IV; American Psychiatric Association [APA], 1994), neither ASD nor PTSD can be diagnosed without establishing sufficient (i.e., direct and/or proximal) exposure to a qualifying event. We sought to examine the limits of this expectation in our ongoing investigation of emotional, cognitive, and social responses to the terrorist attacks of September 11, 2001. We suspected that indirect and/or "low dose" exposure to this event could be very traumatic, and that we might see its psychological impact far beyond the directly affected communities. We sought to examine acute and posttraumatic stress responses among individuals who could not meet the clinical precondition of exposure, but might nonetheless share its symptomatology. Relatively few studies have examined the national and indirect impact of disasters before September 11th (e.g., the Oklahoma City attack: Pfefferbaum et al., 2000; the Kennedy assassination: Smith, Rasinski, & Toce, 2001; the Space Shuttle Challenger explosion: Terr et al., 1999).

While several other research teams conducted early national studies of the impact of the September 11th terrorist attacks (see Schlenger et al., 2002; Schuster et al., 2001; Smith et al., 2001), our prospective longitudinal study is one of the first attempts to recruit a national probability sample of individuals shortly after a major traumatic event and systematically follow them over time, and the only one to continue to do so since 9/11. Using an anonymous Web-based survey methodology, we have collected stress and coping data from a sample approximately 9-14 days after the attacks and at several intervals since then. Mental health and health care utilization data collected prior to 9/11 are available on most of these individuals. Thus, our study addresses many methodological limitations of prior research on community disasters (see Norris et al., 2001; North & Pfefferbaum, 2002). Its overall aims have been to: (a) investigate the psychological and social processes that help explain individual differences in response to a national traumatic event; (b) identify early predictors of long-term adjustment to both the attacks and subsequent events that may occur; and (c) investigate prospectively the psychological and social processes that help explain variability in responses to highly stressful life events more generally.

OVERVIEW OF METHODS

In collaboration with Knowledge Networks (KN), a survey research organization that maintains a nationally representative, Web-enabled research panel of potential respondents, we have administered Web-based surveys at several points in time since 9/11 to a national sample of U.S. residents (see Silver, Holman, McIntosh, Poulin & Gil-Rivas, 2002; Silver, Holman, McIntosh, Gil-Rivas & Poulin, in press, for a fuller description of the methods, sampling strategy, participation rates, etc.). The KN panel is developed using traditional probability methods for creating national survey samples and is recruited using stratified random-digit-dial (RDD) telephone sampling. RDD provides a known non-zero probability of selection for every U.S. household having a telephone, and the distribution of the KN panel closely tracks the distribution of census counts for the U.S. population on age, race, Hispanic ethnicity, geographical region, employment status, income, and education. KN provides households in the panel with free Web access and an Internet appliance, which uses a telephone line to connect to the Internet and uses the television as a monitor. In return, panel members participate in brief Internet surveys three to four times a month. The panel does not respond significantly differently over time to surveys than more "naïve" survey respondents (Dennis, 2001, 2003). Surveys are confidential, self-administered and accessible any time of day for a designated period, and participants can complete a survey only once.

Pre-9/11 mental health was assessed on our sample with a health survey completed by most KN panel members between September, 2000 and September, 2001. Sixty percent of our sample completed these measures before December 31, 2000. Respondents reported whether they had ever suffered from an Anxiety Disorder (Obsessive Compulsive Disorder, Generalized Anxiety Disorder) or Depression, and whether they received such a diagnosis from a medical doctor.

DATA COLLECTION IN THE YEAR FOLLOWING 9/11/01

Knowledge Networks administered an initial survey between September 20 and October 4, 2001 to identify acute stress symptoms experienced in the immediate aftermath of 9/11. The survey included a modified version of the Stanford Acute Stress Reaction Questionnaire (SASRQ; Cardena, Koopman,

Classen, Waelde, & Spiegel, 2000), a measure often used to assess ASD (APA, 1994). Items on the SASRQ were modified to read at a 6.5 grade Kincaid reading level, and respondents reported whether they "experienced" or "did not experience" acute stress symptoms *specific* to the 9/11 attacks. A random sample of 3,496 adult KN panel members was invited to participate in the survey, and 2729 completed it (a 78% participation rate). Over 75% of respondents who completed this survey did so within the first few days (9-14 days post-attacks); the remainder completed it the following week.

At approximately one year post-9/11 (between September 20 and October 24, 2002), another survey was fielded to the Wave 1 sample. Because the SASRQ is specifically tailored to assess ASD symptoms within a month following event exposure, the PTSD Checklist (PCL; Weathers, Litz, Herman, Huska, & Keane, 1993) was used to assess posttraumatic stress symptoms one year after the attacks. The PCL is a well-validated 17-item self-report measure of intrusion, avoidance, and arousal symptoms with excellent reliability. Respondents indicated how distressed or bothered they were by symptoms related to the 9/11 attacks over the prior 7 days using a scale ranging from 1 (not at all) to 5 (extremely).

We were successful in obtaining a representative sample of the US population at both waves of data collection with respect to key demographic characteristics. Most differences were within sampling error, although middle-income households tend to be overrepresented in our sample (see Silver et al., 2002; in press). Overall, 75% ($N = 2,033$) of all eligible adults completed the one-year anniversary data collection (see Silver et al., in press). Individuals who completed the anniversary survey were not significantly different from the non-respondents on pre-9/11 mental and physical health indices, gender, marital status, race/ethnicity, education, or their immediate reactions to the 9/11 attacks. Attrition analyses indicated that people who dropped out of the study were significantly younger ($M = 41$ yrs) than those who completed it ($M = 49$; $t(2,727) = 11.27, p < .001$).

OVERVIEW OF ANALYTIC STRATEGY

The following statistical analyses were conducted with STATA version 7.0, a program designed to handle weighted analyses of complex longitudinal survey data and provide the necessary adjustments of standard errors for these analyses. Data were weighted to adjust for differences in the probabilities of selection and non-response both within and between households. In addition, the post-stratification weights are calculated by deriving weighted sample distributions along various combinations of age, gender, race/ethnicity, region, metropolitan status, and education. Similar distributions are calculated using the most recent U.S. Census Bureau's CPS data and the KN panel data. Cell-by-cell adjustments over the various univariate and bivariate distributions are calculated to make the weighted sample cells match those of the U.S. Census and the KN panel. This process is repeated iteratively until there is convergence between the weighted sample and benchmark distributions.

Analyses were designed to address the relation between exposure to the 9/11 attacks and patterns of acute stress (at two weeks post-attacks) and posttraumatic stress (at 12 months post-attacks), adjusting for relevant demographics and whether or not respondents had pre-September 11th physician-diagnosed mental health problems (none, anxiety or depression, or both). Exposure to the attacks was assessed both as geographic distance from the World Trade Center (WTC) and as the means by which individuals experienced the attacks. Only respondents who completed both the Wave 1 and one-year anniversary surveys and who had non-missing data on all variables were included in these analyses to minimize missing data, yielding a final sample of 1906.

The weighted percentages of individuals reporting acute and posttraumatic stress symptoms were examined using descriptive analyses of SASRQ and PCL symptoms. Individuals experiencing high levels of acute stress were identified using DSM-IV criteria B (three or more dissociative symptoms), C (one or more reexperiencing/intrusive symptoms), D (one or more avoidance symptoms), and E (one or more arousal/anxiety symptoms) for ASD (APA, 1994). Because we did not assess all DSM-IV criteria (e.g., feelings of fear, horror or helplessness; duration of symptoms), respondents were not assumed to have ASD. In addition to this dichotomous (high versus not-high acute stress) variable, we calculated the total number of acute stress symptoms reported by each individual.

We also calculated a dichotomous index of high vs. not-high posttraumatic stress from the PCL data. Symptoms were considered positive if respondents reported having been at least moderately distressed by them in the prior week (2 on a 0-4 point scale) (Mollica et al., 2001). Individuals experiencing high posttraumatic stress were identified using DSM-IV criteria B (one or more reexperiencing symptoms), C (three or more avoidance symptoms), and D (two or more arousal symptoms) for PTSD (APA, 1994). Because we did not assess all DSM-IV criteria (e.g., degree of functional impairment, duration of symptoms), and because respondents did not meet the basic requirement for direct exposure, they were not assumed to have PTSD. The total number of posttraumatic stress symptoms was also calculated by counting the number of symptoms that respondents reported were at least "moderately" distressing.

STATA's "svylogit" procedure for population-averaged logistic regression was used to estimate odds ratios (OR's) for predictors of dichotomized (high versus not-high) levels of acute and posttraumatic stress following the attacks. STATA's "svypois" procedure for population-averaged Poisson regression was used to estimate incidence rate ratios (IRR's) for predictors of the total number of acute and posttraumatic stress symptoms across all symptom categories (e.g., avoidance and arousal).

The analyses addressing the relation between exposure and stress symptoms all examined predictors from three blocks of variables entered sequentially into the regressions: (a) demographics, (b) pre-September 11th mental health history, and (c) September 11th related exposure and distance from the WTC. Significant predictors from each of these blocks were retained while non-significant variables were removed from analyses to provide the most parsimonious model.

EXPOSURE TO THE ATTACKS AND ACUTE AND POSTTRAUMATIC STRESS SYMPTOMS

Based on responses to several individual questions in the surveys people completed in the 12 months following the September 11th attacks, individuals were categorized as belonging to one of three categories of exposure: *direct exposure*, including being in the WTC or Pentagon, seeing or hearing the attacks in person, or being close to someone in the targeted buildings during the attacks (i.e., meeting criterion A1 for ASD and PTSD) ($n = 57$); *live media exposure*, or watching the attacks unfold live on television ($n = 1225$); and *no live exposure*, or only seeing or learning of the attacks after they had occurred ($n = 624$). Using their residential zip codes, individuals were also categorized by azimuth distance from the WTC, with the assumption that such distance could represent a test of the dose-response relationship (similar to an earthquake, with lessening impact as distance from the "epicenter" increased). (For specific categories employed and number of individuals in each category, see Table 1.) Exposure and distance were both dummy coded, with the reference group for exposure being direct exposure and the reference group for distance being less than 25 miles from the WTC.

ACUTE STRESS SYMPTOMS

High Acute Stress. Individuals who met DSM-IV criteria B, C, D and E for ASD were classified as having "high" levels of acute stress. These individuals

TABLE 1. 9/11-Related Acute Stress (Wave 1; 2 Weeks Post 9/11) and 9/11-Related Posttraumatic Stress (at One Year Anniversary) by Degree of 9/11 Exposure and Proximity (N = 1906)

	Weighted % with High Levels of Acute Stress	Mean No. of Acute Stress Symptoms (Weighted)	Weighted % with High Levels of Posttraumatic Stress	Mean No. of Posttraumatic Stress Symptoms (Weighted)
Degree of 9/11 Exposure				
Directly exposed n = 57	9.3%	6.31	11.2%	3.27
Watched attacks on live television n = 1225	12.8%	5.32	4.7%	1.61*
No live exposure n = 624	10.4%	4.45*	3.4%	1.08**
Distance from WTC				
< 25 miles n = 71	21.0%	6.46	3.8%	2.24
25-100 miles n = 124	12.7%	5.14	5.0%	1.32
100-500 miles n = 428	11.7%*	4.99	4.8%	1.32
500-1000 miles n = 524	9.9%**	4.99*	5.0%	1.61
1000+ miles n = 759	12.6%*	5.03*	3.8%	1.44

*p < 0.05; ** p < 0.01

Note: The reference group for the exposure variables was direct exposure; the reference group for the distance variables was within 25 miles of the World Trade Center (WTC).
The Wave 1 data represent the proportion of participants reporting high levels of 9/11-related acute stress (i.e., DSM-IV Criteria B, C, D, and E for Acute Stress Disorder–3 or more dissociative symptoms, one or more reexperiencing symptoms, one or more avoidance symptom(s), and one or more arousal symptom(s)). The One Year Anniversary data represent the proportion of participants reporting *high levels* of 9/11-related posttraumatic stress (i.e., DSM-IV Criteria B, C, and D for PTSD–one or more reexperiencing symptom(s), three or more avoidance symptoms, and two or more arousal symptoms). All analyses adjust for relevant demographics and pre-September 11th physician diagnosed mental health status.

were present at all levels of exposure and across the nation, with 10.4% of those with no live exposure and 12.6% of those who lived over 1,000 miles from the WTC reporting high levels of acute stress at Wave 1. Distance from the WTC was significantly associated with high acute stress, with those between 100 and 500 (OR = 0.41, 95% CI 0.20-0.87), 500 and 1,000 (OR = 0.31, 95% CI 0.15-0.65), and over 1,000 (OR = 0.42, 95% CI 0.20-0.87) miles away less likely to report high acute stress than those within 25 miles of the WTC. Variables associated with high acute stress beyond exposure or distance included mental health status before September 11th (OR = 1.72, 95% CI 1.32-2.24), female gender (OR = 1.56, 95% CI 1.12-2.19), and age (OR = 0.98, 95% CI 0.97-0.99). Degree of exposure was not associated with high acute stress.

Number of Acute Stress Symptoms. Degree of exposure was associated with the number of acute stress symptoms respondents reported, with individuals who had no direct exposure (IRR = 0.76, 95% CI 0.59-0.98) reporting fewer symptoms than those who had direct exposure. Distances of 500 to 1,000 miles (IRR = 0.77, 95% CI 0.61-0.98), or more than 1,000 miles (IRR = 0.79, 95% CI 0.63-0.99) from the WTC, predicted fewer symptoms than being within 25 miles. Significant non-exposure predictors again included history of pre-September 11th mental health disorders (IRR = 1.31, 95% CI 1.21-1.42), female gender (IRR = 1.38, 95% CI 1.25-1.52), and younger age (IRR = 0.99, 95% CI 0.99-0.99).

Posttraumatic Stress Symptoms

High Posttraumatic Stress. Individuals who met DSM-IV criteria B, C, and D for PTSD were classified as having "high" levels of posttraumatic stress. High acute stress was strongly predictive of high posttraumatic stress (OR = 2.44, 95% CI 1.32-4.49). At one year post-attacks, high posttraumatic stress was reported primarily among those directly exposed to the attacks, with 11.2% of these individuals reporting such levels. Nonetheless, controlling for demographic factors, pre-September 11th mental health history, and high levels of Wave 1 acute stress, high posttraumatic stress was not significantly more likely among the directly exposed subsample than among the other two subsamples (see Table 1).[1] Similar findings were obtained for distance from the WTC, with high posttraumatic stress not differing significantly across distance categories. Variables predicting high posttraumatic stress beyond the effects of high acute stress included bachelor's degree or greater education (OR = 0.33, 95% CI 0.15-0.71), income (OR = 0.89, 95% CI 0.82-0.97), and prior mental health diagnoses (OR = 1.82, 95% CI 1.19-2.80).

Number of Posttraumatic Stress Symptoms. The number of acute stress symptoms reported was a significant predictor of posttraumatic stress symptoms reported at the one-year anniversary (IRR = 1.10, 95% CI 1.09-1.13). Degree of exposure to the attacks was also related to the number of posttraumatic stress symptoms reported at the one-year anniversary, beyond the influence of number of Wave 1 acute stress symptoms. Individuals who had no direct exposure (IRR = 0.57, 95% CI 0.38-0.90) or only observed the attacks on live television (IRR = 0.65, 95% CI 0.44-0.95) reported fewer posttraumatic stress symptoms than those individuals who were directly exposed to the attacks. Beyond exposure and acute stress symptoms, African American ethnicity (IRR = 1.77, 95% CI 1.23-2.56) and pre-September 11th mental health diagnoses (IRR = 1.27, 95% CI 1.07-1.50) predicted a greater number of posttraumatic stress symptoms. A bachelor's degree or more education predicted fewer symptoms (IRR = 0.57, 95% CI 0.44-0.74). Distance from the WTC was not a significant predictor of the number of posttraumatic stress symptoms reported at the one-year anniversary.

CONCLUSIONS AND IMPLICATIONS

The unparalleled impact of the September 11th terrorist attacks, combined with the representative nature of our national sample, the pre-September 11th assessment of mental health histories, and the early collection of emotional responses to these events, has provided us with a remarkable opportunity to examine longitudinally how individuals across the U.S. have coped with a major traumatic event. We have found significant psychological reactions across the U.S. after the September 11th attacks; our findings strongly suggest that the effects of these terror attacks were not limited to communities directly affected. Instead, our data show that substantial effects of the events of September 11th rippled throughout the country. Posttraumatic stress symptoms clearly declined over the first year post-9/11. Nonetheless, many individuals who were not directly exposed to the attacks reported symptoms both acutely and over the year afterwards at levels that were comparable to those individuals who experienced the attacks proximally and directly. We acknowledge that by not including clinically significant impairment or dysfunction in our criteria (Criterion F for both ASD and PTSD), we are unlikely to have measured psychopathological symptomatology and may not have identified individuals who warrant psychological intervention. Nonetheless, our data suggest quite clearly that indirect and/or low dose exposure to a community disaster can be very traumatic, and heretofore such levels of exposure have tended to be excluded from discussions of the traumatic impact of such events (cf. Norris, Phifer, & Kaniasty, 1994).

Importantly, the degree of psychological response to the September 11th attacks was not explained simply by degree of exposure or proximity to the trauma. Many individuals who lived hundreds of miles from the attacks or had low levels of exposure (i.e., individuals who watched the attacks live on TV and those who reported no direct exposure at all) reported high levels of symptomatology. In addition, there was great variability in acute and posttraumatic response among individuals who observed the attacks directly or lived within the directly affected community.

These findings suggest that relying on unfounded assumptions about who will be affected by a traumatic event is not useful. It is important that health care providers be sensitive to and aware of the enormous variability in response, both immediately and over time, following a major national trauma. It is also important that these professionals avoid pathologizing "normal" responses to an abnormal event (Silver et al., 2002). Most importantly, health care providers and others must recognize that the impact of terrorist events is likely to go far beyond those directly exposed, and one should not expect a simple dose-response relationship between exposure and psychological impact (see also Kroll, 2003). Instead, one must examine other risk factors that may help explain posttraumatic responses to national disasters, such as preexisting mental conditions, coping strategies employed (Silver et al., 2002), prior traumatic life experiences (Silver et al., in press), or individual difference variables (Bowman, 1997), among others.

Together, the findings from this research challenge some basic assumptions about coping with highly stressful events. Broadly, it is clear that psychological outcomes are multiply determined, and that there are social and psychological factors beyond mere exposure to the event that predict outcomes. Our work also suggests the importance of documenting responses over time (North & Pfefferbaum, 2002). Ultimately, it is our hope that information collected in this effort can illuminate the coping process more generally so as to advance future conceptual work in this area. The absence of an expectation that a traumatic stress response can occur among individuals who were thousands of miles from a traumatic event has hampered investigations of which indirectly exposed individuals might be most affected by national traumas and why.

Ultimately, we hope our national longitudinal research effort can further the understanding of the normal course of responses to terrorism. We also hope that our research can assist public health officials in the identification of individuals in the community who may be at particular risk for the psychological aftereffects of terrorism or other national disasters. Our data can guide educational and intervention efforts with evidence-based information so that they are better informed, more cost-effective and more sensitive to the needs of the country's residents.

NOTE

1. All analyses were conducted two ways: with exposure and distance entered together, and with these sets of variables entered separately. Statistics reported are with both sets of variables entered together, but no findings were altered substantially when exposure and distance were examined separately.

REFERENCES

American Psychiatric Association. (1994). *Diagnostic and statistical manual of mental disorders* (4th ed.). Washington, DC: Author.

Bowman, M. (1997). *Individual differences in posttraumatic response: Problems with the adversity-distress connection.* Mahwah, NJ: Erlbaum.

Cardeña, E., Koopman, C., Classen, C., Waelde, L. C., & Spiegel, D. (2000). Psychometric properties of the Stanford Acute Stress Reaction Questionnaire (SASRQ): A valid and reliable measure of acute stress. *Journal of Traumatic Stress, 13,* 719-734.

Dennis, J. M. (2001, Summer). Are internet panels creating professional respondents? The benefits of online panels far outweigh the potential for panel effects. *Marketing Research,* 34-38.

Dennis, J. M. (2003). *Panel attrition impact: A comparison of responses to attitudinal and knowledge questions about HIV between follow-up and cross-sectional samples.* Menlo Park, CA: Knowledge Networks.

Kroll, J. (2003). Posttraumatic symptoms and the complexity of responses to trauma. *Journal of the American Medical Association, 290,* 667-670.

Mollica, R. F., Sarajlic, N., Chernoff, M., Lavelle, J., Vukovic, I. S., Massagli, M. P. (2001). Longitudinal study of psychiatric symptoms, disability, mortality, and emigration among Bosnian refugees. *Journal of the American Medical Association, 286,* 546-554.

Norris, F. H., Byrne, C. M., & Diaz, E. (2001). *50,000 disaster victims speak: An empirical review of the empirical literature, 1981-2001.* The National Center for PTSD and The Center for Mental Health Services.

Norris, F. H., Phifer, J. F., & Kaniasty, K. (1994). Individual and community reactions to the Kentucky floods: Findings from a longitudinal study of older adults. In R. J. Ursano, B. G. McCaughey, & C. S. Fullerton (Eds.), *Individual and community responses to trauma and disaster: The structure of human chaos* (pp. 378-400). Cambridge: Cambridge University Press.

North, C. S., & Pfefferbaum, B. (2002). Research on the mental health effects of terrorism. *Journal of the American Medical Association, 288,* 633-636.

Pfefferbaum, B., Seale, T. W., McDonald, N. B., Brandt, E. N., Rainwater, S. M., Maynard, B. T. et al. (2000). Posttraumatic stress two years after the Oklahoma City bombing in youths geographically distant from the explosion. *Psychiatry, 63,* 358-370.

Schlenger, W. E., Caddell, J. M., Ebert, L., Jordan, B. K., Rourke, K. M., Wilson, D. et al. (2002). Psychological reactions to terrorist attacks: Findings from the National Study of Americans' Reactions to September 11. *Journal of the American Medical Association, 288,* 581-588.

Schuster, M. A., Stein, B. D., Jaycox, L. H., Collins, R. L., Marshall, G. N., Elliott, M. N. et al. (2001). A national survey of stress reactions after the September 11, 2001 terrorist attacks. *The New England Journal of Medicine, 345,* 1507-1512.

Silver, R. C., Holman, E. A., McIntosh, D. N., Poulin, M., & Gil-Rivas, V. (2002). Nationwide longitudinal study of psychological responses to September 11. *Journal of the American Medical Association, 288,* 1235-1244.

Silver, R. C., Holman, E. A., McIntosh, D. N., Gil-Rivas, V., & Poulin, M. (in press). Coping with a national trauma: A nationwide longitudinal study of responses to the terrorist attacks of September 11. In T. Smith (Ed.), *Social, psychological, and political impact on the American public of the September 11th terror attacks.* New York: Russell Sage.

Silver, R. L., & Wortman, C. B. (1980). Coping with undesirable life events. In J. Garber & M. E. P. Seligman (Eds.), *Human helplessness: Theory and applications* (pp. 279-340). New York: Academic Press.

Smith, T. W., Rasinski, K.A., & Toce, M. (2001). *America rebounds: A national study of public response to the September 11 terrorist attacks.* Chicago, IL: National Opinion Research Center.

Terr, L. C., Bloch, D. A., Michel, B. A., Shi, H., Reinhardt, J. A., & Metayer, S. (1999). Children's symptoms in the wake of Challenger: A field study of distant-traumatic effects and an outline of related conditions. *American Journal of Psychiatry, 156,* 1536-1544.

Weathers, F. W., Litz, B. T., Herman, D. S., Huska, J. A., & Keane, T. M. (1993, October). *The PTSD Checklist: Reliability, validity, and diagnostic utility.* Paper presented at the meeting of the International Society for Traumatic Stress Studies, San Antonio, TX.

Wortman, C. B., & Silver, R. C. (1989). The myths of coping with loss. *Journal of Consulting and Clinical Psychology, 57,* 349-357.

Wortman, C. B., & Silver, R. C. (2001). The myths of coping with loss revisited. In M. S. Stroebe, R. O. Hansson, W. Stroebe, & H. Schut (Eds.), *Handbook of bereavement research: Consequences, coping, and care* (pp. 405-429). Washington, DC: American Psychological Association.

Yehuda, R. (2002). Post-traumatic stress disorder. *The New England Journal of Medicine, 346,* 108-114.

Somatization and Terrorism

Carol S. North

SUMMARY. Few systematic data pertaining to somatization following terrorism are available to guide intervention workers and policymakers in response to terrorist events. Somatization is a well-known but poorly understood phenomenon presenting enormous difficulties in clinical management as well as research investigation. It is a heterogeneous concept that is inconsistently defined in research on traumatic events. This article summarizes the somatization field and applies the principles to recommendations for disasters and terrorism research and interventions related to somatization in the postdisaster setting.

KEYWORDS. Somatization, disasters, terrorism, bioterrorism, medically unexplained complaints, diagnostic validation

Address correspondence to: Carol S. North, MD, MPE, Department of Psychiatry, Washington University School of Medicine, 660 South Euclid Avenue, Campus Box 8134, St. Louis, MO 63110 USA (E-mail: NorthC@psychiatry.wustl.edu).

This research was supported by National Institute of Mental Health Grant MH40025 to Dr. North.

[Haworth co-indexing entry note]: "Somatization and Terrorism." North, Carol S. Co-published simultaneously in *Journal of Aggression, Maltreatment & Trauma* (The Haworth Maltreatment & Trauma Press, an imprint of The Haworth Press, Inc.) Vol. 9, No. 1/2, 2004; and: *The Trauma of Terrorism: Sharing Knowledge and Shared Care, An International Handbook* (ed: Yael Danieli, Danny Brom, and Joe Sills) The Haworth Maltreatment & Trauma Press, an imprint of The Haworth Press, Inc., 2005.

Somatization is a heterogeneous phenomenon with conceptual difficulties, inconsistent definitions, and research plagued by methodological problems. Few studies have examined somatization in the context of disasters and even fewer in the context of terrorism and bioterrorism. This article reviews definitions and methodological issues in somatization and then examines its relationship to extreme trauma and terrorism. The article concludes with recommendations for the research field studying somatization and terrorism and suggestions for disaster mental health intervention workers and policymakers.

SOMATIZATION: NOT A UNIFIED CONSTRUCT

The root "soma" (i.e., involving the physical body) refers to health-related complaints. The term has been variously applied as a noun (*somatization*), verb (*somatize*), and adjective (*somatic* or *somatoform*), often paired with the word "symptom." *Somatic* refers to physical complaints, regardless of etiology. *Somatoform* symptoms, however, are defined by *DSM-IV-TR* (American Psychiatric Association [APA], 2000) as physical symptoms superficially resembling medically-based problems but without full medical explanation, a process termed somatization. Too often, medically unexplained *somatoform* symptoms are not distinguished from the broader category of *somatic* symptoms encompassing both unexplained and medically-based complaints.

Somatization disorder is a severe and disabling psychiatric disorder, occuring predominantly in women and defined as a longstanding pattern of ongoing multiple recurring, medically unexplained symptoms widely distributed throughout the body. Replacement of the pejorative label "hysteria" with the term "somatization disorder" in *DSM-III* (APA, 1980) reflects the definitional focus on the classic severe, pervasive pattern of multiple recurrent medically unexplained physical complaints. This definition is descriptive and atheoretical, avoiding scientifically untestable assumptions of psychological etiology (Guze, 1975) and outdating the older term "psychosomatic" (Guze, 1984).

Somatization disorder is the lead diagnosis in *DSM-IV-TR*'s (APA, 2000) somatoform disorders category and the only disorder of its category validated by the 17th century English physician Sydenham's methods for validation of diagnostic criteria for medical disorders. This validation method was first applied to psychiatry by Robins and Guze in the 1970s (Feighner et al., 1972; Guze, 1975). Diagnostic validation by this method entails five phases: (a) describing the syndrome's core features, (b) establishing exclusion criteria to differentiate the syndrome from other known disorders, (c) identifying laboratory markers of the syndrome, (d) documenting familial transmission, and (e) demonstrating stability over time in follow-up studies showing continued presence of the symptoms without evolution into a different entity (Robins & Guze, 1970).

The population prevalence of somatization disorder in women has been estimated at 1-2 percent (Farley, Woodruff, & Guze, 1968). By definition, onset is before age 30, but it most frequently begins in the decade following puberty (North & Guze, 1998). Although the specific cause of somatization disorder is unknown, a genetic role is well established and early environment and parental modeling also contribute (Craig, Boardman, Mills, Daly-Jones, & Drake, 1995; Guze, 1993).

Somatizing patients also complain of many symptoms of psychiatric disorders they do not have along with many symptoms of other medical disorders they also do not have. They complain of as many or more symptoms of major depression, anxiety disorders, and schizophrenia as patients with these disorders (Lenze, Miller, Munir, Pornoppadol, & North, 1999; Liskow, Penick, Powell, Haefele, & Campbell, 1986). Thus, somatization disorder is not only a *somatoform* condition (defined as complaining of many symptoms of physical disorders not present) that mimics many physical disorders, but also a *psychoform* syndrome (defined as complaining of psychological symptoms of psychiatric disorders not present), simulating psychiatric disorders along with other medical problems (North & Guze, 1998).

The dimensional construct of somatization outside the context of the disorder bearing its name, as a collection of medically unexplained symptoms with assumed psychological origins, signifies the field's quest for additional tools to understand a heterogeneous concept. Outside of somatization disorder, however, somatization symptoms are poorly understood.

MEASURING SOMATIZATION

Methodological problems inherent in studying somatization include inconsistent definitions, non-detection, non-differentiation of diagnosis from symptoms, and failure to separate medically unexplained (somatoform) symptoms from medically-based symptoms. Studying somatization in reference to an event also faces difficulties of differentiating new from pre-existing symptoms.

A fundamental feature of somatization assessment is its dependence on excluding medically-based symptoms. Only when medically explained symptoms are confidently dismissed can symptoms legitimately be considered somatoform (medically unexplained) in either dimensional or categorical systems.

Categorical Measurement (Somatization Disorder). The characteristic poor reliability of patients prone to somatization contributes to difficulty in detecting cases (duGruy, Columbia, & Dickinson, 1987). Somatizers rarely provide sufficient detail of their extensive medical histories in a single interview for definitive diagnosis, portraying their symptoms as medically-based, either as illegitimate parts of genuine medical illness or as legitimate symptoms of avowed but spurious medical illness (Martin, 1988; North & Guze, 1998).

Somatizing patients characteristically present symptoms with a changing focus, selectively unfolding complaints to multiple medical specialists over time. They present symptoms pertaining to the medical specialty of the current visit and downplay, omit, or deny extensive symptoms they have presented to other physicians, including previous chief complaints (Murphy, 1982). Reliance on a single patient interview for diagnosis underestimates prevalence of somatization disorder by several magnitudes (Deighton & Nicol, 1985; Miller, North, Clouse, Alpers, & Wetzel, 2001).

Inability to identify cases has led some practitioners to dismiss the concept of somatization disorder as unduly restrictive, although assessment method, rather than definition, appears to be the problem. Frustrated with the low yield of cases, some researchers have argued for lowering the diagnostic threshold, forming an abridged construct to identify more patients who somatize and overutilize medical treatment (Deighton & Nicol, 1985; Escobar et al., 1998). Relaxed or abridged somatization definitions yield much of the full somatization disorder's characteristic correlations with psychiatric and other health problems, disability, functional impairment, psychiatric comorbidity, family dysfunction, and health care utilization and costs (Escobar, Rubio-Stipec, Canino, & Karno, 1989; Kroenke, Spitzer, deGruy III, & Swindle, 1998) and are likely to include undetected somatization disorder cases not acknowledging their full panoply of symptoms. Identifying greater numbers of cases by lowering diagnostic thresholds, however, may only serve to magnify poor-resolution data.

Dimensional Approaches to Measurement of Somatization. Other researchers have discarded diagnostic approaches in favor of dimensional models of somatization, which maximize statistical power by representing ranges of values. The dimensional approach is far simpler, counting symptoms rather than assessing full diagnostic criteria. In dimensional models, number of somatoform symptoms is linearly associated with disability indicators (days in bed, decreased activities, functional impairment, and self-reported health ratings) (Katon et al., 1991) and inversely proportional to comorbid depression and anxiety.

Because exclusion of medical explanation lies at the essence of somatization, studies that do not differentiate medically explained and unexplained symptoms cannot address somatization, nor can they discriminate somatoform from depressive and anxiety disorders and symptoms. A problem with dimensional measurement is that individual symptoms disarticulated from empirically established nosology lack demonstrated validity and utility of established nosology (Mojtabai & Reider, 1998). Questionnaires and scales such as the popular Symptom Checklist (SCL-90-R), General Health Questionnaire, and Cornell Medical Index that assess somatization symptoms dimensionally after stressful events neither measure somatization nor differentiate medically based from unexplained symptoms (Kaplan et al., 1998) and correlate poorly with clinician assessments (Kass, Skodol, Buckley, & Charles, 1980). Further, many measures lack corrections for biases of response sets and social desirability (Crowne & Marlowe, 1960), and the time periods of symptom assessment fail to address critical time intervals for diagnosis or relationship to an event.

STUDIES OF SOMATIZATION, TRAUMA, AND PTSD

Various studies have reported associations of somatization with trauma and posttraumatic symptoms (Davidson, Hughes, Blazer, & George, 1991; van der Kolk et al., 1996), including high rates of unexplained syndromes and symptoms after collective traumatic experiences of refugees and military veterans, fainting or dizziness and hallucinations among tortured Bhutanese refugees (Van Ommeren et al., 2001), and undifferentiated somatoform complaints among Persian Gulf War military personnel performing body handling functions (Labbate, Cardeña, Dimitreva, Roy, & Engel, 1998). Although these associations may suggest etiological factors in somatization, the possibility cannot be ruled out that predisposition to somatization may be confounded with tendencies to report torture, or biased with relation to selection of individuals for body handling work.

The association of somatization with PTSD may be somewhat nonspecific, with similar associations found between somatization and many other psychiatric diagnoses (Swartz, Landerman, George, Blazer, & Escobar, 1991). Most somatization disorder patients without PTSD in one study exceeded pathological scores on Keane's MMPI (PK) scale (Wetzel et al., 2000). Highly somatizing patients may endorse PTSD symptoms indiscriminately along with their many other psychiatric and medical symptoms.

A consistent and robust finding is that complaints of physical symptoms are associated with endorsement of distress, psychopathology, and reports of traumatic events within individuals. At least part of the association of somatization with multiple other disorders, symptoms, and difficulties is likely to be a byproduct of the polysymptomatic, highly endorsing profile of those who somatize the most, thereby reducing the meaning of specific associations with somatization.

Research on somatization in the context of extreme trauma is complicated by the additional task of differentiating post-event symptoms from problems present before the event. This task is critical for interpretation of causal directionalities. For example, a well-documented history of severe functional headaches dating continuously back to early adolescence would indicate that headache complaints with no discernable medical basis presenting to medical care after a traumatic event are a part of the pre-existing functional headache problem, not a direct result of the event during recent adult life. Obtaining a reliable history of pre-existing functional symptoms may be difficult in some individuals who have experienced traumatic events that present readily available and attractive external etiologic sources for their current complaints.

The literature on somatization in relation to traumatic events in the community is fraught with problems of sampling bias. Traumatized populations have pre-existing characteristics conferring risk for traumatic events (Breslau, 1998; Cottler, Compton, Mager, Spitznagel, & Janca, 1992). These pre-existing characteristics are significantly associated with mental health outcomes, which confounds attempts to understand psychological effects of the traumatic events themselves. Studies of disasters avoid some of the problems of sampling bias, because disasters tend to pick their victims more randomly with less reliance on pre-existing characteristics of the people selected. Sampling from treatment settings is further confounded with psychopathology and somatization. Therefore, studies of treatment samples or traumatized populations in communities may produce associations with somatization not observed in populations affected by disasters and terrorism.

STUDIES OF DISASTERS AND TERRORISM: CLARIFYING RELATIONSHIPS

Somatization disorder is not a reported outcome of major disasters and terrorist incidents. The natural history of somatization disorder with typical onset in the teenage years is inconsistent with theories of traumatic origins in mature adults. Most literature describing psychiatric effects of extreme trauma in adults lacks mention of somatization, although numerous studies have examined reports of symptoms and health complaints. Many such studies have examined strictly physical issues such as health outcomes, need for treatment, laboratory markers, and nonspecific ("somatic") symptoms (Murphy, 1984), none of which delineate medically unexplained from medically-based complaints (Viel, Curbakova, Eglite, Zvagule, & Vincent, 1997). Studies of survivors of catastrophic experiences including torture victims, prisoners of war, and concentration camp victims have been criticized (Merskey, 1995) for failing to consider the potential for confounding of reported symptoms with medical conditions resulting from maltreatment during captivity.

Comparison groups represent a difficult, yet important aspect of studying somatization and disasters. Selection of adequate comparison groups is typically difficult or impossible to achieve in disaster research, due either to contamination of the comparison group by various levels of exposure because of proximity or to fundamental differences of the comparison group unrelated to the disaster exposure.

Without comparisons of pre/postdisaster status with an otherwise comparable but unexposed group, interpretations cannot be offered, whether postdisaster characteristics of the affected population are caused by the event, represent an inherent feature of the population exposed, or relate to some other intervening forces in the population. Therefore, critical to examining the role of traumatic events in the etiology of somatization are pre-/post-event comparisons of exposed and unexposed populations documenting that somatization associated with events is *new* (*incident*) after the event, rather than pre-existing. The ideal study of somatization in the disaster setting would involve a prospective design comparing postdisaster with predisaster levels of medically unexplained symptoms in disaster-exposed and unexposed groups assessed for complaints.

Two studies capitalized upon serendipity to study disaster-exposed populations using structured diagnostic interviews before and after the disaster compared to unexposed groups. The population prevalence of psychiatric disorders was studied in Puerto Rico as part of an epidemiologic research project a year before a natural disaster (torrential rains and mudslides) (Bravo, Rubio-Stipec, Canino, Woodbury, & Ribera, 1990). Postdisaster somatoform symptoms were compared with predisaster symptoms with reference to an unexposed comparison group. Disaster exposure was found to be statistically associated with new (incident) medically unexplained gastrointestinal and pseudoneurological symptoms not present prior to the disaster, but not clinically significant due to the small magnitude of the symptom effects (slopes of 0.05 to 0.07; Bravo et al., 1990). The small but statistically significant associations may have resulted from a few extreme individuals or disaster-related medical disorders or unsanitary conditions.

Another series of disasters including dioxin contamination in Times Beach, Missouri occurred a year after the Epidemiologic Catchment Area Study obtained structured diagnostic interviews of the population (Robins et al., 1986). Prospectively examined somatization symptoms were compared with postdisaster rates. Only one case of somatization disorder was identified, found in the unexposed comparison group, with onset prior to disaster. Somatization symptoms were uncommon, and new symptoms were not evident.

THE SPECIAL CASE OF BIOTERRORISM

The political goal of terrorism is to disrupt society and create widespread fear and confusion in its members (Stern, 1999). The affected population extends far beyond those targeted directly. Bioterrorist attacks may create uncertainties about personal exposure status, the conclusion of the danger, and the potential for future illness. Large numbers of frightened individuals may overwhelm health care facilities demanding treatment, compromising medical care of those physically injured. Risk communication becomes a critical part of the social intervention in order to reduce unexposed people's fears and perceptions of contamination. An attack on Tokyo subways with deadly sarin gas was associated with reported symptoms of headache, muscle stiffness, eye symptoms, and fatigue for several years among patients hospitalized for treatment (Kawana, Ishimatsu, & Kanda, 2001). Further systematic studies of medical and psychological symptoms are needed after bioterrorist incidents. Until then, further insight may be gained by extrapolating from experience with mass psychogenic illnesses following toxic contamination accidents or threats and from epidemics.

For example, an incident of suspected toxic gas exposure in a military barracks resulted in new symptoms in 55% of 1,800 American military recruits in the area. Twenty-five percent reported new onset of cough, lightheadedness, dizziness, chest pain, shortness of breath, headache, or sore throat, and 18% received medical evaluation for the symptoms (Struewing & Gray, 2004). Following a radiological contamination accident in Brazil with four fatalities and several hundred casualties, more than 10,000 people sought medical evaluation for feared contamination and symptoms including vomiting, diarrhea, and rashes of the face and neck (Petterson, 1998). Bartholomew and Wessely (2002) provided a comprehensive review of such incidents.

MANAGEMENT OF SOMATIZATION IN TRAUMATIZED PATIENTS

The first task in clinical management of apparently unexplained physical complaints is to document a reasonable effort to establish or rule out medical explanations, consulting the level of medical expertise needed for such determinations. The second task is to identify somatoform disorder, completion of which depends on the first task. Physical symptoms cannot be determined somatoform until medical explanations have been satisfactorily ruled out. The third task is to identify psychiatric comorbidities and place them into the context of the somatization to determine whether the physical complaints are part of a preexisting or concurrent somatoform disorder or a manifestation of another psychiatric disorder. Then, somatization disorder and other psychiatric disorders are treated by established protocols. Unrecognized somatoform disorders complicate medical and psychiatric treatment.

Only rarely does the passage of time prove medically unexplained symptoms presenting as part of established somatization disorder to be harbingers of occult medical conditions. Uncertainty increases, however, when the presentation of unexplained physical complaints departs from recognized diagnostic categories, which is when the likelihood of undetected medical disease increases. Additionally, when the medical and psychiatric history lack typical characteristics of somatization disorder (multiple symptom complaints in multiple organ systems; multi-problem social histories and interpersonal relationships; familial somatization, sociopathy, or substance abuse; and dysfunctional family dynamics), patiently withholding judgment until additional information accrues is prudent.

Some patients with somatoform complaints subthreshold for the somatization diagnosis may represent undetected cases, providing insufficient information for the diagnosis. The known unreliability of highly somatizing patients makes outside corroboration imperative in order to confirm the reported medical basis of symptoms and collect a complete history of the array of symptoms presented to various health care providers (Martin, 1988; Murphy, 1982). When history from other health care providers is unavailable, prospective observation may be required to accumulate a complete symptom database of the patient's evolving complaints over time.

When somatization presents in the context of traumatic events, the clinician is urged to resist patients' causal interpretations and pause to absorb the larger clinical picture. Common assumptions hold somatic complaints to represent state-related behavior generated by traumatic events or stress. Interventions designed to address these assumptions attempt to heal the psychological injury believed causal by discussing the traumatic experience and associated emotions. A problem with this logic is that it presupposes an etiology to the symptoms that cannot be established in any given case. The symptoms may be part of an as-yet undeclared medical disorder, or they may be part of a lifelong pattern of complaints. Unexplained symptoms are most effectively managed by observation over time while maintaining an agnostic attitude toward the etiology of the symptoms until the diagnosis is clarified. Attributing the symptoms to traumatic events and eliciting emotional responses may be countertherapeutic for these patients whose difficulties may already include excessive emotionality and in-ability to take responsibility for their part in their difficulties.

Treatment of unexplained symptoms starts with simple reassurance that the symptom does not demonstrate medically serious disease and that it can be managed. Therapy then proceeds to help redirect the patient's concerns to-ward applying appropriate problem-solving, coping, and interpersonal skills. The somatoform disorder patient may fail to heed the reassurance or resist these therapeutic efforts, perseverating on the symptom and/or subsequently displaying other somatoform symptoms in different medical contexts, further supporting the possibility of a somatoform disorder.

In the context of disasters and terrorism, somatoform symptoms usually arise in the absence of somatization disorder. Here is it especially important to be circumspect in assuming origins of symptoms, again maintaining an agnos-tic stance. Similarly, research in this setting must be especially careful to rule out medical origins of symptoms and demonstrate temporal occurrence of new symptomatology after events of interest exceeding the incidence in unexposed groups.

To reduce the likelihood of health care systems being overwhelmed by large numbers of people fearing exposure to toxic or infectious agents, atten-tion to risk communication is recommended. Elements of good risk communi-cation pertaining to containment of mass fears of physical illness include learning the public's fears, common myths, and rumors; timely disclosure of appropriate information through honest and trusted sources willing to admit the limitations of knowledge; and providing useful information about things people can do to increase their safety (Covello, Peters, Wojteki, & Hyde, 2001). Education of medical professionals about somatization should improve health care management of populations affected by disasters and terrorism.

REFERENCES

American Psychiatric Association. (1980). *Diagnostic and statistical manual of mental disorders* (3rd ed.). Washington, DC: Author.

American Psychiatric Association. (2000). *Diagnostic and statistical manual of mental disorders* (4th ed., text rev.). Washington, DC: Author.

Bartholomew, R. E., & Wessely, S. (2002). Protean nature of mass sociogenic illness: From possessed nuns to chemical and biological terrorism fears. *British Journal of Psychiatry, 180,* 300-306.

Bravo, M., Rubio-Stipec, M., Canino, G. J., Woodbury, M. A., & Ribera, J. C. (1990). The psychological sequelae of disaster stress prospectively and retrospectively evaluated. *American Journal of Community Psychology, 18,* 661-680.

Breslau, N. (1998). Epidemiology of trauma and posttraumatic stress disorder. In R.Yehuda (Ed.), *Psychological trauma* (pp. 1-29). Washington, DC: American Psychiatric Press.

Cottler, L. B., Compton, W. M., Mager, D., Spitznagel, E. L., & Janca, A. (1992). Posttraumatic stress disorder among substance users from the general population. *American Journal of Psychiatry, 149*(5), 664-670.

Covello, C. T., Peters, R. G., Wojteki, J. G., & Hyde, R. C. (2001). Risk communication, the West Nile virus, and bioterrorism: Responding to the challenges posed by the intentional or unintentional release of a pathogen in an urban setting. *Journal of Urban Health, 87*, 382-391.

Craig, T. K., Boardman, A. P., Mills, K., Daly-Jones, O., & Drake, H. (1995). The South London somatisation study. I. Longitudinal course and the influence of early life experiences. *British Journal of Psychiatry, 163*, 579-588.

Crowne, D. P., & Marlowe, D. (1960). A new scale of social desirability independent of psychopathology. *Journal of Consulting Psychology, 29*, 349-354.

Davidson, J. R. T., Hughes, D., Blazer, D. G., & George, L. K. (1991). Post-traumatic stress disorder in the community: An epidemiological study. *Psychological Medicine, 21*, 713-721.

Deighton, C., & Nicol, A. (1985). Abnormal illness behavior in young women in a primary care setting: Is Briquet's syndrome a useful category? *Psychological Medicine, 15*, 515-520.

duGruy, F., Columbia, L., & Dickinson, P. (1987). Somatization in a family practice. *Journal of Family Practice, 25*, 45-51.

Escobar, J. I., Gara, M., Cohen Silver, R., Waitzkin, H., Holman, A., & Compton, W. (1998). Somatization disorder in primary care. *British Journal of Psychiatry, 173*, 262-266.

Escobar, J. I., Rubio-Stipec, M., Canino, G., & Karno, M. (1989). Somatic symptom index (SSI): A new and abridged somatization construct. *Journal of Nervous and Mental Disease, 177*, 140-146.

Farley, J., Woodruff, R. A., & Guze, S. B. (1968). The prevalence of hysteria and conversion symptoms. *British Journal of Psychiatry, 114*, 1121-1125.

Feighner, J. P., Robins, E., Guze, S. B., Woodruff, R. A., Winokur, G., & Muñoz, R. (1972). Diagnostic criteria for use in psychiatric research. *Archives of General Psychiatry, 26*, 57-62.

Guze, S. B. (1975). The validity and significance of the clinical diagnosis of hysteria (Briquet's syndrome). *American Journal of Psychiatry, 132*, 138-141.

Guze, S. B. (1984). Psychosomatic medicine: A critique. *Psychiatric Developments, 2*, 23-30.

Guze, S. B. (1993). Genetics of Briquet's syndrome and somatization disorder: A review of family, adoption, and twin studies. *Annals of Clinical Psychiatry, 5*, 225-230.

Kaplan, C. P., Miner, M. E., Mervis, L., Newton, H., McGregor, J. M., & Goodman, J. H. (1998). Interpretive risks: The use of the Hopkins Symptom Checklist 90-Revised (SCL-90-R) with brain tumour patients. *Brain Injury, 12*, 199-205.

Kass, F., Skodol, A., Buckley, P., & Charles, E. (1980). Therapists' recognition of psychopathology: A model for quality review of psychotherapy. *American Journal of Psychiatry, 137*, 87-90.

Katon, W., Lin, E., Von Korff, M., Russo, J., Lipscomb, P., & Bush, T. (1991). Somatization: A spectrum of severity. *American Journal of Psychiatry, 148,* 34-40.

Kawana, N., Ishimatsu, S., & Kanda, K. (2001). Psycho-physiological effects of the terrorist sarin attack on the Tokyo subway system. *Military Medicine, 166,* 23-26.

Kroenke, K., Spitzer, R. L., deGruy, R. V., III, & Swindle, R. (1998). A symptom checklist to screen for somatoform disorders in primary care. *Psychosomatics, 39,* 263-272.

Labbate, L. A., Cardeña, E., Dimitreva, J., Roy, M. J., & Engel, C. C. (1998). Psychiatric syndromes in Persian Gulf War veterans: An association of handling dead bodies with somatoform disorders. *Psychotherapy and Psychosomatics, 67,* 275-279.

Lenze, E. L., Miller, A., Munir, Z., Pornoppadol, C., & North, C. S. (1999). Psychiatric symptoms endorsed by somatization disorder patients in a psychiatric clinic. *Annals of Clinical Psychiatry, 11,* 73-79.

Liskow, B., Penick, E. C., Powell, B. J., Haefele, W. F., & Campbell, J. L. (1986). Inpatients with Briquet's syndrome: Presence of additional psychiatric syndromes and MMPI results. *Comprehensive Psychiatry, 27,* 461-470.

Martin, R. L. (1988). Problems in the diagnosis of somatization disorder: Effects on research and clinical practice. *Psychiatric Annals, 18,* 357-362.

Merskey, H. (1995). *The analysis of hysteria: Understanding conversion and dissociation* (2nd ed.). London: Gaskell.

Miller, A., North, C. S., Clouse, R. E., Alpers, D. H., & Wetzel, R. D. (2001). Irritable bowel syndrome, psychiatric illness, personality, and abuse: Is somatization disorder the missing link? *Annals of Clinical Psychiatry, 13,* 25-30.

Mojtabai, R., & Reider, R. O. (1998). Limitations of the symptom-oriented approach to psychiatric research. *British Journal of Psychiatry, 173,* 198-202.

Murphy, G. E. (1982). The clinical management of hysteria. *Journal of the American Medical Association, 247,* 2559-2564.

Murphy, S. A. (1984). Stress levels and health status of victims of a natural disaster. *Research in Nursing and Health, 7,* 205-215.

North, C. S., & Guze, S. B. (1998). Somatoform disorders. In S. B. Guze (Ed.), *Washington University: Adult psychiatry* (pp. 269-283). St. Louis: Mosby.

Petterson, J. (1998). Perception vs. reality of radiological impact: The Goiania model. *Nuclear News, November,* 84-90.

Robins, E., & Guze, S. B. (1970). Establishment of diagnostic validity in psychiatric illness: Its application to schizophrenia. *American Journal of Psychiatry, 126,* 983-987.

Robins, L. N., Fishbach, R. L., Smith, E. M., Cottler, L. B., Solomon, S. D., & Goldring, E. (1986). Impact of disaster on previously assessed mental health. In J. H. Shore (Ed.), *Disaster stress studies: New methods and findings* (pp. 22-48). Washington, DC: American Psychiatric Association.

Stern, J. (1999). *The ultimate terrorists.* Cambridge: Harvard University Press.

Struewing, J. P., & Gray, G. C. (2004). An epidemic of respiratory complaints exacerbated by mass psychogenic illness in a military recruit population. *American Journal of Epidemiology, 132,* 1120-1129.

Swartz, M., Landerman, R., George, L. K., Blazer, D. G., & Escobar, J. (1991). Somatization disorders. In L. N. Robins & D. A. Regier (Eds.), *Psychiatric disor-*

ders in America: The epidemiologic catchment area study (pp. 220-257). New York: Free Press.

van der Kolk, B. A., Pelcovitz, D., Roth, S., Mandel, F. S., McFarlane, A., & Herman, J. L. (1996). Dissociation, somatization, and affect regulation: The complexity of adaptation to trauma. *American Journal of Psychiatry, 153*, 83-93.

Van Ommeren, M., de Jong, J. T., Sharma, B., Komproe, I., Thapa, S. B., & Cardeña, E. (2001). Psychiatric disorders among tortured Bhutanese refugees in Nepal. *Archives of General Psychiatry, 58*, 475-482.

Viel, J. F., Curbakova, E., Eglite, M., Zvagule, T., & Vincent, C. (1997). Risk factors for long-term mental and psychosomatic distress in Latvian Chernobyl liquidators. *Environmental Health Perspectives, 105*, 1539-1544.

Wetzel, R. D., Clayton, P. J., Cloninger, C. R., Brim, J., Martin, R. L., Guze, S. B. et al. (2000). Diagnosis of posttraumatic stress disorder with the MMPI: PK scale scores in somatization disorder. *Psychological Reports, 87*, 535-541.

FINDINGS FROM AROUND THE WORLD

Short and Long-Term Effects
of Terrorist Attacks in Spain

Enrique Baca
Enrique Baca-García
María Mercedes Pérez-Rodríguez
Maria Luisa Cabanas

SUMMARY. This article illustrates the effects of terrorism on its victims. We conducted a study on a sample of 2,998 Spanish victims of terrorism (1997-2001). Victims were evaluated with the General Health Questionnaire (28-item version). A much higher prevalence of psychiatric symptoms (mainly anxiety and psychosomatic symptoms) among the victims than in the general population was found. This was maintained over time. There was a correlation between the degree of harm due to the attack and the severity of the psychopathology. We conclude that terrorist attacks are risk factors that will affect some of their victims for a lifetime.

Address correspondence to: Enrique Baca, MD, Servicio de Psiquiatría, Clínica Puerta De Hierro, San Martín de Porres, Madrid 28020, Spain.

[Haworth co-indexing entry note]: "Short and Long-Term Effects of Terrorist Attacks in Spain." Baca, Enrique et al. Co-published simultaneously in *Journal of Aggression, Maltreatment & Trauma* (The Haworth Maltreatment & Trauma Press, an imprint of The Haworth Press, Inc.) Vol. 9, No. 1/2, 2004; and: *The Trauma of Terrorism: Sharing Knowledge and Shared Care, An International Handbook* (ed: Yael Danieli, Danny Brom, and Joe Sills) The Haworth Maltreatment & Trauma Press, an imprint of The Haworth Press, Inc., 2005.

KEYWORDS. Terrorism, violence, psychopathological sequelae, comorbidity, victims, post traumatic stress disorder

The major psychological and medical consequences of armed conflicts and other large-scale catastrophes have been known for more than a century. Studies conducted on combatants in the Korean and the Vietnam wars documented a syndrome of symptoms often seen in soldiers and others exposed to high levels of war zone stress, and revived the interest of the scientific community in the consequences of both man-made and natural disasters. This led to the development of the new psychiatric category named Posttraumatic Stress Disorder (PTSD). Originally created to explain a specific constellation of symptoms suffered by soldiers, the boundaries of this disorder have been widened and its diagnostic criteria elaborated upon to describe a syndrome that is more prevalent in the general population than was previously believed.

However, this renewed interest in the consequences of disaster did not lead to an increase in research in certain fields heretofore neglected by most scientists. One such neglected area is the link between the psychopathological consequences of an act of aggression and the circumstances and characteristics of the aggression itself, and the mechanisms and determinants through which the victim's psychopathology arises and evolves. We studied the short- and long-term consequences of terrorism in Spain, in an attempt to shed some light on and enrich the understanding of the victims' psychiatric sufferings. The studies we have conducted provide a unique opportunity to confront a problem with such high impact as terrorism, which has repeatedly been rated in nationwide surveys among the major worries of Spanish society.

Although relatively neglected until after the events of September 11, 2001 (Schlenger, 2002), the study of the victims of terrorist attacks had yielded some interesting results. Most of the papers published on the subject referred to the Northern Ireland conflict (Lyons, 1974) or were focused on the development of PTSD (Curran, 1990). Many studies have shown that victims of terrorist attacks have worse mental health than the general population (Baca & Cabanas, 1997). In addition to stress-related disorders, such as PTSD, they have also exhibited symptoms of anxiety and depression. This symptomatology has often been found to evolve toward chronicity (Abenhaim, Dab & Salmi, 1992; Curran, 1988; Giner, 2000).

The main goal of this article is to document the prevalence of clinically significant psychiatric symptomatology following exposure to terrorist attacks in Spain, relative to the time elapsed since the attack. To illustrate the short and long-term psychiatric consequences of terrorism in Spain, we refer to a study we conducted from 1997 to 2002 on a Spanish sample (Baca, Cabanas, & Baca-Garcia, 2002). The study was part of a larger project called the "Phoenix Project," which includes a registry of all those affected by terrorist actions in Spain, and is sponsored by the Association of Victims of Terrorism (AVT) (Baca, Cabanas, & Baca-Garcia, 2003).

THE ASSOCIATION OF VICTIMS OF TERRORISM AND THE PHOENIX PROJECT

The AVT was created in 1981 by the victims of terrorist attacks and their relatives, in an attempt to provide administrative, social, psychological, economic and legal assistance to those affected by terrorism. Currently there are 8,000 associates, who are either direct victims of terrorist attacks, or first-degree relatives of direct victims.

The Phoenix Project was conceived to gain knowledge about the psychosocial and psychopathological consequences of terrorist attacks on the victims and their relatives. It was named after the mythological phoenix bird, which was reborn from its ashes. The main aim of this project is to gather information about the long-term consequences of terrorist attacks at all levels, including the mental health status and quality of life of the affected individuals. The Phoenix registry includes all victims of terrorist attacks in Spain, and the majority of the attacks are perpetrated by the Basque separatists.

Victims

We will first review the concept of "victim" and the various forms in which it may appear. There are primary (i.e., direct) victims, who are directly affected by the traumatic event, and secondary (i.e., indirect) victims, who witnessed the aggression. Secondary victims can be related to the victim (i.e., relatives) or to the event (i.e., policemen, firemen, emergency services staff). It was traditionally believed that the last kind of indirect victims (those related to the event because of their profession) had a high degree of resilience due to their career selection, their preparedness and experience, the fewer injuries they suffered, and post-disaster mental health interventions (North, 2002). However, this assumption has been proven wrong after the 9/11 terrorist attacks, in which firemen who were affected developed high levels of mental diseases.

In this study we included not only direct victims (DV), but also the victims' family members. We did this because we hypothesized that the relatives of the victims (DVR) suffer the consequences of the attack, regardless of whether the victim actually survives the aggression or not. This hypothesis turned out to be very fruitful. Some of the direct victims were also relatives of other victims (DVDVR).

The preliminary hypotheses were as follows: (a) It was assumed that the mental health of victims of terrorist attacks is worse than that of the general population of Spain. Among the victims, we hypothesized that the degree of harm from the attack is an important determinant of the victim's subsequent mental health (direct victims will therefore have a worse quality of life than their relatives who were not involved in the attacks); and (b) It was also assumed that the differential factor of the group studied, with regard to the general population, was the terrorist attack in which they had been direct victims or in which close relatives had been injured. Thus, we hypothesized that the differences between this and the general population, concerning their probability of being a psychiatric case, could be attributed to their having been affected by these attacks, and that this effect was maintained over time.

METHODS

We prepared an interview which asked participants to respond on issues related to socio-demographic data (except personal identification data), the person's relation to the attack (victim, relative, or both at the same time), degree of kinship with the victim, site, type and consequences of the attack, time elapsed since the attack at the time of the survey, current place of residence (as opposed to place of residence at the time of the attack), perceived support by the society as a whole (institutions, relatives, and AVT), estimation of mental health level, and estimation of quality of life. The participants' mental health level was calculated by establishing the probability of being a psychiatric case, measured with Goldberg's General Health Questionnaire (GHQ-28; Goldberg & Williams, 1996). A Spanish version of the GHQ has been validated for use in Spain and it has an extensive bibliography, both on its psychometric properties (i.e., validity, reliability and sensibility), results obtained from the normal Spanish population, and from different types of pathological situations. The GHQ-28 measures the probability of the patient's symptomatology being labelled or diagnosed as a psychiatric case. This is defined as a person who requires some type of support or professional help due to psychological difficulties or problems. The GHQ-28 provides a global index of caseness (i.e., presence of clinically significant psychological symptomatology) and also four specific subscales: (a) Subscale A, which includes somatic symptoms that are common among people who report high levels of psychological distress; (b) Subscale B, which includes symptoms of anxiety; (c) Subscale C, which includes symptoms related to difficulties or dysfunction in social relationships; and (d) Subscale D, which includes symptoms of depression.

To determine if the person interviewed could be classified as a psychiatric case, we set the cutoff point at more than 5 affirmative responses. This cutoff point produced a 77% sensitivity and a 78% specificity in a study in which the Spanish version of the questionnaire was validated (Lobo, Pérez-Echevarría, & Artal, 1998). A total of 2,998 persons belonging to 544 family units agreed to be interviewed from January 1997 to January 2001.

Participants

The interviews were performed by a team, and took place in the victims' homes in one or two sessions in which all family members were gathered. Seventy-three percent of the subjects were relatives of a victim (DVR; $n = 2,188$), 17.6% were direct victims (DV; $n = 533$), 5.4% direct victims and relatives of the victim (DVDVR; $n = 161$), and 3.8% were related to the family but not to the attack (Others; $n = 115$, mostly children who were born after the traumatic event).

Age. The ages of the subjects at the time of the interview did not follow a normal distribution, so we divided the sample into the following age groups: (a) children and adolescents (under 18 years), (b) young adults (18-35 years), (c) adults (35-65 years), and (d) elders (over 65 years). Half of the DVR group were young adults (49.2%) while 80.7% of the DV were between 35 and 65 years.

At the time of the attack, 52.6% ($n = 90$) DV were young adults and 41.5% ($n = 71$) were adults. The DVR were younger, 36.6% ($n = 274$) were young adults and 35.9% were adolescents ($n = 269$). Almost 3% of the DVR were born after the attack (2.9%; $n = 22$). The DVDVR were located in a middle band between DVR and DV, one fourth (25.0%; $n = 18$) being youngsters, one-third (31.9%; $n = 23$) young adults, and 43.1% ($n = 31$) adults.

Gender. Gender distribution was different for each group. The "others" followed the same distribution as the Spanish population, in which there is almost the same proportion of men (49%) and women (51%), according to data from the National Institute of Statistics (2003). However, women outnumbered men in the DVR group (69.5%) and the DVDVR group (61.0%). Conversely, most of the members of the DV group were males (81.6%).

Profession. Among the DV, the most frequent professions were policemen (63.4%, $n = 108$) and civil servants (i.e., elected politicians, university professors and city council workers; 8.4%, $n = 15$). Among the DVDVR, 22.1% ($n = 17$) were housewives, 23.4% ($n = 18$) employees, and 18.2% ($n = 14$) students.

Finally, almost one-third (29.7%; n = 239) of the DVR group were house-wives, 23.7% (n = 191) were employees, and 18.9% (n = 152) were students.

The distributions shown indicate that more than half of the victims belong to the police and armed forces (68.3%; n = 122) but there is also a substantial number of civilians (almost one third) who suffer the direct consequences of the attacks.

RESULTS

A total of 426 attacks had affected these 544 families. The most frequently used methods of attack were explosives aimed at specific persons (n = 180; 42.3%) and shooting (n = 170; 40.1%). The results of the attacks were: (a) fa-talities (306; 71.8%), wounded persons with physical sequelae (n = 245; 57.5%), wounded persons without physical sequelae (n = 149; 35.0%) of the attacks, and material damage to the victim's properties in 115 (27.0%) of them. Ninety-four percent (402) of the attacks were recognized as such by the registry of the Department of Justice. The data on the deceased victims were provided by their closest relatives. Death occurred in 254 instances involving the direct victims (47.1%) and in 24 instances (14.7%) involving individuals who were at the same time both direct victims and relatives of another victim. Obviously, the data of the deceased were not included in the study.

Bivariate associations between exposure group and other study variables were assessed with Student's t test and analysis of the variance for a factor with post-hoc analysis or with the Student-Newman-Keuls test for categorical vari-ables. Confidence intervals (CI; 95%) are also provided for prevalence and other estimates.

The GHQ-28 was adequately answered by 36.1% (n = 1,094) of the people interviewed. Seventy-three percent of the participants who responded to the GHQ-28 were relatives of the victims (DVR; n = 806), 16.4% were direct vic-tims (DV; n = 179), 7.0% were both direct victims and relatives of the victim (DVDVR; n = 77), and 2.8% were related to the family but not to the attack (Others; n = 31). These frequencies do not differ significantly from those of the total group of the interviewed persons.

Mental Health

The prevalence of emotional problems, measured as "the probability of classifying as a psychiatric case," was calculated on the basis of the scores obtained in the General Health Questionnaire of Goldberg (GHQ) in its 28-item version validated in Spain by Lobo et al. (1988). According to the cri-teria used in the previous study (Baca & Cabanas, 1997) 39.6% of the sample studied (n = 434 cases) were in need of psychological-psychiatric care (Table 1).

Compared with the figures of general morbidity, that is, with the general population's risk of suffering emotional disorders that require professional care or intervention detected by the same procedure and with the same instrument in studies carried out in Spain (Herrera, Antonell, Spagnolo, Domenech, & Martín, 1987; Seva & Civera, 1982; Vazquez-Barquero, Diaz Manrique, & Peña, 1987), we found that any terrorist victims present a probability that ranges from two to four times that of the general Spanish population to suffer this type of disorder. The psychiatric morbidity obtained from the general Spanish population range from 11.5% to 20.9%, implying a serious risk of suffering emotional problems. This fact has, in our opinion, no other differential causal factor than the circumstance of having been direct or indirect victims of a terrorist attack.

A statistically significant association was found between the probability of classifying a psychiatric case and the degree of involvement in the attack ($\zeta^2(3) = 29.31$, $p < 0.001$); it was also observed that the mean scores on the GHQ-28 were different in the 4 groups ($F(3) = 12.53$; $p < 0.001$) (see Table 2). The DVD/VR presented greater risk of psychiatric classification as 54.5% exceeded the cutoff and the mean score was 7.87 (CI 6.10-9.63). Regarding the DV, 52.0% were a possible case, the mean score being 8.72 (CI 7.49-9.95). These figures decreased for the DVR in which 36.4% scored on the level of psychiatric pathology and the mean score on the GHQ-28 was 5.61 (CI 5.14-6.09). Finally, the "others" group approached the general population levels with 16.1% of them being at risk of having a psychiatric disorder and a mean score lower than the cutoff 3.19 (CI 1.44-4.95) (see Table 2).

TABLE 1. Probability of Being a Psychiatric Case and Degree of Involvement in Attack

	Not a psychiatric case		Psychiatric case		Total
		CI 95%		CI 95%	
DVR *	513	63.6% 61-67%	293	36.4% 33-40%	806
DV **	86	48.0% 41-55%	93	52.0% 45-59%	179
DVDVR ***	35	45.5% 35-57%	42	54.5% 43-66%	77
Others	26	83.9% 68-93%	5	16.1% 6-26%	31
Total	660	60.4% 58-64%	433	39.6% 35-44%	1093

* DVR = Relatives of the victims
** DV = Direct victims
*** DVDVR = Direct victims and relatives of the victim

Furthermore, within those groups of people who were not direct victims of the attack, it was also verified that there were frequency differences according to the family relationship degree ($\zeta^2(3) = 24.87$; p < 0.001). Parents (47.7%) and spouses (45.6%) were more affected than children (34.2%) and siblings (32.0%).

The four groups presented different mean scores on the GHQ-28 subscales: subscale A of somatic symptoms of psychological origin ($F(3) = 6.90$; $p <$ 0.001), subscale B of anxiety symptoms ($F(3) = 8.01$; $p < 0.001$), subscale C of symptoms related with social dysfunction ($F(3) = 14.18$; $p < 0.001$) and subscale D of depression symptoms ($F(3) = 9.20$; $p < 0.001$) (see Tables 3 and 4). The group with the worst (highest) scores was DV, followed by the DVDVR group. Both of them doubled the mean scores of the "others" group in each of the scales. The maximum scores were reached in B and A subscales (see Table 3). The cross-sectional approach of the study also captured the victims at different periods of time since the attacks. Regardless of the time elapsed since the exposure to the terrorist attack, the prevalence of psychiatric symptoms was higher than in the general population (see Tables 5 and 6).

DISCUSSION

Findings from this study document a much higher prevalence of clinically significant symptoms, and therefore need for treatment, among persons exposed, directly or indirectly, to terrorist attacks than in the general population. Based on the GHQ-28 subscales, the disorders most frequently suffered by DVR, DV, and DVDVR were anxiety disorders and psychosomatic symptoms. It was also found that this greater prevalence of psychiatric cases among the victims was maintained over time, and that the temporal distance between

TABLE 2. Mean Scores and Standard Deviation on the GHQ Scale and Degree of Involvement in Attack (Global Scores)

	n	M	SD	95% Confidence Interval	
DVR *	806	5.61	6.84	5.14	6.09
DV **	179	8.72	8.34	7.49	9.95
DVDVR***	77	7.87	7.78	6.10	9.63
Others	31	3.19	4.78	1.44	4.95
Total	1093	6.21	7.24	5.78	6.64

* DVR = Relatives of the victims
** DV = Direct victims
*** DVDVR = Direct victims and relatives of the victims

TABLE 3. Mean Scores and Standard Deviation on the GHQ Scale and Degree of Involvement in Attack (Subscales A and B)

	n	M	SD	95% Confidence Interval	
Subscale A: Somatic symptoms					
DVR *	806	1.64	2.16	1.49	1.79
DV **	179	2.35	2.42	1.99	2.70
DVDVR ***	77	2.17	2.30	1.65	2.69
Others	31	1.06	1.95	0.35	1.78
Total	1093	1.78	2.22	1.64	1.91
Subscale B: Anxiety symptoms					
DVR *	806	1.9826	2.4095	1.8160	2.1492
DV **	179	2.7598	2.7444	2.3550	3.1646
DVDVR ***	77	2.7662	2.6051	2.1749	3.3575
Others	31	1.1935	1.9903	0.4635	1.9236
Total	1093	2.1427	2.4946	1.9947	2.2908

* DVR = Relatives of the victims
** DV = Direct victims
*** DVDVR = Direct victims and relatives of the victims

TABLE 4. Mean Scores and Standard Deviation on the GHQ Scale and Degree of Involvement in Attack (Subscales C and D)

	n	M	SD	95% Confidence Interval	
Subscale C: Dysfunctional social symptoms					
DVR *	806	1.13	1.80	1.01	1.26
VD **	179	2.09	2.31	1.75	2.43
DVRVD***	77	1.61	2.15	1.12	2.10
Others	31	0.64	1.28	0.18	1.11
Total	1093	1.31	1.94	1.19	1.42
Subscale D: Depressive symptoms					
DVR *	806	0.86	1.71	0.74	0.98
VD **	179	1.53	2.17	1.21	1.84
DVRVD***	77	1.32	2.00	0.87	1.78
Others	31	0.29	0.82	−0.01	0.59
Total	1093	0.98	1.82	0.88	1.09

* DVR = Relatives of the victims
** DV = Direct victims
*** DVDVR = Direct victims and relatives of the victims

TABLE 5. Confidence Intervals at 95% of the Proportion of Psychiatric Cases (%) Among DVR, DV and DVRV According to the Time Passed Since the Attack (Years 0-14)

Years	GROUP	%	CI at 95%	
0-2	DVR *	40.0	29	53
	DV **	66.7	42	85
	DVDVR ***	75.0	30	95
3-5	DVR *	41.9	31	54
	DV **	61.9	41	79
	DVDVR ***	60.0	23	88
6-8	DVR *	41.1	31	51
	DV **	56.5	37	75
	DVDVR ***	65.2	45	81
9-11	DVR *	32.4	22	43
	DV **	48.1	31	66
	DVDVR ***	50.0	32	68
12-14	DVR *	31.2	24	40
	DV **	48.4	32	65
	DVDVR ***	50.0	15	85

* DVR = Relatives of the victims
** DV = Direct victims
*** DVDVR = Direct victims and relatives of the victims

the time of the study and the occurrence of the traumatic event did not decrease the occurrence of psychiatric cases.

Another conclusion was that there is a positive correlation between the degree of harm suffered as a result of the attack and the severity of the psychopathological consequences suffered by the victims. This study shows how, in the short-term, the individuals most directly affected by an attack (DV and DVDVR) have more mental health problems. As time passes, though, all the groups (both the direct victims and their families) have similar mental health levels. This is consistent with the findings of many previous studies. One additional finding of the study was that the relatives of the victims who had not been exposed to the attacks also had higher levels of psychopathology than the general population.

These findings are consistent with those of previous research. For instance, regarding the short-term consequences of terrorism, several studies in France have found that the victims' degree of harm as a result of the attack influenced the rate of PTSD (8.3% in those mildly affected to 30.7% in those affected

TABLE 6. Confidence Intervals at 95% of the Proportion of Psychiatric Cases (%) Among DVR, DV and DVRV According to the Time Passed Since the Attack (Years > 15)

Years	GROUP	%	CI at 95%	
15-17	DVR *	41.7	32	53
	DV **	58.3	32	80
	DVDVR ***	50.0	9	91
18-20	DVR *	35.7	29	43
	DV **	37.0	22	56
	DVDVR ***	37.5	14	70
21-23	DVR *	29.4	18	43
	DV **	55.6	27	81
> 24	DVR *	26.9	14	46
	DV **	50.0	19	81

*DVR = Relatives of the victims
** DV = Direct victims
*** DVDVR = Direct victims and relatives of the victims

with a certain severity) (Abenhaim et al., 1992). Other French prospective studies have also concluded that the consequences of terrorist attack are maintained over time (Jehel, Duchet, Paterniti, Consoli, & Guelfi, 2001; Jehel, Paterniti, Brunet, Duchet, & Guelfi, 2003). Jehel et al. (2001) reported that 41% of the participants met PTSD criteria at six months, 34.4% of them had PTSD at 18 months, and 25% of them still had PTSD at 32 months.

A study by Japan's National Police Agency (Kawana, Ishimatu, & Kanda, 2001) reportedly showed that more than half of the survivors of the sarin gas terrorist attack on Tokyo's underground system in 1995 had symptoms consistent with PTSD four years after the attack. The respondents complained of nightmares, flashbacks, and had panic attacks when they boarded trains. The most common complaint of the victims was weakened vision. In this particular case, a lack of knowledge about the long-term effects of the exposure to the gas was a major source of anxiety for the victims (Kawana et al., 2001; see also Hall, Norwood, Fullerton, Gifford, & Ursano, this volume, and Engdahl, this volume).

A long-term follow-up study of adolescent survivors of a 1974 terrorist attack in Israel indicated that adjustment was impaired in adult years and was mediated by the extent of the injuries experienced (Desivilya, Gal, & Ayalon, 1996a, 1996b). The severity of injuries was positively associated with the severity of post-traumatic stress symptoms seventeen years after the incident.

Without discounting the broader effects of terrorism, it seems that the extent of immediate life threat accounts for substantial variance in how these events are experienced or what kinds of effects they have (Baum & Dougall, 2002). Studies following the Oklahoma City bombing and the September 11 attacks are described in articles by North, Pfefferbaum et al., and Schlenger in this volume.

Terrorist attacks are the traumatic experiences which are most related to the development of PTSD (Amir, Kaplan, & Kotler, 1996; Tucker, Dickson, Pfefferbaum, McDonald, & Allen, 1997). Some authors have shown how the selectivity of terrorist actions (i.e., attacks of specific victims previously chosen) influences their impact on the victim's social sphere. That is, the less indiscriminate an attack is, the more it affects the victim's social relationships (Curran, 1988). In our sample, the quantity and quality of emotional and social relationships become affected to a substantial degree in both the marital/familial and in the professional/social contexts (Baca et al., 2003).

As the prevalence of psychiatric disorders among the victims remains high after the attack, a series of questions arises, awaiting future research: Is there a temporal relationship to the type of psychic disorder that the DVR, DV and DVDVR suffer? Once DVR, DV and DVDVR suffer a psychiatric disorder due to an attack, do they become sensitized, and thus have a greater vulnerability to develop these disorders and suffer relapses? Are terrorist attacks going to cause disorders in almost all people affected by them and will their personal characteristics make the diseases show up at different periods of time?

The study also has a number of limitations. First, the post-only, cross-sectional, one-group design limits substantially the basis for causal inferences. Rather, the findings from this study are better thought of as hypothesis *generating* than hypothesis *testing*. Second, the external validity depends on both the comprehensiveness of the registry of victims from which the study sample was drawn and on the response rate among registry members included in the study. As noted, only about one-third of those selected for the sample actually participated, and no adjustments for non-response were made. Third, the GHQ is a screening instrument, not a comprehensive clinical evaluation, but its relationship to clinically-identified cases has been well documented empirically in a variety of population-based studies. Fourth, the GHQ screens for non-specific distress, much of which may not be related to exposure to terrorism or other traumatic events and may in fact predate the exposure(s). Finally, the bivariate analyses reported here do not take account of within-family clustering of responses, and as a result the size of the bivariate relationships may be overestimated. Taking into account the methodological limitations explained above, the main conclusion of this study is that terrorist attacks are risk factors that will affect some of their victims for a lifetime.

REFERENCES

Abenhaim, L., Dab, W., & Salmi, L. R. (1992). Study of civilian victims of terrorist attacks (France 1982-1987). *Journal of Clinical Epiaiolology, 45*,103-109.

Amir, M., Kaplan, Z., & Kotler, M. (1996). Type of trauma, severity of posttraumatic stress disorder core symptoms, and associated features. *Journal of General Psychology, 123*(4), 341-51.

Baca, E., & Cabanas M. L. (1997). Niveles de salud mental y calidad de vida en las víctimas del terrorismo [Mental health status and quality of life in victims of terrorism]. *Archivos de Neurobiología, 60*(4), 283-296.

Baca, E., Cabanas, M. L., & Baca-Garcia, E. (2002). Impacto de los atentados terroristas en la morbilidad psiquiátrica a corto y largo plazo [Short- and long-term effects of terrorist attacks on psychiatric morbidity]. *Actas Españolas de Psiquiatría, 30*(2), 85-90

Baca, E., Cabanas, M. L., & Baca-García, E. (2003). El "Proyecto Fénix." Un estudio sobre las víctimas del terrorismo en España [The "Phoenix Project." A study of victims of terrorism in Spain]. In E. Baca, & M. L. Cabanas (Eds.), *Las víctimas de la violencia [The victims of violence]* (pp. 139-187) Madrid, Spain: Triacastela Ed.

Baum, A., & Dougall, A. L. (2002). Terrorism and behavioral medicine. *Current Opinion in Psychiatry, 15*(6), 617-621.

Curran, P. S. (1988). Psychiatric aspects of terrorist violence: Northern Ireland 1969-1987. *British Journal of Psychiatry, 153*(4), 470-5.

Curran, P. S., Bell, P., Murray, A., Roddy, R. J., & Kee, M. (1990). Psychological consequences of the Enniskillen bombing. *British Journal of Psychiatry, 156,* 479-482.

Desivilya, H. S., Gal, R., & Ayalon, O. (1996a). Long-term effects of trauma in adolescents: Comparison between survivors of a terrorist attack and control counterparts. *Anxiety Stress Coping, 9,* 135-150.

Desivilya, H. S., Gal, R., & Ayalon, O. (1996b). Extent of victimization, traumatic stress symptoms, and adjustment of terrorist assault survivors: A long-term follow-up. *Journal of Traumatic Stress, 9,* 881-889.

Engdahl, B. (2004). Integrating international findings on the impact of terrorism. *Journal of Aggression, Maltreatment, & Trauma, 9*(1/2/3/4), 265-276.

Giner, J. (2000). El proceso de medicalización de la víctima [The victim's medicalization process]. *Archivos de Neurobiología, 63*(3), 287-296.

Goldberg, D., & Willians, P. (Ed). (1996). *Cuestionario de Salud General GHQ.* Barcelona: Masson.

Hall, M. J., Norwood, A. E., Fullerton, C. S., Gifford, R., & Ursano, R. J. (2004). The psychological burden of bioterrorism. *Journal of Aggression, Maltreatment, & Trauma, 9*(1/2/3/4), 293-305.

Herrera, R., Antonell, J., Spagnolo, E., Domenech, J., & Martín, S. (1987). Estudio epidemiológico en salud mental en la comarca del Baix Llobregat, Barcelona [Epidemiological study on mental health in the Baix Llobregat region]. *Informaciones Psiquiátricas, 107,* 12-40.

Jehel, L., Duchet, C., Paterniti, S., Consoli, S. M., & Guelfi, J. D. (2001). Evaluation of post-traumatic stress disorders among victims, after a terrorist attack: A prospective study. *Encephale, 27*(5), 393-400.

Jehel, L., Paterniti, S., Brunet, A., Duchet, C., & Guelfi, J. D. (2003). Prediction of the occurrence and intensity of post-traumatic stress disorder in victims 32 months after bomb attack. *European Psychiatry, 18*(4), 172-176.

Kawana, N., Ishimatsu, S., & Kanda, K. (2001). Psycho-physiological effects of the terrorist sarin gas attack on the Tokyo subway system. *Military Medicine, 166*(suppl 12), 23-26.

Lobo, A., Pérez-Echevarría, M. J., & Artal, J. (1998). Validity of the scaled version of General Health Questionnaire (GHQ-28) in Spanish population. *Psychological Medicine, 16*, 135-140.

Lyons, H. A. (1974). Terrorist's bombing and the psychological sequelae. *Journal of the Irish Medical Association, 67*, 15-19.

Muñoz, P. E., Tejerina, M., & Cañas, F. (1996). Estudio de validación predictiva del GHQ en población general urbana. Memoria. Beca FIS 93/0905 (inédito) [Study of predictive validation of the GHQ in a general urban population. FIS 93/0905 Grant]. In D. Goldberg, & P. Willians (Eds.), *Cuestionario de salud general [General health questionnaire]*. Barcelona: Masson.

North, C. S., Tivis, L., McMillen, J., Pfefferbaum, B., Spitznagel, E. L., Cox, J., Nixon, S. et al. (2002). Psychiatric disorders in rescue workers after the Oklahoma City bombing. *American Journal of Psychiatry, 159*(5), 857-859.

Schlenger, W. E., Caddell, J. M., Ebert, L., Jordan, B. K., Rourke, K. M., Wilson, D. et al. (2002). Psychological reactions to terrorist attacks: findings from the National Study of Americans' Reactions to September 11. *Journal of the American Medical Association, 288*(5), 581-588.

Seva, A., & Civeira, J. M. (Ed.) (1982). *Análisis higiénico-sanitario de la salud mental en Soria [Hygienic-sanitary análisis of mental health in Soria]*. Soria: Diputación Provincial de Soria

Tucker, P., Dickson, W., Pfefferbaum, B., McDonald, N. B., & Allen, G. (1997). Traumatic reactions as predictors of posttraumatic stress six months after the Oklahoma City bombing. *Psychiatric Services, 48*(9), 1191-1194.

Vazquez-Barquero, J. L., Díaz Manrique, J. F., & Peña, C. (1987). A community mental health survey in Cantabria: General description of morbidity. *Psychological Medicine, 17*, 227-242.

Voice:
Spain:
The ETA Enigma

Al Goodman

When I think of a particularly gutsy Spaniard, I think of Edurne Uriarte. A political science professor with raven black hair and a ready smile, she was the intended target of a powerful package bomb left in an elevator that she frequently uses at the University of the Basque Country. Her bodyguard spotted the suspicious package, averting a tragedy for Uriarte and many others on campus that December 18, 2000.

A university professor with a bodyguard? Sadly yes. In today's bitterly divided northern Basque region, it's not just the teachers. Several thousand town councilors, lawyers, journalists, even a priest, who have been outspoken about the outlawed Basque separatist group ETA, dare not step outside without one or two hefty gun-toting shadows. These are frequently plainclothes police officers, or private security guards.

It is just one telling reaction to ETA, which poses special danger in the Basque region, but is also a threat that extends to practically every corner of Spain. Even architect Frank Gehry's famed Guggenheim Museum in Bilbao, the largest Basque city, was an ETA target, just before it opened in 1997, and a police officer died.

Address correspondence to: Al Goodman, Edificio Sogecable, Avenida de los Artesanos, 6, 28760 Tres Cantos, Madrid, Spain (E-mail: al.Goodman@turner.com).

[Haworth co-indexing entry note]: "Voice: Spain: The ETA Enigma." Goodman, Al. Co-published simultaneously in *Journal of Aggression, Maltreatment & Trauma* (The Haworth Maltreatment & Trauma Press, an imprint of The Haworth Press, Inc.) Vol. 9, No. 1/2, 2004; and: *The Trauma of Terrorism: Sharing Knowledge and Shared Care, An International Handbook* (ed: Yael Danieli, Danny Brom, and Joe Sills) The Haworth Maltreatment & Trauma Press, an imprint of The Haworth Press, Inc., 2005.

Yet the bodyguards are not infallible. Uriarte was spared, and has not stopped her criticism of ETA; but 10 months earlier, on February 22, 2000, while out for a walk, Basque politician Fernando Buesa and his bodyguard were killed by an ETA bomb. Within hours of that massacre, thousands of Spaniards were on the streets to protest the violence. The protests have become routine, intertwined with the grief after each fatal ETA attack and, for many Spaniards, one of the noblest responses to ETA's methods of seeking an independent Basque homeland.

My closest known brush was in January 2001, when our CNN crew was at a cemetery in the town of Zarautz to cover a posthumous homage for a Basque town councilman shot dead by ETA. Politicians mingled with his relatives. We later learned that despite police sweeps of the cemetery, ETA had placed a bomb in a flowerpot by the man's tomb. The bomb didn't explode due to a technical problem.

The letters ETA, in the Basque language, stand for Basque Homeland and Freedom. ETA is listed as a terrorist organization by the United States and the European Union, of which Spain is a member. Officials blame ETA for killing more than 800 people and wounding several thousand during the past 35 years.

This is not to say that Spain looks like a battle zone. To the contrary, visitors to bustling, dynamic Spain might not even know ETA exists, unless they're unlucky enough to get wounded in an attack, as seven European students were on July 22, 2003 in a hotel bombing in Alicante, on the Mediterranean coast.

Which gives one pause, and leads to some sensible precautions. Since police stations are often targets (just look at the barricades outside them), I try to steer clear unless I have business there. And you can't help remembering when you pass by the scenes of previous ETA bombings, like the narrow pedestrian street between two department stores in central Madrid whose windows were blown out. You wonder whether you, or your loved ones, might get caught in a bombing. You don't stop going outside, but you try to be aware of your surroundings.

The protests against ETA have adopted various symbols over the years. One of the most notable, hands painted white or covered with a white glove, was started by university students to show their hands were clean, not bloodied like ETA's.

The pro-independence camp, while a minority, also does not forget its own, whom it considers victims as well. There are small, weekly protests in support of ETA prisoners in Spanish jails (569 prisoners on December 3, 2003, including 479 men and 90 women who had either been convicted or were awaiting trial). In many Basque villages, sheets or banners hang from balconies in support of the prisoners.

The conflict between centrist-oriented Spaniards in Madrid and the Basques goes back centuries. One enduring flashpoint was in April 1937 during the Spanish Civil War, when Franco ordered the bombing of the Basque town of Guernica, a horror Picasso depicted on canvas for the world.

Today in democratic Spain, the Basque region has a parliament, police force, and other home-rule powers. Spain, France, and the European Union have all said they don't want a Basque nation. Polls show not even a majority of Basques themselves want independence. Yet, far-left independence groups, as well as moderate Basque leaders who support independence, but not ETA's violence, still want to put independence to a vote.

Some Spaniards insist that dialogue is the only long-term solution. Secret talks between the government and ETA in 1989 and in 1999 produced no results. The conservative administration of Prime Minister Jose Maria Aznar took a hard-line stance during its two terms, betting on a police crackdown and other pressure to stifle ETA in 1996.

No one in Spain with whom I've ever talked, whether high official or ordinary citizen, was willing to predict when ETA's violence would really end. The indelible mark of this violence on Spain might best be seen through Jessica Lopez Rodriguez. The 16-year-old was a victim of ETA even before her birth. Her pregnant mother worked as a cashier at a Barcelona department store, which was bombed by ETA in 1987. The blast's shock waves, doctors later determined, affected Jessica in the womb. She was born deaf.

Her mother survived but 21 people died that day. Jessica, now attending high school near Barcelona and wearing a hearing aid, knows that Spaniards refuse to remain silent when it comes to ETA. But no one has figured out yet how to silence ETA's violence.

Northern Ireland:
The Psychological Impact
of "The Troubles"

Andrea Campbell
Ed Cairns
John Mallett

SUMMARY. Maintained by the desires of the Catholic community to see Northern Ireland unified with the rest of Ireland and the Protestants' desire to remain part of the United Kingdom, violence in Northern Ireland lasted for 30 years, causing 3,585 deaths. This violence impacted people's lives through mental health and intergroup relations. While some individuals were deeply scarred by "the troubles," most learned to cope partly by habituation, distancing, and/or denial. The impact on intergroup relations has been subtler but more damaging. Segregation in housing and education is widespread. This in turn has made it harder to reach a long-term settlement.

Address correspondence to: Ed Cairns, PhD, FBPsS, School of Psychology, University of Ulster, Coleraine Campus, N. Ireland, BT52 1SA.

The authors are grateful to Stephanie McGaughey for editorial assistance.

[Haworth co-indexing entry note]: "Northern Ireland: The Psychological Impact of "The Troubles." Campbell, Andrea, Ed Cairns, and John Mallett. Co-published simultaneously in *Journal of Aggression, Maltreatment & Trauma* (The Haworth Maltreatment & Trauma Press, an imprint of The Haworth Press, Inc.) Vol. 9, No. 1/2, 2004; and: *The Trauma of Terrorism: Sharing Knowledge and Shared Care, An International Handbook* (ed: Yael Danieli, Danny Brom, and Joe Sills) The Haworth Maltreatment & Trauma Press, an imprint of The Haworth Press, Inc., 2005.

KEYWORDS. Northern Ireland, conflict, violence, mental health, memories, forgiveness

BACKGROUND

In Northern Ireland there are two versions of everything: "green" and "orange." For example, in the 1990s, a series of ceasefires by paramilitary groups on both sides led to a political agreement known to Catholics as "The Good Friday Agreement" and to Protestants as "The Belfast Agreement." It led to the setting up of a local assembly and a power-sharing government that embraced all the major political parties. The government is still "in suspension" at the time of this writing and faces both political and military challenges. Dissidents in both communities maintain an almost daily, both cross- and intra-community, litany of violence, including beatings, arson, and pipe bombs. Therefore, while it could be argued that the war has (almost) ended, the conflict goes on.

At its most basic, this conflict is a struggle between those who wish to see Northern Ireland remain part of the United Kingdom (Protestants) and those who wish to see the island of Ireland unified (Catholics). The conflict is, in turn, underpinned by historical, religious, political, economic, and psychological elements, which have fuelled the violence. Here we will discuss the major impact that violence has had on the people of Northern Ireland and, in particular, the resulting deaths and injuries, the increased community divisions, and the impact on mental health (Cairns & Darby, 1998).

DEATHS AND INJURIES

The 30 years from 1968 onwards have been colloquially referred to as "The Troubles." During this period, 3,585 people in Northern Ireland were killed and 40,000 injured (Smyth, 1998). These figures may not appear too startling, as these are much lower rates than those of murder and assault in many American cities. However, the total population of Northern Ireland barely exceeds 1.6 million, and the close-knit nature of community life ensures that a considerable number of people have had indirect experience of the violence, such as witnessing a friend or relative being killed or being near a bomb explosion (Cairns, Wilson, Gallagher, & Trew, 1995).

Additionally, the violence in Northern Ireland has varied along the dimensions of intensity, location, and nature. First, there has been a considerable variation in the intensity of the violence, as measured by the number of deaths and injuries during different stages of the troubles. For example, a total of 13 people were killed in 1969 compared to 467 in 1972 (Cairns & Wilson, 1993). Second, the majority of violence occurred in the larger cities of Belfast and Derry, although smaller towns have also been targeted. Finally, the nature and type of violence has varied widely from street rioting and demonstrations to bombs and assassination attempts. The seemingly random and unpredictable nature of the violence carried with it the implication that everyone living in Northern Ireland was at some degree of uncontrollable risk (Cairns et al., 1995).

MENTAL HEALTH

First attempts to understand the relationship between political conflict and mental health relied almost exclusively on psychiatric admission, referral rates, and evidence from clinical case studies. We will not review this work because it tended to use relatively simplistic research approaches whose conceptual and methodological precisions are open to debate (Cairns & Darby, 1998). By the 1980s, community-based studies became the predominant means of assessing the mental health effects of political violence. The information obtained from these community studies led to a subsequent interest in "coping strategies" such as denial, distancing, and habituation.

Community-Based Studies of Children. During the height of the troubles, four main community-based studies examined the effects of political violence on children. The first two, carried out by Fee (1980, 1983) in 1975 and 1981, involved 5,000 and 7,000 children, respectively. Results revealed that approximately 15% of children scored above the cut-off point for psychopathology in 1975 compared to 9% of children in 1981. Fee (1983) suggested that this decrease in the percentage of disturbed children corresponded to a decrease in political violence during the same period. Comparison of the prevalence rate in Belfast for these two years with that from similar populations indicates a substantially higher rate of disturbed cases in Belfast (Cairns & Wilson, 1993).

A third community-based study (McWhirter, 1983) involved a stratified sample of 1,000 children from "troubled" and relatively "peaceful" areas of Northern Ireland. These children were then compared to a sample of 210 children from the north of England. Results indicated no difference in measures of trait anxiety between Northern Irish children and British and American norms or the English. Additionally, no differences were observed between children from "troubled" and "peaceful" areas in Northern Ireland.

The last study (McGrath & Wilson, 1985) examined the relationship between children's stress levels and their actual exposure to political violence, using a random sample from the general population. No significant relationship was found between depression and experiences of political violence, although the observed levels of depression were slightly higher than those for British children in other surveys. However, a significant correlation was observed between exposure to political violence and manifest anxiety. Specifically, children were more likely to report symptoms of anxiety when their friends or relatives were injured or killed as a result of the troubles or when they perceived their area to be unsafe.

Overall, these community studies suggest that the majority of children in Northern Ireland do not suffer from serious psychological problems, at least with respect to depression. However, variations in the level of anti-social behavior appear to parallel variations in level of political violence. This has been a recurring finding with young people in Northern Ireland. Muldoon and Trew (2000) have provided evidence that reinforces the possibility that experiencing political violence may be causally related to externalizing and delinquent behaviors. Their study also illustrates that, while children in Northern Ireland were not exposed to political violence to the same extent as children caught up in all-out war, many did experience such things as rioting or witnessing a shooting. For example, almost 60% of their sample of 8 to 11 year olds reported being caught up in a bomb scare. A follow-up study indicated changes in the centrality of these events, which interacted both with gender and denomination (Muldoon, 2003).

Community-Based Studies of Adults. Virtually all work in this area utilized the General Health Questionnaire (GHQ), a widely used measure of psychiatric morbidity validated in Northern Ireland by Cairns, Wilson, McClelland, and Gillespie (1989). For example, a survey conducted in 1984 questioned people about the level of violence in the area where they lived and of safety levels in general. Multiple regression analyses indicated employment status as the best predictor of psychiatric morbidity. However, perceptions of the violence and safety levels contributed significantly to an increase in the total explained variance. This suggests that although socio-demographic characteristics are the most important correlates of mild psychiatric morbidity, perceptions of violence and safety levels are other important factors (Cairns & Wilson, 1993).

Cairns and Wilson (1993) provided further evidence confirming the relationship between political violence and mental health. They compared two towns, matched for socio-demographic characteristics but having experienced contrasting levels of violence during the previous 10 years. Participants completed a 30-item version of the GHQ and indicated their perception of the level of violence in their area and how safe they considered their area to live in. As expected, those who lived in the town with a higher level of violence scored at a significantly higher level on the GHQ. The results also revealed a significant interaction between objective and perceived levels of violence. Specifically, individuals living in a violent area that accurately recognized the area to be relatively violent displayed higher levels of disorder compared to those who perceived little or no violence.

Overall, the evidence from these community studies suggests that the majority of people in Northern Ireland were able to cope with low levels of stress associated with political violence. This, of course, is not true for those involved in the most serious incidents, such as the bombing involving civilians at Enniskillen (Curran, Bell, Murray, Loughrey, Roddy, & Rocke, 1990) or Omagh (Gillespie, Duffy, Hackmann, & Clarke, 2002). Indeed, the Omagh bomb led to PTSD not just for those directly involved but also for health care staff working with the survivors (Luce, Firth-Cozens, Midgley, & Burges, 2002).

Coping Processes. Given this evidence, a series of studies set out to attempt to isolate the particular coping mechanism or mechanisms at work. The first suggestion (McWhirter, 1987) was that people had simply habituated to the daily drip, drip of political violence and the relatively low levels of stress it invoked, and Cairns and Wilson (1993) proposed the coping mechanism of denial and adapted subscales from the Lazarus and Folkman (1984) Ways of Coping Questionnaire to test it in a community survey. They found that those who perceived the violence to be less serious tended to use more "distancing" strategies (Cairns, Wilson, Gallagher, & Trew, 1995).

INTERGROUP RELATIONS

In Northern Ireland, segregation leading to limited contact between the Catholic and Protestant communities is apparent in many different areas of social life. In this section we will examine the data on segregation, not because we believe it to be the cause of intergroup conflict, but because we believe it plays a major role in maintaining conflict between the two communities.

According to Niens, Cairns, and Hewstone (2003), the types of segregation that have received most attention in Northern Ireland are educational, residential, personal, and matrimonial. Other types of segregation (e.g., at work, sport, and leisure) have also been identified but have received less attention in the research literature (Smyth, 1995).

Educational Segregation. In Northern Ireland, virtually all elementary and secondary education is segregated. Both communities back this school system even though surveys show the majority of the population claims they would support integrated education (see Hughes & Carmichael, 1998). Because segregation in education in Northern Ireland was almost total, particularly at the primary or elementary level, in 1987 the government introduced Education for Mutual Understanding (EMU), which promotes cross-community school activities. At about the same time, integrated schools involving pupils from both sides were established. In 1989, there were only about 10 integrated schools. Currently, there are 46 integrated schools, consisting of 17 integrated second level colleges and 29 integrated primary schools. However, the integrated sector still educates only a small minority of the total pupil population (about 5%).

Residential Segregation. Since total segregation does not exist in Northern Ireland, it cannot be concluded that educational segregation is simply a product of residential segregation (Cairns & Hewstone, 2002). Whyte (1990) has estimated that "about 35 to 40 percent of the population live in segregated neighbourhoods" (p. 34), which means that more than 50% of the population live in mixed neighborhoods. Segregated living appears to have increased during the period of the "troubles." Indeed, some local commentators have suggested that this segregation is set to increase more rapidly in a "peaceful" Northern Ireland, which they believe is now entering a period of "benign apartheid."

Personal Segregation. Despite the conflict and the associated violence, and the educational and residential segregation, surprisingly, cross-community friendships do exist in Northern Ireland. However, evidence from surveys over the past 30 years indicates that such friendships are the exception rather than the rule. The majority of respondents report that all or most of their friends are from their own community (Cairns & Hewstone, 2002). An even more important way to measure intimacy across community lines might be to look at cross-community marriages. For the last 30 years, endogamy has been around 5% (Niens et al., 2003). More recently, however, data from the Northern Ireland Life and Times Survey (NILT, 2000) have indicated an increase to around 11% in cross-community marriages.

WHEN THE WAR IS OVER: POST-CEASEFIRE RESEARCH

Despite some ongoing residual tension from the troubles, the ceasefires of August 1994 have provided researchers on Northern Ireland with a unique opportunity to examine the possibility that there have been long-term psychological costs of 30 years of sectarianism and social violence.

Mental Health. O'Reilly and Stevenson (2003) interviewed a random sample of 1,700 adults to assess mental health using the General Health Questionnaire. Two questions measured the effects of the troubles, the first on the respondent's area, the second on the participant or his or her family. The researchers found that 21.3% of participants reported that the troubles had either "quite a bit" or "a lot" of impact on their lives or the lives of their family, and just over 25% reported a similar impact on their local area. They concluded that, even after accounting for socioeconomic or demographic factors, political violence placed an additional toll on mental health (O'Reilly & Stevenson, 2003). Similarly, in a random sample of 1,000 adults, Cairns, Mallett, Lewis, and Wilson (2003) reported that psychological well-being, as measured by the GHQ, was lower for those who simply considered themselves victims of the troubles. Indeed, recent evidence indicates that victims and their relatives may continue to suffer psychologically for years after a particularly traumatic event such as Bloody Sunday (Shevlin & McGuigan, 2003).

Memories of the Troubles. There is also evidence (Cairns et al., 2003) that the political violence of the past still remains a prominent feature in the minds of the Northern Irish population. People were asked to list two events that had occurred in the past 50 years that they considered important. Most of the memories reported were concerned with the conflict. Over half were related to a violent aspect of the conflict and 41% to some aspect of the peace process.

Evidence for a link between memories of the troubles and mental health in the post-troubles era emerged in a study by Cairns and Lewis (1999). This study looked at the long-term effects of one of the most salient incidents in Northern Ireland involving civilian mass casualties, the result of a bomb exploding in the centre of a small town (Enniskillen), injuring 63 people and killing 11. Interviews there and at a neighboring town found that relatively few people included the Enniskillen bomb when asked to mention two Northern Irish events or changes that had taken place over the past 50 years that "come to mind as important to you." Further, the majority of these came from Enniskillen and were Protestants (as were all of the casualties). Significantly, Protestants and respondents from the neighboring town who mentioned the bomb scored at a significantly higher level on the General Health questionnaire (indicating poorer mental health).

FORGIVENESS

Faced with this evidence, McLernon, Cairns, Lewis, and Hewstone (2003) concluded that a major stumbling block to peace in Northern Ireland is that memories of conflict, both current and from the distant past, are easily activated in Northern Irish society; that if the historical cycle of violence and revenge is to be brought to an end, the issue of forgiveness will have to move further up the agenda.

A series of surveys explored the correlates of intergroup forgiveness in the context of sectarian conflict in Northern Ireland (Hewstone, Cairns, Voci, McLernon, Niens, & Noor, in press). One major conclusion is that forgiveness is probably best thought of as a socio-political rather than a religious construct. This is because religion was found to be a weak predictor of forgiveness, whereas in-group identification and especially out-group attitude were very strong predictors. Also, as might be expected, the more the respondents in the surveys had actually experienced the troubles, the less forgiving they tended to be.

CONCLUSIONS

It is clear that the troubles have left "most families touched in some way" (Cairns & Darby, 1998, p. 754). This is because so many people have been victims of violence, either directly (e.g., being a victim of a violent event, and perhaps suffering injury) or indirectly (e.g., having a family member or close relative killed or injured).

The research we have highlighted in this chapter suggests that "the troubles" did not have the major impact on the mental health of the Northern Irish population (adults or children) that was originally anticipated. Where severe impact has occurred has either been to individuals directly exposed to the violence or to larger groups but only for relatively short periods of time.

This conclusion would appear to fit the evidence that the ceasefires have brought no appreciable improvement in psychological well-being in Northern Ireland. Of course, a range of factors, of which the troubles is just one, influences psychological health, and until these other (social) factors also change, no dramatic improvements can be expected.

That the troubles would have an impact on the social fabric of Northern Ireland was not originally anticipated. In fact, this is where the major impact seems to have been. It has taken the form of increased residential segregation and only little decease in educational segregation, which is still almost complete. There are some signs that the intergroup marriage rate may be increasing. It could further be argued that the overall impact is likely to be long-lasting; that, in turn, will impact negatively on the attempts to move Northern Ireland to a more peaceful society through processes of forgiveness and reconciliation.

REFERENCES

Cairns, E., & Darby, J. (1998). The conflict in Northern Ireland: Causes, consequences and controls. *American Psychologist, 53*(7), 754-760.

Cairns, E., & Hewstone, M. (2002). Northern Ireland: The impact of peacemaking on intergroup behaviour. In G. Salomon & B. Neov (Eds.), *Peace education: The concept, principles, and practices around the world* (pp. 217-228). Mahwah, NJ: Lawrence Erlbaum Associates.

Cairns, E., & Lewis, C. A. (1999). Collective memories, political violence and mental health in Northern Ireland. *British Journal of Psychology, 90*(1), 25-33.

Cairns, E., Mallett, J., Lewis, C. A., & Wilson, R. (2003). *Who are the victims? Self-assessed victimhood and the Northern Irish conflict.* Belfast: Northern Ireland Statistics & Research Agency.

Cairns, E., & Wilson, R. (1993). Stress, coping and political violence in Northern Ireland. In J. P. Wilson & B. Raphael (Eds.), *International handbook of traumatic stress syndromes* (pp. 365-377). New York: Plenum Press.

Cairns, E., Wilson, R., Gallagher, T., & Trew, K. (1995). Psychology's contribution to understanding conflict in Northern Ireland. *Peace and Conflict: Journal of Peace Psychology, 1*(2), 131-148.

Cairns, E., Wilson, R., McClelland, R., & Gillespie, K. (1989). Improving the validity of the GHQ30 by rescoring for chronicity: A failure to replicate. *Journal of Clinical Psychology, 45*(5), 793-798.

Curran, P. S., Bell, P., Murray, A., Loughrey, G., Roddy, R., & Rocke, L. (1990). Psychological consequences of the Enniskillen bombing. *British Journal of Psychiatry, 156*, 479-482.

Fee, F. (1980). Responses to a behavioural questionnaire of a group of Belfast children. In J. Harbison & J. Harbison (Eds.), *A society under stress: Children and young people in Northern Ireland* (pp. 31-42). Somerset, England: Open Books.

Fee, F. (1983). Educational change in Belfast school children 1975-81. In J. Harbison (Ed.), *Children of the troubles: Children in Northern Ireland* (pp. 44-57). Belfast: Stranmillis College Learning Resources Unit.

Gillespie, K., Duffy, M., Hackmann, A., & Clarke, D. M. (2002). Community-based cognitive therapy in the treatment of post-traumatic stress disorder following the Omagh bomb. *Behaviour Research and Therapy, 40*(4), 345–357.

Hewstone, M., Cairns, E., Voci, A., McLernon, F., Niens, N., & Noor, M. (in press). Intergroup forgiveness and guilt in Northern Ireland: Social psychological dimensions of "The Troubles." In N. R. Branscombe & B. Doosje (Eds.), *Collective guilt: International perspectives.* New York: Cambridge University Press.

Hughes, J., & Carmichael, P. (1998). Community relations in Northern Ireland: Attitudes to contact and segregation. In G. Robinson, D. Heenan, A. M. Gray, & K. Thompson (Eds.), *Social attitudes in Northern Ireland: The seventh report* (p. 8). Aldershot, England: Gower.

Lazarus, R. S., & Folkman, J. (1984). *Stress, appraisal, and coping.* New York: Springer Publishing.

Luce, A., Firth-Cozens, J., Midgley, S., & Burges, C. (2003). After the Omagh bomb: Posttraumatic stress disorder in health service staff. *Journal of Traumatic Stress, 15*(1), 27–30.

McGrath, A., & Wilson, R. (1985, September). *Factors which influence the prevalence and variation of psychological problems in children in Northern Ireland.* Paper presented at the Annual Conference of the Developmental Section of the British Psychological Society, Belfast.

McLernon, F., Cairns, E., Lewis, C. A., & Hewstone, M. (2003). Memories of recent conflict and forgiveness in Northern Ireland. In E. Cairns & M. Roe (Eds.), *The role of memory in ethnic conflict* (pp. 125-143). London: Palgrave Macmillan.

McWhirter, L. (1983, October). *How "troubled" are children in Northern Ireland compared to children who live outside Northern Ireland?* Paper presented at the Annual Conference of the Psychological Society of Ireland, Athlone, Ireland.

McWhirter, L. (1987). Psychological impact of violence in Northern Ireland: Recent research findings and issues. In N. Eisenberg & D. Glasgow (Eds.), *Recent advances in clinical psychology* (pp. 119-146). London: Gower.

Muldoon, O. T., & Trew, K. (2000). Children's experience and adjustment to political conflict in Northern Ireland. *Peace and Conflict: Journal of Peace Psychology, 6,* 157-176.

Muldoon, O. T. (2003). Perceptions of stressful life events in Northern Irish school children: A longitudinal study. *Journal of Child Psychology and Psychiatry, 44*(2), 193-201.

Niens, U., Cairns, E., & Hewstone, M. (2003). Contact and conflict in Northern Ireland. In O. Hargie & D. Dickson (Eds.), *Researching the Troubles: Social science perspectives on the Northern Ireland conflict* (pp. 123-140). London: Mainstream Publishing.

Northern Ireland Life and Times Survey. (2000). Retrieved April 1, 2002, from http://qub.ac.uk/ss/csr/nilt

O'Reilly, D., & Stevenson, M. (2003). Mental health in Northern Ireland: Have "the Troubles" made it worse? *Journal of Epidemiology and Community Health, 57*(7), 488-492.

Shevlin, M., & McGuigan, K. (2003). The long-term psychological impact of Bloody Sunday on families of the victims as measured by The Revised Impact of Event Scale. *British Journal of Clinical Psychology, 42,* 427-432.

Smyth, M. (1995, November). *Limitations on the capacity for citizenship in post cease-fires Northern Ireland.* Paper presented at The Inaugural Meeting of the European Observatory on Citizenship, University College, Cork, Ireland.

Smyth, M. (1998). *Half the battle: Understanding the impact of the troubles on children and young people.* INCORE: Londonderry.

Whyte, J. (1990). *Interpreting Northern Ireland.* Oxford: Clarendon Press.

Voice:
Brave Little Man

Tony Maddox

The boy could have been no more than ten years old, maybe a little younger. But he looked every inch the smart young man. Dressed in a dark suit, white shirt, and dark tie, you could not look at him without breaking into a little smile. It was his big day, and he knew it. He was going to have to be the man of the family.

Why? Because a couple of days before, his dad had been shot through the head as he walked down the street.

It was another terrorist act. Not even especially shocking. Not in Ulster, where the pain threshold had been forced up to unnatural levels.

And so the boy began his walk behind his father's coffin. His mother was overwhelmed by grief. Unable to walk alone, relatives had to support her. His sisters, younger than him, were confused, crying, with more friends and relatives there to hold their hands, and carry them. Throughout the formalities the boy was stony faced, being brave, like his uncles, grandparents, like his dad's friends.

Such a brave little man.

But he wasn't really. He was a little boy who loved his dad. And now his dad was dead, his mum was broken-hearted, and his life would never be the same again.

Address correspondence to: Tony Maddox, 1 CNN Center, Atlanta, GA 30303 USA (E-mail: Tony.Maddox@turner.com).

[Haworth co-indexing entry note]: "Voice: Brave Little Man." Maddox, Tony. Co-published simultaneously in *Journal of Aggression, Maltreatment & Trauma* (The Haworth Maltreatment & Trauma Press, an imprint of The Haworth Press, Inc.) Vol. 9, No. 1/2, 2004; and: *The Trauma of Terrorism: Sharing Knowledge and Shared Care, An International Handbook* (ed: Yael Danieli, Danny Brom, and Joe Sills) The Haworth Maltreatment & Trauma Press, an imprint of The Haworth Press, Inc., 2005.

And then, in a matter of just a few seconds, reality bit. The brave face crumpled into a mass of tears. His grief took voice from the bottom of his lungs and he cried, and cried, and cried.

I witnessed the scene, as I did most of the action during my spell in Northern Ireland, in an edit suite. I had been called in by a producer, who wanted me to take a look at a sequence we were cutting for that night's show.

As the death toll had built over years of conflict, the British Broadcasting Corporation (BBC) had developed a policy of covering the funeral of every victim of "the Troubles." We had editors who had cut hundreds of funerals.

The cameraman and the reporter had latched onto the little boy early in the day, and made sure they stayed with him. Between them, they had also covered far too many funerals.

But once in a while, one slipped through. The emotional armor plating they had developed had a chink, and this lad got through it. There was a stony silence in the edit suite. There were tears in eyes.

A few deep breaths. We discussed which parts of footage we should use, and we used nearly all of it. Then I was called away to some other matter, and although the footage was never far from my mind for the rest of the day, other stuff came along and I did not get back to the package until it went out in the show.

A newsroom when the nightly show is going out is always an interesting place to sit. A bit of low-level chatter, people going quiet when their piece is on, then making fun of another reporter's story. Phones still need to be answered, and there is the odd cry for help from the transmission gallery. It takes a lot to make it go silent.

But the funeral story did. And there were tears. And it was a very short post-programme debrief. No one had much to say.

In the years since I have left Northern Ireland, I have reflected on why this story had the impact it did.

I lived there between 1995 and 1998. I was the head of news and current affairs, one of the "suits." Across radio and TV, there were more than a hundred news professionals, the vast majority from Northern Ireland. Many of them had grown up through "the Troubles," while some of the more experienced members of the staff had spent a career covering them.

They had developed a sceptical attitude, in some cases a profound cynicism, as they were exposed on a daily basis to a grinding conflict, which was fed on a regular diet of death and devastation.

A dark sense of humour developed–it was without question the wittiest newsroom I have ever worked in–and everyone developed coping mechanisms. For many, there was a real life away from work, more so than in other newsrooms I have known.

There was a determination that this was "their" story, and they were going to stick with it. And, by and large, they did.

But it was at a price, and the little boy who was not ready to be a little man, called them on it.

As journalists, camera operators, and editors, we witness suffering and hardship, and often we do not get the chance to look away. But we do move on. There are other stories to tell, and it does not pay to dwell.

For me, and I suspect a few others that day, it was the close-up grief of this child. And tough as it makes our lives, we should give thanks that every once in while, often when we least expect it, some story will get through and will hurt like hell.

Voice:
"So What Is It Like Now That Your Country Is Run by a Terrorist?"

Brandon Hamber

In 1997, I was a visiting fellow at the University of Ulster in Northern Ireland on sabbatical from the Centre for the Study of Violence and Reconciliation in South Africa. At the time, a group of community activists from across the political spectrum living in Derry (or Londonderry, depending on your politics) were preparing for a trip to South Africa. I was asked to give the group a brief orientation. South Africa was a place they had all heard much about with its iconic status of all that is appalling and hopeful in this world wrapped into one, but most knew little of what to expect.

I cannot remember exactly what I said to the group that wintry night. I am sure I spoke about the positive changes in South Africa. I certainly mentioned the Truth and Reconciliation Commission (TRC), a process I was working closely with at the time.

I opened the floor to questions; I expected the usual: "Does Northern Ireland need a De Klerk-like figure?" or "Do you think Northern Ireland needs a truth commission?" But that night was different. No sooner had I asked for

Address correspondence to: Brandon Hamber, 23 University Street, Belfast BT7IFY, Northern Ireland.

[Haworth co-indexing entry note]: "Voice: 'So What Is It Like Now That Your Country Is Run by a Terrorist?'." Hamber, Brandon. Co-published simultaneously in *Journal of Aggression, Maltreatment & Trauma* (The Haworth Maltreatment & Trauma Press, an imprint of The Haworth Press, Inc.) Vol. 9, No. 1/2, 2004; and: *The Trauma of Terrorism: Sharing Knowledge and Shared Care, An International Handbook* (ed: Yael Danieli, Danny Brom, and Joe Sills) The Haworth Maltreatment & Trauma Press, an imprint of The Haworth Press, Inc., 2005.

questions when a man leapt to his feet and blurted: "So what is it like now that your country is run by a terrorist?"

I was astounded. I could not remember when last someone even vaguely equated Mandela with terrorism, a discussion that had long since slipped from the political landscape. The only response I could muster was that I personally felt it was fine. More to the point, and at the risk of dragging up an old cliché, I commented that he needed to remember that one person's terrorist was another person's freedom fighter.

Over the next year, I completed my fellowship and returned to South Africa. When in 2001 I moved back to Northern Ireland, I realized that the question was a preliminary taster of the differences between the two societies.

In Northern Ireland, the word 'terrorist' is frequently heard, even today. The word has gained new life since the events of 11 September 2001 in the US. The "war on terror" has given it global legitimacy once again. Some use it as a qualifier as to why Sinn Féin, the largest elected Republican party in Northern Ireland, with its association with the IRA, should be excluded from the power-sharing government. It is used sometimes to describe anyone from a paramilitary background regardless of his/her current politics or approach. It is rarely used to describe state atrocities.

Conversely, in South Africa "terrorism" is a term that steadily began to die out from 1990 onwards following the peace process. Prior to that, it was ubiquitous. I grew up in a South Africa where the government wanted us to believe that the "terrorist" *rooi/swart gevaar* (red/black danger) was pervasive. The world, including the US government, supported this view well into the 1980s.

This is not to say the liberation forces in South Africa did not commit violent, terror-inducing acts; indeed, there were many. But it remained a glaring irony that, despite their rhetoric, the monopoly over acts of terror resided with the apartheid state. This somewhat obvious contradiction became increasingly evident as the peace process unfolded. This led to the eradication of the word from the South African political lexicon.

Another factor in its disappearance was the TRC. Within its framework, "terrorism" as a word largely proved meaningless. It was at best a descriptor (i.e., it described acts that caused terror). For us, it was only significant to peace-building when it was contextualized and accompanied with explanations as to why certain acts took place by combatants or the state, and if we could use it to learn from the past and prevent future violence.

In Northern Ireland, things are changing. There is little doubt that it is a safer place than before. That said, the peace process lurches between moments of profound progress and hiatus. There has not been a wholesale change of political power as there was in South Africa. The political forces remain fairly evenly balanced. Northern Ireland finds itself facing more of a stalemate than South Africa ever did.

In this context, words such as "terrorism" still have currency. Unlike in South Africa, the past of certain individuals, especially former paramilitaries regardless of their political mandate or contemporary politics, continues to be used as the major reason for halting the peace process. Calling someone a "terrorist" poses as a one-word explanation as to why her/his voice should be silenced.

Clearly, as a descriptive label "terrorism" and how we use it is deeply linked with debates about the legitimate use of violence by the state and combatants. The people of Northern Ireland and the British State still have to reckon with this.

When making peace, a new vocabulary is needed in which past atrocities are not only described in detail in all their abject awfulness, but at the same time the context, causes, and nature of all acts by all players need to be better understood and lessons learned. This is a tall and ambitious order, but living in two violent societies has taught me that genuine peace-building is embedded through efforts at explanation and not just descriptive words that pretend to explain.

On the personal front, from time to time, my wife (who is from Northern Ireland) and I both still catch each other glancing at an empty car on a lonely street or an unattended bag in a public place. Thousands of miles apart we both grew up with the lurking threat of bomb-blasts. But these little fragments of personal history will mean little to our children if we never find the words to articulate and *fully* explain the context in which our seemingly odd little paranoias were born.

The Long-Term Effects of Terrorism in France

Louis Jehel

Alain Brunet

SUMMARY. France has been subjected to terrorism for the past 15 years. Several epidemiological studies have pointed to the high prevalence and severity of PTSD symptoms among the victims. Terrorism-related injuries and time elapsed since the trauma were associated with a negative prognosis. Since 1997, these findings led to the development of a medico-psychological intervention network accompanying the traditional emergency medical team, and giving pre-hospital psychological emergency care to provide secondary prevention. Specialized hospital-based psychiatric services were developed to complement this front-line network, offering an innovative system of care. Studies are needed to examine the effectiveness of this system in reducing trauma-related disorders.

Address correspondence to: Louis Jehel, MD, PhD, (E-mail: louis.jehel@tnn.ap-hop-paris.fr).

Alain Brunet acknowledges the financial support (salary award) of the *Fonds de Recherche en Santé du Québec (FRSQ)*.

[Haworth co-indexing entry note]: "The Long-Term Effects of Terrorism in France." Jehel, Louis, and Alain Brunet. Co-published simultaneously in *Journal of Aggression, Maltreatment & Trauma* (The Haworth Maltreatment & Trauma Press, an imprint of The Haworth Press, Inc.) Vol. 9, No. 1/2, 2004; and:*The Trauma of Terrorism: Sharing Knowledge and Shared Care, An International Handbook* (ed: Yael Danieli, Danny Brom, and Joe Sills) The Haworth Maltreatment & Trauma Press, an imprint of The Haworth Press, Inc., 2005.

KEYWORDS. Acute intervention network, risk factors, PTSD, specialized consultation, professional association

When terrorist acts are committed, politicians and media react above all as a function of the number of dead and wounded. Once the crisis is over and media coverage of the emotional reactions has died down, the fate of the injured falls most often into social indifference. This is even more true for the psychologically wounded who do not have physical lesions and whose suffering remains largely ignored.

Acts of terrorism in France affect mostly people living in the capital, Paris, but also people living in regions agitating for independence from France, in particular the Basque region and Corsica. In these two regions the targets are primarily public buildings and the number of victims has remained small. The psychological consequences of these acts of violence on the people remain unknown.

In France, the real awakening to the importance of post-traumatic problems of the direct victims of terrorism arose from the second wave of terrorist attacks occurring in 1995 in the Paris area. Following these acts, a small number of epidemiological studies showed the importance of post-traumatic after-effects, and the health and political authorities put in place a unique plan of intervention. In this article, we first present the principal epidemiological studies conducted in France on the psychological impact of terrorist acts on the affected victims and, second, the kinds of healthcare and interest group responses currently occurring in France.

EPIDEMIOLOGICAL STUDIES

Since September 15, 1974, when a bomb blast in a downtown Parisian store killed two people and injured 32, about thirty additional attacks have occurred in metropolitan France, injuring 400 and killing 60. The first epidemiological study conducted on this subject, by Dab, Abenhaim, and Salmi (1992), was launched in 1987 and included 254 persons involved in terrorist attacks between 1982 and 1987. The first problem these authors confronted was the definition of victim. To be considered a victim, the person had to be listed in the police registers. The study excluded those injured from the police or army. Between 1982 and 1987, 346 victims of terrorism were listed. A battery of questionnaires accompanied by a consent form was addressed to 326 persons and the response rate was 78% ($N = 254$). In that survey population, 18% of the participants exhibited Post-Traumatic Stress Disorder (PTSD) as defined by the criteria of the DSM-III-R. The principal risk factors identified were the presence of initial physical wounds and the time elapsed since the attack. Serious physical wounds were reported in 40% of this population.

Bouthillon-Heitzmann, Crocq, and Julien (1992) found that among 43 victims of an attack perpetrated in a large Parisian store on September 17, 1986, 13 persons (30%) had PTSD 3 years later. Furthermore, they underlined that in this sample 25% of the victims were unable to return to their previous professional activities. Among the victims, 58% were treated with psychotropic drugs after the attack.

Rouillon and Hautecouverture (2003) studied 286 victims from seven attacks committed between 1995 and 1996 in which 12 persons died and 544 were wounded. The participation rate in this study was very high (86%). More than a third of the victims had had a severe initial physical wound (i.e., burn, fracture, amputation) and half had initially been hospitalized. Two to 3 years after the attacks, two victims out of every three suffered from tinnitus (ringing in the ears). One out of three complained of the effect on his or her physical appearance and its repercussions on relationships. The authors noted that 42% still suffered from bothersome pains in their daily activities, and 25% regularly used analgesics and anti-inflammatories. It was reported that 31% exhibited PTSD and 49% significant depressive symptoms. The relationships with their family, friends and associates were disturbed for 25% of the persons and 10% had separated from their spouses, presumably as a consequence of the attack. This study also confirmed the link between current psychological problems and the severity of initial physical lesions; half of the victims sought psychological help from a doctor or a psychologist.

PROSPECTIVE STUDIES

On December 3, 1996, a gas canister filled with powder and nails exploded on the platform of the RER (commuter train) B line in the Port-Royal station in Paris. The attack killed 4 and wounded 128. For several months, intelligence services had been concerned about the rebuilding of networks giving aid to the GIA (Armed Islamic Group) on French soil. The investigators examined carefully the claims of responsibility arriving via the media but concentrated on the trail of the Algerian GIA. The Vigipirate Plan was reactivated, putting soldiers on the street. Concerning health services, the emergency aid plans were immediately acted upon with, for the first time in France, the implementation of specific units with the CUMPs (Cellule d'Urgence Médico-Psychologique; emergency medico-psychological unit), which will be discussed below.

Upon arrival of the medico-psychological team, we found the wounded to be in a dazed shock, but that some victims had already left in a state of psychomotor agitation. Beyond the immediate reactions of stress that led to the creation of the emergency medico-psychological unit and its official establishment on French territory by the decree of May 1997, we had wanted to follow, through research, the evolution of the psychological problems of the victims of this event.

The main objective of our study (Jehel, Duchet, Paterniti, Consoli, & Guelfi, 2001; Jehel, Paterniti, Brunet, Duchet, & Guelfi, 2003) was to assess the degree of psychopathological repercussions of this deadly attack over the long-term by following longitudinally the direct victims. Another objective was to identify in this population the characteristics constituting the risk factors of developing persistent post-traumatic psychological troubles.

The first step consisted of a psychometric evaluation 6 months after the attack. The second was an evaluation 18 months after the attack, and the third, 32 months after the attack, was proposed to all those who had initially agreed to participate in this survey. Some responded at 32 months without having done so at 18 months. The set of questionnaires and the consent form was sent by courier to the home address initially provided by the victims.

This survey was conducted between May 1997 and June 1999. In it, a diagnosis consistent with DSM-III-R nomenclature was derived from a French language self-report version (Brunet & Boyer, 1995) of the PTSD-Interview (Watson et al., 1991), renamed the autoquestionnaire de l'état de stress post-traumatique (Questionnaire of Posttraumatic Stress; QSPT; Jehel, Duchet, Paterniti, & Louville, 1999). In addition, a French version of the Impact of Event Scale (Horowitz, Wilner, & Alvarez, 1979) was used to derive a PTSD symptom score. Particular interest was paid to the coping style used and the links with the evolution of PTSD symptoms and diagnosis among the survivors of that attack.

According to the QSPT, the percentages of participants showing PTSD at 6 and 18 months were 41% and 34%, respectively. It dropped to 25% at 32 months. For the group evaluated at 18 months, of the 14 participants who had PTSD at 6 months, 8 still had PTSD at 18 months. On the other hand, in this group, among the 16 participants who were unscathed by PTSD at 6 months, 3 met the criteria for PTSD at 18 months.

At 6 months, based on the Impact of Event Scale, there was a trend for persons physically injured during the attack to have a lower PTSD symptom score than the others ($p = 0.09$), particularly if they were hospitalized after the attack for more than 48 hours ($p = 0.04$). At 18 months, these differences were no longer significant. Finally, in addition to PTSD symptomatology, at 18 months 32 participants (50%) had pathological scores of psychological distress (> 3) as measured by the General Health Questionnaire (GHQ-12; Goldberg & Hillier, 1979).

The professional position (management or non-management) and the consumption of psychotropic drugs before the attack predicted the severity of PTSD symptoms measured by the Impact of Event Scale at 32 months (see Table 1). The average PTSD symptom scores were higher at 32 months for those who had a diagnosis of PTSD (based on the QSPT) at 6 months, or who had physical injuries from the attack.

As indicated in Table 2, the analysis by linear regression confirms the importance of pre-attack use of psychotropic drugs, the professional position, and the presence of physical injuries from the attack as independent variables explicative of the intensity of PTSD symptoms at 32 months in this population.

We sought to examine the preferred coping styles of the victims to find out whether this preference could act as a predictor of the development of PTSD. Indeed, a strong correlation appeared between an emotion-centered coping style (as opposed to the problem-solving coping style) and PTSD symptom score. However, it appears that this coping style is a marker of the victim's emotional state rather than a trait; when it is adjusted for anxiety level, the coping style no longer has any value for predicting PTSD symptoms (Jehel et al., 2003).

HEALTH SERVICES IN FRANCE

The occurrence of several terrorist attacks in France in 1995 and 1996 mobilized the political authorities as well as mental health professionals. Political decision-makers and the media thus recognized the existence of psychological injuries. The need to add an emergency medico-psychological unit (CUMP) to the already existing emergency medico-surgical aid became clear, just as it had long been military practice to have psychiatrists with their personnel (Crocq, Sailhan, & Barrois, 1983). A first circular, dated May 28, 1997, laid the foundations for a national emergency medico-psychological intervention network in the event of catastrophe. This network was reinforced by the circular of May 20, 2003, which increased to 34, from the initial 7, the number of permanent intervention teams on French territory. These units were activated by the well-established emergency medical aid service intervening outside hospitals at the site of catastrophes (called the SAMU). Each CUMP team is made up of a psychiatrist, a psychologist, and nurses. Once the victims are brought back to the hospital, emergency hospital psychiatric teams then take over for these teams (for more details, see Garnier, Louville, & Crocq, 1997).

TABLE 1. Relation Between Socio-Demographic Characteristics, Clinical Variables, and Severity of PTSD Symptoms 32 Months After a Terrorist Attack (N = 32)

	PTSD Symptom Score**			
	M *(SD)*	*t*-test	df	*p*-value
Gender Male Female	29.0 (30.1) 35.1 (28.4)	0.59	30	0.56
Professional Position Management Other	13.1 (20.0) 43.4 (28.6)	3.42	28	0.002
Marital Status Single/Other Living in Couple	24.4 (17.0) 34.5 (32.4)	1.14	27	0.26
Physical Injuries* No Yes	23.1 (21.1) 37.6 (32.6)	1.53	30	0.14
Pre-Attack Psychotropic Use No Yes	18.6 (21.4) 60.4 (22.5)	5.05	30	0.001
PTSD at 6 Months§ No Yes	25.9 (26.7) 47.1 (29.0)	1.90	23	0.07

*Physical injuries from the terrorist attack.
**Impact of Event Scale (Horowitz et al., 1979).
§Measured by the QSPT (Jehel et al., 1999); six values missing for this variable.

Over the last 2 years, specialized consultations in caring for psychological traumas have been developed and structured in several hospitals in France. Those specialized consultations care for victims of terrorist acts, but also for migrant populations (e.g., refugees) victimized in their country of origin, as well as for victims of sexual assault and motor vehicle accident victims. This specialized consultation team is composed of nurses, social workers, psychologists and psychiatrists. A close collaboration has developed between the judiciary system, the police and the associations helping victims of terrorism.

FRENCH ASSOCIATIONS HELPING VICTIMS OF TERRORISM

Parallel to the official health services network, a strong association network has developed in France since 1986, in particular with SOS attentats (SOS Attack), an association created by victims for victims. A network of aid-to-victim professionals was also built, federated into the Institut national d'aide aux

TABLE 2. Stepwise Linear Regression Predicting the Intensity of PTSD Symptoms 32 Months After a Terrorist Attack (N = 32)

	Adjusted R^2	R^2	F	df	p<	F change p-value	Step 1 β	Step 2 β	Step 3 β
Step 1 Psychotropic Use*	0.41		21.5	1	0.001		0.66	0.54	0.45
Step 2 Professional Position**	0.48	0.07	14.3	2	0.001	0.04		−0.31	−0.44
Step 3 Physical Injuries*§	0.56	0.08	13.1	3	0.001	0.02			0.32

*Psychotropic drug use and injuries: 1 = yes, 0 = no.
**Professional Position: 1 = management, 0 = non-management.
§ Physical injuries from the attack.

victimes et de mediation *or* INAVEM (National Institute of Aid to Victims and of Mediation). The purpose of this Institute is to coordinate the social and judicial support for all victims. These associations actively participated in the creation of the Fonds de garantie des victimes (Victims Guarantee Fund). The fund was created on July 6, 1990 to help the victims of terrorist acts and other crimes. Written applications for compensation in case of crime are sent to the nearest Commission d'indemnisation des victimes d'infractions, CIVI (Crime Victims Compensation Board). These boards sit at each Tribunal de grande instance (Departmental Courts; France is divided into departments). The Victims Guarantee Fund compensates all victims, regardless of nationality, for acts of terrorism occurring in France starting January 1, 1985. For acts of terrorism occurring abroad, the guarantee fund compensates only victims of French nationality. The Procureur de la république (State Prosecutor) in France or the diplomatic or consular authority abroad informs the Guarantee Fund of an attack and of the victims' identities. In such a case, the Guarantee Fund contacts the victims directly to provide for their compensation. Any person who feels that she or he has been the victim of an act of terrorism can send an application for compensation to the Guarantee Fund. If the requisite conditions are met, the compensation covers the physical damages of the injured person and, for deceased persons, moral and economic damages of the successors in title. This is done within an allotted time and in accordance with an out-of-court procedure stipulated by law.

CONCLUSION

The fact that terrorism can yield posttraumatic stress symptoms and disorders has been increasingly recognized and accepted in France over the last 10 years.

The increasing awareness of the pathological consequences of terrorist acts in France since 1995 has mobilized the political and social-medical systems to develop new specialized services for the victims of such acts. During that period, a growing scientific literature has emerged. The unique model of the CUMP (emergency medico-psychological units) developed in France appears to be largely used and appreciated by the population. Our goal for the future will be to validate scientifically the usefulness of such an approach, which has become increasingly sought in the aftermath of potentially traumatic situations.

REFERENCES

Abenhaim, L., Dab, W., & Salmi, L.R. (1992). Study of civilian victims of terrorist attacks (France 1982-87). *Journal of Clinical Epidemiology, 45,* 103-109.

Bouthillon-Heitzmann, P., Crocq, L., & Julien, H. (1992). Stress immédiat et séquelles psychiques chez les victimes d'attentats terroristes [Immediate stress and psychic sequelae among victims of a terrorist attack]. *Psychologie Médicale, 24,* 465-470.

Brunet, A., & Boyer, R. (1995, May). *Évaluation de la version française auto-administrée du PTSD-i* [Evaluation of the French self-administered version of the PTSD-i]. Paper presented at the IVth European Conference on Traumatic Stress, Paris.

Crocq, L., Sailhan, M., & Barrois, C. (1983). Névroses traumatiques (névroses d'effroi, névroses de guerre) [Traumatic Neuroses (Fright neuroses, war neuroses)]. *Encyclopédie Medico-chirurgicale.* Éditions techniques, Paris.

Garnier H., Louville, P., & Crocq, L. (1997). Integration of a psychiatric team to emergency care in catastrophe situation. *Presse Médicale, May 24, 26(17),* 814-817.

Goldberg, D. P., & Hillier, V. F. (1979). A scale version of the General Health Questionnaire. *Psychological Medicine, 9,* 139-145.

Horowitz, M. J., Wilner, N., & Alvarez, W. (1979). The Impact of Event Scale: A measure of subjective distress. *Psychosomatic Medicine, 41,* 209-218.

Jehel, L., Duchet, C., Paterniti, S., Consoli, S. M., & Guelfi, J. D. (2001). Étude prospective de l'état de stress post-traumatique parmi des victimes d'un attentat terroriste [Prospective study of PTSD among vicitms of a terrorist act]. *L'Encéphale, XXVII,* 393-400.

Jehel, L., Paterniti, S., Brunet, A., Duchet, C., & Guelfi, J. D. (2003). Prediction of the occurrence and intensity of Posttraumatic Stress Disorder in victims 32 months after bomb attack. *European Psychiatry, 18,* 172-176.

Jehel, L., Duchet, C., Paterniti, S., & Louville, P. (1999). Construction et étude de validité d'un autoquestionnaire de l'état de stress post-traumatique issu du PTSD-Interview: le QSPT [Development and validation of a self-report questionnaire for PTSD derived from the PTSD-i: the QSPT]. *Revue Française de Psychiatrie et de Psychologie Médicale, 24,* 203-205.

Watson, C. G., Juba, M. P., Manifold, V., Kucala, T., Anderson, P. E. D. et al. (1991). The PTSD Interview: Rationale, description, reliability, and concurrent validity of a DSM-III based technique. *Journal of Clinical Psychology, 47,* 179-188

Rouillon, F., & Hautecouverture, S. (2003, March 20). Communication orale [Oral presentation]. *Journée de Psychotraumatisme de l'AP-HP,* Paris, France.

Psychological Effects of Terrorist Attacks in Algeria

Noureddine Khaled

SUMMARY. Since 1990, Algerians have suffered from the effects of radical Islamist terrorism. The official estimate of 150,000 massacred terrorism victims seems low and includes only direct victims. Epidemiological research conducted in 1999-2000 found that the Algerian population has suffered enormously. A random sample of the adult population showed 91.9 percent of these adults were victims of a traumatic event. Of those, 39.5 percent suffered from posttraumatic stress disorder, 23.3 percent from a mood disorder (depression), 38.5 percent from an anxiety disorder (e.g., panic disorder or phobia), and 8.7 percent from somatoform disorder. Healing would necessitate a concerted, collaborative effort, with much greater resources and leadership provided by governmental and civil institutions.

KEYWORDS. Terrorism, psychological effects, mental health, traumatic events, psychiatric disorders, psychosocial interventions

Address correspondence to: Noureddine Khaled, PhD, 27, Rue du boulodrome, Dely Ibrahim, 16320 Algiers, Algeria (E-mail: sarp@wissal.dz) or (nourkhaled@hotmail.com).

The content of this article is largely inspired by Ait Sidhoum, M. A., Arar, F., Bouatta, C., Khaled, N., & El Masri, M. (2002). Terrorism, traumatic events and mental health in Algeria. In Joop De Jong (Ed.), *Trauma, war and violence. Public mental health in socio-cultural context*. New York: Kluwer Academic/Plenum Publishers.

[Haworth co-indexing entry note]: "Psychological Effects of Terrorist Attacks in Algeria." Khaled, Noureddine. Co-published simultaneously in *Journal of Aggression, Maltreatment & Trauma* (The Haworth Maltreatment & Trauma Press, an imprint of The Haworth Press, Inc.) Vol. 9, No. 1/2, 2004; and: *The Trauma of Terrorism: Sharing Knowledge and Shared Care, An International Handbook* (ed: Yael Danieli, Danny Brom, and Joe Sills) The Haworth Maltreatment & Trauma Press, an imprint of The Haworth Press, Inc., 2005.

HISTORICAL CONTEXT

In 1962, after a long struggle for liberation, Algeria gained its independence from France, which had colonized the country for 130 years. Since then it has been governed by the National Liberation Front (FLN), with a succession of elected presidents, most of whom were colonels during the war of liberation. The government followed a one-party socialist system until 1988, when the riots in Algiers and the constitutional referendum of 1989 opened the way to a multiparty system. Since then, many political parties with different orientations have appeared and disappeared. Three main poles characterize Algerian politics. The first is the conservative pole, represented by the old party FLN and the recently-formed RND (National Democratic Assembling). They still hold power and seek Arabization of culture and education and moderate Islamization of the country. The second is the Islamic pole, represented by a range of parties seeking the creation of a radical Islamic state in Algeria: the FIS (Islamic Front for Salvation), Hammas, and Nahdha. Finally, the democratic pole, which is represented mainly by FFS (Socialist Front Forces) and RCD (Assembling for Culture and Democracy), calls for a democratic civil society.

A century and a half of French colonial rule has created an ambivalent, strongly polarized relationship with the West and Western culture and has made French culture an essential component of the identity and social structure. Paradoxically, Algerian nationalism has been fostered by the confrontation with French colonial rule and has been based on Islamic concepts and relations with a wider Arab-Islamic world. In Algeria, there are two conflicting philosophies of society: the democratic, which recommends a secular state, opening to the modern world, political pluralism, and recognition of women's rights; and the Islamic and theocratic, which favors a return to the Koran and to Islam's ancestral values, which rejects laicity, democracy, and women's rights.

On October 5, 1988, riots started in Algiers. They rapidly spread to other parts of the capital and to other cities, such as Oran and Annaba, largely surpassing the capacities of the security forces to stop the protests. Two indicators foreshadowed the importance of this popular revolt: the state of emergency declared six days before the first riots and the building up of security forces to disperse the crowds and stop the destruction and looting of public institutions. According to official estimates, this intervention resulted in 159 deaths and 3,500 arrests. The impact of the events of October 1988 was high both at the political and the social level. First, the revolt opened the political field to a multiparty system, marking the end of FLN supremacy. Second, it allowed a critical review of the socialist ideology so far considered a taboo. These changes have been explicitly introduced in the 1989 constitution. It is important to underline that this new constitution clearly prohibits creating a political party on the basis of religion, ethnicity or language.

The Formation of the First Armed Islamic Group. Islamic fundamentalists began their activities well before October 1988, when they focused on controlling the mosques and building new ones where they could ensure the loyalty of *imams* of their choice. With the arrival of the Islamists in Iran, they started reproaching their chiefs for focusing a lot more on preaching in the mosques than on action (Rouadjia, 1991). Mustapha Bouyali was the first to start by creating in 1982 his own group, the Armed Islamic Algerian Movement (MAIA). MAIA committed itself to using force against security forces, attacking several targets until Bouyali himself was killed during an exchange of fire with the security forces in 1987. On June 20, 1987, 202 members, thought to belong to Bouyali's group, were brought to trial. Three weeks later, four of them were sentenced to death, four to life sentences, and seven to 20 years of criminal imprisonment.

Evolution of Events in Algeria from 1988 to 1992. The period after October 1988 was marked by a rapid evolution in the Algerian political situation. In June 1990, FIS won 55 percent of the vote by utilizing, some felt, intimidation and pressure. In December 1991, the first general elections were held in the context of a multiparty system, with the FIS winning 45 percent of seats in Parliament. In January 1992, Parliament was dissolved, President Chadli resigned, and a five member High State Council was appointed. In March 1992, the Supreme Court ordered the FIS dissolved. Three months later, President Boudiaf was assassinated.

Evolution of Terrorist Activities. According to the report of the United Nations Panel in June 1998, published in the daily newspaper *El Watan* on September 17, 1998, the terrorist movement went through four stages differentiated by the nature of objectives targeted by the terrorist attacks. In the first stage, the FIS and its popular armed groups targeted only the security forces and public service employees, i.e., all persons representing the authority of the State. Partially, it was the absence of a strong legitimate state that made a segment of the population lean toward supporting fundamentalism. The FIS, drawing from its divine legitimacy, had the advantage of attracting a large number of unsatisfied people. FIS gave them the hope of breaking with a painful past, which was replaced with the illusion of a just future.

In the second stage, the FIS considered it necessary to attack every person who attempted to encourage the population to take a critical stand toward the archaic maneuvers used to manipulate the crowds emotionally. Intellectuals were especially targeted by the terrorists. Sometimes youngsters no older than 15 were recruited to participate in the assassination of a large number of intellectuals, scientists, media professionals or simply citizens who had a certain credibility among the population and who refused to advocate religious fundamentalism. The expansion of organized violence gradually led to spreading doubt concerning the validity of the fundamentalist cause and to the first breaks in popular support for it.

The third stage was the effort to destroy the country's infrastructure. They used all available means to subjugate the State, even if they had to destroy the whole country and its economic and social structures (bridges, vehicles, factories, schools, local administration settings, and healthcare facilities).

The impact of this massive destruction on the citizens, whose lives became impossible, seriously harmed the fundamentalist movement. The popular support for the terrorists began to decline. This made the toughest of them angry, and they thus decided to launch the first "punishing operations" against some areas. These were to serve as examples against any failure in the support that the population was expected to provide. To justify these operations and to involve the population, they promulgated a *fatwa* that considered any person showing resistance to them as a renegade, committing a serious fault with regard to religion. However, contrary to the terrorists' expectations, the results of these operations led to the fourth phase of massive killings.

The inhabitants of some isolated areas were really frightened when the first population massacres occurred. Those who had the means began leaving their homes, while others asked public authorities to give them arms so they could defend themselves. In another context, conflicts took place between different armed groups and their political representatives. The reduction of popular support was sometimes interpreted as a result of help to a rival group. Consequently, the punishing operations increased and took new forms. With the rapid decline of support for the fundamentalist groups, the scope of this reactive punishment broadened. The number of collective massacres counted by the National Observatory of Human Rights (ONDH) was 299 through 1996 (cited in Benyoub, 1999).

These massacres claimed the lives of hundreds of people at a time. The brutality of killing and mutilations, the secretly told incidents of rape, and the horror of children having witnessed the killing of their own parents are beyond description. In all massacres, some maimed people and children were left alive to tell the stories and deliver the message that this will be the punishment of those who betray.

Through the situation described above, we can see that the type of violence in Algeria is not the same as that in Israel, where there is an armed conflict between two communities with disproportionate means at war. It is also not the same as in New York on September 11, 2001, where attacks came from abroad by an Islamist organization which considers the USA a sworn enemy of Islam, due, in part, to its unconditional support of Israel. In Algeria, Islamist terrorism has penetrated into the society, growing insidiously in the institutions of the Republic: in the schools, universities, mosques, and also in families. It lived on the economic misery of the population, on identity crises of youth who have no future prospects, and on the general dissatisfaction of the population toward corrupt and incompetent people in power.

The similarities in all these kinds of violence, whatever the country or the context, are feelings of deep injustice and the despair of those who involve themselves in the terrorist organizations to make themselves human bombs within extremists' grasp executing irretrievable and unjustifiable acts.

THE IMPACT OF THE TRAGEDY: SOME EPIDEMIOLOGICAL RESEARCH RESULTS

This section assesses the impact of the tragedy by drawing upon the results of an epidemiological survey conducted with a team from the Algerian Society for Research in Psychology (SARP; Khaled, 2000). The survey sampled two representative areas in the department of Algiers, Sidi Moussa and Dely Ibrahim. The total sample of 652 was equally divided, with 50 percent from the area of Sidi Moussa and the other 50 percent from Dely Ibrahim. Two thousand addresses were randomly selected from local government lists of the area. Only 42 percent of people on the list of addresses were approached because the names of people on the remainder of the addresses did not match with the names of the persons living there. Of the 850 persons approached, 652 (76.7 percent) agreed to participate.

Sidi Moussa is a semi-rural area located 20 kilometres southeast of Algiers. It has lived through a decade of permanent terrorism and in 1996 was a theatre of many extreme violent events, in which more than 400 persons were massacred during the night. Dely Ibrahim is a suburban district of Algiers that was not very affected by terrorism, although the population lived during the "black decade" with the fright and the stress of terrorism, as did other places in Algeria.

Exposure to Traumatic Situations. The main themes in exposure to traumatic stress were death, threat, and loss (see Table 1). Nearly all respondents reported deaths or murders. In Sidi Moussa, 73 percent of the respondents reported the death of a family member or a friend, and 35.5 percent actually witnessed the killing of strangers. Although the situation was less dramatic in Dely Ibrahim, the corresponding figures are 62.5 percent and 20 percent. Considering the total number of deaths, 38.5 percent of those reported deaths in Dely Ibrahim and 55.5 percent in Sidi Moussa were attributed to the violence.

TABLE 1. Exposure to Trauma (Epidemiological Survey, SARP, 1999-2001)

	Sidi Moussa (n = 326) Percent exposed			Dely Ibrahim (n = 326) Percent exposed		
	Male	Female	*Total*	Male	Female	*Total*
Loss and deprivation:						
Lack of food or water	30	40	*35.0*	14	11	*12.5*
Ill health	20	29	*24.5*	5	8	*6.5*
Lack of shelter	23	18	*20.5*	8	14	*11.0*
Lost house or land	16	9	*12.5*	2	3	*2.5*
Lost job or employment	32	11	*21.5*	17	19	*18.0*
Lost means of livelihood	11	6	*8.5*	5	2	*3.5*
Lost personal belongings	16	15	*15.5*	4	5	*4.5*
Imprisonment and torture:						
Imprisonment	15	1	*8.0*	8	1	*4.5*
Torture	11	2	*6.5*	9	1	*5.0*
Witnessed torture	11	4	*7.5*	11	6	*8.5*
Solitary confinement	6	2	*4.0*	7	0	*3.5*
Death:						
Death of family member or friend	53	44	*48.5*	53	48	*50.5*
Murder of family member or friend	31	18	*24.5*	19	5	*12.0*
Witnessed murder of strangers	47	24	*35.5*	31	9	*20.0*
Threatening situations:						
Caught in combat situation	56	60	*58.0*	30	23	*26.5*
Witnessed curfew searching	78	83	*80.5*	52	32	*42.0*
Was close to death	65	63	*64.0*	46	27	*36.5*
Serious injury	20	11	*15.5*	22	12	*17.0*
Separation from family:						
Separated from family	18	7	*12.5*	10	6	*8.0*
Witnessed other events	45	40	*42.5*	28	17	*22.5*

Grief over the loss of human lives is prevalent everywhere. This survey of sampled households points to the fact that three of four households in Sidi Moussa, and two of three in Dely Ibrahim, suffered the tragic loss of at least one family member or close friend.

Exposure to threatening situations, like witnessing massacres and terrorist attacks (i.e., caught in combat situation), witnessing the murder of people, or the sight of decapitated and mutilated bodies (close to death), was reported by nearly everyone in Sidi Moussa and more than two of three of the respondents in Dely Ibrahim.

Regarding the loss of material resources, in Sidi Moussa 12.5 percent of the respondents reported loss of their house, 8.5 percent loss of source of livelihood (shops, stocks, jobs) and 15.5 percent loss of personal belongings. It is interesting to note that Dely Ibrahim, which was considered a relatively safe town spared from massacres, also witnessed high rates of losses and life-threatening events.

Psychological Distress. The survey used the SCL-90-R (Derogatis, 1977), a psychological assessment instrument that measures the degree of current psychological distress. Results show that the degree of distress was high, with 38 percent of residents in Sidi Moussa and 27 percent in Dely Ibrahim scoring high on the Global Severity Index (GSI, assessing degree of distress). Distress was especially high in women and those of younger age. Most at risk were people exposed to traumatic separations from their family or to threatening situations and those deprived of basic resources.

The characteristic responses of women in this sample were feelings of sadness, loneliness, and hopelessness and crying easily, accompanied by self-blame and feelings of guilt. Males complained very frequently of sleeping problems, poor concentration, nervousness and irritability, and inability to trust others. Multiple somatic symptoms were frequent in both males and females.

The Prevalence of DSM-IV Psychiatric Disorders. The survey used an adapted Arabic translation of the CIDI 2.1 (Composite International Diagnostic Interview; World Health Organization, 1993) to measure the lifetime prevalence of psychiatric disorders using the DSM-IV criteria (American Psychiatric Association, 1994). The results are alarming (De Jong et al., 2001; Khaled et al., 2001).

There is an evident high lifetime prevalence of all disorders, especially PTSD and major depressive disorder. Phobias are very prevalent, with high rates of morbid fears of all sorts: natural, blood, situational (included in Specific Phobic Disorder). This was especially evident in young females exposed to threatening situations (see Table 2). The high prevalence of PTSD reflects the wide exposure to many types of traumatic situations. In general, females had higher lifetime prevalence of most disorders than males. Widows, divorced and separated women had even higher rates.

Given the size of the population in both areas, one can imagine the enormity of the problem faced by mental health workers. In Sidi Moussa alone, with a population of 300,000 people, there would be more than 40,000 women who suffered from PTSD and 21,000 from a major depressive disorder. Further calculations, taking co-morbidity into consideration, point to the fact that at any time, around 20,000 women in Sidi Moussa would have a current diagnosis of PTSD, and half of them would have an associated major depressive disorder. These two disorders, usually chronic or recurrent, have been shown to be asso-

TABLE 2. Prevalence of DSM-IV Psychiatric Disorders (Epidemiological Survey, SARP, Algeria, 1999-2000)

DSM IV diagnosis	Sidi Moussa			Dely Ibrahim		
	Male	*Female*	*Total*	*Male*	*Female*	*Total*
Posttraumatic Stress Disorder	41	58	**48.5**	22	33	**27.5**
Major Depression	23	36	**29.5**	13	23	**18.0**
Specific Phobic Disorder	22	44	**31.5**	17	37	**27.0**
Social Phobia	4	7	**5.5**	2	2	**2.0**
Agoraphobia	4	20	**12.0**	4	9	**6.5**
Panic Disorder	5	6	**5.5**	1	3	**2.0**
Generalized Anxiety Disorder	1	1	**1.0**	1	1	**1.0**
Obsessive Compulsive Disorder	1	3	**2.0**	1	5	**3.0**
Any somatoform disorder	5	22	**13.5**	3	6	**4.5**

ciated with a high degree of distress and disability, making the sufferers more vulnerable to further loss and suffering (Wells et al., 1989). The association between depression and grief was first noticed by Freud (1895). The rates described here exceed most rates reported in population studies on depression (Robins & Regier, 1991) but are comparable to rates reported for some third world countries that went through civil wars or conflicts (Weissman et al., 1996).

PSYCHOSOCIAL AND SOCIAL INTERVENTIONS
PROVIDED BY THE SIDI MOUSSA CENTER (CAP)

The Centre d'Aide Psychologique aux victimes (CAP) in Sidi Moussa was created in an area deeply affected by violence. This area witnessed two of the very first and largest scale massacres. In Ben Talha, more than 400 people were murdered in only one day. This massacre had a profound effect on the social structure and life in general. In Rais, another village in Sidi Moussa, a second massacre that was widely publicized for the brutality of the killings and mutilations took place. In addition to these massacres, for 10 long years, this area has been under constant threat of assassinations, kidnappings, and intimidation. Although many families have escaped from Sidi Moussa, the majority remained, enduring threats and losses simply because they had no other place to go.

At the Center, treatment is provided free of charge for all clients, the majority of whom have lost one or more family members. Most of them are very poor and deprived of resources. They have lost their homes, land, and work because they had to leave for safer areas or because of the destruction of the infrastructure. Many of the families have lost the father or breadwinner. The majority of the clients are therefore women and children of rural or semi-rural origin, many of whom are illiterate or have only limited education. Since its opening in April 2000, the Center has received some 1,000 individual patients; of those patients, 130 asked for many kinds of help at the same time (social, medical, psychological and legal advice), 590 for social help, and 275 for specific psychological therapy. Four hundred and five persons, 204 children or adolescents and 201 adults (131 women and 70 men), have received psychotherapy.

The clients are usually aware of the relation between their symptoms and the events they experienced during the crisis. The Center provides a wide variety of interventions at the individual, group, and family levels. Children and adolescent groups usually employ an art therapy or psychodrama approach. Therapy groups for women allow them to support each other and exchange experience and information. Until now, individual consultation has been predominant. However, there is a need and tendency to use group and family interventions in order to be able to deal with the size and nature of the problems presented.

In many cases, the therapists realize the need for social interventions. Since May 2000, a large proportion of the clients (720) have asked for and received social assistance. The problems presented to the social worker are:

- Administrative problems, usually presented by women with little education, who have to deal with administrative and legal offices in order to receive assistance.
- Children who are dismissed from schools after having failed.
- Material needs and financial problems, such as the lack of jobs or homes. In these cases, the social worker orients and accompanies the clients to the appropriate organizations and associations.
- Undiagnosed or untreated medical illnesses. Here, the social worker refers clients to hospitals or other organizations for treatment. She has developed an outreach service (home visits and networking) in which she visits families known to have problems, such as child abuse, and patients needing medical or therapeutic care.

Usually the problem is presented to therapists as a family problem. Table 3 shows different motives for consulting a psychologist. For children, 53 percent cited difficulties at school with memory and language disorders and 25 percent cited anxiety and fear with nightmares. These symptoms are, for the

TABLE 3. Motive for Consultation (SARP, CAP, 2000-2003)

Motives/age	Children and adolescents N %		Adults N %		TOTAL N %	
Anxiety, fear, insecurity	50	25	120	60	170	42
School difficulty	90	44	0	0	90	22
Memory and language disorders	19	9	8	4	27	7
Psychiatric disorders	3	1	20	10	23	6
Somatic pains	2	1	21	10	23	6
Depression	1	1	20	10	21	5
Mental retardation	11	5	2	1	13	3
Jealousy	9	4	2	1	11	3
Timidity	6	3	2	1	8	2
Family problems	7	3	0	0	7	2
Enuresis	5	2	0	0	5	1
Insomnia, nightmares	1	1	3	1	4	1
Motor instability	0	0	3	1	3	1
TOTAL	204		201		405	

most part, related to the traumatic events. For adults, we can mention first anxiety, fears, and feelings of insecurity (60 percent) and secondly mood disorders, depression, and multiple somatic pains and aches.

The Center is developing its network of partners in the educational, health, and legal systems. We realized that such a network is not only a complementary but also an integral part of the service. The Center is compiling an inventory of associations and organizations that can be approached for awareness raising, training, and collaboration.

CONCLUSION

Algeria is witnessing a bloody civil and political conflict. The rise and decline of fundamentalism has been associated with a severe fragmentation of the infrastructure of the country and the social values and individual well-being of its inhabitants. The reactions at different levels form a vicious cycle in which loss and grief lead to vulnerability and further loss. Communities, families, and individuals are entangled in the meshes of conflict and violence, and gravitate down the scale of well-being to a state of poverty, misery, and depression.

The loss of resources, sense of insecurity, and guilt-ridden grief characterize the psychological effects on the population. Both males and females of all age groups have shown measurable psychological distress. The effect of the violence on the social structure and functioning of Algerian society is immense: lack of trust, feelings of hopelessness, and decline in social cohesion and support threaten to become the long-term after-effects of the crisis on the population. Recently, mental health professionals have directed their attention to the impact of the tragedy. Classical psychodynamic and individual-oriented interventions proved unsuccessful in the face of the size and nature of suffering and mental illness in the exposed communities. The complexity and extent of exposure and reactions make clear that interventions with communities affected by terrorism cannot be the responsibility of any single agency. There is a need for a concerted and collaborative effort from all concerned.

The reaction of the governmental and civil institutions to the impact of this tragedy has been disoriented and scattered and has suffered from lack of resources and coordination. SARP, in collaboration with Transcultural Psychosocial Organization (TPO), has launched a mental health program to deal with the consequences of trauma at the community, family, and individual levels. Starting from its own resources of professionals, training, research and clinical interventions, and drawing upon potential resources in the professional and public communities in Algeria, SARP has been able to initiate a model that is acceptable to other professionals and institutions requiring services. Both the change in conceptualization and modes of intervention and the increasing demands pose a challenge to the professionals of SARP; on the one hand, they aim at expanding and disseminating the model through training and sensitization, and on the other, they realize the need to evaluate and monitor the interventions that were introduced and increase their efficacy.

REFERENCES

Ait Sidhoum, M. A., Arar, F., Bouatta, C., Khaled, N., & El Masri, M. (2002). Terrorism, traumatic events and mental health in Algeria. In J. De Jong (Ed.), *Trauma, war and violence. Public mental health in socio-cultural context.* New York: Kluwer Academic/Plenum Publishers.

American Psychiatric Association. (1994). *Diagnostic and statistical manual of mental disorders* (4th ed.). Washington, DC: Author.

Benyoub, R. (1999). *Annuaire politique de l'Algérie* [Political yearbook of Algeria]. Alger: Entreprise Nationale des Arts Graphiques.

De Jong, J. T. V. M., Komproe, I. H., Van Ommeren, M., El Masri, M., Mesfin, A., Khaled, N. et al. (2001). Lifetime events and post-traumatic stress disorder in four post-conflict settings. *Journal of the American Medical Association, 286*(5), 555-562.

Derogatis, L. R. (1977). *The SCL-90 manual.* Baltimore: Johns Hopkins University School of Medicine.

Freud, S. (1895). General theory on neuroses. In A. Freud (Ed.), The standard edition of the complete psychological works of Sigmund Freud. London: Hogarth Press.

Khaled, N. (2000). Recherche-action sur la santé mentale d'une population longtemps exposée aux événements traumatiques: Considérations méthodologiques et résultats de terrain [Action research on the mental health of a population exposed to the traumatic long-term events: Methodological considerations and field results]. *Psychologie SARP, 8,* 37-51.

Khaled, N., Bouatta, C., Arar, F., El Masri, M., Boukhaf, M., Tadjine, S. et al. (2001). Evénements traumatiques et santé mentale. Résultats d'une recherche épidémiologique [Traumatic events and mental health: Results of epidemiological research]. *Psychologie SARP, 9,* 11-139.

Robins, L. N., & Regier, D. A. (1991). *Psychiatric disorders in America: The epidemiologic catchment area study.* New York: The Free Press.

Rouadjia, A. (1991). *Les frères et la mosquée* [The brothers and the mosque]. Alger: Bouchene.

Wells, K., Steward, A., Hays, R., Burnam, A., Rogers, W., Daniels, M. et al. (1989). The functioning and well-being of depressed patients: Results from the Medical Outcomes Study. *Journal of the American Medical Association, 262,* 914-919.

Weissman, M. M., Bland, R. C., Canino, G. J., Faravelli, C., Greenwald, S., Hwu, H. G. et al. (1996). Cross-national epidemiology of major depression and bipolar disorder. *Journal of the American Medical Association, 276,* 293-299.

World Health Organization. (1993). *Composite International Diagnostic Interview.* Geneva: Author.

Voice:
Nadia, a Victim/Survivor
of a Terrorist Massacre
# of Her Family in Algeria

Noureddine Khaled

I am a 24-year-old woman, who comes from a family of 12 persons who lived in a semi-rural area about 50 km southwest of Algiers, in Algeria. I have two married sisters, five younger sisters, and a five-year-old brother.

In 1996, terrorists, many of them our neighbors, asked my father to give them two of his daughters (myself and my sister) to marry. My father flatly refused. To the terrorists, his refusal was a betrayal of their cause.

On a winter's dark night, a group of six terrorists came and attacked my family. They massacred all the adults, my father, my mother, and my grandmother. I ran away with my sisters in this dark night calling for help, forgetting my brother who was sleeping at home. The terrorists wanted to pursue us, but one of them ordered them to go off. Later, my brother joined us with a neighbor. He was safe and sound, but seemed shocked and had blood stains all over his body.

We were all shocked by this big violence. We felt totally confused; we did not know what to do and where to go. We were only sure that we did not want

Address correspondence to: Noureddine Khaled, PhD, 27, Rue du boulodrome, Dely Ibrahim, 16320 Algiers, Algeria (E-mail: sarp@wissal.dz or nourkhaled@hotmail.com).

[Haworth co-indexing entry note]: "Voice: Nadia, a Victim/Survivor of a Terrorist Massacre of Her Family in Algeria." Khaled, Noureddine. Co-published simultaneously in *Journal of Aggression, Maltreatment & Trauma* (The Haworth Maltreatment & Trauma Press, an imprint of The Haworth Press, Inc.) Vol. 9, No. 1/2, 2004; and: *The Trauma of Terrorism: Sharing Knowledge and Shared Care, An International Handbook* (ed: Yael Danieli, Danny Brom, and Joe Sills) The Haworth Maltreatment & Trauma Press, an imprint of The Haworth Press, Inc., 2005.

to stay in this accursed house. With my young brother and my five sisters, we were left on our own. We ran away from the family home and wandered about the streets, finding temporary refuge in many public-lodging centers. Our relatives (uncles and married sisters) stayed aloof from us because I think it is very difficult to take charge of seven persons, and they also were afraid that the terrorists would come back searching for us. Everybody tried to convince us to return home, but even until now, it is very difficult to look to that solution. Finally, after two years of wandering, I was accepted with my brother and sisters for indeterminate duration in a center for abandoned children.

Suddenly, I found myself responsible for a family, without any preparation. In this very difficult situation, I could not think of myself. My only concern was to take care of my brother and sisters. Since we lodged in this center, the stress began to go down. I could take care of myself and begin to feel my problems. In this center, I heard about a psychologist who helps children with problems. I decided to come for consultation and agreed to talk about my own experiences. I felt very tired and suffered many difficulties in life. I am a very emotional woman and have big trouble sleeping. When I sleep, I often have nightmares, and when I am aware, I often see the same scene of the massacre of my family. I also feel myself persecuted by everybody and feel myself in danger anywhere. I have a deep sense of injustice and despair. However, I try to talk with a psychologist about my experiences and try to cope with my difficulties. Sometimes, I pass through depressive moments of withdrawing into myself and being discouraged and tempted to drop everything. Often, I ask myself if someone can do anything for me and my family and if I must spend all my life in this center. I have serious doubts about my future.

Short- and Long-Term Effects on the Victims of Terror in Sri Lanka

Daya Somasundaram

SUMMARY. Due to two decades of ethnic war in Sri Lanka, victims of terror have been profoundly affected psychologically and socially. The impact is seen at the individual, family, and community levels. Epidemiological surveys show that civilians have experienced widespread traumatization, with high levels of somatization, anxiety, depression, Posttraumatic Stress Disorder (PTSD), relationship problems, and alcohol abuse. At the community level, the cumulative effect of terror is collective trauma, with a general tendency to mistrust, dependence, silence, withdrawal, passivity, and lack of motivation. Socially, there is evidence of deterioration in values and ethics with marked increases in child abuse, violence against women, crime, and brutalization.

address: <docdelivery@haworthpress.com> Website:

Address correspondence to: Daya Somasundaram, MD, Department of Psychiatry, Faculty of Medicine, University of Jaffna, Sri Lanka. (E-mail: d_somasundaram@ yahoo.com).

[Haworth co-indexing entry note]: "Short- and Long-Term Effects on the Victims of Terror in Sri Lanka." Somasundaram, Daya. Co-published simultaneously in *Journal of Aggression, Maltreatment & Trauma* (The Haworth Maltreatment & Trauma Press, an imprint of The Haworth Press, Inc.) Vol. 9, No. 1/2, 2004; and: *The Trauma of Terrorism: Sharing Knowledge and Shared Care, An International Handbook* (ed: Yael Danieli, Danny Brom, and Joe Sills) The Haworth Maltreatment & Trauma Press, an imprint of The Haworth Press, Inc., 2005.

KEYWORDS. War trauma, psychosocial problems, torture, South Asia, Tamils, PTSD, collective trauma

The recent ethnic war in Sri Lanka is a good example of the modern use of terror on a mass scale. All parties in conflict have resorted to the use of terror tactics. The Sri Lankan state, the various Tamil militants, who have for over 20 years fought to create an independent state, the Sinhala Janatha Vimukthi Perumana (JVP), an ultra leftist militant group that made two attempts to violently overthrow the government, and India, during its short intervention in the island (1987-90), have all used mass terror to control the population, win over loyalty and suppress dissent. But in the scale, duration, and sheer numbers of victims, it is the Sri Lankan state that is most guilty of the massive use of terror. The use of internal terror by the Tamil militants, particularly the Liberation Tigers of Tamil Eelam (LTTE), the Indian intervention, and the JVP and counter terror by the state in the South, has been described elsewhere (Hoole, 2001; Hoole, Somasundaram, Thiranagama & Sritharan, 1988; Somasundaram, 1998; Somasundaram & Jamunananthan, 2002). This article will deal mainly with the psychosocial effects of state terror on the Tamil population living in the north of Sri Lanka, specifically in the Jaffna peninsula.

Gradually, state terror became institutionalized into the very laws of the land (Amnesty International, 1996), structures of society and mechanisms of governance. Arbitrary detention, torture, massacres, extrajudicial killings, disappearances, rape, forced displacements, bombings, and shelling became common. The minority Tamil community, especially in the north and east of Sri Lanka, encompassing 17,624 square kilometers with an estimated population of 2,600,000 (the total area of Sri Lanka is 65,610 square kilometers, with a total population of 19,000,000), experienced the brunt of the terror. The effects were seen on the individual, family, and community levels.

NEGATIVE EFFECTS OF WAR

Individual Trauma. According to Somasundaram and Sivayokan (1994), epidemiological surveys of the general population in war-affected areas of Sri Lanka show that the population has faced a variety of war-related stressors like injury, detention, arrest, torture, deaths of relatives, destruction of property, witnessing violence and displacement (see Table 1) and consequent psychosocial problems (see Figure 1).

As culturally expected, those affected did not seek help for the psychological traumatization per se, but presented with somatic complaints to the health

TABLE 1. Distribution of war stress in the community

Stress factors Direct stress	Community (n = 98)	OPD[1] (n = 65)
Death of friend/relation	50%	46%
Loss of property	46%	55%
Injury to friend/relation	39%	48%
Experience of bombing/shelling/gunfire	37%	29%
Witness violence	26%	36%
Detention	15%	26%
Injury to body	10%	9%
Assault	10%	23%
Torture	1%	8%
Indirect stress		
Economic difficulties	78%	85%
Displacement[2]	70%	69%
Lack of food	56%	68%
Unemployment	45%	55%
Ill health[3]	14%	29%

1. Outpatient department (OPD) of a general hospital.
2. After the 1995 mass displacement when the figure would have reached almost 100%.
3. Ill health due to war-related injuries, including amputations caused by landmine blasts, epidemics like malaria, reduced resistance to infections (due to stress and malnutrition), and septicemia had debilitating mental effects.

sector including: (a) hospital out patient departments (OPDs), (b) general practitioners, and (c) traditional healers. For example, in Jaffna, the largest city in the Tamil area, the level of traumatization and symptom formation was higher among OPD patients than in the general population (Somasundaram, 2001). The mean stress score for the OPD attendees (41.4) was significantly higher than in the general population (36.2). The implications of these findings for the time and cost of inappropriately treating these large numbers in the OPD and the need to address their real difficulties properly, such as through counseling, relaxation exercises and socio-economic rehabilitation, should be realized.

Noteworthy, in the above research, is the finding that 1% of the study population had been tortured, but the figure reached 8% in the OPD patients. Torture was used as a routine procedure carried out on all those detained. Studying 168 ex-detainees, Doney (1998) found that all had been subject to torture. Eighty-six percent of the ex-detainees were found to suffer from Post Traumatic Stress Disorder (PTSD). Notably, different and opposed parties use

FIGURE 1. Psychosocial and psychiatric problems in the OPD compared to the community

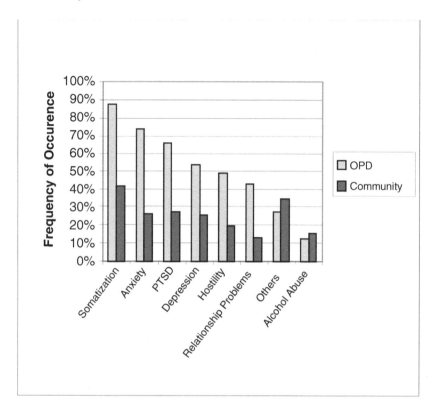

the very same methods of torture, even on their own cadres, such as beating with plastic pipes filled with sand, putting chili powder into eyes, nostrils or genitalia, suffocating with a 'shopping' bag filled with petrol, and driving pins under the nails. In *Dharmachakra' (wheel of righteousness),* a new method, also called *'jujuyekebab'* (fried chicken) in Iran, the victim's wrists are tied together just below the bent knees, so that a pole can be passed simultaneously through the crook of the bent knees in front of the elbows. The pole is then suspended and, when rotated rapidly like a wheel, there is intense pain to the body but the only evidence will be healing abrasions at the wrist (Fernando, 2001). The person becomes confused and breaks down (with loss of resistance). The curious use of the Buddhist spiritual term *Dharmachakra* for this type of torture is psychologically revealing (Gunasekara, 2001). Many individuals do not survive torture, but those who do are released in a broken condition. The maimed bodies of the ones who do not survive are conspicuously exhibited as a warning to others. Torture developed into a physical and psychosocial tool to break the individual personalities of those who try to resist as well as an encompassing method to coerce a community into submission. It became one aspect of institutionalized violence and laws were passed, such as the Prevention of Terrorism Act and Emergency Regulations, which facilitate prolonged incommunicado detention without charges or trial, in locations at the discretion of the Security Forces, and allowing for the disposal of bodies of victims without judicial inquiry. In turn, this legislation legitimizes the use of torture and death in custody (Amnesty International, 1986).

A more recent epidemiological survey (Vivo, 2003) carried out in the Vanni, an area in the north of Sri Lanka, found that 92% of primary school children had been exposed to potentially terrorizing experiences including combat, shelling, and witnessing the death of loved ones. In 57% of the children, the effects of these experiences were interfering considerably with their daily life (e.g., social withdrawal and weakening school performance). About 25% were found to suffer from PTSD.

Family Trauma

Due to close and strong bonds and cohesiveness in nuclear and extended families in the Tamil culture, the families tend to function and respond to external threat as a unit rather than as individual members. During times of terrifying experiences, the family will come together as a unit to face the threat and provide mutual support and protection. Due to the ongoing war, the extended and nuclear family systems have been weakened or shattered by displacement, separation, migration, death, detention, and the disappearance of family members. Children are now socialized in a war milieu with direct experiences of violence, emotions of terror, grief and hatred and militant role models. The role of the mother has also undergone momentous change with increasing non-traditional responsibilities and activities. The uncertainty and grief about missing family members add to the ensuing maladaptive family dynamics. The loss of the essential unifying role of a missing member may cause disruption and disharmony. From the loss of one or both parents, separations and traumatization, pathological family dynamics can adversely affect each remaining member, particularly the children. A common situation is where the father has been detained, "disappeared," or been killed but the family members are not sure of his fate. They are caught in a "conspiracy of silence" where further inquiries may lead to more problems for the father were he still alive and the mother may not be able to share the truth with the child. The family itself often becomes ostracized by society. The child then presents with behavioral problems. Having the mother share her fears and feelings with the child can be helpful. This is particularly difficult for a family where the male has been "disappeared" by the Tamil militants, where the social situation compels the remaining members to keep silent and makes it extremely difficult for them to receive social support. They often have to suppress the memory of the person altogether. In addition, the mother has to adapt to all the negative implications of being a "widow" in Tamil society.

In the Jaffna peninsula, there are close to 20,000 female-headed households. The effect on the families, the widows (Kumerandran et al., 1998) and the children has been immense. Jeyanthy et al. (1993) assessed the impact of displacement on the functioning of the family system. Psychological disturbances, particularly depressive symptoms, were much more common in displaced families than in those living in their own homes. Separation anxiety, cognitive impairment, conduct disorders, and sleep disturbances were common in displaced children. Disturbances in family dynamics, particularly disputes and quarreling between father and mother, were attributed to economic stress, lack of privacy, and interference of others in overly crowded camps.

Community Trauma

The war has had a tremendous impact on the community or village. During the current war whole communities or villages have been targeted for total destruction, including their way of life and their environment. The village traditions, structures, and institutions were the foundation and framework for daily life. In the Tamil tradition, a person's identity is defined to a large extent by their village of origin (Daniel, 1984), but all of this has been irrevocably changed (Council of NGOs, 1998; National Peace Council & Marga, 2001).

Apart from direct attacks, entire villages of all communities have been disrupted, displaced and uprooted due to the ongoing conflict. Fishermen have been at increased risk of death, disappearance, detention, or injury, due to the nature of their work that takes them into the sea, a highly contested area in the war. As a result, the highest numbers of widows are from this community. Many have shifted to other occupations; some are still unemployed, living off government rations, while others have left the area. They have lost their way of life and culture and yearn for the former days of peace. It has been a similar tale with farmers, many of whom have been displaced from their traditional lands, and have lost all their equipment. Some are unable to cultivate their land, as it is located in so-called High Security Zones or mined areas. The Muslims, who were a very prosperous business community as well as specializing in trades like tailoring, tinkering, and leather work, have lost their occupations and way of life after being forced to leave their homes in the north. The Sinhalese were well-known bakers in the north and east, but now all have left.

Some villages have ceased to exist. Due to dislocation, people have been separated so that the network of relationships, structures, and institutions has been lost. Erikson (1976) described it as a *"loss of communality."* A very good example of the collective effect of displacement was the mass exodus from Valikamam in 1995 (University Teachers for Human Rights, Jaffna, 1995). Even when people have returned to their villages, as happened in Jaffna in 1996, the village was not the same. There were numerous newcomers. The old structures and institutions were no longer functioning. The protective environment provided by the *uur* (village) was no longer there.

Similarly, in the life of Tamils, their house (*veedu*) and its history are very important. The dead ancestral relations continue to have connections with the house. They are remembered and considered as if they were present in the house, especially when rituals are performed. When people leave the house for long periods (e.g., displacement, going abroad), it is as if a biological link breaks. This affects the mental condition in several ways. People believe that ghosts or demons will occupy houses that are left alone for a long time. People who returned to their houses after displacement felt a change in the organic bond; they could not re-establish the relationship with their houses.

The ubiquitous presence of buried landmines creates a pervasive apprehension in the back of the minds of people, making them ever vigilant, cautious about walking freely on the land, afraid of putting a wrong foot somewhere. Some developed nightmares of being the victim of an exploding landmine. The once beloved land itself becomes a source of terror (Gunaratnam et al., 2003).

Collective Trauma

The cumulative effect of terror on the community can be described as collective trauma, which goes beyond the individual. In fact, given the widespread nature of the traumatization due to war, the individual's psychosocial reactions may have come to be accepted as a normal part of life. But at the community level, manifestations of the terror can be seen in its social processes and structures, as in the prevailing cultural coping strategies. People have learned to survive under extraordinarily stressful conditions.

However, some coping strategies that may have had survival value during intense conflict may become maladaptive during reconstruction and peace. For example, the Tamils have developed a deep suspicion and mistrust of others. People have learned simply to attend to their immediate needs and survive to the next day. Any involvement or participation carried considerable risk, particularly because the frequent changes in those in power entailed recrimi-nations, false accusations, revenge, and killings. These happened, for exam-ple, in 1987 (Indian Peace Keeping Force; IPKF), 1990 (Liberation Tigers of Tamil Eelam; LTTE), 1996 (Sri Lanka Army; SLA), and again in 2002-3 as the LTTE took over the society in Tamil areas. Gradually, those with leader-ship qualities, those willing to challenge and argue, the intellectuals, the dis-senters and those with social motivation, were weeded out, either intimidated into leaving, silenced, or killed. Gradually, people became very passive and submissive. These qualities have become part of the socialization process, where children are now taught to keep quiet, not to question or challenge, and to accept the situation, as too forward a behavior carries considerable risk.

The repeated displacements and disruption of livelihood have made people dependent on handouts. People have lost their self-reliance, earlier the hall-mark of the Tamil. They have lost their motivation for advancement, progress, or betterment. There is a general sense of resignation to fate. They have devel-oped dependence on help from outside sources, on relief, on handouts. Fur-ther, they have lost their trust in their fellow human beings as well as in the world order. They no longer trust the security forces, including the police; their experiences have taught them otherwise. Instead of trust in and respect for law and order, and belief in their legitimacy, there is terror.

Brutalization of Personality

Apart from the militarization of all aspects of life and the pervasiveness of the 'gun culture' is the long-term effect on thinking and behavior patterns. Witnessing the horrifying death of loved ones, friends or strangers, or killings, seeing many mutilated or dismembered bodies, the decaying and bloated re-mains, is bound to saturate the consciousness with images of death (Lifton, 1967) and brutalize the personality. Similarly, watching with trepidation the destruction of a till-then permanent structure, like a home, or having to aban-don it under forced circumstances, inevitably results in the collapse of every-thing secure and strong, creating a vacuum that can never be filled. With time, people have become habituated to such scenes and experiences. They have be-come immunized to the worst aspects of the war. However, they have also lost the sensitiveness of being human. The natural helping hand, sympathy, kind-ness for a kindred soul in distress, is fast disappearing. A good example is from the health sector where, until recently, there was a spirit of service. Medical staff would stay with their patient, sometimes sacrificing their own well-being for the interests of the patient. The collective experience of what happened at General Hospital, Jaffna on Theepavali day in 1987 has made most staff lose their altruism. During that fateful period, staff decided to stick to the hospital and patients despite considerable risk. When the Indian Army entered and massacred both patients and staff, this last bit of service ideal died, too. Staff now look after their self-interests first. At the slightest hint of trouble, they abandon the hospital, their responsibilities, and patients, as happened during the intensification of the conflict in May 2000.

Abnormal personality development in children and personality disorders, particularly anti-social ones, are well-known, long-term consequences of war (APA, 1994). Increased irritability, poor impulse control, and unpredictable explosions of aggressive behavior have been described frequently in war veterans (Andreason, 1985). An increase in juvenile delinquency among children under war conditions has been noted (Lewis, 1942). Paranoid personality was common among the militants, more marked in the higher ranks, where they showed deep suspicion and intolerance, particularly for rival groups. Many of the youthful militants initially had a "soft," amiable personality with altruistic and humanitarian concern for their society. In time, these militants became hardened and rigid in their thinking, probably due to the indoctrination and brutalizing effect of the acts they had to perform.

Social Deterioration

The signs of the effects of collective trauma can be seen in all social institutions, structures, and organizations in present day Jaffna. There is a general ennui. Most have left their houses and property neglected in disrepair. Once a hard-working society dominated by a strong work ethic, its output has now declined considerably, since most people are not inclined to work. They spend most of their effort obtaining relief items, rations, incentive payments, and risk allowances. There is a crisis of leadership. No one comes forward to take positions like the chairmanship or presidency; most are thus filled by default. There is a complete lack of quality in all aspects of society, partly due to the crippling brain drain, but also the devastating effect of the war. As in adolescents (Geevathasan et al., 1993; Sivashanmugarajah et al., 1994), marked impairment in cognitive functioning can be discerned in adults.

There is a marked deterioration in social values, demonstrated both with regard to sexual mores (i.e., medical personnel report increased unwanted pregnancies, teenage abortions, and child sexual abuse in the refugee camps in Vavuniya and society in general) and to social ethics (i.e., robberies of the houses and property of those displaced, now claimed as a right; increase in crime rates). When the army took over Thenmarachi in 1996, widespread looting by the public was indulged in even by the most socially respectable teachers. There is currently a dramatic increase in the number of incidents of child abuse, including sexual abuse, reported to the District Child Protection Committee (see Figure 2) at the General Hospital in Jaffna.

This could be due to increased awareness of the problem (child abuse always existed in Tamil society, but is only now coming to light) but is also due to the war. Many families are displaced from their familiar surroundings and natural habitat where they had the support and protection of extended family and friends in the village. They now have to live in crowded camps or accommodations in strange and new places. Parents have to go out to attend to various urgent requirements like fetching relief and meeting authorities. Some families are without their men. In some, the mother has started another relationship. This is compounded by the aforementioned general deterioration in social values and principles, a reduction in restraints and even disinhibition. There is also a noticeable increase in violence against women.

POSITIVE EFFECTS OF WAR

In contrast to the overwhelming negative consequences of the sustained terror on the community, there have been a few positive developments described below.

Emerging Community Organizations. Some new community grass roots organizations have emerged such as those for widows and the disappeared. Leadership by women of many of these organizations is particularly noteworthy. New religious movements, particularly the charismatic, emotive ones, have become popular, attesting to the community's need for the emotional support, fellowship, leadership, and meaning to events they provide. *Villipu kulus,* community vigilante organizations, have started functioning in vil-

FIGURE 2. Child Abuse in 2001, 2002 and 2003

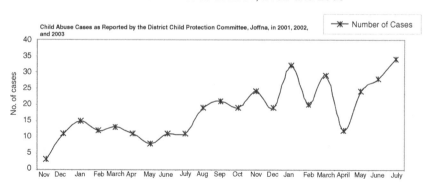

lages, for example, in Kopay, to control anti-social activity and to carry out other community functions such as sports, cultural shows, and education. However, it should be noted that, even though apparently permitting more space for these organizations, the authorities do not allow any such movement to be effective past a certain point. For example, the LTTE totalitarian system tolerates no independent organization.

Decline of Caste Structure. The caste system, one of the strongly embedded institutions within the Hindu sociocultural system, has been responsible for considerable covert violence throughout history. Its highly hierarchical structure depends on social controls that keep the various castes, particularly the lower ones, in their place. When the hierarchical system is transgressed, violence can become overt. Before the war, Jaffna society was very much under the caste system (i.e., the lower castes were suppressed by the higher). Though there had been some loosening of the system due to modernization, education, economic progress, and leftist agitation, it was the current war that made considerable inroads into it. During the mass displacements, people could not observe the usual caste exclusions as they were thrown together in unexpected circumstances, which created many relationships across caste lines. There were some rare exceptions where, even under the threat of death, people held onto caste distinctions, for example, by refusing to stay in certain refugee camps with lower castes. In the various Tamil militant movements, particularly in the leftist leaning movements, caste has become a non-issue. Thus, with the progress of the war, caste has lost its tight hold on society, though it lingers on, for example, in marriage arrangements. Whether it will come back once the war is over is difficult to say but in all probability it will not have the same stranglehold it once had.

Changing Status of Women. Similarly, Tamil society had always suppressed women into a subservient position. During the colonial period, modern education began to loosen this to some extent and some women managed to get free. However, it was the war that played a crucial role in liberating women. Some males left to seek jobs and other opportunities abroad. The males who initially joined the militants, were killed, migrated or left the area out of fear, seeking asylum in foreign countries. The women were left behind to shoulder the responsibility of family and home and to keep the society functioning (Sivachandran, 1994). While men left their wives and children behind, women did not (with the exception of Middle East housemaid jobs). They were left to face the trauma of war alone. They looked after their families single-handedly, filling in for the absent male in what had been until then traditional male roles. They rode bicycles, went to the shops, met and argued with authorities, took their children to schools and temples, and generally "kept the home fires burning." As a result, women were forced to take a more leading role, thereby furthering their freedom.

Some women have also joined the militants. Factors inducing them to leave society were the tight control, the nature of their domestic life and facing a bleak future. Joining the militants was a liberating act, promising them more freedom and power (Balasingham, 2001; Trawick, 1999). Some families, too poor to afford a good dowry for their daughters, actively encouraged them to join.

CONCLUSIONS

The psychosocial effects of the continuous reign of terror on the community in Sri Lanka can be seen on the individual, family and community levels. In addition to the discernable individual psychiatric disorders, PTSD in particular, it is the more subtle but pernicious development of pathology in social structures and functioning that will need to be addressed if society is to recover. Community level approaches and interventions should reverse some of the worse effects of collective trauma. Thus, awareness programs (i.e., psychoeducation for the general and specific vulnerable populations); training for grass-roots workers in simple, basic psychosocial skills to help those in the community; networking with governmental and non-governmental organizations to rebuild community structures, institutions, and processes; efforts to address issues of social justice, reconciliation, individual human and socio-cultural rights; and socio-economic rehabilitation and non-violent conflict resolution strategies will go a long way in restoring war-torn societies (Somasundaram & Jamunanantha, 2002).

REFERENCES

American Psychiatric Association. (1994). *Diagnostic and statistical manual of mental disorders* (4th ed.). Washington, DC: Author.

Amnesty International. (1986). *Sri Lanka disappearances* (AI Index: ASA 37/08/86). London: Author.

Amnesty International. (1996). *Sri Lanka: Wavering commitment to human rights* (ASA 37/08/96). London: Author.

Andreason, N. (1985). Posttraumatic stress disorder. In A. I. Kaplan, A. M. Preddman, & E. T. Sodock (Eds.), *Comprehensive textbook of psychiatry* (4th ed., Vol 1, pp. 918-924). Baltimore, MD: Williams & Willkins.

Balasingham A. (2001). *The will to freedom*. London: Fairmax Publishing Ltd.

Council of NGOs, Jaffna District. (1998). *Review of resettlement and rehabilitation programme-Jaffna Peninsula*. Jaffna: Author.

Daniel, V. E. (1984). *Fluid signs: Being a person the Tamil way.* Berkeley, CA: University of California Press.

Doney, A. (1998). Psychological after effects of torture. In D. J. Somasundaram (Ed.), *Scarred minds* (pp. 256-287). New Delhi: Sage Publications.

Erikson, K. T. (1976). Loss of communality at Buffalo Creek. *American Journal of Psychiatry, 135*(3), 330-335.

Fernando, R. (2000). *Medico legal aspects of torture.* Colombo: Family Rehabilitation Centre.

Geevathasan, M. G., Somasundaram, D. J., & Parameshwaran, S. V. (1993, August). *Psychological consequence of war on adolescents.* Paper presented at the Ninth Annual Scientific Sessions, Jaffna Medical Association, Jaffna, Sri Lanka.

Gunaratnam, H. R., Sinothaya, S., & Somasundaram, D. J. (2003). The psychosocial effects of landmines in Jaffna. *Medicine, Conflict, & Survival, 19*, 223-234.

Gunasekara, L. (2001, July 15). The Dharmachakara as a form of torture. *Sunday Observer,* p. 7.

Hoole, R. (2001). *Sri Lanka: The arrogance of power, myths, decadence, and murder.* Colombo: University Teachers for Human Rights (Jaffna).

Hoole, M. R., Somasundaram D. J., Thiranagama R., & Sritharan K. (1988). *Broken palmyra.* Claremont, California: Harvey Mudd College Press.

Jeyanthy, K., Loshani, N. A., & Sivarajini, G. (1993). *A study of psychological consequences of displacement on family members.* III MBBS Research project, Dept. of Community Medicine, University of Jaffna.

Kumerandran, B., Pavani, A., Kalpana, T., Nagapraba, S., Kalamgagal, T., Thayanithi, S., Sivashankar, R., & Somasundaram, D. J. (1998, September). *A preliminary survey of psychosocial problems of widowhood and separation among women in Jaffna.* Paper presented at the Jaffna Medical Association 10th Annual Sessions, Jaffna, Sri Lanka.

Lewis, A. (1942, August 15). Incidence of neurosis in England under war conditions. *The Lancet,* pp.175-185.

Lifton, R. J. (1967). *Death in life: Survivors of Hiroshima.* New York: Random House.

National Peace Council & Marga. (2001). *Cost of the war.* Colombo: National Peace Council.

Sivachandran, S. (1994). Health of women and the elderly. In K. Arulanantham, S. Raatneswaran, & N. Sreeharan (Eds.), *Victims of war in Sri Lanka* (pp. 48-50). London: Medical Institute of Tamils.

Somasundaram, D. J. (1998). *Scarred minds.* New Delhi: Sage Publications.

Somasundaram, D. J. (2001). War trauma and psychosocial problems: Patient attendees in Jaffna. *International Medical Journal, 8*, 193-197.

Somasundaram, D. J., & Jamunanantha, C. S. (2002). Psychosocial consequences of war: Northern Sri Lankan experience. In J. T. V. M. De Jong (Ed.), *Trauma, war and violence: Public mental health in socio-cultural context* (pp. 205-258). New York: Plenum Press.

Somasundaram, D. J., & Sivayokan, S. (1994). War trauma in a civilian population. *British Journal of Psychiatry, 165*, 524-527.

Trawick, M. (1999). Reasons for violence: A preliminary ethnographic account of the LTTE. In S. Gamage & I. B. Watson (Eds.), *Conflict and community in contempo-*

rary Sri Lanka: 'Pear of the East' or the 'Island of tears' (pp. 139-163). New Delhi: Sage Publications.

University Teachers for Human Rights (Jaffna). (1995). *Exodus from Jaffna*. Colombo: Author.

VIVO [Victims' Voice]. (2003). *Epidemiological survey of children's mental health in the Vanni region*. Colombo: German Technical Cooperation.

Voice:
Sri Lanka:
The Destruction
of South Asia's Most Developed Society

Barbara Crossette

While I remember the terrible moments, some chillingly ironic, they added up to more. I was on a peaceful hilltop above Colombo, the capital, talking with Tamil and Sinhala Catholic priests about their inter-communal work, when the dull thud of a large explosion sent me down into town and into the center of blood and gore, as a bomb devastated the central bus station. I can still picture one driver, his windshield gone and his crazed and bloody face frozen by fear, driving as fast as he could in his empty bus to get out of there, to anywhere else, scattering cars, and people. Reporting from Sri Lanka between 1985 and 1991, I saw Buddhists slaughtered in their holy city of Anuradhapura. I sat in a Colombo hospital with a women coughing blood as she told me how her son had died as they rode toward the city on a shopping trip. "He saw them get on the bus wearing uniforms, and then he saw their rubber sandals and he said, 'Mummy, these are not soldiers.'" In a second, the boy was dead and she was badly wounded. I never knew whether she survived. Multiply those stories many times over: families searching for the bodies of children, parents and friends

Address correspondence to: Barbara Crossette, P.O. Box 250, Upper Black Eddy, PA 18972 USA (E-mail: bcrossette@aol.com).

[Haworth co-indexing entry note]: "Voice: Sri Lanka: The Destruction of South Asia's Most Developed Society." Crossette, Barbara. Co-published simultaneously in *Journal of Aggression, Maltreatment & Trauma* (The Haworth Maltreatment & Trauma Press, an imprint of The Haworth Press, Inc.) Vol. 9, No. 1/2, 2004; and: *The Trauma of Terrorism: Sharing Knowledge and Shared Care, An International Handbook* (ed: Yael Danieli, Danny Brom, and Joe Sills) The Haworth Maltreatment & Trauma Press, an imprint of The Haworth Press, Inc., 2005.

along beaches after hearing rumors they had been dumped in rivers or at sea, a university vice-chancellor assassinated, it seemed, for being a reasoning intellectual.

It was one of the nastiest and most bloodthirsty conflicts of the late 20th century, but the civil war in Sri Lanka, at one point two simultaneous, equally ugly wars, somehow was never studied as widely as it should have been. With tens of thousands dead from a poisonous mix of linguistic chauvinism, embattled ethnicities, and thoughtless power politics, Sri Lanka perfected suicide bombing, necklacing with burning tires, forced recruitment of children, urban explosions and rural massacres of astonishing cruelty for a land of theoretically peaceful Buddhists and Hindus. While one group or another specialized in particular horrors, Tamil suicide bombers, for example, and Sinhalese butchery that left streams choked with blood and bodies, the cataclysmic descent of South Asia's most civilized, literate and developed society on one of the world's most beautiful islands should have sent up warning flares. Strangely, the conflicts remained far away and barely understood.

Sri Lanka's longest civil war, between Tamils in the north and east and the country's Sinhalese majority in the south and central areas, leaving aside for the moment an important Muslim minority on both east and west coasts, was rooted in efforts after independence from Britain in 1948 to reassert native identities. To simplify, the Sinhalese (who are mostly Buddhists but with a significant Christian component) felt that under British rule the Tamils of the Jaffna peninsula and parts of the northeast (mostly Hindus but also Christians educated and converted by American missionaries) had been favored at the expense of Sinhalese. This culminated in the 1950s with an aggressive get-even policy by Sinhalese-led governments that resulted in the downgrading of Tamil language and culture, and a bias against Tamil employment in government service. It became acceptable to treat Tamils as second-class citizens. Add an astonishingly short-sighted insensitivity and lack of public conscience or accountability in the Sinhalese ruling class, a select number of families who dominated the political system for decades.

Tamil rights organizations grew over the 1970s, eventually spawning the lethal Liberation Tigers of Tamil Eelam, the LTTE, which systematically murdered its liberal Tamil opponents and controlled an area it ruled with utter, terrifying totalitarianism. As a reporter, I had seen nothing like this closed, cowed society since Cambodia in the wake of the Khmer Rouge. The Tiger leader, Vellupillai Prabhakaran, was, indeed, sometimes compared with Pol Pot, if only for his reductionism and single-minded rebuilding of a society. Years of guerrilla wars between the disciplined LTTE and the ill-led Sri Lankan army followed. Both sides engaged in atrocities, but the Tigers, as they became known, were cold, master killers with no concern for any civilian life.

They bombed buses, office buildings and political rallies, and killed university professors with the same single mindedness as they killed soldiers.

That war has now apparently run its course as Western nations, belatedly and in the wake of their experience with the Taliban and Al Qaeda, decided that the festering sore Sri Lanka had become to its own people might also harbor contagion that could affect outsiders. Moreover, during that Tamil-Sinhala war, efforts to reach peace agreements provoked vicious reactions from fringes of the Sinhalese majority who wanted nothing less than the annihilation of the Tigers and as many other Tamils as possible. This give-no-quarter lobby included both Buddhist nationalists and a resurgent Sinhalese leftist movement once as absolutist and terror-prone as the Tigers.

Throughout the quarter-century beginning in 1978, Sri Lanka's most painful loss, to an outsider who had not suffered directly, may be the destruction of its civility. Politics coarsened visibly and steadily. A culture of guns and corruption flourished everywhere. A generation of credible political leaders, both Tamil and Sinhalese, were assassinated, mostly by the Tigers, who also killed the country's leading human rights lawyer, Neelan Tiruchelvam, a Tamil intellectual known worldwide for his efforts toward peace and reconciliation. The Muslim minority was pushed and pulled, and also experienced extreme violence. Muslims are now angry, fearful of Tamil militants and distrustful of a Sinhalese-led government.

In such an environment, faith in institutions, certainly in politicians, and in fellow Sri Lankans eroded dangerously. Sri Lanka was not alone. In Cambodia, for example, society is still stunted a generation or two after the Khmer Rouge. In Iraq, the dictatorship of Saddam Hussein and his two monstrous sons wrought their horrors to lasting negative effect. Buildings can be rebuilt, and fortifications removed, but repairing a whole people will take a very long time, and outsiders must learn to understand this better in an era of civil conflict.

Observations on the Impact on Kenyans of the August 7, 1998 Bombing of the United States Embassy in Nairobi

Samuel B. Thielman

SUMMARY. The August 7, 1998 bombing of the American embassy in Nairobi affected a large number of people, both Kenyan and American. The bombing led to a large-scale response from the Kenyan mental health community and to collaboration between American and Kenyan responders. Kenyans affected by the bombing frequently expressed their psychological distress in terms of somatic complaints. Case histories and written narratives illustrate the way an African worldview shaped survivors' interpretation of the bombing and its consequences.

KEYWORDS. Counseling, cross-cultural comparison, disasters, explosions, Kenya, stress disorders, post-traumatic, terrorism

Address correspondence to: Samuel B. Thielman, MD, PhD, 2401 E Street, N.W., Washington, DC 20522 USA (E-mail: thielmansb@state.gov).

The ideas and opinions expressed in this paper are the author's own and do not represent any position or policy of the United States Department of State.

[Haworth co-indexing entry note]: "Observations on the Impact on Kenyans of the August 7, 1998 Bombing of the United States Embassy in Nairobi." Thielman, Samuel B. Co-published simultaneously in *Journal of Aggression, Maltreatment & Trauma* (The Haworth Maltreatment & Trauma Press, an imprint of The Haworth Press, Inc.) Vol. 9, No. 1/2, 2004; and: *The Trauma of Terrorism: Sharing Knowledge and Shared Care, An International Handbook* (ed: Yael Danieli, Danny Brom, and Joe Sills) The Haworth Maltreatment & Trauma Press, an imprint of The Haworth Press, Inc., 2005.

On August 7, 1998, Al Qaeda operatives destroyed the U.S. Embassy build-ings in Nairobi, Kenya and Dar Es Salaam, Tanzania with coordinated truck bomb attacks. Although the U.S. had experienced a similar bombing of the U.S. Embassy in Beirut in 1983, the magnitude of the psychological impact of the East Africa bombings was much greater, in part because in Nairobi the bombings killed 201 Kenyans and 12 U.S. diplomatic staff and injured 5000 (the destruction in Dar Es Salaam was less extensive). Psychiatrists with the State Department from South Africa, India, and Europe became involved in efforts to assist U.S. government employees, both Kenyan and American, who were affected by the bombing. I arrived in Nairobi in January of 2000 and was responsible for supervising the on-site support for both Americans and more than 200 Kenyans who had survived the bombing, arranging for and, in many instances, delivering psychiatric care to the Kenyans. Eventually I became in-volved in assisting in the ongoing mental health program for Kenyan victims of the bombing that was sponsored by the United States Agency for Interna-tional Development (USAID), and was able to observe the reactions of a large number of people from two different cultures to a single catastrophic event.

THE KENYAN RESPONSE

Kenya's public mental health infrastructure is low on the priority list of the Kenyan government. A number of psychiatrists, most affiliated with the Uni-versity of Nairobi, maintain busy private practices. At the time of the 1998 bombing, Kenya had something over 50 psychiatrists; Tanzania had perhaps thirteen.

Kenya is ethnically and religiously diverse. The country has more than 70 ethnic groups, although about 70% of the population belongs to one of five largest groups (East Africa Living Encyclopedia, n.d.). Approximately 7% of the population is Muslim, and the Muslim community on the coast of Kenya is very old, dating back at least to the twelfth century, and probably before. An-other 12% of the population are African traditional religionists, but the major-ity of Kenyans (79%) are Christian and belong to a variety of Christian denominations (Barrett, Kurian, & Johnson, 2001).

The initial mental health response to the bombing was organized by Ken-yans for Kenyans. Psychiatry exists in the East African setting and, in fact, Kenya and Uganda have university training programs that are active both in-tellectually and clinically. The psychiatrists in Nairobi were very knowledge-able and patriotic, and some are also well connected with the international psychiatric community. However, psychiatrists in Kenya, as in much of the world, are overworked, poorly funded, and collect and discuss much more information than they ever publish. A prominent Kenyan psychiatrist, Dr. Frank Njenga, initiated a mental health response to the bombing, Operation Recovery, which was organized under the auspices of the Kenyan Medical Association. This effort involved an extensive program of education and counseling to ameliorate the negative psychiatric effects of the bombing. They trained some 700 counselors and treated some 7000 people (exact statistics were not kept; USAID, 2001). Operation Recovery used an educational approach to inform victims of potential symptoms. They organized large group debriefings, visited and treated wounded survivors in local hospitals, and then scheduled follow-up visits. Workers visited schools and went to outlying areas of the country where many relatives of the deceased lived (Kenya Medical Association, 2001).

Although their methods of treatment used the western PTSD framework and counseling approaches as a starting point for dealing with problems, Kenyan mental health care providers adapted western knowledge to the local African situation. In fact, the circumstances in Kenya mandated that significant modifications be made to accommodate local cultural and economic realities. Dr. Njenga, in particular, made use of the local media to educate people about the psychological effects of trauma, a strategy that was particularly helpful. As he wrote later, victims of disasters in developing countries are often poorly informed about what has happened, and in an event such as the 1998 Nairobi bombing, the psychological impact spreads far beyond the area of the blast (Njenga, Nyamai, & Kigamwa, 2003). He and others used the media to explain the psychological symptoms of such a disaster and tried to help viewers accept the negative emotions they were feeling. They hosted call-in shows that fielded questions about religion and terrorism, vented anger, and worked for a conciliatory attitude toward the diverse elements of Kenyan society.

U.S. GOVERNMENT ASSISTANCE

Following the bombing, most Kenyans looked to the international community for aid. Although the Kenyan press was very belligerent toward the U.S., little attention was given to the Kenyan government's inability to respond effectively to the crisis. Likewise, victims of the bombing looked to the U.S. rather than the Kenyan government for aid. U.S. government efforts to assist the Kenyans in providing mental health care were hampered in a variety of ways. Congress had appropriated $37 million to assist Kenyans in recovering from the bombing, and many who came to the U.S.-sponsored counseling program came for financial aid rather than mental health counseling. Many families had suffered the loss of a breadwinner and were experiencing a financial crisis. Parents came asking for school fees, money for housing, and a variety of other things. In fact, the counselors, at least in the beginning of the program, found themselves explaining frequently that they were not there to assist in that way. This led to the obvious question of whether or not the money used for mental health care might not have been better spent on direct financial aid to families affected by the bombing. In fact, USAID did sponsor a very substantial program that paid school fees for children of people who died in the bombing. The mental health program was something that had been initiated by Kenyans and run by Kenyans. Further, both Operation Recovery and the subsequent USAID program highlighted the need for more education about and treatment of depression, post-trauma symptoms, and other mental health problems. Both programs also enhanced the stature of mental health providers in Nairobi and other urban areas in Kenya. Eventually, funds were exhausted and the programs ended.

The Kenyans collected a large amount of data, but as of now have been unable to analyze and present it. Although Operation Recovery reported that 60% of patients they surveyed found that their psychological symptoms improved after speaking with a mental health counselor, it is difficult to know what such statistics really mean (Kenya Medical Association, 2001).

Perhaps more instructive are the findings of a Kenyan psychiatrist who tried to evaluate the effects of this approach and discovered that their interventions really had not been the primary factor, or even a major factor, in improvement for most people. One year after the bombing, Kigamwa, Njenga, and Nyamai (n.d.) surveyed a convenience sample of 52 people, most of whom (96%) had been injured by the blast. Of this group, 85% had received some form of counseling. They were asked what was "most useful" for coming to terms with the bombing. The most helpful was religion, prayer, and faith in God (20%), followed by family support (12%), group therapy (9%), counseling (6%), and personal resourcefulness (3%). Clearly, counseling people to rely on themselves, or using messages focusing on autonomy such as "you're normal" or "draw on the resources within you" would have missed the mark with this group, since most found religious or relational influences to have been the most helpful.

CLINICAL ISSUES

A pressing question for Westerners involved in the mental health response was the extent to which culture shaped the nature, extent, and course of post-trauma symptoms (see Engdahl, this volume; Nader & Danieli, this volume). Somatically oriented presentations for psychological symptoms were common, as is the case in much of the world (Kirmayer, 2001; Ohaeri & Odejide, 1994). My three and a half years experience in Kenya convinced me that the cultural issues surrounding the identification and treatment of psychiatric problems in a non-western culture were somewhat less daunting than I had initially supposed. Kathuku and his colleagues screened 453 survivors of the bombing who had been evaluated at Kenyatta National Hospital for problems related to the bombing (Kathuku, Othieno, Ndetei, & Dech, 1999). Six months after the event, 17% of patients suffered from mixed anxiety/depression, 13% from depression alone, 7% from anxiety alone, and 7% from psychosis, a profile of problems perhaps not that different from what one might see after a similar event in the U.S. or Europe (Marsella, Friedman, Gerrity, & Scurfield, 1996; see also Engdahl, this volume).

Dr. David Ndetei (personal communication, 2000) reported that one of the primary complaints of men suffering from PTSD following the bombing was sexual impotence. A number of men came to psychiatric attention complaining of impotence, and with further questioning, they reported symptoms consistent with PTSD and depression. Dr. Ndetei reported that treatment with imipramine or a similar antidepressant (selective serotonin inhibitors, though available, are unaffordable for most Kenyans) often improved or resolved such symptoms. In fact, a USAID program that funded treatment for Kenyan victims of the bombing discovered that a significant portion of the budget for medications for victims was going to the purchase of Viagra, a month's supply of which cost about as much as the monthly wage of a low level Kenyan laborer.

Shortly after beginning my work in Nairobi, I noticed that of the more than two hundred Kenyans who worked for the embassy and were affected by the bombing, none failed to return to work solely because of psychological symptoms related to the stress of the bombing. Quite a few could not work who had injuries that were complicated by depression, posttraumatic stress disorder, or cognitive impairment resulting from a head injury. A number had psychological problems that came to my attention. Among these problems were depression and psychosis. But of those affected, none failed to continue working as a result of the bombing.

WORLDVIEW AND TRAUMA RESPONSE

Perhaps the most striking contrast between the patients I treated in the U.S. and the Kenyans was the difference in worldview. Fatalism tended to shape the clinical response of many of the victims. Among the many Kenyan survivors and rescuers with whom I had contact, expressions of survivor guilt were virtually nonexistent. This was not true for the American survivors, who not uncommonly wondered why the bombing had happened to them or why they had been spared while someone else died. In fact, there is some evidence that guilt as a symptom of depression (and presumably of other psychiatric disorders) is a culture-dependent symptom (Stompe, Ortwein-Swoboda, Chaudhry, Friedman, & Schanda, 2001).

The Kenyans who reflected on the meaning of the bombing, whether Muslim, Christian, or Hindu, more often than not viewed what had happened as God's will. In a series of recollections about the bombing written for the second anniversary, many spoke of "God's will." Some noted their "good luck" in surviving. Many expressed anger at the terrorists, but none at the deity. Since survivor guilt and anger at God have come to be seen as "normal" in western descriptions of reactions to disaster, this absence was striking.

Certainly, the African view of life is fatalistic in many ways. Christianity, Islam, and African traditional religion (ATR) see God as a benevolent, all powerful creator, although in ATR God is considered unknowable (Mbiti, 1991). In a society where one in 10 people is infected by HIV, crime and poverty are ubiquitous, and social services are sparse, a newly hired policeman makes $45 per month. Expectations of what God or society owe victims are different than in the industrialized world.

On the other hand, Kenyans did sometimes express guilt about their own actions at the time of the bombing. A case in point is a woman in her early 30s who had started muttering things to herself at work, hitting things near her for no particular reason, and whose work performance had declined precipitously after years of diligent service in an embassy-related job. When I interviewed the woman, she said that she had had a premonition that something bad was going to happen at the embassy and she believed that she had not done enough to warn people at the embassy of the impending doom. She had most of the vegetative signs of depression and I treated her with an antidepressant and talked to her about her experience and her feelings. Over a period of several months, I saw her periodically, though she frequently skipped our appointments saying she had forgotten them. She continued the medication I gave her for a time and, I learned, attended a Pentecostal church where church members prayed for her regularly. She stopped the medicines I had given her, but would come by to see me every few weeks to report on her progress at my request. With the talking, the church support, and possibly the medication (what she was taking, exactly, was difficult to establish), she returned to her job and improved markedly. She resumed her old pattern of work, her agitation disappeared, and did well for about a year and a half prior to my departure in June 2003. Guilt over a perceived failure to fulfill a responsibility to those who had died led to dramatic psychological symptoms that resolved with psychological support and African religious intervention.

Kenyans constructed their responses around other themes as well. Some considered themselves "lucky." One Kenyan writing about his experience two years after the bombing organized his experience around the number seven, a number that among his tribe, the Kamba, holds special significance similar to its significance to westerners (Lindblom, 1920): "Seven has always been a lucky or sacred number and was given to all manner of grouping [sic] in antiquity. . . . I also am associated with some SEVENS; after all I was born on the SEVENTH day of May. On the SEVENTH day of August, I had an occasion to witness a life threatening incident from which I have learned a lot in life" (*Recollections of foreign service nationals of the August 7, 1998 bombing of the American Embassy in Nairobi*, 2000). In his account of the bombing, collected two years after the event, he talked about his luck in surviving. He has done quite well since the bombing, and continues to work as a financial manager for one of the substantial U.S. government entities with a branch in Kenya.

A number of Kenyans felt they had been spared by God, often with the implication that he was sparing them for a purpose. They mourned the deaths of their colleagues, but rarely asked why the colleagues had died. Many, however, believed that God had spared their lives for a reason. Wrote one, "GOD HAD A REASON FOR SAVING YOUR LIVES. IT IS TIME YOU ASK GOD WHAT HE HAS IN STORE FOR YOU" (*Recollections of foreign service nationals*, 2000). Another wrote, "I was bitter at our attackers. Why [had] our colleagues . . . fallen? Why us, etc.? Later, I thank God for each new day and believe I must go on and make the best of each new day that God gives me, for I do not know whether I will live to see the end of this day. Death comes without warning" (*Recollections of foreign service nationals*, 2000).

The impact of the event on several of the Kenyans has persisted with great intensity throughout the five years since the bombing. At the third anniversary, one of the leaders of the Kenyan employees remarked in a commemorative speech, "I stand before you with fresh memories. I stand before you with a heart full of sorrow. My eyes are full of tears. My heart is heavy and my legs weak. . . . Three years down the road, the memories of the 1998 August 7th bombing are as fresh as if it happened yesterday. I can still see clearly my colleagues struggle under the rubble. I can still hear their cries in the choking smoke. I can still feel the bodies of those who could not make it. I can still hear the cries of those trapped under collapsed walls." He was not alone. Many Kenyans felt the same, though others seemed to have been able to move beyond the worst of their pain. We owe a great debt to the Kenyan mental health community and to the survivors of the bombing for their efforts to use the experience of the bombing to enhance our understanding of the nature of the human response to trauma in a non-Western setting.

REFERENCES

Barrett, D. B., Kurian, G. T., & Johnson, T. M. (2001). *World Christian encyclopedia: A comparative survey of churches and religions in the modern world* (2nd ed.). New York: Oxford University Press.

East Africa Living Encyclopedia. Kenya–Ethnic groups. Retrieved March 1, 2004 from University of Pennsylvania, African Studies Center Website: http://www.africa. upenn.edu/NEH/kethnic.htm

Engdahl, B. (2004). Integrating international findings on the impact of terrorism. *Journal of Aggression, Maltreatment & Trauma,* 9 (1/2/3/4), 265-276.

Kathuku, M. D., Othieno, C., Ndetei, M. D., & Dech, H. (1999). *The pattern of psychiatric morbidity among the survivors of the Nairobi bomb blast: Six months after the event.* Unpublished manuscript.

Kenya Medical Association. (2001). *Operation Recovery Report: The mental health response to the August 7th 1998 Nairobi bombing. A project of the Kenya Medical Association.* Unpublished manuscript, Nairobi, Kenya.

Kigamwa, P., Njenga, F., & Nyamai, C. (n.d.). *1 year follow-up of victims of the 1998 Nairobi U.S. embassy bombing.* Unpublished manuscript.

Kirmayer, L. J. (2001). Cultural variations in the clinical presentation of depression and anxiety: Implications for diagnosis and treatment. *Journal of Clinical Psychiatry, 62*(Suppl 13), 22-28; discussion 29-30.

Lindblom, G. (1920). *The Akamba in British East Africa; An ethnological monograph* (2nd ed., enlarged.). Uppsala, Sweden: Appelbergs boktryckeri aktiebolag.

Marsella, A. J., Friedman, M. J., Gerrity, E. T., & Scurfield, R. (1996). *Ethnocultural aspects of post-traumatic stress disorders: Issues, research, and clinical applications.* Washington DC: American Psychological Association.

Mbiti, J. S. (1991). *Introduction to African religion* (2nd ed.). Nairobi, Kenya: East African Educational Publishers, Ltd.

Nader, K., & Danieli, Y. (2004). Cultural issues in terrorism and in response to terrorism. *Journal of Aggression, Maltreatment & Trauma,* 9(1/2/3/4), 399-410.

Njenga, F. G., Nyamai, C., & Kigamwa, P. (2003). Terrorist bombing at the USA Embassy in Nairobi: The media response. *East African Medical Journal,* 80(3), 159-164.

Ohaeri, J. U., & Odejide, O. A. (1994). Somatization symptoms among patients using primary health care facilities in a rural community in Nigeria. *American Journal of Psychiatry, 151*(5), 728-731.

Recollections of foreign service nationals of the August 7, 1998 bombing of the American Embassy in Nairobi. Unpublished manuscript (2000).

Stompe, T., Ortwein-Swoboda, G., Chaudhry, H. R., Friedman, A., Wenzel, T., & Schanda, H. (2001). Guilt and depression: A cross-cultural comparative study. *Psychopathology, 34,* 289-298.

United States Agency for International Development. (2001). *Up from the ashes: Lessons learned from the bombing of the United States Embassy, Nairobi, Kenya.* Unpublished manuscript, Nairobi, Kenya.

Voice:
We Are Asked to Do Anything and Everything Except Be Victims

Nairobi, Kenya. August 7, 1998, 10:38 a.m. A loud explosion. I turn toward the windows but my childhood training stops me, explosions and windows don't mix. I learned that as a teenager in Laos from 1963 to 1969, Vietnam war time. Someone says it's the Embassy. Can't be, this is Nairobi, not Beirut. But it is. With the Embassy gone, that means our building, United States Agency for International Development (USAID), will be the command post. I prepare for what I know will be a long, long workday, week, and month(s).

Satellite phone is up and running. There is no 911 to call, no serious police or fire service, virtually no ambulances, and the hospitals are overwhelmed. Embassy colleagues flee the building, make sure they are alive, and then go back in to pull out their dead and injured colleagues. Some try to establish a perimeter line with the guns on hand. Our doctor and three nurses blessedly survive. They set up triage. Next door is even worse. An eight-story building has collapsed and it's carnage in the 22-story bank behind the Embassy. People ran to the window after the terrorists initially threw a grenade. Their faces were all up on the glass when the bomb went off.

Address correspondence to: Lee Ann Ross, 3062 NW Underhill Place, Bend, OR 97701 USA (E-mail: rossleeann@yahoo.com).

[Haworth co-indexing entry note]: "Voice: We Are Asked to Do Anything and Everything Except Be Victims." Ross, Lee Ann. Co-published simultaneously in *Journal of Aggression, Maltreatment & Trauma* (The Haworth Maltreatment & Trauma Press, an imprint of The Haworth Press, Inc.) Vol. 9, No. 1/2, 2004; and: *The Trauma of Terrorism: Sharing Knowledge and Shared Care, An International Handbook* (ed: Yael Danieli, Danny Brom, and Joe Sills) The Haworth Maltreatment & Trauma Press, an imprint of The Haworth Press, Inc., 2005.

The Ambassador arrives and asks for a volunteer to run the operations center. I raise my hand, I know our building, and I know what our staff can do. We try to make a list of the dead and injured. It's very hard. Our phone list is out of date. Someone suggests the radio call list. Someone else calls Paris to send us the Kenyan embassy employees' payroll list.

I dispatch our Kenyan employees to the hospitals and the morgue to look for our dead and injured. Others work the phones to tell distressed relatives who is alive and who is dead. Volunteers only, I could never order anyone to do this, knowing the trauma they are about to experience. I call all the counselors I know in town, all five or six of them, and ask them to help us. Two regional State Department psychiatrists arrive the next day. One runs a Critical Incident Stress Debriefing. No one wants to attend. I found it grueling, but incredibly useful.

All told, 213 dead including 12 US employees and 34 Kenyan employees from our embassy. My best friend is among them. It takes a day and a half to find her. Her husband calls me every hour to see if we have any news. When she's been identified, I can't give him the news, I don't take his last calls. I send a counselor to his house. His daughter has been with my daughter all this time. I call my husband and tell him to take Karen home.

I'm in total denial. Can't understand why I can't breathe right. I do pretty well for a week or two. Adrenaline keeps me going. Then the nightmares start; I can't sleep. Playing golf, the flashbacks from the war in Laos start. I can get through the third hole but then the movies in my head begin. The rest of the round I'm in Laos in living color. Aerial bombings, being shot at, coups, counter coups, high school friends dying, some dads dying, no memorial services, and no acknowledgement that this is crazy. Denial is the antidote.

We're offered an extra R & R. I don't really want to go, but I need to sleep. I'd like the movies to stop. I see a counselor in town. She wants me to get out of town. I suggest a golf tournament in Uganda. Not good enough, she suggests the States for a few weeks. I go. A friend hooks me up with a counselor in Oklahoma City. We talk several times. She wants to know how I feel. I tell her I don't feel anything; I am working overtime on not feeling. I tell her I'm fine, it's already been six weeks, so I'm sure I'm about through this. I don't really need help. What little I know.

Back in Kenya we design a disaster relief package for the Kenyan victims and argue with Congress to get money. We only have the Ambassador's Disaster Fund to work with, $25,000. It takes until December to get any more money. Tragic. The Kenyans can't believe that we can't be more responsive. We can't either. Tensions run high.

Somehow many see us at fault. It's as if they think we blew ourselves up. We are never viewed as victims. We are asked to do anything and everything, except be victims. Later, some of the Kenyan victims sue Bin Laden while most of the American victims sue the State Department in federal court alleging the Embassy didn't do enough to protect them.

What can go wrong will go wrong. The head Washington psychiatrist comes out after four months. After eight months, a temporary psychiatrist has been posted and in January 1999, a psychiatrist is permanently assigned. The implicit message has been pretty clear, Foreign Service Officers are not supposed to be affected by trauma. Great theory, but it just doesn't seem to be working. No system of counseling was ever set up for the US personnel. The phone numbers of the few Western oriented counselors in town were circulated. One had to pay for counseling oneself, or more exasperating still, get Office of Workers' Compensation Programs to pay for it. Somehow it was okay to design a mental heath program for the Kenyan victims but not for us.

It's been five years. I worked in Kenya for two years following the bombing. Between the bombing, carjacking, and crime, it was time to go. I spent a year in USAID Washington as a policy advisor on international terrorism. I wasn't able to move the bureaucracy forward very far. Embassies will be bombed again. We need a pre-established plan on how we are going to care for our employees. We can't make it happen. Incredibly frustrating.

I retired three years after the bombing. Had enough, and moved to Oregon. I'm back on antidepressants, have a lot of somatization, and I'm seeing a counselor again. Finally paid by workers comp five years and a month following the bombing. At last, I'm starting to deal with the Nairobi trauma. The State Department has blessedly instituted a mental health policy position in June, 2003.

Terror and Trauma in Bali: Australia's Mental Health Disaster Response

Beverley Raphael
Julie Dunsmore
Sally Wooding

SUMMARY. On October 12, 2002, the island of Bali experienced a horrific terrorist attack in which 202 people, 88 of them Australian, died; many of the victims were young people on holiday. This article chronicles the authors' experience as policy makers, administrators, and clinicians responding to the bombing. It focuses on the immediate and continuing needs of those involved and the complex challenges faced by a systems response in the acute and ongoing phases. Survivors' narratives, reflecting the enduring difficulties experienced by both individuals and systems, are included. The article highlights issues of mental

---

Address correspondence to: Emeritus Professor Beverley Raphael, MD, Centre for Mental Health, New South Wales Health Department, Locked Mail Bag 961, North Sydney, 2059, Australia (E-mail: BRAPH@doh.health.nsw.gov.au).

Dr. Bill McNeil was holidaying in Bali and assisted in the wake of the two bombings. He has provided valuable feedback for this article and has contributed generously his own account of the immediate and ongoing impact of October 12, 2002 (see his Voice, this volume).

[Haworth co-indexing entry note]: "Terror and Trauma in Bali: Australia's Mental Health Disaster Response." Raphael, Beverley, Julie Dunsmore, and Sally Wooding. Co-published simultaneously in *Journal of Aggression, Maltreatment & Trauma* (The Haworth Maltreatment & Trauma Press, an imprint of The Haworth Press, Inc.) Vol. 9, No. 1/2, 2004; and: *The Trauma of Terrorism: Sharing Knowledge and Shared Care, An International Handbook* (ed: Yael Danieli, Danny Brom, and Joe Sills) The Haworth Maltreatment & Trauma Press, an imprint of The Haworth Press, Inc., 2005.

health aspects of disaster victim identification and responses to the variously affected groups.

KEYWORDS. Terrorism, disaster, mental health response, trauma, bereavement

The responses of Australians to the terrorist bombing in Bali brought shock, courage, compassion, horror, anger, and grief. There were and are specific issues about the ethos and meaning of the events that occurred in Bali; the particular groups who were there and were directly or indirectly affected; the responses of health and other systems to the attack and its consequences; and the emergency, immediate, and long-term mental health interventions and consultation in response to the psychological needs in the acute phase and in the aftermath.

A range of studies and experiences with response to terrorism and disaster provides guidance about the impact of such incidents, their mental health consequences and what can be done to respond to them. This literature is well encompassed by a number of resources that inform this article, but are not quoted in detail (see National Institute Mental Health [NIMH], 2002; New South Wales [NSW] Health Department, 2000; Norris, Friedman, Watson, Byrne, Diaz, & Kaniasty, 2002; Ursano, Fullerton, & Norwood, 2003; Zatrick, 2003). They include Ursano et al.'s excellent 2003 volume on terrorism and disaster, and also reports from Project Liberty, the New York community mental health program following September 11 (see Felton, 2002). Their translation into the implementation of mental health response, such as that described here, forms a background that clearly highlights how much more work needs to be done to understand, respond to, and prevent or manage the mental health consequences of terror, trauma, and loss.

Bali is a tourist resort island that has been very popular with Australians: popular because of its people with their gentle and welcoming culture, popular because of its beautiful beaches and relaxed atmosphere, and popular as a symbol of getting away, letting go in a "foreign" place but one that is close to home. Many Australians of different backgrounds holiday in this "island paradise," as it has often been called. This context is very relevant in terms of those who were in Bali at the time of the bombing, shattering this image of a safe and beautiful place.

Another background is the Australian experience with terrorism. Despite significant major national and other disasters, such as transportation accidents (Granville rail disaster; see Raphael, 1977) and mass shootings (such as at Port Arthur, Tasmania), Australia has perceived itself as "innocent" of this type of violence. This was part of the national perception and response to Bali: "we have lost our innocence."

On the evening of October 12, 2002, two bombs were detonated at a bar and nightclub frequented by Australians and other westerners. As this terrorist attack occurred in another country, there were special complexities in terms of response. These included the difficulties of mobilizing a medical disaster response on the Indonesian island of Bali; how the Australian government and other agencies would deal with the response in an appropriate relationship with Indonesia, which to some degree, especially in Bali, is seen as a developing country; the issues of the care for the injured in limited hospital and health care settings; the transport back to Australia for ongoing medical care (e.g., intensive burns and other traumatic injuries); management of the bodies and identification of the deceased; the repatriation of Australians back to Australia; the concern for and response to the Balinese people who were killed, injured or otherwise affected; the response to other nationalities injured in the blasts; the recognition of overwhelming impact on all directly and indirectly involved; and the difficulties of knowing those who were victims, both direct and indirect, of this terrorist attack.

Mobilizing a mental health response both in the emergency and long-term took place in these contexts. Those affected were widely dispersed throughout Australia and their principal contacts were through Federal police liaison officers and the Red Cross. These systems were variously linked to each State's mental health response system.

EMERGENCY AND ACUTE PHASE

The voice of a young doctor holidaying in Bali (Bill McNeil) tells of dealing with the injured in circumstances where physical resources were inadequate for the extent and severity of the wounds and numbers affected. He describes patients, "most burned beyond that which I thought possible to survive," how they were "piled with the dead," and how they "all bore their suffering with great dignity."

The words of those who were there vividly describe the experiences of those who survived. The accounts provided in this section have been obtained from documentary news reports (Belsham, 2003).

John and Tracey went to Bali for a family holiday with their daughter Angela and son Michael. They went to the Sari Club that night but left their daughter with friends as they went back together to their hotel not far away. They heard the blast, saw the fire, and ran toward the club, against the crowd who was fleeing and many of who were burnt or bleeding. John ran: "I was screaming and screaming, looking for Angela, knowing that she was there . . . just hoping she had got out . . . you just scream . . . lifting up sheets of metal . . . just sifting through whatever trying to find her."

John describes what he saw when he got to the Sari Club: "I just saw–dead people everywhere. Dead people in any shape or form you can imagine." He went on to explain "Oh just body parts, people's eyelids blown off, just staring at you . . . young people, meat everywhere. . . . Then I looked into the flames and I just knew she was dead."

There are many other descriptions of the horror and chaos. Many people were in Bali as part of a family or group holiday, such as young men from football clubs, from rural or metropolitan centers, celebrating the end of the sporting seasons. There were young women in groups of friendship and support after weddings, some young mothers, sisters, daughters, some girls and their friends.

People affected, and Australia as a whole, were given clear messages by both State and National Governments via the media and other response agencies, that every possible assistance would be provided. This ensured strong and ongoing recognition of the suffering and response to address the needs of those affected and reinforced community strengths in adversity. A further parallel process that has significance for mental health was the need to address the anxieties of the general population as there had been no previous experience of this degree of malevolent attack "so close to home" since the bombing of Darwin in the Second World War. The National Government's development of a greater focus on security and a media campaign to educate the population to be "alert not alarmed," represented a new focus. There were significant anxieties in the general population regarding the potential for a future attack.

STATE GOVERNMENT MENTAL HEALTH RESPONSE AND SERVICE DELIVERY

Government response commenced with the news of the attack and, in the authors' home state of New South Wales, followed existing defined and structured disaster response plans (NSW Health Department, 2000). Of the 88 Australians killed in Bali, 42 were from New South Wales (23 women and 19 men). The State's response plan had been formulated by the primary author of this article and implemented as a component of the preparation for the 2000 Olympic Games in Sydney.

Mobilization of response to the Bali attack in *all* Australian states led to preparations for returning families and the establishment of programs of support and psychological first aid. For instance, a time was established at the Sydney Airport for a variety of agencies (such as Red Cross, Department of Health and Mental Health and the Federal Police) to be present to meet returning flights of families brought back from Bali.

Those with severe burns and other injuries were medically evacuated after initial treatment. However, in general the rest of the returning Australians had minor injuries, were shocked, or just were desperate to return to the safety of their homeland. As one person said, "it's so good to have your feet on Australian soil again, it was horrific, chaos, we couldn't wait to get out and I saw things I can't speak about now–I don't want to–I'm just glad to be home." People were met by loved ones and were offered support and opportunities for later follow-up by mental health services. An operational debriefing for all service agencies (e.g., Emergency Service personnel, Community Mental Health clinicians, airport officers) was held some weeks later, and at this meeting services such as Customs officers and the Federal Police noted the value of the presence of mental health professionals: "we knew we had the support if we needed it."

MENTAL HEALTH RESPONSE

The nature and difficulties associated with mental health response are discussed below and particularly draw upon reports of participants. Significant issues include: the difficulty of identifying and accessing the wide variety of those affected; the variation in traumatic experience; and the timing of intervention. Also significant was the resistance to issues of mental health and the subsequent reticence and delay in seeking help.

Responding to the Acutely Bereaved

In the wake of the bombing and as the extent of needs of those likely to be bereaved became clearer, programs were put in place to respond to their diverse issues, which built on understanding the complexity of these traumatic bereavements and the need for assessment and care from the earliest stages (Raphael & Martinek, 1997; Raphael & Wooding, 2004). Initial responses focused on available empirical evidence advocating psychological first aid and to first "do no harm." Stress debriefing was inappropriate and not recommended in these circumstances in line with the current evidence-based recommendations (Litz, Gray, Bryant, & Adler, 2002; NIMH, 2002; Raphael & Wilson, 2000).

There were bereaved people who were with family members or friends in Bali, and others who had flown to Bali to try to find their loved ones, desperate to see if they were alive. They had actively searched and reported having experienced the traumatic stressors of the bombing and its aftermath in addition to the loss.

There were also those returning home who had, to some degree, seen and acknowledged that their loved ones were among the dead. This in itself was often extremely psychologically traumatic, as it had involved searching among multiple bodies in the heat and with little formal mortuary process or preservation. Misidentification occurred, as with one man who thought (incorrectly) that he had found his wife. The need for formal forensic identification was soon established but, while giving accuracy, this involved delay and other complex processes that were also stressful for those bereaved.

Where possible, Federal authorities arranged for families to return on the same flight as their deceased family member with support and full recognition of the deceased and the family on arrival in Australia. For example, Australian flags were placed upon coffins. Customs and quarantine formalities were shaped to these needs. Coroners agreed not to conduct further examination as formal processes that had established causes of death and identities of the deceased had been conducted in Bali. Nevertheless, there were extensive questions to be responded to regarding the identification; DNA and related Disaster Victim Identification (DVI) matters were also involved before the bodies of the deceased could be returned to their families. Skilled bereavement counselors trained in both formal processes and appropriate support for those who were both acutely traumatized and bereaved worked with these families through this immediate process. These were skilled team members attached to the city morgue.

For those bereaved where there was a longer time of uncertainty, prolonged searching, and growing recognition that their loved one must have died in the bombing, this was a profoundly challenging period. There was a more prolonged time without specialized support, potentially aggravating their despair and distress. Nevertheless, eventually all deaths were formally listed and the rituals of community recognition and family mourning took place. Longer-term follow-up of bereaved people was also provided in response to need.

Identifying and Contacting Populations Who Were Exposed to Psychological Trauma

While it was recognized that many were exposed through witnessing or experiencing the explosions, or being present in Bali in the horror of the aftermath, identifying and making contact with these people was complex and many who were "unrecognized" victims (e.g., medical staff) presented over the following months. Many Australians rushed home in the wake of the bombing, wanting only to see their home and family and avoiding official channels of recording and contact.

As discussed, mental health response was built on experience and evidence of what was most likely to be of benefit in the immediate and longer term (NIMH, 2002). Wherever possible, those who were known to have been at the sites of the explosions in Bali were contacted on their return to Australia. Their initial relief and denial meant that many felt that they did not need help, and appeared to be coping well. Others who were not at the site but close by were not likely to be identified as victims, yet some of these people came forward 6-9 months later identifying symptoms of Post Traumatic Stress Disorder (PTSD), or more general symptoms of depression, anxiety, or behavioral problems. A further group are those who were not in Bali at the time, but went there during the immediate aftermath to join or find friends or family, or to help.

The young men who were in Bali, or who returned there were, on the whole, not likely to readily see themselves as needing psychological help. They were often part of a young group focussed on sport, physical activity, and drinking alcohol for release. Many people had never had contact with a mental health professional and felt that seeking or accepting assistance may indicate that they were weak or "crazy." As a result, they made contact later during the mental health outreach program (provided in collaboration with other agencies) or through other family and group contacts.

One method of outreach designed both to deliver intervention and to provide access for others (friends, siblings) affected was the information evenings that were held in communities where there had been a significant number of deaths. This outreach program was advertised only to survivors and bereaved and was held in partnership with key agencies such as the Australian Federal Police, Red Cross (who also provided financial assistance for counseling), State Departments of Health (Mental Health), and the Department of Community Services.

Information about the investigation of the terrorist attack, how to access available financial assistance, and information on coping with stress, trauma, grief, and loss was provided. These evenings received a very positive response and provided an environment that normalized any difficulties with coping. Attendees often stayed behind to talk to therapists, to find out more information on when and where to go to get help. Many expressed relief that they were not 'going crazy' and that others were experiencing similar emotions. They spontaneously showed photos of their lost loved ones and began to discuss their feelings with therapists and with other families and survivors.

It is recognised that this outreach was not as systematic as would have been ideal in terms of accessing all those likely to be affected. This article is intended to reflect the obstacles and complexities of system and clinical response in such contexts. One of the most significant difficulties experienced in this case was contacting those who may have been affected to provide information on mental health issues.

INTERVENTION FRAMEWORK FOR MENTAL HEALTH RESPONSE

There are significant and very real obstacles in providing interventions during and subsequent to such a challenging environment. In this case, therapeutic approaches were built on frameworks of existing evidence-based grief and trauma counseling techniques, cognitive behavior therapy (CBT), and other appropriate therapeutic approaches, and were delivered in both individual and group modalities. For instance, many young men chose group formats after having undergone earlier individual counseling; some of these brought a friend to their first session before continuing individually. Others preferred the format of a group information evening prior to individual counseling.

Clinical Issues and Reported Outcomes

Whether in an individual or group, commonly reported phenomena among those traumatized included profound symptoms of psychological traumatization such as dissociation and flashbacks. Insomnia and nightmares with images and re-experiencing from the blast continued to disturb those affected for many months. Others reported relationship breakdown, impulsivity, aggression and substance abuse, suicidality, and increased motor vehicle or workplace accidents.

Although initially reticent, a number of young people have now utilized the mental health counseling outreach program provided by the State Health Department and reported it to be of benefit. The majority report they have been able to return to work and to participate in their relationships and communities. They have also reported the value of group and community support. Group therapy with young men and also for bereaved mothers has been a component of the response system and reported by participants as very helpful. As with most traumatic circumstances, many have also demonstrated resilience and drawn upon existing support networks, thereby enhancing their sense of mastery while still allowing their distress, sadness, and grief.

Children and Families

There were children, young people, and families affected by the loss of loved ones, and the horror and trauma. Support and outreach were offered, but were variously taken up, perhaps because many had such positive support from their networks. Psychological impacts may include traumatic stress, grief, depression, anxiety, and behavioral problems presenting more subtly or at a later time. Children may be identified by different systems, for instance, education and family medicine (see Pfefferbaum, 2003; Wooding & Raphael, in press).

Workers

Workers in such settings face enormous stresses. Those responding in Bali included Australian embassy staff, aircrews evacuating victims to Australia, and doctors, nurses, and police both at the site and in the responding area, as well as in Australia. The deaths and the horrific injuries and burns had profound impacts. Formal and informal support systems were available through their organizations.

For the longer-term care, counselors involved in all aspects of mental health response need to have ready review and supervision mechanisms. Caring for the rescuers and carers needs to be further developed (Danieli, 2001). The clinical framework of case supervision is a model not only of support, but can also contribute to mitigating the workers own responses to such attacks, acknowledging achievements, and building active mastery and personal growth as well as skills for the future.

OFFICIAL STRUCTURES FOR RECOVERY

As indicated above, formal response systems to this emergency and its aftermath were complex as they are in most settings where such events take place. Federal Police coordinated the follow-up of Australians and put in place family liaison officers. The Australian Red Cross provided financial relief and was the coordinating agency for free counseling services, with psychologists or other providers funded for their time by the Australian government. In addition, a telephone help line, the "Bali help line," was established as a call center and funded by the State Government. It was staffed by mental health professionals who, after providing some immediate support, triaged callers to established systems of mental health care.

Memorialization at focal points, such as Christmas and at the 6- and 12-month anniversaries following the bombing, also brought affected people together, facilitating discussion and sharing of experience, but at the same time acknowledging loss and the value of those who had died. Memorial processes occurred both spontaneously in the community and memorials were also organised by the Government. Political support and leadership recognized community and individual strengths, resilience, and the Australian spirit of "mateship" through times of adversity. Throughout the year following the bombing, information and outreach kept those who had been identified as victims informed of both what was happening, and what resources and services were available through various agencies, including community services. These processes were perceived as positive and supportive.

CHALLENGES OF IMPLEMENTATION AND IMPLICATIONS FOR FUTURE POLICY AND PRACTICE

As noted above and reported at the recent Consensus Workshop on Early Intervention (NIMH, 2002), there is a limited evidence base for response to those affected by terrorist attacks. In terms of service delivery, a number of important issues emerged:

1. People have been resilient and supportive of one another; indeed, many may not seek or need intervention. Nevertheless, many have reported ongoing mental health impacts and that some of these had not been detected or treated. This indicates that systematic outreach does not reach all who need it. Suggestions to improve outreach approaches include (a) outreach coordination by lead disaster response agencies to link in and support mental health outreach; and (b) routine contact and follow-up with all identified victims; outreach to groups through specific other channels, such as the media.
2. While traumatic experiences occurred with the impact, there were many other traumatic aspects that appeared over time (e.g., for observers and helpers). It is not easy to identify all those who may be at risk through exposure to psychologically traumatic experiences. Improved identification of those at risk must consider the breadth of those affected and tailor ongoing systems of ready access, assessment, and care.

The experiences of the bereaved were complex. While their needs were supported via counselors working for the Coroner's office in the acute and shorter timeframe, they had multiple and evolving needs over time. Bereavement programs should (a) commence with notification of the event and introduce information, support, assessment, and supportive counseling through DVI processes; (b) include staged follow-up and counseling that deal with both trauma and grief complexities for those identified as at risk (Raphael & Wooding, 2004; Stroebe, Hannson, Stroebe, & Schut, 2001); (c) acknowledge the role and need for memorials and their varied impact; and (d) where possible, be tailored to suit cultural beliefs/requirements such as body viewings (a male relative or a mother only); or the gender of the doctor (e.g., a male doctor dealing with a female's body).

3. Part of the healing process includes the individual's and society's search for meaning, which is often a focus for those struggling with the loss and trauma. Questions about terrorism evolve over time, with differing patterns of adaptation to actual or possible threat. Identification of the perpetrators and management of the trials is likely to have been helpful, but should not be seen as giving resolution. Social and psychological aspects of the search for meaning and justice need to be taken into account.
4. Specialized interventions may be effective in preventing or treating morbidity, but how these may be implemented and who receives and responds to them are not well documented or evaluated. More formal research and evaluation is needed into the short- and long-term impacts, optimal methods of outreach, and the nature of effective interventions.
5. There is often a convergence of multiple agencies in such situations. Issues that arose in response to the Bali terrorist attack have led to formal planning, exercises, and review to ensure effective response for the future in a range of terrorist or other scenarios. Coordination, planning, and evaluation by key agencies at operational reviews provide opportunities for active learning and optimize planning for future response.

As Ursano et al. (2003) conclude, there have been significant advances in knowledge and understanding but "each event must be faced and dealt with . . . while at the same time promoting further understanding of the human response to the traumatic events which mark our time" (p. 338).

REFERENCES

Belsham, B. (2003, September 15). *After Bali. 4 Corners television program*. Sydney, Australia: Australian Broadcasting Commission.

Danieli, Y. (Ed.) (2001). *Sharing the front line and the back hills: International protectors and providers, peacekeepers, humanitarian aid workers and the media in the midst of crisis*. Amityville, NY: Baywood Publishing Company.

Felton, C. J. (2002). Project Liberty: A public health response to New Yorkers' mental health needs arising from the World Trade Center terrorist attacks. *Journal of Urban Health, 79*(3), 429-433.

Litz, B. T., Gray, M. J., Bryant, R. A., & Adler, A. B. (2002). Early intervention for trauma: Current status and future directions. *Clinical Psychology: Science and Practice, 9*, 112-134.

National Institute of Mental Health. (2002). *Mental health and mass violence: Evidence-based early psychological intervention for victims/survivors of mass violence. A workshop to reach consensus on best practices.* Washington, DC: U.S. Government Printing Office. Available online from, http://www.nimh.nih.gov/research/massviolence.pdf

New South Wales Health Department. (2000). *Disaster mental health response handbook.* Sydney, Australia: NSW Health and the Centre for Mental Health. Available online from, http://www.nswiop.nsw.edu.au/Resources/Disaster_Handbook.pdf

Norris, F. H., Friedman, M. J., Watson, P. J., Byrne, C. M., Diaz, E., & Kaniasty, K. (2002). 60,000 disaster victims speak: Part I. An empirical review of the empirical literature, 1981-2001. *Psychiatry, 65*, 207-239.

Pfefferbaum, B. (2003). The children of Oklahoma City. In R. J. Ursano, C. S. Fullerton, & A. E. Norwood (Eds.), *Terrorism and disaster: Individual and community mental health intervention* (pp. 58-70). New York: Cambridge University Press.

Raphael, B. (1977). The Granville train disaster: Psychological needs and their management. *The Medical Journal of Australia, 1*, 303-305.

Raphael, B., & Martinek, N. (1997). Assessing traumatic bereavement and posttraumatic stress disorder. In J. P. Wilson & T. M. Keane (Eds.), *Assessing psychological trauma and PTSD* (pp. 373-395). New York: Guilford Press.

Raphael, B., & Wilson, J. P. (Eds.) (2000). *Psychological debriefing: Theory, practice and evidence.* Cambridge: Cambridge University Press.

Raphael, B., & Wooding, S. (2004). Early mental health interventions for traumatic loss in adults. In B. T. Litz (Ed.), *Early intervention for trauma and traumatic loss* (pp. 147-178). New York: Guilford Press.

Stroebe, M. S., Hannson, R. O., Stroebe, W., & Schut, H. (Eds.). (2001). *Handbook of bereavement research: Consequences, coping, and care.* Washington, DC: American Psychological Association.

Ursano, R. J., Fullerton, C. S., & Norwood, A. E. (Eds.). (2003). *Terrorism and disaster: Individual and community mental health intervention.* New York: Cambridge University Press.

Wooding, S., & Raphael, B. (in press). Psychological impact of disasters/terrorism on children and adolescents: Experiences from Australia. *Prehospital and Disaster Medicine.*

Zatrick, D. (2003). Collaborative care for individual victims of individual and mass trauma: A health services research approach to developing early intervention. In R. J. Ursano, C. S. Fullerton, & A. E. Norwood (Eds.), *Terrorism and disaster: Individual and community mental health intervention* (pp. 189-208). New York: Cambridge University Press.

Voice:
Memories of Bali

Alan Atkinson

It was the glass. I couldn't understand why there was so much of it. As I ran in the dawn light to find the bombsite, I saw Balinese shopkeepers, grim-faced, trying to sweep it up. Where had the smiles gone? I'd already passed sullen soldiers on the sea front. Everyone seemed in shock. An anxious tourist on the beach told me there'd been a fireball in the night sky. He'd seen it from a kilometer away.

Within minutes, I'd joined the silent crowd beside Paddy's Bar. Everything was black: tables, chairs, a stump, a hand, and a skull. They were bringing the bits out on twisted sheets of corrugated iron. Some were carefully wrapped, some not. I counted fifty full bodies, but more were coming. Black bodies, inside white sheets. The smell was sickening.

My heart was beating fast, but I knew I had to try to keep a cool head. I pushed into the Macaroni Club and met Howard, a Canadian, who was without sleep, white, and sweating. There were bodies everywhere, he said. People without limbs, and so many dead. And the Sari Club was just for Westerners. He was in tears. I grabbed a phone and asked him to speak to Australia. It was the first of many calls that went to air as those back home were rising for another lazy Sunday.

Address correspondence to Alan Atkinson, P.O. Box 69, Belair, South Australia 5052, Australia. (E-mail: atkinson.alan@abc.net.au).

[Haworth co-indexing entry note]: "Voice: Memories of Bali." Atkinson, Alan. Co-published simultaneously in *Journal of Aggression, Maltreatment & Trauma* (The Haworth Maltreatment & Trauma Press, an imprint of The Haworth Press, Inc.) Vol. 9, No. 1/2, 2004; and: *The Trauma of Terrorism: Sharing Knowledge and Shared Care, An International Handbook* (ed: Yael Danieli, Danny Brom, and Joe Sills) The Haworth Maltreatment & Trauma Press, an imprint of The Haworth Press, Inc., 2005.

At the morgue, a doctor took me into the hallway. Here the dead were not covered; many were unrecognizable as people. I tripped on severed limbs.

I looked into the doctor's eyes for help. "If you can work in here so can I," I thought, but not for long.

"Come with me," he said, "I'll show you the list: 182 so far."

Outside, gulping for clear air, I met two Western women, Bali residents. They'd called all their friends, asking for blood, bandages, anything. Many more will die, they told me. Bali has no burns unit. They, too, spoke on the phone for me to Australia. One asked why I was there. I was on holiday, I said. She hugged me. No one knew what to say, except sorry.

How did I get through that first day, filing radio reports from dawn until after midnight? As I recall, it was as if everything was happening at one remove, yet, I knew what was going on was real and I was in the middle of it. That sense of disconnectedness, while at the same time being totally, intimately involved, stayed with me and helped me through as I stumbled from bombsite to morgue to airport, somehow keeping an open line to the newsroom in Australia.

But first and foremost, I had a job to do. I was not just a bystander. If I had been simply a witness, without the enforced focus and discipline of putting it down in words, I would probably have been a mess very quickly. To have a learned capacity to observe, study, analyze, record, and report certainly helped me cope both with the awful scenes and also the emotions, both my own and the raw grief of relatives, which at times threatened to overwhelm, even from a distance.

Secondly, after the first long hours of reporting alone I was part of an Australian Broadcasting Corporation (ABC) reporting team. Even if we didn't have time to talk much in between assignments, we were all seeing the same bad stuff. Thirdly, and so importantly, I had not lost a loved one. Luckily, my family and I had gone back to our hotel from Legian Street early. I was able to send them home in one piece.

I'm aware that if any of those three elements (the reporting, teamwork, and a safe family) had been different I would have been much less effective in doing my job. Indeed, it might have been impossible.

And there are the beginnings of perspective. I can look back and be right there, in the middle of that stinking mess at Sanglah Hospital watching exhausted volunteers putting their own lives on the line to try to save others. Sometimes I wake at night and remember a face, someone in tears, or the young Balinese girl from the surf shop singing Ave Maria to a silent crowd in the street in memory of her lost colleague. But now, back at work, among familiar surroundings, and with the loving support of friends and family, the shocking scenes are starting to fade a little, though the deep sadness I feel for the Balinese and for all those who lost so much is easily stirred.

In August 2003, I returned to Bali on a private visit. It helped to share stories with others who had been there. A friend took me to the bombsites, now two vacant blocks, one planted with banana trees. We stood for a while, reading the messages on the fence. My friend wept. All around, the shops and clubs are rebuilt and repainted and the tourists are drifting back to a new Paddy's along the street.

While the Balinese have held their cleansing ceremonies and believe the souls of the dead have passed on, there is, of course, still great personal pain. At my hotel, a young porter, just 20, shyly asked if I was Australian and promptly told me how sad he was, how he missed his older brother who had died in the Sari Club. He stood, in tears, at my door, then recovered, apologized profusely, and hurried back to work. And later on at the beach, I remembered the day after the bombing when I'd joined a ceremony at which Balinese and Westerners had scattered petals into the sea. It was one of the few occasions I'd allowed myself to cry.

I took off my shoes, the same tough old shoes I'd worn on October 13, shoes that had walked in blood and trodden on body parts. I left them there and watched as the sea washed over them. I don't know why I did it. I suppose it was a little ritual of my own.

Back home I have built a small stone lantern among the eucalypts beside the garden path. It's modeled on one that lit the path to our hotel room in Ubud. When I turn it on, it reminds me of those who died, and also of the Bali I love.

Voice:
A Baptism of Fire in Bali

Bill McNeil

I was a 28-year-old Australian male doctor. On the night of October 12th, 2002 in Kuta, Bali, Islamic fundamentalist militants with links in Malaysia and Afghanistan exploded a massive car bomb, killing 202 people almost instantly, while horrifically scarring many hundreds more.

A suicide bomber detonated on the dance floor of Paddy's Irish pub to draw rescuers from the much more crowded Sari Club on the opposite side of the street. Outside, there had been a parked 10-seat minibus modified to carry a fertilizer bomb with the explosive power of one ton of dynamite. Aluminum powder was added to create a metallic napalm effect, to increase the burning.

I saw the effects up close on the cars in the street, on the cinderblock and glass buildings, and on the people streaming from the site. A circle of destruction extended for a kilometer where tornadoes of pressure and fire had been.

Further on, when I felt the comfort of futility, I turned tail and beat a tactical retreat. Eventually, I found myself working the night shift in Sanglah Hospital in Denpasar where all of the seriously ill were sent. I had been assured that everything was under control and there was no need for me to come in, which I did not believe for a second. The scene was one of misery piled on horror, and I have no intention of making any sort of recovery.

Address correspondence to: Bill McNeil, c/o Centre for Mental Health, New South Wales Health Department. Locked Mail Bag 961 North Sydney, 2059, Australia (E-mail: SAWOO@doh.health.nsw.gov.au).

[Haworth co-indexing entry note]: "Voice: A Baptism of Fire in Bali." McNeil, Bill. Co-published simultaneously in *Journal of Aggression, Maltreatment & Trauma* (The Haworth Maltreatment & Trauma Press, an imprint of The Haworth Press, Inc.) Vol. 9, No. 1/2, 2004; and: *The Trauma of Terrorism: Sharing Knowledge and Shared Care, An International Handbook* (ed: Yael Danieli, Danny Brom, and Joe Sills) The Haworth Maltreatment & Trauma Press, an imprint of The Haworth Press, Inc., 2005.

Things rapidly went from almost normal to inferno. Many people were walking from the Kuta end of the street, looking okay, but a bit confused. Then there was a wave of people. The zombies. Glass was everywhere. Murderous shards of plate glass were suspended from frames, guillotines, and spread all over the road. The two story glass shop fronts lining Jalan legian were all blasted to pieces. What if you were sitting under the window like everyone did? Where were the people who had been in the shop fronts?

I zigzagged up the street screening the zombies, covered with nicks and scratches, and deaf from punctured eardrums and blast ravished hair. Most barefoot, walking oblivious with lacerated feet over hundreds of meters of glass. Their blank faces most alarming.

It was very difficult work. My mind kept bouncing all over the place, flooded with data. There was still a chance to run away; after all, I wasn't doing much. New ways of dying kept occurring to me.

"Australian doctor."

"Doctor over here."

I looked at their heads, their eyes, pupil size, and their bodies. Was any one spurting blood? Everyone was dazed and looking at me blankly. Closer, they were almost a wall of bodies singly and in groups. What could I do? I was the only one going in against this wall. It was terribly lonely.

"Over here," quietly, not an urgent call, much to my disappointment. Finally, something respectable to do. I preened myself and strode up straight to the footpath where a small, sorry looking crowd had gathered. Feeling warmed by a babble of accents.

"What's going on?" I asked with authority.

Everyone was looking down. More at the ground than her.

"She might need a doctor," in the earnest European voice of a backpacker alpha male.

"Hello, my name is Bill, I am an Australian doctor." "Hello," she replied with a gentle, German twist. She told me her name (I forget), her age (was it 24?) and that she was German.

Half on the footpath, legs over the gutter and onto the road she lay, cradled in the lap and arms of a man. Another held her body. Someone else rested his hand gently on her. Others stood attentive to her every breath, seeming ready to drop to their knees every now and again to just touch her, caress her. She was a lovely, gorgeous, and young woman with blue eyes and blonde hair. The sort of woman that you would like to meet in other circumstances to charm and flirt with.

All the blood had drained from her body through a 2cm wound just over the appendix from which an offending piece of bowel was protuberant. Her pallor made her translucent and in the quiet fading voice of her death she seemed transcendent too.

I did doctor-like things. Told of the wound, I called for scissors; there may have been some dramatic need to cut off her clothes. I pulled down her shorts a little and there it was. Her pulse was extremely fast and very weak. She was not bleeding from anywhere. I imagined the kind of resuscitation and exploratory surgery she required.

She was looking at me; I am horrified to say, with hope. Her eyes, my passion and anguish. I wish now that I had kissed her and held her tight against me, as was my first impulse at the time. I wish that I could have lain next to her, like the others, and held her and touched her until she died. I wish I could have curled up with those lovely kind people and cried my soul to death.

I hated palliative medicine. It is very grim. Like offering cigarettes to blokes with tracheotomy tubes. It is, though, very important. It would be nice to be better at it.

Futility! Just the sort of thing that I must avoid. I told them that they must not leave her, and that they must make her comfortable. I held her by the arms, close to me, and then drew away.

Looking into her eyes, I saw them drift into focus and said very clearly: "I am so sorry there is nothing that I can do for you."

I let her sink back into the stranger's lap and I stood up as tall as I could to shake off the filth of this moment, and I walked off looking ahead.

It is late now and I have an early appointment with my psychologist tomorrow. I think I will just finish off this bottle of vodka and then try and get some sleep. . . .

International Findings
on the Impact
of Terrorism

Brian Engdahl

SUMMARY. This article highlights findings on terrorism's impacts in countries outside of the United States. It reviews preceding articles and other published reports, and describes interventions and programs. It introduces the topic of "medically unexplained symptoms" that arise after terrorist attacks to explain some of the wide cultural variation in responses to terrorism. The article concludes with recommendations to expand our understanding of the impacts of terrorism: (a) adopt a broader framework, (b) increase emphases on studies of intervention and program development, and (c) recognize and seek to enhance resilience and the potential for growth in the aftermath of terrorism.

KEYWORDS. Terrorism, PTSD, cultural factors, somatic symptoms, resilience

---

Address correspondence to: Brian Engdahl, PhD, Psychology Section (116B), U.S. Department of Veterans Affairs Medical Center, Minneapolis, MN 55417 USA (E-mail: brian.engdahl@med.va.gov).

[Haworth co-indexing entry note]: "International Findings on the Impact of Terrorism." Engdahl, Brian. Co-published simultaneously in *Journal of Aggression, Maltreatment & Trauma* (The Haworth Maltreatment & Trauma Press, an imprint of The Haworth Press, Inc.) Vol. 9, No. 1/2, 2004; and: *The Trauma of Terrorism: Sharing Knowledge and Shared Care, An International Handbook* (ed: Yael Danieli, Danny Brom, and Joe Sills) The Haworth Maltreatment & Trauma Press, an imprint of The Haworth Press, Inc., 2005.

CLINICAL REPORTS AND EPIDEMIOLOGICAL STUDIES

Terrorism creates such diverse and complex destruction that a multidimensional, multi-disciplinary integrative framework will ultimately be required to describe it (see Danieli, Brom, & Sills, this volume; Danieli, Engdahl, & Schlenger, 2003). To date however, most worldwide literature flows from a western academic framework, is predominately descriptive, and consists primarily of clinical reports, epidemiological surveys of varying quality, and quasi-experimental designs. As such, the work, although fragmentary, generally converges, at least in the domains defined by objective measures of pathology and formal psychiatric diagnoses.

In India, three days after a 1996 terrorist bombing of a bus, 11 of 31 survivors studied had diagnosable psychiatric disorders (acute stress reaction, depression, and dissociative amnesia). The most common symptoms were depersonalization (interpersonal detachment), feeling things were not real, sleep disturbances, loss of appetite, nightmares, situational anxiety, depression, irritability, dulled feelings, self blame, guilt, loss of interest, suicidal ideas, and worry about money, spouse, work, and children (Gautam, Gupta, Batra, Sharma, Khandelwal, & Pant, 1998).

In Nairobi, Kenya, a survey of 500 school children after the 1998 United States embassy bombings found that their exposure was mostly indirect. Over 40% denied impaired functioning as a result. Ninety percent had experienced other crimes or human-caused violence. Greater numbers of traumatic events other than the bombings, dissociation at the time of *any* trauma, and stronger posttraumatic reactions to all trauma predicted bomb-related posttraumatic stress (Pfefferbaum, this volume; Pfefferbaum, North, Doughty, Gurwitch, Fullerton, & Kyula, 2003). The authors were struck by the apparent resilience of these children as indicated by their relatively low level of bombing-related functional impairment, despite their trauma histories and the generally dismal economic conditions in which they lived. The authors suggested that assessing protective factors is important and that mental health interventions in developing countries need to consider the disaster's context and the characteristics of the population and recovery environment. (See also Thielman, this volume, for more on the survivors of the 1998 embassy bombing and their care.)

In Spain, Baca, Baca-García, Pérez-Rodriguez, and Cabanas (this volume) used a standard measure of general psychopathology (the General Health Questionnaire) in a large sample of citizens exposed to terrorist attacks. They examined the correlates of the negative effects and found all exposed groups had higher rates of distress than the general Spanish population. The degree of exposure predicted negative effects, and victims' parents and spouses were more distressed than their children or siblings were. Time elapsed since trauma exposure ranged from zero to twenty years and bore little relationship to distress levels, illustrating the persistence of terrorism's impact. Similarly, 17 years after an attack by Palestinian guerillas, where 120 Israeli children were taken hostage and 20 killed, the survivors were still experiencing many PTSD symptoms, especially those who were physically injured (Desivilya, Gal, & Ayalon, 1996).

IMPACTS ON FAMILIES, COMMUNITIES, AND SOCIETIES

Published work that describes terrorism's impact at broader levels (e.g., families, community) is scarce, but common themes are identifiable. Somasundaram (this volume) provides a broad view of terrorism's impact on Sri Lanka. Starting with the western-style psychiatric variables, he quickly advances to a detailed consideration of terrorism's impact on families and communities. He refers to collective trauma (the cumulative effect of terror on the community) as leading to deep suspicion and mistrust, passiveness and submissiveness, and a brutalization of society. Perhaps most importantly, he discusses social deterioration, indexed by declines in sexual mores and social ethics, and increased child abuse and suicide rates. He highlights the "subtle but pernicious development of pathology in social structures and functioning that will need to be addressed if society is to recover" (p. xx).

Campbell, Cairns, and Mallett (this volume) summarize psychiatric effects of the violence between the Protestant and Catholic factions that dominated Northern Ireland over the last 30 years with tremendous impact on families and communities. Segregation has grown at the personal, residential, and educational levels. Austin (1989) examined how Filipinos have reacted to the continuing presence of terrorist violence (i.e., ambush, murder, kidnapping, and property destruction). The influence of terrorism on the basic social institutions was scrutinized. A typology of adaptations to terrorism was offered, reflecting a variety of role stresses resulting from living in a hostile region.

The literature on the effects of terrorism in Israel is large, going well beyond descriptions of psychiatric symptoms and disorders (see articles in this volume). For example, Nuttman-Shwartz and Lauer (2002) reported that terrorist-injured Israelis had difficulties coming to terms with terrorism in group therapy. These difficulties paralleled and interacted with Israeli society's difficulties in coming to terms with terror. Group cohesion and a sense of empowerment developed, but members could not cope with their terrorism-related fear, humiliation, and helplessness, nor mourn their losses. They clung to their shared identity as terrorism victims, helpless and isolated from others. The authors likened the group members' fixity to this identity as comparable to Israeli society's fixity to a parallel identity. Their analyses may apply to other societies, especially those that are less individualistic and more collectivistic. Such may be true in Japanese society, where the consequences of the Tokyo sarin gas attack were described as not only a personal trauma for those directly affected, but as a *national* trauma (Bowler, Murai, & True, 2001).

In a sample of 50 Israeli bus commuters, Gidron, Gal, and Zahavi (1999) examined the relationship between anxiety from terrorism and three coping strategies: (a) emotion-focused coping (calming-distraction); (b) problem-focused coping (checking behavior); and (c) denial (reduced perceived vulnerability). Anxiety over terrorism predicted less frequent commuting and more problem-focused coping. Further analyses suggested that moderate levels of problem-focused coping, emotion-focused coping, and minimizing perceived vulnerability ("healthy denial") may reduce anxiety from terrorism. In contrast, Bleich, Gelkopf, and Solomon (2003) reported that social support and *active* coping (seeking accurate information about loved ones' safety) were protective factors among Israelis exposed to terror attacks. In a nationally representative sample, rates of direct and indirect exposure were high (16.4% and 37.3%, respectively). Distress levels were also high, as was a reduced sense of safety, but the estimated rate of PTSD was moderate (9.17%).

What is striking is how coping with recurrent attacks and threats of attacks can in a sense become a way of life. Living under a continuous threat of terrorist attack can lead to "emergency routine" (see Yellin, this volume) where one conducts necessary daily tasks with an ever-present sense of danger, characterized by tension, apprehension, and distress, changing society's definitions of "normal." Psychiatric casualties are less likely to be stigmatized or ignored. They typically suffer from an acute stress disorder, and are referred to in the media as anxiety or shock casualties. Hyperarousal and hypervigilance during the post-attack period are seen not only as normal, but as desirable functional behaviors. Avoidance that reduces the chance of becoming a casualty is interpreted as functional coping.

INTERVENTIONS AND PROGRAM DEVELOPMENT

Reports that take a broader view of terrorism's impacts usually include descriptions of intervention efforts, perhaps because the authors frequently take active roles not only in research and writing, but also in interventions and advocacy. Jehel and Brunet (this volume) address the negative effects of terrorist attacks on French citizens and France's response. In addition to summarizing multiple studies documenting substantial and persistent posttraumatic stress, they describe the formation and function of a specialized health services network, victim self-help groups, and aid-to-victim professional groups, all of them vital in helping their society to heal. They highlight a major concern: social indifference that descends once a crisis is over and media coverage of emotional reactions has faded (also known as the conspiracy of silence; see Danieli et al., this volume). The fate of the injured, especially the psychologically injured, remains largely ignored. Because recovery in the aftermath of terrorism has a longer time dimension, one concept that can unite these elements is adaptation (Danieli, Engdahl, & Schlenger, 2004). There is obviously no single "quick fix" for these problems.

Campbell et al. (this volume) report that forgiveness (in the socio-political, not religious sense) has been sought in Northern Ireland. It has been more difficult to achieve among those most affected by the violence. Cairns and Toner (1993), however, suggested that hatred and ideological rifts can be transformed into a force for reconciliation. They described a program in which discussion of ideological differences takes place within the context of developing peer relationships.

Gillespie, Duffy, Hackmann, and Clark (2002) provided community-based cognitive therapy to Omagh, Ireland bombing survivors and documented a reduction in PTSD severity. One quarter of the doctors involved in the care of the Omagh bombing victims in 1998 were found to have PTSD (Firth-Cozens, Midgley, & Burges, 1999).

Kilpatrick, Best, Smith, and Falsetti (2002) evaluated services provided to family members affected by the Pan Am 103 terrorist bombing. These services included an international toll-free telephone number and informational hotline, a secure Internet Web page to provide updates about the trial, funding for mental health services, travel funds to attend the trial, assistance with travel arrangements, and a Lockerbie trial handbook. The most frequently used resources were the trial handbook and Web page. These innovative services allowed accurate information to be disseminated to large numbers of people. Although the family member's death was traumatic and nearly half of the family members reported emotional or behavioral problems serious enough to consider seeking therapy, only about one-third of them used mental health services. Reasons for this low utilization included beliefs that they could handle their difficulties on their own with the support of friends, family, and clergy, the stigma associated with obtaining services, and the lack of funds. However, 90% of the survivors who did use such services evaluated them positively.

Weine, Danieli, Silove, Van Ommeren, Fairbank, and Saul (2002) published guidelines for training in mental health and psychosocial interventions for trauma-exposed populations in the international arena. They recommend promoting the use of culturally-appropriate interventions in community settings. As an example, among survivors of a South African church congregation massacre, religious beliefs and practices were used to construct a meaningful retrospective narrative of the massacre (Ogden, Kaminer, Van Kradenburg, Seedat, & Stein, 2000). Lykes (1994) described a community-based group process aimed at child survivors of terrorism in Guatemala. It included drawing, story telling, collage, and dramatization, relying heavily on existing cultural traditions (e.g., story telling) and resources (nature, plants). Although they use mainstream mental health interventions to care for survivors of terror attacks in Israel, Adessky and Freedman's (this volume) interventions are at times dominated by their culture, a culture defined by the high probability of exposure to future terrorist attacks.

Even when culture-specific, data-based research on interventions is inadequate, providers have collected data and simultaneously used it to inform their service delivery. Khaled (this volume) describes such a mental health model initiated by the Algerian Society of Research in Psychology. Seeking to alleviate distress caused by ongoing terrorism in the absence of systematic research, they were limited to data provided by the daily work of their team, but were able to use it methodically to direct and improve their clinical efforts.

POSITIVE EFFECTS IN RESPONSE TO TERROR

Trauma may act as a catalyst for personal and societal transformation. As an example of direct positive effects at the societal level, the violence in Sri Lankan society has led to the emergence of community organizations, a decline in the grip of the caste system, and the increased liberation of women (Somasundaram, this volume). The war on terrorism in Afghanistan has also improved conditions for women: 25% of their national council must be made up of women and there is a growing realization of women's rights, particularly the right to education.

Antonovsky and Bernstein (1986) called for a shift in focus from pathogenesis, the process by which trauma exposure leads to only negative outcomes, to "salutogenesis," the process by which trauma exposure can lead to successful, that is, healthy outcomes. Such studies are rare, despite the fact that up to 90% of individuals exposed to some form of trauma report that they have experienced some benefits from coping with the aftermath of trauma, an experience termed "posttraumatic growth" (Tedeschi & Calhoun, 1996). The changes include positive developments in interpersonal relationships and one's spiritual life, a sense of personal strength, new pathways for one's life, and changes in personal philosophy. No reports to date have assessed survivors of terrorism for possible posttraumatic growth, nor have studies searched for predictors of successful coping with the impact of terrorism outside of the United States.

THE IMPACT OF TERRORISM:
CROSS-CULTURAL CONSIDERATIONS

The diagnostic construct of PTSD does not encompass the wide range of effects seen around the globe in the wake of terrorist attacks. De Jong (2002) has gone further and argued that diagnostic categories as defined in the DSM-IV or ICD-10 (World Health Organization, 1992) are often not even appropriate in non-western cultures. He called for a worldwide inventory of traumatic stress reactions that would yield a continuum. Because the response to threat is hardwired into human biology, one end of this continuum would be anchored by a common core of neurobiological alterations. The other end of this continuum would consist of a wide range of culturally-influenced behavioral and sociological phenomena. He urged investigators to use a phenomenological approach that combines qualitative and quantitative research methods applied within the sociocultural context being studied.

Using exactly that approach, Norris and her colleagues studied trauma exposure and its consequences in Mexico (Norris, Murphy, Baker, Perilla, Rodriguez, & Rodriguez, 2003). They demonstrated that PTSD encompasses features that transcend cultural differences. Because theirs was an investigation in a developing country, they conducted extensive qualitative research to identify emotional reactions among trauma survivors using unstructured interviews. Of the 17 PTSD symptoms, 14 were mentioned with little or no prompting by the investigators. Participants also used many expressions (e.g., always live with the fear, ill from fright) that suggested that the concept of trauma, broadly defined, was relevant for Mexican trauma survivors.

SOMATIC SYMPTOMS AFTER TERRORIST ATTACKS

The long-term effects of an episode of chemical or biological attack, real or suspected, are likely to be as damaging as the acute ones, if not more so (Wessely, Hyams, & Bartholomew, 2001). Mass panic, marked by nonsocial and nonrational flight as depicted in disaster movies, is a rare response to disaster. However, mass anxiety and the outbreak of somatic symptoms are common (Pastel, 2001). They may be the main threat in the face of a bioweapons attack (Moscrop, 2001; Hall, Norwood, Fullerton, Gifford, & Ursano, this volume). Immediately following the Tokyo sarin gas attack, psychological casualties outnumbered physical casualties by approximately four to one (Kawana, Ishimatsu, & Kanda, 2001; also see Lifton, this volume). Even five years later, psychological and somatic symptoms remained among survivors.

Some have suggested that somatic symptoms are the "idioms of distress" in developing countries (Nichter, 1981) and that non-westerners express their distress through somatic rather than psychological symptoms. Thielman (this volume) notes that Kenyans affected by the 1998 U.S. Embassy bombing often expressed psychological distress through somatic symptoms. However, somatic symptoms are common among trauma survivors around the globe. For example, a recent study of UK servicemen from 1854 onward who had been awarded war pensions for stress disorders found that body pains, heart palpitations, feeling faint, and fatigue were the most prominent post-combat symptoms (Jones et al., 2003). Varying proportions of trauma survivors, regardless of their culture, have difficulty articulating their symptoms. Those who have suffered both physical and psychological injuries after a terrorist attack may manifest their distress primarily through somatic symptoms. They may therefore seek treatment for symptoms that can be heavily influenced by ethnocultural variables, specifically cultural norms as to how one is to respond to trauma (Jones et al., 2003).

North (this volume) notes that somatic symptoms (but not somatoform *disorders*) develop after exposure to terrorist attacks. Acutely, people may experience what has been termed *hypochondriacal worry*, worry that is probably related to anxiety and a catastrophizing cognitive style (Kirmayer, 1996). Hypochondriacal worry arises in situations where attention is focused on the body, or where people feel vulnerable or uncertain. Such worry also often involves physiological disturbances aggravated by anxiety or depression and by cognitive misattributions; people attribute common sensations to illness, or are unable to generate normalizing explanations for distress.

Survivors appear to be served best when they learn through public health messages that most somatic and psychiatric symptoms experienced after terroristic attacks are self-limited. Clauw, Engel, Aronowitz, Jones, Kipen, and Kroenke (2003) provided an expert consensus statement on the characteristics of these symptoms and guidelines for intervention. They recommended that clinicians treat these patient concerns respectfully, viewing them as legitimate from the outset. (North [this volume] advocates an initial "agnostic" stance). Sufferers should not be trivialized as "the worried well." Public statements, research practices, and clinical care should be formulated with their direct input (Clauw et al., 2003).

If the acute problem of hypochondriacal worry fails to resolve, patients are then often said to be *somatizing*, or described as presenting with *medically unexplained symptoms*. Such may have been the case in the aftermath of the Tokyo sarin gas attack (Kawana, Ishimatsu, & Kanda, 2001, noted above). Somatic complaints may congeal into *symptom complexes*. These symptom complexes include multifocal pain, fatigue, cognitive or memory problems, and psychological distress. Ill-defined symptom complexes such as "Gulf War Syndrome" and "World Trade Center Syndrome" challenge patients, clinicians, scientists, and policymakers. Chronic somatic symptoms are common sequelae when catastrophic events last for a prolonged period or are accompanied by long-term worry or fear (Clauw et al., 2003).

CONCLUSION AND RECOMMENDATIONS

Although we are just beginning to study the impact of terrorism, an emerging understanding is obvious when one reads this volume. International collaboration, as difficult as that is to accomplish, will enhance intervention, research, and policy development recommended below.

1. *Adopt a broader framework*: A multidimensional, multidisciplinary framework (see Danieli et al., this volume) provides the perspective needed to move beyond the starting points provided by symptom checklists and psychiatric diagnoses. Only then will we have the broader understanding that is needed to improve research, interventions, education, and public policy.

A broad view of terrorism's consequences must recognize that many survivors develop temporary or persistent symptom complexes that do not meet "full criteria" for established medical and psychiatric diagnoses. This may contribute to observed cultural differences in the effects of terrorism. Although such symptom complexes may be "sub-syndromal," they merit our attention and should not be ignored by health care providers, researchers, or policy makers.

2. *Increase emphases on intervention studies and program development*: Many writers have provided recommendations for prevention, practice, and policy regarding the impact of terrorism and other severe trauma (De Jong, 2002; Green et al., 2003). Among the multitude of recommendations are the following:

a. Study the impact of interventions in many different cultures, especially group-and community-level interventions. Too few studies have been conducted and there is little agreement on outcome indicators and methods of assessing impact.

b. Train and use indigenous practitioners in psychosocial interventions whenever possible. As appropriate, involve community elders, tribal chiefs, and organizations such as the media, churches, and community groups in rehabilitation efforts. See Thielman (this volume) for examples from Kenya.

c. Inform legislators in affected countries about psychosocial problems faced by terrorism survivors, and encourage funding of services that include outreach and research.

d. Study terror-related health and psychosocial problems and interventions among survivors, including ill-defined and poorly understood symptom complexes observed in many survivors (i.e., joint pain, fatigue, headaches, memory loss, skin problems, etc.).

3. *Recognize and study resilience and the potential for growth in the aftermath of terrorism.* There is an encouraging increase in studies that assess coping strategies and other factors that can buffer against the negative effects of terrorism (e.g., Baum, this volume). Resilience and positive outcomes are only beginning to be studied in their own right, and merit increased attention.

REFERENCES

Adessky, R., & Freedman, S. A. (2004). Treating survivors of terrorism while adversity continues. *Journal of Aggression, Maltreatment, & Trauma, 9*(1/2/3/4), 443-454.

Antonovsky, A., & Bernstein, J. (1986). Pathogenesis and salutogenesis in war and other crises: Who studies the successful coper? In N. A. Milgram (Ed.), *Stress and coping in times of war: Generalizations from the Israeli experience* (pp. 52-65). New York: Brunner/Mazel.

Austin, W. (1989) Living on the edge: The impact of terrorism upon Philippine villagers. *International Journal of Offender Therapy and Comparative Criminology, 33,* 103-119.

Baca, E., Baca-García, E., Pérez-Rodríguez, M., M., & Cabanas, M., L. (2004). Short-and long-term effects of the terrorist attacks in Spain. *Journal of Aggression, Maltreatment, & Trauma, 9*(1/2/3/4), 157-170.

Baum, N. (2004). Building resilience: A school-based intervention for children exposed to ongoing trauma and stress. *Journal of Aggression, Maltreatment, & Trauma, 9*(1/2/3/4), 487-498.

Bleich, A., Gelkopf, M., & Solomon, Z. (2003). Exposure to terrorism, stress-related mental health symptoms, and coping behavior among a nationally representative sample in Israel. *Journal of the American Medical Association, 290,* 612-620.

Bowler, R., Murai, K., & True, R. (2001). Update and long-term sequelae of the sarin attack in the Tokyo, Japan subway. *Chemical Health and Safety, 8,* 53-55.

Cairns, E., & Toner, I. (1993). Children and political violence in Northern Ireland: From riots to reconciliation. In L. Leavitt & N. Fox (Eds.), *The psychological effects of war and violence on children* (pp. 215-229). Hillsdale, NJ: Lawrence Erlbaum.

Campbell, A., Cairns, E., & Mallett, J. (2004). Northern Ireland: Impact of the Troubles. *Journal of Aggression, Maltreatment, & Trauma, 9*(1/2/3/4), 175-184.

Clauw, D. J., Engel, C. C., Jr., Aronowitz, R., Jones, E., Kipen, H. M., & Kroenke, K. (2003). Unexplained symptoms after terrorism and war: An expert consensus statement. *Occupational & Environmental Medicine, 45,* 1040-8.

Danieli, Y., Brom, D., & Sills, J. (2004). Introduction. *Journal of Aggression, Maltreatment & Trauma, 9*(1/2/3/4), 1-17.

Danieli, Y., Engdahl, B., & Schlenger, W. E. (2003). The psychological aftermath of terrorism. In F. M. Moghaddam & A. J. Marsella (Eds.), *Understanding terrorism: Psychological roots, consequences, and interventions* (pp. 223-246). Washington, DC: American Psychological Association.

De Jong, J. T. V. M. (2002). Public mental health, traumatic stress and human rights violations in low-income countries. In: J. T. V. M. De Jong (Ed.). *Trauma, war, and violence: Public mental health in socio-cultural context* (pp.1-92). New York: Kluwer Academic/Plenum Publishers.

Desivilya, H., Gal, R., & Ayalon, O. (1996). Extent of victimization, traumatic stress symptoms and adjustment of terrorist assault survivors: A long-term follow-up. *Journal of Traumatic Stress, 9*, 88-89.

Firth-Cozens, J., Midgley, S., & Burges, C. (1999). Questionnaire survey of post-traumatic stress disorder in doctors involved in the Omagh bombing. *British Medical Journal, 319*,1609.

Gautam, S., Gupta, I., Batra, L., Sharma, H., Khandelwal, R., & Pant, A. (1998). Psychiatric morbidity among victims of bomb blast. *Indian Journal of Psychiatry, 40*, 41-45.

Gidron, Y., Gal, R., & Zahavi, S. (1999). Bus commuters' coping strategies and anxiety from terrorism: An example from the Israeli experience. *Journal of Traumatic Stress, 12*, 185-191.

Gillespie, K., Duffy, M., Hackmann, A., & Clark, D. (2002). Community based cognitive therapy in the treatment of posttraumatic stress disorder following the Omagh bomb. *Behavior Research and Therapy, 40*, 345-357.

Green, B., Friedman, M., de Jong, J., Solomon, S., Keane, T., Fairbank, J. et al. (Eds.) (2003). *Trauma interventions in war and peace: Prevention, practice, and policy.* New York: Plenum Press.

Hall, M. J., Norwood, A. E., Fullerton, C. S., Gifford, R., & Ursano, R. J. (2004). The psychological burden of bioterrorism. *Journal of Aggression, Maltreatment & Trauma, 9*(1/2/3/4), 293-305.

Jehel, L., & Brunet, A. (2004). The long-term effects of terrorism in France. *Journal of Aggression, Maltreatment & Trauma, 9*(1/2/3/4), 193-200.

Jones, E., Vermaas, R., McCartney, H., Beech, C., Palmer, I., Hyams, K. et al. (2003). Flashbacks and post-traumatic stress disorder: The evolution of a 20th century diagnosis. *British Journal of Psychiatry, 182*, 158-163.

Kawana, N., Ishimatsu, S., & Kanda, K. (2001). Psycho-physiological effects of the terrorist sarin gas attack on the Tokyo subway system. *Military Medicine, 166*(Suppl. 2), 23-26.

Khaled, N. (2004). Psychological effects of terrorist attacks in Algeria. *Journal of Aggression, Maltreatment & Trauma, 9*(1/2/3/4), 213-214.

Kilpatrick, D., Best, C., Smith, D., & Falsetti, S. (2002). Lessons from Lockerbie: Service utilization and victim satisfaction after the Pan Am 103 terrorism bombing. *The Behavior Therapist, 25*, 40-42.

Kirmayer, L. (1996). Confusion of the senses: Implications of ethnocultural variations in somatoform and dissociative disorders for PTSD. In A. Marsella, M. Friedman, E. Gerrity, & R. Scurfield (Eds.), *Ethnocultural aspects of posttraumatic stress dis-*

order: Issues, research, and clinical applications. (pp. 131-164). Washington, DC: American Psychological Association Press.

Lifton, R. J. (2004). Aum Shinrikyo: The threshold crossed. *Journal of Aggression, Maltreatment & Trauma, 9*(1/2/3/4), 57-66.

Lykes, M. (1994). Terror, silencing and children: International, multidisciplinary collaboration with Guatemalan Maya communities. *Social Science and Medicine, 38,* 543-52.

Moscrop, A. (2001). Mass hysteria is seen as main threat from bioweapons. *British Medical Journal, 323,* 1023.

Nichter, M. (1981). Idioms of distress: Alternatives in the expression of psychosocial distress: A case study from India. *Culture, Medicine, and Psychiatry, 5,* 379-408.

Norris, F., Murphy, A., Baker, C., Perilla, J., Rodriguez, F., & Rodriguez, J. (2003). Epidemiology of trauma and posttraumatic stress disorder in Mexico. *Journal of Abnormal Psychology, 112,* 646-656.

North, C. (2004). Somatization and terrorism. *Journal of Aggression, Maltreatment & Trauma, 9*(1/2/3/4), 143-155.

Nuttman-Shwartz, O., & Lauer, E. K. (2002). Group therapy with terror injured persons in Israel: Societal impediments to successful working through. *Group, 6,* 5-16.

Ogden, C., Kaminer, D., Van Kradenburg, J., Seedat, S., & Stein, D. (2000). Narrative themes in response to trauma in a religious community. *Central African Medical Journal, 46,* 178-84.

Pastel, R. (2001). Collective behaviors: Mass panic and outbreaks of multiple unexplained symptoms. *Military Medicine, 166*(Suppl. 2), 44-46.

Pfefferbaum, B. (2004). Review of psychological impact of terrorism on children and families. *Journal of Aggression, Maltreatment & Trauma, 9*(1/2/3/4), 143-155.

Pfefferbaum, B., North, C., Doughty, D., Gurwitch, R., Fullerton, C., & Kyula, J. (2003). Posttraumatic stress and functional impairment in Kenyan children following the 1998 American embassy bombing. *American Journal of Orthopsychiatry, 73,* 133-140.

Somasundaram, D. (2004). Short-and long-term effects on the victims of terror in Sri Lanka. *Journal of Aggression, Maltreatment & Trauma, 9*(1/2/3/4), 215-226.

Tedeschi, R. G., & Calhoun, L. G. (1996). The Posttraumatic Growth Inventory: Measuring the positive legacy of trauma. *Journal of Traumatic Stress, 9,* 455-471.

Thielman, S. B. (2004). The effects on Kenyan employees of the attacks on the American embassies in East Africa. *Journal of Aggression, Maltreatment & Trauma, 9*(1/2/3/4), 233-240.

Weine, S., Danieli, Y., Silove, D., Van Ommeren, M., Fairbank, J., & Saul, J. (2002). Guidelines for international training in mental health and psychosocial interventions for trauma exposed populations in clinical and community settings. *Psychiatry, 65,* 156-164.

Wessely, S., Hyams, K., & Bartholomew, R. (2001). Psychological implications of chemical and biological weapons. *British Medical Journal, 323,* 878-879.

World Health Organization. (1992). *International statistical classification of diseases and related health problems, tenth revision (ICD-10).* Geneva: Author.

Yellin, D. (2004). Ten years later. *Journal of Aggression, Maltreatment & Trauma, 9*(1/2/3/4), 605-607.

Traumatic Loss, Complicated Grief, and Terrorism

Ilona L. Pivar
Holly G. Prigerson

SUMMARY. The experience of losing loved ones is an inevitable outcome of acts of terror. In assessing mental health outcomes in survivors of such acts, researchers have frequently not measured the distress of bereavement even when losses occur. This article defines current concepts of complicated and traumatic grief and reviews the progress researchers have made in measuring the full extent of distress caused by violent and traumatic events. The authors suggest that measurement of complicated and traumatic grief must be included in research and assessment protocols within cultural contexts in order to develop successful treatments for survivors of terrorist acts.

KEYWORDS. Bereavement, violent deaths, genocide, Holocaust, collective grief, gender, culture

Address correspondence to: Ilona L. Pivar, Mailbox 352E117 (MPD), Department of Veterans Affairs, Palo Alto Health Care System, 3801 Miranda Avenue, Palo Alto, CA 94304 USA (E-mail: Ilona.Pivar@med.va.gov).

[Haworth co-indexing entry note]: "Traumatic Loss, Complicated Grief, and Terrorism." Pivar, Ilona L., and Holly G. Prigerson. Co-published simultaneously in *Journal of Aggression, Maltreatment & Trauma* (The Haworth Maltreatment & Trauma Press, an imprint of The Haworth Press, Inc.) Vol. 9, No. 1/2, 2004; and: *The Trauma of Terrorism: Sharing Knowledge and Shared Care, An International Handbook* (ed: Yael Danieli, Danny Brom, and Joe Sills) The Haworth Maltreatment & Trauma Press, an imprint of The Haworth Press, Inc., 2005.

Terrorism can rupture the bonds of love and connectedness to family, friends, coworkers, and community, thereby undermining the survivors' sense of trust, security and justice both at individual and collective levels. Those bereaved may be at risk for prolonged suffering, their resiliency impeded by the severity of the event and the perceived malevolence of human beings. This article examines current and recent studies addressing traumatic loss after terrorist-related and other violent deaths. We attempt to educate readers about complicated grief and the importance of including specific assessments of grief in studies of terrorism within a cultural and community context.

COMPLICATED GRIEF AND TRAUMATIC LOSS

The terms traumatic grief, unresolved grief, and complicated grief have often been interchangeable in the literature. An effort to standardize the terminology must be part of the continual process of recognition of distress factors associated with grief. When referring to the clinical dimensions of unresolved and maladaptive grief, we use the term complicated grief (CG).

The symptoms of CG are increasingly recognized as a separate stress syndrome requiring intervention. The term traumatic loss is event-focused and refers to loss experienced from a death taking place under externally traumatic circumstances, which may elicit shock, disbelief, horror, or helplessness, and there is evidence that such grief often remains unresolved over time. Bereavement over traumatic loss then fits the clinical model of CG.

Prigerson et al. (1999) established a model and criterion for CG, defined as particular maladaptive grief symptoms that do not decrease in intensity or frequency after the first 2-6 months (see Table 1). There is evidence that intense, frequent and unremitting grief symptoms that continue more than 6 months may affect mental and physical health indicating CG as a distinct distress syndrome (Prigerson et al., 1997). Unexpected separation from a significant person, even due to natural causes, may result in CG, depending upon the nature of the relationship and the circumstances surrounding the loss. In a violent death, feelings and images of fear, horror, and helplessness further compound separation anxiety, especially in the absence of effective intervention. For example, unresolved grief was found in 70% of the sample of Vietnam veterans with PTSD (Pivar, 2000).

Development of adequate treatments for the survivors suffering sequalae of terrorism and related events requires a specific focus upon the interplay of grief with co-morbid distress syndromes (Marwitt, 1996; Raphael & Martinek, 1997). Researchers have been intrigued by the interaction of loss with levels of PTSD, depression, and other psychological symptoms. However, with rare exceptions, specific measures and assessments of grief have not been included in studies of traumatic events and their aftermath.

FOUNDATIONS OF A CONCEPTUAL MODEL OF GRIEF AND TRAUMA

PTSD appears to be a disorder related to the intensity or horror of a fear-provoking exposure. Horowitz, Weiss, and Marmar (1987) considered grief a stress syndrome similar to PTSD. By contrast, Prigerson et al. (1999) conceptualized CG as an attachment disturbance more a function of separation/loss anxiety than of PTSD. Although some overlap in symptoms appears to exist between CG and PTSD (e.g., intrusive thoughts, sense of futility about the future, numbness/detachment/disbelief, irritability), some of the core symptoms of CG are absent in PTSD (yearning, pining, searching, feeling a part of oneself has died with the deceased) (American Psychiatric Association, 2000). Prigerson et al. (2002) revealed that kinship to the deceased (e.g., parents/spouses vs. siblings and second-degree relatives) heightened the risk of having CG. Prigerson, Maciejewski, and Rosenheck (2000) have found the quality of the relationship to the deceased (e.g., closeness and dependency) is among the best predictors of poor health and functioning and greater health service use and health care costs and, more specifically, of CG (as cited in Prigerson et al., 1997).

GRIEF AND TERRORISM: A REVIEW OF RECENT STUDIES

Researchers have begun to recognize the interaction of loss with Posttraumatic Stress Disorder (PTSD). A few have begun to measure specific symptoms of CG

TABLE 1. Criteria for Complicated Grief

- Criterion A: Person has experienced the death of a significant other. The response involves 3 of 4 symptoms experienced: at least sometimes intrusive thoughts of the deceased; yearning for the deceased; searching for the deceased; loneliness as a result of the death.
- Criterion B: In response to the death, 4 of the 8 following symptoms as mostly true: Purposelessness or feelings of futility about the future; subjective sense of numbness, detachment or absence of emotional responsiveness; difficulty acknowledging the death; feeling life is empty or meaningless; feeling that part of oneself has died; shattered world view (loss of sense of security, trust, control; assumes symptoms or harmful behaviors of the deceased person; excessive irritability, bitterness, or anger related to the death.
- Criterion C: Duration of disturbance (symptoms listed) beyond a minimum of 2-6 months.
- Criterion D: The disturbance causes clinically significant impairment in social, occupational, or other important areas of functioning.

as it exists co-morbidly with PTSD and recognize the communal impact of losses resulting from these events.

Oklahoma City Bombing. In the aftermath of the 1995 bombing in Oklahoma City, Pfefferbaum et al. (1999) performed a clinical assessment to identify middle school and high school aged students who were in need of formal evaluation for posttraumatic response symptoms. The assessment instrument was administered to 3,218 (grades 6 through 12) students seven weeks after the bombing. Posttraumatic stress symptoms were significantly associated with exposure through knowing someone who was injured or killed, gender, and bomb-related television viewing. Knowing someone who was killed predicted higher PTSD scores, pointing to the interaction of traumatic loss and PTSD. The study points to the wide range of the people affected as well as the importance of loss as a factor. Over 1000 students knew someone who was killed.

North et al. (1999) emphasized the impact of loss by studying direct adult survivors of the bombing in Oklahoma City. Forty-three percent reported loss of a friend or family member and 92% personally knew someone who was injured or killed. Predictors of bombing-related PTSD included secondary exposure through loss of loved ones by death. They did not expand the study by including a specific measure of grief.

Recognition of the interaction of loss and PTSD prompted Pfefferbaum et al. (2001) to include a specific grief measure in the aftermath of the Oklahoma City bombing. The study describes CG in 40 adults who suffered losses. The authors administered several measures including the Texas Revised Inventory of Grief (TRIG), safety concerns, and functioning. A strong association was found between posttraumatic stress symptoms and grief. The relationship between grief and difficulty functioning was stronger at higher levels of posttraumatic stress than at lower levels. Grief was a stronger predictor of PTSD stress symptomology than initial self-reported psychological reactions. Six months after the event, grief scores persisted at high levels indicating a potential for developing CG. Grief accounted for 49% of the variance in intrusive symptoms.

9/11 Attacks. Silver, Holman, McIntosh, Poulin, and Gil-Rivas (2002) utilized an Internet-based national probability sample by a web-based survey research company. The survey took place in three time periods from 9 days to 6 months post-9/11. They assessed severity of 9/11-related loss but confounded the loss variable by scoring 0 as no loss, 1 as the property loss of someone close, 2 as personal property loss, 3 as injury of someone close, 4 as death of someone close, and 5 as personal injury in the attack. Severity of loss experienced in the attacks predicted higher levels of global distress. Nevertheless, the definition of the variable "loss" was confusing and no specific grief measure for addressing the loss of relationship was included.

Kenya. Pferfferbaum et al. (2003) studied PTSD symptoms in Kenyan children following the 1998 American embassy bombing. She found that the severity of posttraumatic stress symptoms was related to grief.

Karachi, Pakistan. Closeness of relationship appears to supercede violence in predicting complicated grief. In a recent study of psychiatric outpatients exposed to frequent terrorist attacks in Karachi, Prigerson et al. (2002) found that death of the significant other by violent means ("dacoity," bandits' attacks) did not heighten the risk of CG, whereas the kinship relationship to the deceased did.

THE INTERACTION BETWEEN GRIEF AND TRAUMA

Studies addressing traumatic grief and loss in terrorism, while increasing, are small in number. Other accounts of survivors of violent deaths can serve to emphasize the need for more research.

Grieving Deaths from Accidental and Intentional Violence. Green and colleagues (2001) examined psychological outcomes of traumatic loss in a group of young women with experiences of "no trauma assault." No trauma assault is defined as a single physical assault upon their person while "traumatic loss" is defined as the loss of a parent, sibling or very close friend by suicide, homicide or accident. The "traumatic loss" group experienced significantly higher rates of acute stress disorder including intrusion symptoms, impaired school performance, and problems with overall adjustment, compared to the no-trauma and assault groups.

Kaltman and Bonanno (2003) assessed PTSD symptoms in 87 persons over time following the death of a spouse, using violence and suddenness of loss as potential outcome predictors. Compared to natural deaths, violent deaths (i.e., fatal motor vehicle accidents, suicide, murder) predicted PTSD symptoms, especially avoidance of thoughts of the deceased and persistence over time of depression. The authors conclude that results support including "the violent death of a loved one among the broader category of events producing PTSD" (p. 142). Unfortunately, no grief measure was used in the study to differentiate more fully PTSD from bereavement symptoms. Several other studies suggest that traumatic losses from violent deaths are associated with higher levels of general distress and impaired functioning (Dyregrov, Nordanger, & Dyregrov, 2003; Rynearson, 1993).

MASS DEATHS, COLLECTIVE GRIEF, AND THE RESPONSE OF COMMUNITIES

Grief responses to individual deaths are compounded in situations of mass death. The meaning and implications of collective (as well as individual) mourning become highly relevant in healing or prolonging bereavement. Lifton (1973) described the importance of renewing human connectedness for survivors of the Holocaust and the Hiroshima bombing in order to heal the moral wounds of intentional human violence. Sitterle and Gurwitch (1999), in recording their experiences in treating survivors of the Oklahoma City bombing, also documented the importance of a collective and community response, including anniversary and commemorative interventions. Wright and Ursano (1990) observed individual and community responses to an aircraft disaster and concluded that "present models do not adequately describe the complexity, duration and spread of the effect of a disaster across a 'global community'" (p. 136).

Even within the context of group loss in disasters, closeness of the relationship to the deceased is a powerful predictor of grief. In a study of acute (1 week post-disaster) and subsequent (2 months) bereavement in 71 adult members of an Air Force community after the loss of seven crew members and a passenger in a plane crash in 1989, Fullerton, Ursano, Tzu-cheg and Bharaitya (1999) found that "The higher symptoms in subjects reporting greater closeness to the lost crew is consistent with other studies of complicated grief in which a positive association is reported between the closeness of a relationship and acute psychiatric morbidity" (p. 908). Relative to a comparison group, the subjects had higher levels of acute, intrusive and avoidant symptoms, and of depressive symptoms.

Mourning and ritual in response to an Army airline tragedy forms the focus of a study by Katz and Bartone (1998). Multiple mourning rituals by the geographically localized families and surviving soldiers contribute to group and individual recovery by reaffirming solidarity of the unit or community and helping survivors to re-establish a sense of control.

GENOCIDE AND ATROCITIES:
MOURNING VICTIMS
OF POLITICAL VIOLENCE

Tully (1995) examined the impact of political violence on Nicaraguan women whose relatives "disappeared" during the Contra War. The collective silence about the disappeared, continuing socio-political instability within the country, and personal uncertainty over what happened to a family member, presented obstacles to the healing processes of the subjects.

Bolton (2001) examined how Rwandans perceive the mental health effects of the 1994 genocide. The study assessed diagnostic symptoms of depression and posttraumatic stress disorder as results of the genocide. He also looked at "local" symptoms not included in the established diagnostic criteria, yielding a local depression-like illness, and a "mental trauma" syndrome including mostly posttraumatic stress disorder symptoms. Rwandan psychiatrist, Athanase Hagengimana (personal communication to H. Prigerson, October 18, 1998), asserted that "CG symptoms were more apt than PTSD to explain people's distress over genocidal disappearances."

Boehnlein (1987) addressed the problems of Cambodian refugees who had survived mass murders of the 1970s. He found that some symptoms of anxiety and PTSD could be treated with medication but more long-standing symptoms of bereavement and grief remained, especially where ritual expression was no longer available to the refugees in a new culture.

Addressing the needs of victims of the Holocaust as well as other instances of political violence and oppression, Danieli (1992) recognized that social isolation, mistrust, and loneliness may develop when society is in denial and expects the victims to get on with their lives. She suggests that monetary compensation alone is not sufficient and may inflict its own hardships when survivors are asked to put a price on their loss or participate in evaluating their need. The fact that the larger community can be a healing force as well as a distorting factor in the grief process is highlighted in Klein's (1971) study of Holocaust survivor families in a kibbutz. The kibbutz provided a renewed cultural system for mourning, continuation of the family, regeneration of hope among its children, and transition from collective grief to pride in the present.

Al-Krenawi, Graham, and Sehwail (2001, 2002) studied bereavement responses following the Hebron massacre of 1994 in which 53 people were killed in an attack upon a mosque. The Derogatis SCL-90-R was administered to surviving widows, daughters, and sons to assess responses of the bereaved, though a standard measure of grief was not used. Statistically significant results occurred in 3 of 9 subscales including somatization, phobic responses, and anxiety. Girls and adults experienced greater somatic responses. Culturally- and religiously-prescribed gender and familial roles appeared to contribute to the different bereavement response patterns.

Elbedour, Baker, Shaloub-Kevorkian, and Belmaker (1999) conducted another study assessing psychological responses of surviving family members within seven months of the Hebron massacre. Using the Clinician-Administered PTSD scale (CAPS) as its measure, the study found that 34.4% of subjects met criteria for PTSD, and noted that daughters (teenage girls) displayed the highest rate. Sons (teenage boys) harbored the highest rate of hostility. Again, no specific measure of grief was utilized; however, the criteria of hopelessness, depression and helplessness ranked among the highest scores. The authors observed that the low level of expressed survivor guilt may be accounted for by the Islamic belief that God will avenge an injustice. They concluded that there is a "distinct somatization reaction to stress" (p. 30) found in studies of Muslim groups.

Collective mourning in response to political violence is described in Klingman's (2001) survey of Israeli children's reactions to the 1995 assassination of Prime Minister Yitzhak Rabin. He administered the Bar-Ilan Picture Text for Children (a projective measure) to 4th-grade children two days after the event, evaluating grief responses. The prevalence of grief was 79.5% of the subjects, with 27.6% rated high in distribution of anxiety and bereavement. "Grieving was related to emotional expressiveness, coping/adapting, and (moderately to) social support" (Klingman, 2001, p. 40). There were gender group differences with girls expressing higher levels of grieving.

COMBAT LOSSES AND COMPARABILITY OF THE EXPERIENCES OF WAR AND TERRORISM

The effects of combat losses upon survivors have been widely noted and recent studies have empirically addressed CG. Green, Grace, Lindy, Gleser, and Goldine (1990) reported that 70% of veterans with PTSD reported the loss of a buddy, compared to 29% without PTSD. In a study of unresolved grief among Vietnam veterans, Pivar (2000) and Pivar and Field (2003) differentiated grief symptoms from those of both depression and PTSD in a sample of 114 combat veterans. They found that thirty years after the conflict, 70% of these veterans could be diagnosed with CG over the loss of a buddy in combat. Perceived closeness of the relationship to the lost person was the most significant factor predicting CG, and was additionally associated with higher levels of survivor guilt and self-blame. Like survivors of terrorist acts, combat veterans often experienced sudden, horrific deaths, with little opportunity to mourn the remains of the deceased in timely communal ceremonies.

THEMES REQUIRING FURTHER ELABORATION

Although the current data from terrorism are limited, certain themes point to a need for greater elaboration and research.

When grief is measured as a distinct factor, it is found to be a robust predictor of overall distress (Pfefferbaum et al., 2001). Hagengimana (personal communication to H. Prigerson, October, 18, 1998) concluded that CG symptoms were more apt than PTSD to explain the distress of people over disappearances as a result of the Rwandan Genocide.

Even when loss occurs in the context of a traumatic event, closeness of the relationship is the most significant risk factor predicting CG (Fullerton, 1999; Pivar, 2000; Pivar & Field, 2003; Prigerson et al., 1997, 2002).

Individual grief in traumatic loss may interact with cultural and national or historical factors (Sitterle, 1999; Tully, 1995). Culturally- and religiously-proscribed gender and familial roles may contribute to different bereavement response patterns (Al-Krenawi et al., 2001). How somatization (Elbedour et al., 1999) may relate to grief is a topic deserving of further investigation because it would indicate ways to enhance detection and treatment of an underlying grief-related disturbance.

Finally, personality traits such as resiliency have not been sufficiently recognized in bereavement studies (Bonnano, 2004). Resiliency as the "ability to maintain a stable equilibrium" (p. 20) in the face of a close personal loss should not be overlooked in assessing or treating naturally bereaved and/or traumatized survivors.

Neria and Litz (in press) are currently embarking on a web-based study of traumatic grief in victims of 9/11, measuring grief, coping, attachment, past losses, restorations and rituals, locus of control, social support, religious factors and life events. The study promises to produce much needed data that will shape future mental health responses.

CONCLUSION

Researchers have been slow to recognize the importance of measuring grief in the context of terrorism. Because the experience of loss is implicit in the aftermath of terrorist attacks, the risk of complicated bereavement, depression, PTSD and other co-morbid symptomology is high. Assessments in the future will hopefully include a specific validated measure of grief as well as an accounting of personal loss of relationship, and the type and intensity of the relationship that was lost (e.g., close, confiding, hostile, dependent, empathetic, supportive, conflicted), cultural and community factors so that psychological distress can adequately be assessed over time and addressed clinically.

REFERENCES

Al-Krenawi, A., Graham, J. R., & Sehwail, M. A. (2001/2). Bereavement responses among Palestinian widows, daughters and sons following the Hebron massacre. *Omega, 44*(3), 241-255.

American Psychiatric Association. (2000). *Diagnostic and statistical manual of mental disorders* (4th ed., text rev.). Washington, DC: Author.

Bolton, P. (2001). Local perceptions of the mental health effects of the Rwandan geno-cide. *Journal of Nervous & Mental Disorders, 189*(4), 243-248.

Bonanno, G. A. (2004). Loss, trauma, and human resilience. *American Psychologist, 59*(1), 20-28.

Danieli, Y. (1992). Preliminary reflections from a psychological perspective. In T. C van Boven, C. Flinterman, F. Grunfield, & I. Westendorp (Eds.), *The right to resti-tution, compensation and rehabilitation for victims of gross violations of human rights and fundamental freedoms* (pp. 196-213). Netherlands Institute of Human Rights, Special Issue No. 12.

DeLisi, L. E., Maurizio, A., Yost, M., Papparozzi, C., Fulchino, C., Katz, C. et al. (2003). A survey of New Yorkers after the Sept. 11, 2001 terrorist attacks. *Ameri-can Journal of Psychiatry, 160*(4), 780-783.

Dyregrov, K., Nordanger, D. & Dyregrov, A. (2003). Predictors of psychosocial dis-tress after suicide, SIDS and accidents. *Death Studies, 27*(2), 143-165.

Elbedour, S., Baker, A., Shalhoub-Kevorkian, A., Irwin, M., & Belmaker, R. (1999). Psychological responses in family members after the Hebron Massacre. *Depression and Anxiety, 9*, 27-31.

Fullerton, C., Ursano, R. F., Tzu-Cheg, K., & Bharaitya, V. R. (1999). Disaster-related bereavement. *Aviation, Space and Environmental Medicine, 70*(9), 902-909.

Galea, S., Ahern, J., Resnick, H., Kilpatrick, D., Bucuvalas, M., Gold, J. et al. (2002). Psychological sequelae of the September 11 terrorist attacks in New York City. *New England Journal of Medicine, 346*(13), 982-987.

Green, B. L., Grace, M.C., Lindy, J., Gleser, G., & Goldine, C. (1990). Risk factors for PTSD and other diagnoses in Vietnam veterans. *Journal of Anxiety Disorders, 4*(1), 31-39.

Green, B. L., Krupnick, J. L., Stockton, P., Goodman, L., Corcoran, C., & Petty R. (2001). Psychological outcomes of traumatic loss in young women. *American Be-havioral Scientist, 44*(5), 817-837.

Horowitz, M. J., Weiss, D. S., & Marmar, C. (1987). Posttraumatic stress disorder and the perennial stress-diathesis controversy (Commentary). *Journal of Nervous and Mental Disease, 175*(5), 265-266.

Kaltman, S., & Bonanno, G. (2003). Trauma and bereavement: Examining the impact of sudden and violent deaths. *Journal of Anxiety Disorders, 17*(2), 131-147.

Katz, P., & Bartone, P. (1998). Mourning and ritual-Army airline tragedy. *Omega, 36*(3), 193-200.

Klein, H. (1971). Families of Holocaust survivors in the kibbutz: Psychological stud-ies. In H. Krystal & W. G. Niederland (Eds.), *Psychic traumatization: Aftereffects in individuals and communities* (pp. 69-72). Boston: Little Brown.

Klingman, A. (2001). Israeli Children's reaction to the assassination of the Prime Min-ister. *Death Studies, 25*, 33-49.

Lifton, R. J. (1993). From Hiroshima to the Nazi doctors: Evolution of psychoformative approaches to understanding traumatic stress syndromes. In J. P. Wilson & B. Raphael, (Eds.), *International handbook of traumatic stress syndromes* (pp. 11-23). New York: Plenum Press.

Marwit, S. J. (1996). Reliability of diagnosing complicated grief. *Journal of Counsel-ing and Clinical Psychology, 64*(3), 563-568.

Neria, Y., & Litz, B. (in press). Bereavement by traumatic means: The complex syn-ergy of trauma and grief. *Journal of Loss and Trauma.*

North, C. S., & Pfefferbaum, B. (2002). Research on mental health effects of terrorism. *Journal of the American Medical Association, 288*(5), 633-636.

North, C. S., Nixon, S., Shariat, S., Mallonee, S., McMillen, J., Spitznagel, E. L. et al. (1999). Psychiatric disorders among survivors of the Oklahoma City bombing. *Journal of the American Medical Association, 282*(8), 755-762.

Pfefferbaum, B., North, C. S., Doughty, D., Gurwitch, R., Fullerton, C., & Kyula, J. (2003). Posttraumatic stress and functional impairment in Kenyan children following the 1998 American embassy bombing. *American Journal of Orthopsychiatry, 73*(2), 133-140.

Pfefferbaum, B., Call, J. A., Lensgraf, S., Miller, P.D., Flynn, B. W., Doughty, D. et al. (2001). Traumatic grief in a convenience sample of victims seeking support services after a terrorist incident. *Annals of Clinical Psychiatry, 13*(1), 19-24.

Pfefferbaum, B., Nixon, S., Krug, R. S., Tivis, R. D., Moore, V. L, Brown, J. M. et al. (1999). Clinical needs assessment of middle and high school students following the 1995 Oklahoma City bombing. *American Journal of Psychiatry, 156*(7), 1069-1074.

Pivar, I. (2000). Measuring unresolved grief in combat veterans with PTSD. *Dissertation Abstracts International, 61* (6-B), Jan. 2000, 3288. (UMI No. 0419-4217).

Pivar, I. (2001, November). Comparison of war veterans on risk factors of complicated/traumatic grief. In M. Cloitre (Chair), *New developments in traumatic grief.* Symposium conducted at the conference of International Society for Traumatic Stress Studies, New Orleans, LA.

Pivar, I., & Field, N. (in press). Measuring unresolved grief in combat veterans with PTSD. *Journal of Anxiety Disorders.*

Prigerson, H. G., Ahmed, I., Aqueel, N., Jacobs, S. C., Maciejewski, P. K., Saxena, A. et al. (2002). Rates and risks of complicated grief in Karachi, Pakistan. *Death Studies, 26*(10), 781-792.

Prigerson, H. G., Maciejewski, P. K., & Rosenheck, R. A. (1999). The effects of marital dissolution and marital quality on health and health service use among women. *Medical Care, 37*(9), 858-873.

Prigerson, H. G., Maciejewski, P. K., & Rosenheck, R. A. (2000). Preliminary explorations of the harmful interactive effects of widowhood and marital harmony on health, health service use, and health care costs. *Gerontologist, 40*(3), 349-357.

Prigerson, H. G., Maciejewski, P. K., & Rosenheck, R. A. (2001). Combat trauma: Trauma with highest risk of delayed onset and unresolved posttraumatic stress disorder symptoms, unemployment, and abuse among men. *Journal of Nervous and Mental Disorders, 189*(2), 99-108.

Prigerson, H. G., Shear, M. K., Frank, E., Beery, L., Silberman, R., Prigerson J. et al. (1997). Complicated grief: A case of loss-induced trauma. *American Journal of Psychiatry, 154*(7), 1003-1009.

Prigerson, H. G., Shear, M. K., Jacobs, S. C., Kasl, S. V., Maciejewski, P. K., Silverman, G. K. et al. (2000). Grief and its relationship to PTSD. In D. Nutt & J. R. T. Davidson (Eds.), *Post traumatic stress disorders: Diagnosis, management and treatment* (pp. 163-186). New York: Martin Dunitz.

Prigerson, H. G., Shear, M. K., Jacobs, S. C., Reynolds, C. F., Maciejewski, P. K., Davidson, J. R. et al. (1999). Consensus criteria for traumatic grief. *British Journal of Psychiatry, 174*, 67-73.

Raphael, B., & Martinek, N. (1997). Assessing traumatic bereavement and posttraumatic stress disorder. In J. P. Wilson & T. M. Keane (Eds.), *Assessing psychological trauma and PTSD* (pp. 373-395). New York: Guilford Press.

Rynearson, E., & McCreery, J. (1993). Bereavement after suicide: A synergism of trauma and loss. *American Journal of Psychiatry, 150* (2), 258-261.

Schlenger, W., Caddell, J., Ebert, L., Jordan, B., Rourke, K., Wilson, D. et al. (2002). Psychological reactions to terrorist attacks: Findings from the National Study of Americans' Reactions to September 11. *Journal of the American Medical Association, 288*(5), 581-588.

Silver, R., Holman, E., McIntosh, D., Poulin, M., & Gil-Rivas, V. (2002). Nationwide longitudinal study of psychological responses to September 11. *Journal of the American Medical Association, 288*(10), 1235-1244.

Sitterle, K., & Gurwitch, R. (1999). The terrorist bombing in Oklahoma City. In E. Zinner & M. B. Williams (Eds.), *When a community weeps* (pp.160-189). Philadelphia: Taylor and Francis.

Tully, S. R. (1995). A painful purgatory: Grief and the Nicaraguan mothers of the disappeared. *Social Science & Medicine, 40*(12), 1597-1610.

Wright, K., & Ursano, R. J. (1990). Individual and community responses to an aircraft disaster. In M. E. Wolf & A. D. Mosniam (Eds.), *Posttraumatic stress disorder: Etiology, phenomenology, and treatment* (pp. 127-138). Washington, DC: American Psychiatric Press.

Voice:
Theo Was on Pan Am 103

Susan Cohen
Daniel Cohen

Over the years, Susan and I have developed the reputation of being the angriest, fiercest, most uncompromising, and least forgiving of all the Pan Am 103 family members. I have no idea whether this is true, but we are certainly the most outspoken. And this bothers people. In general, we Americans like to be cheerful and optimistic. We talk about "triumph over tragedy," "finding peace" or a "new meaning in life," or at least of "moving on."

"Theo would want you to find peace and forgive," people have told me, people who never knew Theo. I often think of something that happened when she was about five years old. She had been born and spent her earliest years in the country. But when she was ready to go to school, we moved into a nearby town so she could meet more children, and so we would not have to spend half our day chauffeuring her around.

Late one afternoon, I looked out of the window and saw Theo surrounded by a group of neighborhood children. It wasn't serious. She was the new kid on the block and her place in the pecking order had not yet been determined. Kids are like that. Theo was also the shortest kid in the crowd. She was always the shortest kid in the crowd. But this time she had a weapon, a stick, and not an

---

Address correspondence to: Susan and Daniel Cohen, 877 Hand Avenue, Cape May Court House, New Jersey, NJ 08219 (E-mail: BlndgsCast@aol.com).

Adapted from the book *Pan Am 103* (Signet, 2001).

[Haworth co-indexing entry note]: "Voice: Theo Was on Pan Am 103." Cohen, Susan and Daniel Cohen. Co-published simultaneously in *Journal of Aggression, Maltreatment & Trauma* (The Haworth Maltreatment & Trauma Press, an imprint of The Haworth Press, Inc.) Vol. 9, No. 1/2, 2004; and: *The Trauma of Terrorism: Sharing Knowledge and Shared Care, An International Handbook* (ed: Yael Danieli, Danny Brom, and Joe Sills) The Haworth Maltreatment & Trauma Press, an imprint of The Haworth Press, Inc., 2005.

ordinary stick, a piece of lath from a nearby construction site, with a large rusty nail sticking out of the end. And she was swinging it at her tormentors. They backed off, half in jest, but half in fear.

I rushed out and took the nail-studded stick away from her. I said all the good father things. "You could have put someone's eye out." "The next time they bother you, come to me and I'll talk to their parents." But in truth, I was immensely proud of my daughter, and she knew it. Nobody was going to push Theo around, and if they tried, they were going to pay. That's the way she lived her life.

She was murdered by some faceless goons, thousands of miles away, for no reason other than that she was an American. She didn't even have a chance to swing a stick at them. I don't have a stick either, but I have used whatever weapons I could find to get back at them, not for justice, there is no possibility of justice here. I do it just to let them know that I am there, that I have not forgotten, forgiven, or been bought off.

I hope Theo would have been proud of me, as I was of her. I think she would. I owe it to her memory.

Voice:
When You Are Alone, It Is Different

Conny Mus

Working and living under extremely difficult and often dangerous circumstances eventually turns you into a different person. The people around you see the change but you do not. You become a realist, maybe too much of one. And you become indifferent to many things in life that are important to the people around you and had previously been important to you, too. I have come to see things like paying a bill, repairing a leaky faucet or a garden gate, or taking my daughter to the doctor when she has the flu, as unimportant.

When my partner pressures me to take such things seriously, I often shrug them off, tell her that they can wait and ask her why she thinks these things matter. In the same way, I could no longer care less if some fellow driver on the road misbehaves. "Go right ahead," I think. A while back, I would have rolled down my window to say something nasty to him or her.

I am a devoted father to my little daughter, but if she happens to fall or cough, after ensuring that she is eating, drinking, and moving, I do not make a big deal out of it, when sometimes I should. Once she was running a high fever, but seemed to be doing fine otherwise, so I postponed the visit to the doctor for a few days. As it turned out, she was developing pneumonia, and her mother was right that it would have been more sensible to get her to the doctor

Address correspondence to: Conny Mus, Correspondent RTL4 Nieuws, Holland Media Groep, Givat Hayonim 2, P.O. Box 10-003, Jerusalem 93467, Israel (E-mail: rtlconny@netvision.net.il).

[Haworth co-indexing entry note]: "Voice: When You Are Alone, It Is Different." Mus, Connie. Co-published simultaneously in *Journal of Aggression, Maltreatment & Trauma* (The Haworth Maltreatment & Trauma Press, an imprint of The Haworth Press, Inc.) Vol. 9, No. 1/2, 2004; and: *The Trauma of Terrorism: Sharing Knowledge and Shared Care, An International Handbook* (ed: Yael Danieli, Danny Brom, and Joe Sills) The Haworth Maltreatment & Trauma Press, an imprint of The Haworth Press, Inc., 2005.

sooner than we did. Once you have seen as many dead, severely injured, dis-membered bodies as I have, you look at the mundane problems of daily life and think, "What is everyone making such a fuss about?"

The way you cope with your normal emotional reactions to these atrocities is different every time. I usually become very quiet and stare straight ahead, with no desire to talk about what I have experienced. Sometimes I watch a dumb movie or have too many drinks. When I drink with colleagues, a conversation about the difficult events naturally ensues. This is often accompanied by inappropriate jokes, but they do serve a purpose. On one horrific occasion, I was doing my TV song and dance routine at the site of a bombing, a meter away from where people were collecting human brains from the pavement with rubber gloves. "Look out," said a colleague, "take one more step and you'll be standing on it." My crass reply was, "don't worry. I'm crazy about brains, but I just ate." Everybody started laughing and I released my own tension.

If you are ever under gunfire or in a bombing, you had better hope not to be there alone. When your colleagues or some local people are there as well, then it is bearable, because you can decide together where to take cover. But if you are alone, it is a different story.

After a night of missile attacks in Baghdad, I informed my office that I could not take any more and I wanted to leave. Alone in my hotel room with the whole building shaking, the lobby windows lying smashed on the floor, I trembled for hours. I had no one to talk to, no one with whom I could share what I was going through. I could not contact my office because we do not broadcast at night. In such a situation you feel very alone.

How you deal with danger is different each time because the situations are so different from each other. Heroes do not exist. Each of us has to find his own way to deal with the danger and the accompanying fear, and you never, ever, get used to it.

Why do you keep doing it, at least up until the point when you feel that you cannot do it anymore? I have seen many colleagues quit the job. I think it is very sensible to do so if you feel that you cannot cope with it anymore. If you force yourself to continue, both your work and your private life will suffer.

One reason for me to go on after more than 20 years of seeing far more horrors than happy stories is that I think it is important that the news reaches the world. In addition, I feel that so far I can still cope with it. Each time I cope in a different way. Yes, I have changed, but I think it is in a good cause and I still have a very interesting job.

The Psychological Burden of Bioterrorism

Molly J. Hall
Ann E. Norwood
Carol S. Fullerton
Robert Gifford
Robert J. Ursano

SUMMARY. Planning for the public's psychological and behavioral reactions to a bioterrorist attack must address individual and community preparedness, response, and recovery. Bioterrorism raises issues requiring skilled risk communication and education including isolation, quarantine, administering vaccinations and distributing medications. The United States anthrax attacks, the international outbreak of Severe Acute Respiratory Syndrome (SARS), and the U.S. smallpox vaccination program offer useful lessons. The Iraqi missile attacks on Israel and the Tokyo sarin gas attacks highlight challenges of emergency medical evaluation and triage. Early public health interventions should identify symptoms and behaviors linked to psychological distress and suggest strategies to restore well-being.

Address correspondence to: Molly J. Hall, MD, 4301 Jones Bridge Road, Bethesda, MD 20814-4799 USA (E-mail: mhall@usuhs.mil).

[Haworth co-indexing entry note]: "The Psychological Burden of Bioterrorism." Hall, Molly J. et al. Co-published simultaneously in *Journal of Aggression, Maltreatment & Trauma* (The Haworth Maltreatment & Trauma Press, an imprint of The Haworth Press, Inc.) Vol. 9, No. 1/2, 2004; and: *The Trauma of Terrorism: Sharing Knowledge and Shared Care, An International Handbook* (ed: Yael Danieli, Danny Brom, and Joe Sills) The Haworth Maltreatment & Trauma Press, an imprint of The Haworth Press, Inc., 2005.

KEYWORDS. Planning, preparedness, risk communication, public education, psychological distress, psychiatric illness

Although all chemical, biological, radiological, nuclear, and high-yield explosive (CBRNE) weapons are effective at causing terror (Holloway, Norwood, Fullerton, Engel, & Ursano, 1997), biological agents possess uniquely frightening characteristics. They are invisible, odorless, imperceptible to humans, and their effects are delayed and often protracted. Agents such as smallpox that cause disfigurement, deformity and have the potential for person-to-person transmission further amplify horror. The anthrax attacks of October 2001 employed a silent, invisible weapon that produced delayed effects in unexpected places and harmed even those apparently not at risk. Compared to the destruction and loss of life on September 11, 2001, the effects of the anthrax attacks were relatively small. While only five people died and 22 fell ill, thousands of people were placed on medication and the economic, psychological, and social costs were enormous.

Since the 2001 anthrax attacks, there has been progress in the United States' planning for bioterrorism. Communities across the country have conducted mock disaster drills and lessons learned were applied with greater success to the threat of a Severe Acute Respiratory Syndrome (SARS) outbreak in this country (Stolberg & Miller, 2001). While many scientific, public health and medical experts acknowledge that the nation is better prepared, they maintain that the effort is insufficient and that personnel and medical resources do not have the surge capacity needed in the event of an attack ("The Bioterror Threat: Are We Ready?," 2003). Anticipating the psychological and behavioral consequences of a bioterrorist attack is an urgent task facing our government's leaders and our nations' public healthcare system (Hall, Norwood, Ursano, & Fullerton, 2002).

Bioterrorism raises special issues such as coordinating vaccination programs, distributing prophylactic medication, evacuation, isolation, and quarantine, all of which demand skilled psychosocial management. Developing a risk communication and public education program that addresses these concerns is essential to sustain the public's trust and ensure that people will follow directions that help control the spread of disease. Equally important is engaging the public to prepare for a potential attack.

Agroterrorism is a unique bioterrorist threat and many believe our nation's two million farms are highly vulnerable (National Academies of Science, 2002). Contamination of food and water supplies could be highly lethal but even without human casualties, the economic, psychological, and social toll would be severe. The most recent outbreak of Hoof and Mouth disease in Great Britain required the government to destroy nearly 4 million animals to stop the epidemic. Estimated losses to the food, agriculture, and tourist industries exceeded US $10 billion (U.S. General Accounting Office, 2002).

THE PUBLIC'S MENTAL HEALTH: PREPAREDNESS AND RESPONSE

Plans to manage mental health consequences of a bioterrorist attack must take into account preparedness behaviors, disaster event behaviors, and response/recovery behaviors in individuals, institutions, and communities (Fullerton, Ursano, & Norwood, 2003; National Academy of Sciences, 2003). This public health approach to the nation's psychological health requires an expansion of the traditional mental health role of intervention in response to a disaster (Hall, Norwood, Ursano, & Fullerton, 2003). Managing and treating immediate psychological casualties is important, but preparing the nation for terrorism is a larger task requiring an understanding of the public's psychological and behavioral reactions to this unique threat. In a survey conducted in March 2003 by the Harvard School of Public Health (Blendon, 2003), only 10% had made an evacuation plan or prepared to shelter in place.

In the immediate aftermath of a terrorist attack, individuals and communities will respond with a range of behaviors that may be helpful and adaptive. The same can be said for less useful, possibly harmful, behaviors that will appear. A community's social capital, defined as the community members' level of civic participation, reciprocity, and trust in each other (Cullen & Whiteford, 2001), as well as individual and family preparedness, all influence this response. The recent Institute of Medicine Report recommends that public health surveillance for pre-event, event and post-event factors include background rates of behavioral and psychological factors predicting psychological impacts, risk factors for negative outcomes, needs assessments for mental health services, and prevalence of event and post-event consequences (National Research Council of the National Academies, 2002). Knowledge of a community's resilience and vulnerability before a disaster or terrorist event enables leaders and medical experts to talk to the public, promote resilient healthy behaviors, sustain the social fabric of the community, and facilitate recovery. Government and health officials must be prepared to use real time information on distress and coping in order to understand and influence positively behavioral choices of individuals and groups. During the anthrax attacks in Washington, DC, two equally at-risk groups made very different choices regarding continued prophylaxis. In contrast to the federal employees and elected officials on Capitol Hill, workers from the Brentwood Postal Facility declined the anthrax vaccine, and elected continued treatment with antibiotics. The two exposed groups were demographically (socially, racially, and economically) different, and the postal workers' risk had initially been underestimated (Stolberg & Miller, 2001).

The nature of a threat and the public's perception of risk are major determinants of behavioral response. The sniper attacks in the Washington area embodied all of the characteristics of situations we fear most and evaluate as highest risk (Appelbaum, 2002). No one was safe and there was no pattern that would have allowed people to reasonably change behavior to decrease risk. The sniper attacks generated more fear and distress, caused more behavioral change, and had more severe social and economic consequences than the anthrax attacks. Fifty percent of those surveyed about the sniper were very worried or somewhat worried about becoming a victim (Morin & Deane, 2002), while 33% surveyed about anthrax in the Washington area were very or somewhat worried that they would contract anthrax (Blendon et al., 2002). Forty-four percent of people threatened by the sniper altered or eliminated outdoor activities while 34% of people questioned in the wake of the anthrax mailings were taking some precautions opening the mail.

An anxious and mistrustful public may take matters into its own hands if the government and medical response is perceived to be slow, ineffective, or protecting some but not others. Although prosocial behavior is the norm following natural and manmade disasters (Glass & Schoch-Spana, 2002), the risk of panic is heightened when people believe that there is a small chance of escape, that they are likely to become infected, and that there are limited resources available (Holloway et al., 1997). A range of negative outcomes is possible, including a population's refusal to accept preventative measures or treatment regimens such as isolation and quarantine; ineffective or dangerous use of prophylactics; social disruption; and civil violence.

By late July 2003, six months after SARS first appeared, infecting 8,100 people and killing 774, the epidemic was declared under control. In the ensuing six months, three additional cases were identified as a result of ongoing international surveillance: two linked to accidents in research laboratories in Singapore and Taiwan and one case in China, of uncertain origin (Pan, 2004). The effectiveness of tried-and-true public health measures such as case-finding, isolation, and quarantine, the global availability of information, and the willingness to share knowledge prevailed (Brown, 2003). The SARS scare has also frighteningly re-educated the world about the risks of mishandling the public's trust. The Chinese government did not acknowledge, nor did it let the press report, that a mysterious new disease was causing villagers from the Guangdong province to become sick and die. No serious public health interventions were implemented until April 2003 (Grady, 2003). By the last week of April 2003, citizens began fleeing Beijing, a city of 14 million with approximately 700 confirmed cases of SARS, ignoring official appeals for people to avoid travel. People surged into grocery stores, emptying shelves, despite the government's televised reassurances that stocks were not threatened (Eckholm, 2003).

RISK COMMUNICATION AND PUBLIC EDUCATION: UNIQUE CHALLENGES OF BIOTERRORISM

Among the many elements of an effective response to a bioterrorist attack, an incident information management system insures rapid dissemination of accurate information and coordinated recommendations (Barbera & Macintyre, 2002). Credible scientific authority and a clear message from government leaders and media providing the rationale behind difficult decisions are critical to public confidence. At the beginning of the anthrax attacks, Centers for Disease Control scientific advisors were not aware of the benefits of combining antibiotic prophylaxis with vaccination. As a result, timely recommendations could not be forwarded to public and medical personnel. Conflicting recommendations on prophylaxis and vaccination by different jurisdictions in the national capital area were confusing. In contrast, during the SARS outbreak, the World Health Organization (WHO) became the information incident management center by virtue of its instant communications capabilities. WHO's recommendations were followed even though it had no authority to mandate investigation or compliance with its advisories.

Bioterrorism poses a threat that encompasses elements of our highest risk perceptions and the accompanying fear and anxiety are intense. High levels of stress may lead to decision-making that is more impulsive, less willing to consider alternatives and driven to premature closure (Covello, Peters, Wojtecki, & Hyde, 2001). The public must rely on media and opinions from medical and scientific experts who may disagree, thus increasing fear and anger. During the anthrax attacks, the infectivity of the spores differed from what was expected, spread and aerosolization were underestimated and the pulmonary form of the illness responded to treatment in some cases (Brown, 2001). The media can be a vector for propagating distress but an equally powerful resource for public education and recovery. It would have been very helpful, for instance, had the role of nasal swabbing for spores been made clear as the presence of spores was confused with infection.

The US smallpox vaccination program failed to convince the medical community and the public of the need to reintroduce vaccinations to counter a terrorist threat that had not been disclosed in any detail. The first phase of the vaccination program called for 500,000 volunteer healthcare workers to be inoculated in the first 30 days. By the end of the sixth week, only 12,404 healthcare workers had received the vaccine. Hundreds of hospitals and most major unions refused to have their employees vaccinated. Reasons cited include: known serious side effects; worries about litigation; increased risk to family members, pregnant women, infants, and people with certain medical conditions; lack of compensation in the event of adverse effects; and, perhaps of most concern, lack of credible evidence that a bioterrorist attack using smallpox is likely (U.S. General Accounting Office, 2003; "The Bioterror Threat: Smallpox Fiasco," 2003).

Once China acknowledged the extent of SARS within its borders, massive public health measures of quarantine, contact tracing and case isolation were initiated. A combination of China's authoritarian political structure, a culture emphasizing group values, and a large work force is credited with the swift implementation of these strategies. Taiwan, who implemented quarantine during the SARS outbreak as well, also undertook several strategies simultaneously, making it difficult to evaluate the independent effectiveness of a single measure such as quarantine. Of the 131,132 persons quarantined in Taiwan, only 133 were diagnosed with suspect or probable SARS; more than double that number, or 286 people, were fined for violation of quarantine (Centers for Disease Control and Prevention, 2003). Whether other countries in Europe or North America would have been able to mount as extensive a response is questionable (Brown, 2003). On a much smaller scale, the Canadian outbreak was contained through voluntary cooperation with quarantine (McNeil, 2003), but some scientists argue that China's "overkill" response would have been required had the disease become more widespread. Case by case isolation is appropriate in conjunction with separation of individuals known to have been exposed to a contagious infection during the incubation period. Imposing quarantine on large groups with individuals who were not exposed or who are at low risk is usually not feasible. The risk of unintended consequences, driving infected people away from treatment or into hiding, is high, and there are little data to support its efficacy (Barbera et al., 2001).

THE HEALTH CARE SYSTEM AS FIRST RESPONDERS

The most important element of psychological first aid is good medical care (National Institute of Mental Health, 2001). Health care providers and the health care system are first responders in bioterrorist events and a well-organized, effective medical response will instill hope and confidence. Clinical staff and hospital employees are as vulnerable to fear and anxiety as the rest of the public. In the 1994 outbreak of pneumonic plague in Surat, India, 80% of the private physicians fled the city (Garrett, 2000). At the outset of the SARS epidemic, some hospitals in Vietnam and Hong Kong were working with half the staff as nurses and other health care workers stayed at home fearing that they would become sick (Altman, 2003). Absenteeism can result from the conflicted loyalties of the hospital staff, divided between caring for their own families and taking care of patients. Emergency plans should ensure that employees' families will be cared for to reduce possible absenteeism. Demoralization is also a concern if there are high mortality rates and limited ability to provide care for advanced illness.

EARLY MEDICAL MANAGEMENT

There have been a number of disasters, terrorist attacks and the use of novel weapons in the context of war which suggest that the healthcare system may be inundated with patients seeking evaluation and care (Joint Commission on Accreditation of Healthcare Organizations, 2003). Arousal and intense anxiety may be experienced as somatic symptoms in any organ system including palpitations, shortness of breath, nausea, and flushing. Frightened individuals may easily interpret these symptoms to mean they have been exposed. During the Iraqi scud missile attacks on Israel between January and February 1991, over 1,000 people presented for emergency care with only 22% having been directly injured (Karsenty et al., 1991). The overwhelming majority of patients suffered from acute anxiety, side effects of auto-injected atropine, injuries occurring while running to safety, suffocation from incorrect gas mask use or myocardial infarction. Following the 1995 Aum Shinrikyo sarin gas attacks in Tokyo that killed 11 people, over 4,000 people who showed no signs of exposure sought emergency medical care (Ohbu et al., 1997; see also Lifton, this volume).

Identifying patients who are ill from exposure and those with somatic symptoms due to distress is a critical and challenging first step in emergency care. A non-stigmatizing triage labeling system such as high risk, moderate risk, and minimal risk conveys concern and promises continued monitoring which is reassuring to patients whereas a term such as "worried well" is disparaging and dismissive. Psychiatrists working with other mental health professionals should be an integral part of the teams performing screening and triage. Establishing a clinical registry to follow up patients who are anxious about potential exposure is a sound public health intervention as well as a psychological intervention. Patients believe that their concerns are being taken seriously and it facilitates outreach. To groups such as pregnant women or women with young children who may be particularly worried, initial psychological interventions should be focused on well-being and function rather than mental illness. Encouraging sufficient rest and sleep, normalizing eat-sleep-work cycles, and limiting exposure to media reports, traumatizing images and sounds are all measures that facilitate coping and recovery (Uniformed Services University Center for the Study of Traumatic Stress, 2001).

PSYCHIATRIC ILLNESS

Although most people do not develop psychiatric disorders following a disaster or a terrorist attack, some people will. The risk of developing posttraumatic stress disorder (PTSD) is highest in people who are directly exposed to high magnitude, severely disturbing events. These individuals do not necessarily have other risk factors such as a pre-existing psychiatric condition or recent negative life events. Forty percent of directly exposed individuals in the Oklahoma City bombing who developed PTSD and depression had no prior history of psychiatric illness (North et al., 1999). Disorders such as depression, generalized anxiety, panic, and somatization may develop and are more likely to lead to seeking out primary care providers than mental health professionals. Increased alcohol, nicotine, and other substance use as well as family conflict and family violence may occur. People at increased risk to react in these ways are those directly exposed to disastrous events including medical personnel caring for victims of bioterrorism, those who were more vulnerable before the event due to pre-existing mental illness, and those who suffered acute losses and other negative life events after the event. In a follow-up study (Goode, 2003) by the New York Academy of Medicine (see also Ahern, Galea, Resnick, & Vlahov, this volume), people continuing to suffer from PTSD symptoms 15 months after the attack had experienced subsequent stressful events such as divorce or the loss of a family member. Early abandonment of active coping, or an early "giving up" and denial of an ongoing threat, also appears to increase the risk of ongoing distress and PTSD (Silver, Holman, McIntosh, Poulin, & Gil-Rivas, 2002). Primary care clinics should routinely assess the degree of patients' concerns about exposure-related illness regardless of whether a known exposure occurred. A helpful screening question is to ask whether the patient's visit is related to terrorism or bioterrorism concerns. If the answer is "yes," extra time can be devoted to exploring the nature of these concerns and developing recommendations for additional testing, clinic visits, and patient education. Early triage into this level of follow-on care may reduce the development of persistent medically unexplained symptoms such as Gulf War syndrome (Engel & Katon, 1999).

MANAGING DISTRESS

Most people will experience some degree of psychological distress following a disaster or terrorist event including an altered sense of safety, hypervigilance, sadness, anger, fear, decreased concentration, and sleep problems. Others will alter their behavior, travel less, stay at home, keep children out of school, or increase nicotine and alcohol use. Psychological effects are not limited to those experiencing the trauma directly; nationwide, millions of ordinary people suffered as well (Silver, Holman, McIntosh, Poulin, & Gil-Rivas, 2002; see also Silver, Poulin, Holman, McIntosh, Gil-Rivas, & Pizarro, this volume). Several studies conducted after 9/11 documented early high levels of distress in people across the United States (Schuster et al., 2001; Pew Survey, 2001). In a mental health needs assessment by the District of Columbia Department of Mental Health conducted after the Pentagon and anthrax attacks, 70% of 161 focus group participants reported an adverse health impact or psychological symptom for which less than 10% had sought care. Many had not made the connection between the psychological distress they were experiencing and these events (DC Report of Findings, 2001).

Differentiating psychological distress from psychiatric illness is a critical public health intervention (North & Pfefferbaum, 2002). In the days and weeks following a terrorist event, well-planned public education and information campaigns are invaluable. Distress is universal and the accompanying symptoms will abate for most people over several weeks (Ursano, 2002). Educating the public, emphasizing the natural recovery process, and linking anticipated reactions and behaviors provide a measure of individual control and improve coping.

CONCLUSION

Anticipating the psychological impact of bioterrorism requires a broad perspective on mental health and behavioral intervention. Responding to the psychological and mental health needs of affected individuals and groups in a clinical setting is only one facet of a broader preparedness strategy. Pre-event planning requires an understanding of how different people in different communities experience risk and how that is likely to affect their decisions and behaviors. In the event of bioterrorism, effective risk communication and risk management must address the intense emotional responses to an invisible, unpredictable, life-threatening enemy. The post-event recovery process is similarly influenced by multiple variables. Adopting a public mental health perspective that incorporates surveillance of pre-event, event, and post-event factors that address behavioral and psychological impacts will enhance adaptation and coping, thus reducing morbidity and long-term adverse outcomes.

REFERENCES

Ahern, J., Galea, S., Resnick, H., & Vlahiv, D. (2004). Television watching and mental health in the general population of New York City after September 11. *Journal of Aggression, Maltreatment & Trauma, 9*(1/2/3/4), 109-124.

Altman, L. J. (2003, March 21). Asian medics stay home, imperiling respiratory patients. *The New York Times*, p. A6.

Appelbaum, P. (2002, October 15). The mind of the murderer. *The Washington Post*, p. A19.

Barbera, J., & Macintyre, A. G. (2002, December). The reality of the modern bioterrorism response. *The Lancet, 360*(Suppl. 1), s33-s34.

Barbera, J., Macintyre, A., Gostin, L., Inglesby, T., O'Toole, T., DeAtley, C. et al. (2001). Large-scale quarantine following biological terrorism in the United States. *Journal of the American Medical Association, 286*(21), 2711-2717.

Blendon, R. J., Benson, J. M., DesRoches, C. M., Pollard, W. E., Parvanta, C., & Herrmann, M. J. (2002, April 17). The impact of anthrax on the American public. *Medscape General Medicine 4*(2). Retrieved July 15, 2003 from, www.hsph. harvard.edu/press/releases/blendon/report.pdf

Blendon R. J. (2003, April 17). *Harvard School of Public Health project on the public and biological security*. Retrieved July 15, 2003 from, www.hsph.harvard.edu

Brown, D. (2001, December 12). Canadian study shows anthrax's easy spread–One letter could cause many deaths. *The Washington Post*, pp. B1, B5.

Brown, D. (2003, July 20). The SARS triumph and what it promises. *The Washington Post*, p. A27.

Centers for Disease Control and Prevention. (2003, July 25). Use of quarantine to prevent transmission of severe acute respiratory syndrome–Taiwan. *Morbidity and Mortality Weekly Report, 52*, 680-683.

Covello, V., Peters, R. G., Wojtecki, J. G., & Hyde, R. C. (2001). Risk communication, the West Nile virus epidemic, and bioterrorism: Responding to the communication challenges posed by the intentional or unintentional release of a pathogen in an urban setting. *Journal of Urban Health: Bulletin of the New York Academy of Medicine, 78*, 382-91.

Cullen, M., & Whiteford, H. (2001, June 30). *The interrelations of social capital with health and mental health*. Retrieved July 15, 2003 from http://www.mental health.gov.au

District of Columbia: Report of Findings: Terrorism-Related Mental Health Needs Assessment Project. (2001, December 17). Prepared by Resource Development Group, Bowie, Maryland for The District of Columbia Department of Mental Health, Washington, DC.

Eckholm, E. (2003, April 24). Illness's psychological impact in China exceeds its actual number. *The New York Times*. Retrieved January 8, 2004 from, http://www. nytimes.com

Engel, C. C. Jr., & Katon, W. J. (1999). Population and need-based prevention of unexplained symptoms in the community. In Institute of Medicine, *Strategies to protect the health of deployed U.S. forces: Medical surveillance, record keeping, and risk reduction* (pp. 173-212). Washington, DC: National Academy Press.

Fullerton, C. S., Ursano, R. J., & Norwood, A. E., (2003). Trauma, terrorism and disaster. In R. J. Ursano, C. S. Fullerton, & A. E. Norwood (Eds.), *Terrorism and disaster. Individual and community mental health interventions* (pp. 1-20). Cambridge, UK: Cambridge University Press.

Garrett, L. (2000). *Betrayal of trust: The collapse of global public health.* New York: Hyperion.

Glass, T. A., & Schoch-Spana, M. (2002). Bioterrorism and the people: How to vaccinate a city against panic. *Clinical Infectious Diseases, 34*, 217-223.

Goode, E. (2003, February 20). Long-term effects of post-trauma events. *The New York Times*, p. A15.

Grady, D. (2003, April 7). Fear reigns as dangerous mystery illness spreads. *The New York Times*, p. A1.

Hall, M. J., Norwood, A. E., Ursano, R. J., & Fullerton, C. S. (2003). The psychological impacts of bioterrorism. *Biosecurity and Bioterrorism: Biodefense Strategy, Practice, and Science 1*, 139-144.

Hall, M. J., Norwood, A. E., Ursano, R. J., & Fullerton, C. S. (2002). Preparing for bioterrorism at the state level: Report of an informal survey. *American Journal of Orthopsychiatry, 72*, 486-496.

Holloway, H. C., Norwood, A. E., Fullerton, C. S., Engel, C. C., & Ursano, R. J. (1997). The threat of biological weapons: Prophylaxis and mitigation of psychological and social consequences. *Journal of the American Medical Association, 278*(5), 425-427.

Joint Commission on Accreditation of Healthcare Organizations Report. (2003, March 12). *Health care at the crossroads: Strategies for creating and sustaining community-wide emergency preparedness systems.* Retrieved September 10, 2003 from, http://www.jcaho.org/about+us/public+policy+initiatives/emergency+preparedess.pdf

Karsenty, E., J., Shemer, J., Alshech, I., Cojocaru, B., Moscovitz, M., Shapiro, Y. et al. (1991). Medical aspects of the Iraqi missile attacks on Israel. *Israel Journal of Medical Sciences 27*, 603-607.

Lifton, R. J. (2004). Aum Shinrikyo: The threshold crossed. *Journal of Aggression, Maltreatment & Trauma, 9*(1/2/3/4), 57-66.

McNeil, D. (2003, April 20). Wielding a big stick, carefully, against SARS. *The New York Times*, p. A12.

Morin, R., & Deane, C. (2002, October 24). Washington area sniper poll. *The Washington Post*, p. A01.

National Institute of Mental Health Report. (2001, October 29-November 1). *Mental health and mass violence: Evidence-based early psychological intervention for victims/survivors of mass violence. Report of a workshop to reach consensus on best practices.* Retrieved September 10, 2003, from http://www.nimh.nih.gov/research/massviolence.pdf

National Academy of Sciences. (2002). *Countering agricultural bioterrorism.* Washington DC: National Academies Press.

National Academy of Sciences. (2003, July 15). *Preparing for the psychological consequences of terrorism: A public health strategy.* Retrieved September 10, 2003 from, http://www.nap.edu/openbook/0309089530/html/109.html

North, C. S., Nixon, S. J., Shariat, S., Mallonee, S., Mcmillen, J. C., Spitznagel, E. L. et al. (1999). Psychiatric disorders among survivors of the Oklahoma City bombing. *Journal of the American Medical Association, 282*(8), 755-762.

North, C. S., & Pfefferbaum, B. (2002). Research on the mental health effects of terrorism. *Journal of the American Medical Association, 288,* 633-636.

Ohbu, S., Yamashina, A., Takasu, N., Yamaguchi, T., Murai, T., Nakano, K. et al. (1997). Sarin poisoning on Tokyo subway. *Southern Medical Journal, 90*(6), 587-593.

Pan, P. (2004, January 6). New SARS case confirmed. *The Washington Post,* p. A11.

Pew Survey. (2001, September 13-17). *American psyche reeling from terror attacks.* Retrieved July 15, 2003 from, http://people-press.org/reports

Schuster, M. A., Stein, B. D., Jaycox, L. H., Collins R. L., Marshall, G. N., Eliott, M. N. et al. (2001). A national survey of stress reactions after the September 11, 2001, terrorist attacks. *New England Journal of Medicine, 345,* 1507-1512.

Silver, R. C., Holman, E. A., McIntosh, D. N., Poulin, M., & Gil-Rivas V. (2002). Nationwide longitudinal study of psychological responses to September 11. *Journal of the American Medical Association, 288,* 1235-1244.

Silver, R. C., Poulin, M., Holman, E. A., McIntosh, D. N., Gil-Rivas, V., & Pizarro, J. (2004). Exploring the myths of coping with a national trauma: A longitudinal study of responses to the September 11th terrorist attacks. *Journal of Aggression, Maltreatment, & Trauma, 9*(1/2/3/4), 129-141.

Stolberg, S., & Miller, J. (2001, October 24). A nation challenged: The response–Officials admit underestimating danger posed to postal workers. *The New York Times,* p. A1.

Stolberg, S. G. (2003, May 2). The SARS epidemic: Lessons of anthrax attacks help U.S. respond to SARS. *The New York Times,* p. A14.

"The bioterror threat: Are we ready?" (2003, July 13). Editorial. *The Washington Post,* p. B06.

"The bioterror threat: Smallpox fiasco" (2003, July 14). Editorial. *The Washington Post,* p. A20.

U. S. General Accounting Office. (2003, April). *Smallpox vaccination: Implementation of national program faces challenges* (pp. 1-31). (GAO Report-03-578).

U. S. General Accounting Office. (2002, July). Foot and mouth disease: To protect U.S. livestock, USDA must remain vigilant and resolve outstanding issues. (GAO Report 02-808).

Uniformed Services University Center for the Study of Traumatic Stress, Fact Sheets. (2001, September 28). Retrieved July 15, 2003 from http//www.usuhs.mil/psy/disasteresources.html

Ursano, R. J. (2002). Post traumatic stress disorder (Editorial). *New England Journal of Medicine, 346*(2), 130-131.

CHILDREN

Psychological Impact of Terrorism on Children and Families in the United States

Betty J. Pfefferbaum

Ellen R. DeVoe

Jennifer Stuber

Miriam Schiff

Tovah P. Klein

Gerry Fairbrother

SUMMARY. This article reviews the literature on the psychological impact of terrorism on children and families in the United States. It includes studies of the 1993 World Trade Center bombing in New York City and the 1995 bombing of the Alfred P. Murrah Federal Building in

Address correspondence to: Betty J. Pfefferbaum, MD, JD, Paul and Ruth Jonas Chair, Professor and Chairman, Department of Psychiatry and Behavioral Sciences, College of Medicine, University of Oklahoma Health Sciences Center, 920 S. L. Young Boulevard, WP-3470, Oklahoma City, OK 73104 USA (E-mail: betty-pfefferbaum@ouhsc.edu).

[Haworth co-indexing entry note]: "Psychological Impact of Terrorism on Children and Families in the United States." Pfefferbaum, Betty J. et al. Co-published simultaneously in *Journal of Aggression, Maltreatment & Trauma* (The Haworth Maltreatment & Trauma Press, an imprint of The Haworth Press, Inc.) Vol. 9, No. 3/4, 2004; and: *The Trauma of Terrorism: Sharing Knowledge and Shared Care, An International Handbook* (ed: Yael Danieli, Danny Brom, and Joe Sills) The Haworth Maltreatment & Trauma Press, an imprint of The Haworth Press, Inc., 2005.

Oklahoma City, as well as the September 11 attacks. These studies explore the impact of various forms and degrees of exposure to terrorism on children across the development spectrum and on the relationships between parental and child reactions. The article concludes with a framework for future research on children's adaptation following mass trauma.

KEYWORDS. Disaster mental health, disasters, posttraumatic stress, posttraumatic stress disorder, September 11, terrorism, trauma

Based on an extensive literature on the effects of disaster on children, a body of work specifically focused on children's responses to terrorism is emerging. To date, no singular pattern of post-event outcomes has been identified, although responses to multiple kinds of traumatic events including terrorism have been documented. In this paper, we explore the broad effects of terrorism on children in the United States in the first generation of research in this area. The studies to date provide critical information regarding the relationship between exposure and child outcomes and direction for more refined approaches to address developmental, family, and socio-cultural factors in future research. The unprecedented nature of the September 11, 2001 attacks demarcated a new era in the global context of terrorism. Thus, we organize the paper to review studies of incidents that occurred prior to September 11 and then those that specifically address the September 11 attacks. Because we know little about how developmental trajectories, family processes, and socio-cultural factors may affect and be affected by exposure to terrorism, we conclude by offering a framework for considering additional elements that potentially influence children's adaptation following community trauma such as terrorism.

STUDIES OF PRE-SEPTEMBER 11 INCIDENTS

Prior to September 11, 2001, available literature on incidents in the U.S. was limited to studies of the 1993 World Trade Center bombing in New York City and the 1995 bombing of the Alfred P. Murrah Federal Building in Oklahoma City. These studies explored the impact of various forms and degrees of exposure to terrorism on children across the developmental spectrum and, to a lesser extent, effects on their parents, with minimal attention to the socio-cultural factors that may have affected their response.

The 1993 World Trade Center Bombing

The 1993 bombing of the World Trade Center trapped thousands inside the building, killed six, and injured many more. Koplewicz and colleagues (2002) compared 22 elementary school children trapped in the building with 27 children in a community convenience sample who were not at the site. Children and their parents, primarily mothers, were interviewed at three and nine months post-incident. The exposed children were highly symptomatic with moderate posttraumatic stress reactions at both time points. In contrast, children in the comparison group had only mild posttraumatic stress reactions. The exposed children reported significantly greater fear than the comparison group with no significant decline between assessments. This study is one of a few examining children with a high degree of direct exposure to a terrorist incident.

Parents of both groups of children experienced a decrease in their own posttraumatic stress reactions and fears and reported decreased posttraumatic stress reactions and fear in their children at nine months. Parents underestimated the suffering of their children, reporting fewer posttraumatic stress symptoms for their children than the children did for themselves at three months. Parents' reports of their own and their child's trauma symptoms were moderately correlated at both three and nine months. The findings related to parental symptoms illustrate the potentially powerful influence of children's exposure on parents who themselves have not been directly exposed.

The 1995 Oklahoma City Bombing

The 1995 bombing of the Alfred P. Murrah Federal Building in Oklahoma City resulted in the death of 168 people including 19 children. Hundreds were injured. Investigations of this disaster examined children across the developmental spectrum and explored various types of exposure.

Gurwitch and colleagues (Gurwitch, Pfefferbaum, & Leftwich, 2002; Gurwitch, Sitterle, Young, & Pfefferbaum, 2002) described the reactions of 11 preschool children, aged two to six years, attending day care at a nearby YMCA on the morning of the bombing. Many of the children suffered minor injuries and their evacuation and reactions were chronicled by the media. Mothers of the children were interviewed approximately six months after the bombing and the children were observed informally by day care workers and clinicians. Many showed signs of trauma including posttraumatic play, increased arousal, regressive behaviors, and functional difficulties; however, avoidance/numbing symptoms and restricted range of affect were not observed. Parents also reported anxiety, worry, and mood and sleep disturbance. Unfortunately, no information on the relationship between child and parent reactions in this sample has been published.

Pfefferbaum and colleagues (Pfefferbaum, Nixon, & Krug et al., 1999; Pfefferbaum, Nixon, & Tucker et al., 1999) examined various forms of exposure in a self-report survey of over 3,000 Oklahoma City middle and high school students seven weeks after the bombing. Most of the children in this convenience sample were at school on the day of the incident and not physically present at the disaster site, though many heard and/or felt the explosion. More than one-third of the children knew deceased victims and more than 40% knew injured survivors. Two-thirds reported that most or all of their television viewing in the aftermath of the incident was bombing-related. Posttraumatic stress at the time of the assessment was associated with female gender, interpersonal exposure (exposure through relationship with someone directly affected), bombing-related television viewing, and initial fear and arousal.

Investigators also examined a convenience sample of over 1,000 Oklahoma City elementary school children in the same school district during the next academic year, eight to ten months after the bombing (Gurwitch & Sitterle et al., 2002). Like the middle and high school sample, these children experienced high rates of interpersonal exposure. Many reported ongoing distress and almost one-third continued to worry about family members. Female gender, closer relationship to direct victims, and exposure to television coverage were associated with posttraumatic stress.

To examine more remote effects of the bombing, Pfefferbaum and colleagues (2000) studied the relationship between posttraumatic stress reactions and exposure to media coverage, both broadcast and print, in 69 sixth-grade children 100 miles from Oklahoma City two years after the bombing. While many children self-reported posttraumatic stress reactions at two years, few acknowledged deleterious effects on their functioning. Functional impairment, when it was present, was associated with indirect interpersonal exposure (a friend knew someone killed or injured in the explosion) but not with exposure to either broadcast or print coverage.

SEPTEMBER 11 STUDIES

The September 11, 2001 attacks represented the largest human-caused disaster in U.S. history. Over 3,000 people were killed and thousands were injured or evacuated from the World Trade Center complex and the lower downtown area of Manhattan and the Pentagon. Eight children died on the airplanes that crashed and virtually all children at Ground Zero near the World Trade Center fled for safety, experienced difficulty getting home that day, were trapped in their apartments or day care settings, and continued to smell smoke for weeks following the attacks (Hoven, 2002). Approximately one in ten children in Manhattan lost a relative or friend (Stuber et al., 2002), an estimated 40% of children saw a parent crying about the attacks, and approximately one in four watched television for more than four hours per day in the week following the attacks when coverage of the event dominated the media (Stuber et al., 2002). Children across the country also were exposed to the extensive media coverage of the events (Schuster et al., 2001). The large number of direct victims, extensive property damage, prolonged and pervasive media coverage, financial repercussions, and ongoing threat of additional acts raised concern about the mental health of the population at large.

Early data on children's reactions to the attacks were collected three to five days after the event using a nationally representative random-digit dial telephone survey of 560 adults to assess their reactions and, where applicable, their perceptions of their children's (ages 5 to 18 years) reactions. Information was obtained on 170 children. Thirty-five percent of parents reported that their children had at least one of the five stress symptoms measured, and almost one-half said that their children were concerned about their own or a loved one's safety. There was a positive association between parental and child responses using parent report (Schuster et al., 2001).

The significance of parental reactions to the attacks was highlighted in a study of kindergarten through sixth-grade students in two Washington, DC public elementary schools (Phillips, Scheibelhut, & Prince, 2003). Parents were contacted by mail in November 2001. Older children were surveyed in small groups at school and parents were asked to complete a questionnaire. The total sample was comprised of 176 parents (90% mothers) and 47 children (fourth through sixth grade). Both parent and child surveys focused on exposure to the attacks including loss of loved ones, emotional and behavioral responses to the attacks, parent-child communication about the attacks, children's actions following the attacks, and parent actions in support of children's coping following the attacks. Children's exposure in this sample was limited to media coverage and discussion of the events with parents and at school. Negative parental reactions, including greater concern about health problems, job security, and their own and their children's safety, and exposure to media coverage were associated with greater distress among children. Consistent with findings from the 1993 World Trade Center incident (Koplewicz et al., 2002), parents underestimated the degree of negative reactions experienced by their children.

A web-based, nationally representative study of 2,273 adults, completed one to two months after the attacks, focused on adult reactions, but respondents in households that included children younger than 18 years of age (n = 729) were asked if any children in the household were upset by the attacks. Children reported to be upset experienced trouble sleeping; were irritable, grouchy, or easily upset; and feared separating from their parents (Schlenger et al., 2002).

Stuber and colleagues (2002) conducted a telephone survey of a random sample of adult residents of Manhattan one to two months after the attacks. Of the 1,008 adults sampled, 112 were parents of at least one child. Respondents who were parents had greater posttraumatic stress than those who were not. Many parents recalled concern about their children's safety at the time and over one-half were not reunited with their children for more than four hours. Over 20% of the parents indicated that their children had received counseling related to the disaster. Predictors of counseling were male gender, parental symptoms consistent with posttraumatic stress disorder, and having at least one sibling living in the household.

In subsequent analyses based on a random digit-dial representative telephone survey of 434 New York City parents four to five months after the attacks, researchers documented a relationship between posttraumatic stress reactions that parents observed in their children to the receipt of counseling services. Severe or very severe posttraumatic stress reactions were highly predictive of receiving counseling in children, but 83% of children with severe or very severe posttraumatic stress reactions had received no services since the attacks. Among children who received counseling, 44% received services in schools, 36% from medical or professional providers, and 20% from other sources (Fairbrother, Stuber, Galea, Fleischman, & Pfefferbaum, 2003).

Using the same survey of 434 parents, Fairbrother, Stuber, and Galea (2003) assessed predictors of posttraumatic stress reactions in children between the ages of 4 and 17 years. Overall, 18% of children were reported by their parents to have experienced severe or very severe posttraumatic stress reactions and 66% had moderate posttraumatic stress reactions. Exposure of various forms, including parental posttraumatic stress, the parent crying in front of the child, seeing three or more graphic images of the disaster on television, and living in Manhattan, were associated with severe or very severe posttraumatic stress reactions in children.

Comparing the same sample of 434 parents to other adults in New York, researchers also sought to determine whether parents were more vulnerable to adverse outcomes after the September 11 attacks than non-parents. Parents and non-parents had the same level of exposure to the attacks, as did single parents and parents in two-parent households. Parents were no more likely than non-parents to have lost a job or health insurance after the attacks or to have posttraumatic stress disorder or depression. However, single parents, compared to those in two-parent households, were more likely to have lost a job or health insurance after the attacks, to have posttraumatic stress disorder, to be depressed, and to have increased cigarette smoking after the attacks. This vulnerability persisted even after controlling for parental age, gender, borough of residence, race, income, and education (Fairbrother, Stuber, & Galea, 2003).

No studies to date have used a longitudinal design to assess the impact of the September 11 attacks on children. One study used data collected from three cross-sectional random digit-dial telephone surveys of parents conducted 11 months before and four and six months after the attacks to examine behavior problems in children post-September 11. Parents reported fewer behavior problems in their children four months after the attacks compared to pre-September 11 levels, but problems returned to pre-September 11 levels by six months after the attacks. This finding suggests that behavior problems may be dampened, or that parents may not be sensitive to these problems, in the acute aftermath of a traumatic event. Demographic characteristics including the child's race/ethnicity, low income, living in a single parent household, disaster event experiences, and parental reactions to the September 11 attacks were associated with child behavior problems in multivariable models (Stuber et al., in press).

In the largest study of the effects of terrorism on school-age children to date, a representative sample of 8,266 New York City public school children (grades four through twelve) was surveyed six months after September 11 to determine exposure, prior trauma, and post-September 11 adjustment. Recognizing that the psychological impact of terrorism on children may extend beyond symptoms of posttraumatic stress disorder, the investigation assessed an array of probable psychiatric disorders. New York City children had higher than population rates of posttraumatic stress disorder (11%), major depression (8%), generalized anxiety (10%), agoraphobia (15%), and separation anxiety (12%), although the extent to which these disorders were specifically tied to the September 11 attacks cannot be definitely established. Researchers concluded that there may have been differential susceptibility to certain types of psychiatric disorders in response to the disaster by age, gender, ethnicity, and exposure. Older children were more likely than younger children to meet criteria for conduct disorder and depression, whereas younger children were more likely to have posttraumatic stress disorder, agoraphobia, and separation anxiety. Rates of most disorders were higher in girls than boys with the exception of conduct disorder, where boys appeared more susceptible. Children who were personally exposed to the event (e.g., fled the disaster site) or had family exposure (e.g., family member killed, injured, or escaped unhurt) were at greater risk for posttraumatic stress disorder. Hispanics had higher rates of posttraumatic stress disorder, separation anxiety, agoraphobia, and panic attacks than children of other races, although differences by ethnicity were less significant than differences by gender or age. The finding of ethnic differences underscores the critical need to examine further the role of culture in understanding children's responses to trauma (Hoven, 2002).

Although children of all ages were exposed to the September 11 attacks, most studies have focused on school-aged children and adolescents. Preliminary findings from a study of 240 New York City children who were 5 years old or younger on September 11 were consistent with results from Oklahoma City and with research on child trauma in general (DeVoe, Klein, & Marcus, 2003; Klein, DeVoe, & Miranda, 2003). A convenience sample of parents who lived in New York City on September 11 was interviewed 9 to 12 months after the attacks. Parents' retrospective accounts of their children's acute responses indicated that 54% of children expressed themes related to the World Trade Center tragedy in play, 52% experienced sleeping difficulties, and 29% experienced increased separation anxiety. Applying *Zero to Three* (1994) diagnostic guidelines for posttraumatic stress disorder, children were reported to have reexperiencing symptoms (78%), numbing (19%), increased arousal (57%), and other new symptoms including fears (57%). In total, 13% of children met posttraumatic stress disorder criteria.

LIMITATIONS IN CURRENT RESEARCH

The results of the existing studies on children's reactions to terrorism must be interpreted in light of limitations in samples, methodology, and instruments. Most studies to date have examined convenience samples, which may not have been representative (Gurwitch, Pfefferbaum, & Leftwich, 2002; Gurwitch & Sitterle et al., 2002; Koplewicz et al., 2002; Pfefferbaum, Nixon, & Krug et al., 1999; Pfefferbaum, Nixon, Tucker et al., 1999; Phillips, Scheibelhut, & Prince, 2003). Hoven's (2002) study of New York City children is a notable exception that examined a large representative sample with findings that should generalize to this urban environment. Most of the studies have described primarily indirect victimization through interpersonal relationships outside the immediate family and/or exposure to media coverage, rather than examining children who were physically present at the site of an attack (Fairbrother, Stuber, Galea, Fleischman, & Pfefferbaum, 2003; Gurwitch & Sitterle et al., 2002; Pfefferbaum, Nixon & Krug et al., 1999; Pfefferbaum, Nixon & Tucker et al., 1999; Pfefferbaum et al., 2000; Phillips, Scheibelhut, & Prince, 2003; Stuber et al., 2002). Noteworthy, therefore, are the studies by Koplewicz and colleagues (2002) and Gurwitch and colleagues (Gurwitch, Pfefferbaum, & Leftwich, 2002; Gurwitch & Sitterle et al., 2002), which examined directly exposed children. Unfortunately, their samples were small and volunteer but they provided preliminary information about trauma directly experienced in young children, an area not well examined. Studies by DeVoe and colleagues (DeVoe, Klein, & Marcus, 2003; Klein, DeVoe, & Miranda, 2003) have also added to the literature on young children.

A number of studies have relied on parent report (Fairbrother, Stuber, Galea, Fleischman, & Pfefferbaum, 2003; Schlenger et al., 2002; Schuster et al., 2001; Stuber et al., 2002), which is problematic because adults commonly underestimate the distress of children (Koplewicz et al., 2002). There were limitations in the outcome measures of many studies which included, for the most part, symptoms associated with posttraumatic stress disorder (Fairbrother, Stuber, Galea, Fleischman, & Pfefferbaum, 2003; Gurwitch, Pfefferbaum, & Leftwich, 2002; Pfefferbaum, Nixon & Krug et al., 1999; Pfefferbaum, Nixon & Tucker et al., 1999; Stuber et al., 2002) rather than examining a full range of positive and negative results. Most studies have used scales that do not establish diagnosis, thus limiting the determination of clinical significance. Because these scales are not diagnostic tools, the results must not be interpreted to suggest widespread pathology. Instruments in several studies have more closely mirrored diagnostic criteria (Hoven, 2002; Koplewicz et al., 2002). Finally, selection of potential correlates of trauma and of the potential risk and protective factors that may be associated with outcome have been guided by studies of childhood trauma in general. If terrorism presents novel experiences, these correlates must be reconsidered.

DIRECTIONS FOR THE NEXT GENERATION OF STUDIES

Existing research clearly demonstrates that children are not immune from psychological harm following terrorist acts. The potentially diverse responses to terrorism in children can be understood within the context of a transactional-ecological model of developmental psychopathology (Pynoos, Steinberg, & Piacentini, 1999). Within this framework, type (e.g., direct, familial, and media), severity, and accumulation of exposure interact with the individual characteristics of the child and social ecology to influence adaptation. The research to date has been limited but has laid important groundwork for future work in the area.

While posttraumatic stress disorder is the condition most commonly associated with terrorism, other disorders and comorbid conditions are also likely to emerge, including affective and anxiety disorders, aggressive behavior and conduct problems, substance use, and sub-clinical psychological distress. To better understand the impact of terrorism on children and their families, future research should consider these diverse outcomes.

Most existing research on terrorism has focused on the role and characteristics of exposure as the primary predictor of children's reactions with little grounding in a developmental framework. Yet, the developmental context is crucial to understanding the intrinsic and extrinsic factors that influence a child's reaction to trauma. For example, as children develop greater cognitive competence and emotional mastery, they are better able to appraise danger, increasing their effectiveness in managing their emotional and physiological responses to trauma (Pynoos et al., 1999). While exposure to trauma, including terrorist acts, may not always result in developmental harm, it does increase the potential for subsequent negative consequences to the child (Rutter, 1987).

Children's adaptation to trauma is influenced directly and indirectly by the functioning of significant caregivers (Garbarino & Kostelny, 1996; Pynoos, Goenjian, & Steinberg, 1998) who buffer and translate terrorist acts. Because children's development, especially during the formative years, is so intimately tied to parent functioning, parent reactions are key to understanding children's adaptation. While several studies have assessed the impact of terrorist events on parents and the associations between child and parent reactions, too little is known about specific family influences in this area. Even less is known about the factors that may mediate or exacerbate child and parent reactions.

A developmental framework for understanding the impact of terrorism is essential for understanding children's responses to exposure and must include a view of children in the context of their families. Children are greatly affected by parental support and intervention and by the larger "recovery environment" in the aftermath of trauma, including terrorist assault. Over time, parents' ability to manage their own responses and to support their children's processing of events will influence the child's adjustment (Miller, 1996; Pynoos et al., 1998). At the same time, terrorism creates independent health and mental health effects on parents. We know little about how terrorism may alter parenting beliefs and practices, which in turn may influence a child's reaction. More focused examination of the impact of terrorism on the parenting process and the parent-child relationship is an important next step in identifying risks to the developmental process that have both acute and long-term implications for the child. Further, this emphasis has implications for the preparedness of families and for supportive intervention with families in the aftermath of terrorism.

Much more information is needed on the factors that contribute to posttraumatic stress and other adverse reactions to terrorism. Prior traumatic experiences emerge as one such factor. For example, studies from other countries, primarily those in the Middle East, have shown negative effects of cumulative violence associated with political conflict (Garbarino & Kostelny, 1996; Garbarino, Kostelny, & Dubrow, 1991; Gorman-Smith & Tolan, 1998) and posttraumatic stress related to other trauma was the best predictor of post-bombing stress in Kenyan school children after the 1998 American Embassy bombing (Pfefferbaum et al., 2003).

Additional research is needed on factors that may ameliorate the effects of terrorism. Studies of children in the Middle East have examined the role of religion and ideology in buffering children's reactions to terrorism in the context of cumulative political conflict existing in the region, but the results of these studies are inconsistent (Punamäki, 1996; Slone, Adiri & Arian, 1998; Slone & Hallis, 1999). Thus, conclusions about this and other social and cultural issues remain in question.

CONCLUSIONS

Research on the psychological impact of terrorism on children is in its infancy. Children who are directly exposed to a traumatic event are particularly vulnerable to adverse psychological outcomes, but children with less direct exposure are also at risk. Research after the Oklahoma City bombing and following the September 11 attacks has shown an association between exposure to televised coverage of terrorist events and adverse psychological outcomes. Less is known about the extent to which continuing fear and anxiety about terrorism contribute to these outcomes. In the next generation of research on the impact of terrorism on children, it will be useful to broaden the scope of assessment beyond the current construct of exposure, to consider pathways to varied outcomes, including conditions other than posttraumatic stress, and to examine coping and resilience. Age-specific vulnerabilities and competencies including the capacity to appraise danger to self and others and to make sense of a terrorist event, the significance of caregivers in shaping children's post-event adaptation, and the influence of a host of cultural factors warrant further examination.

REFERENCES

DeVoe, E. R., Klein, T. P., & Linas, S. (2003, December). *Helping young children and their parents and caregivers: Lessons from Ground Zero.* Workshop presented at the Zero to Three: 18th National Training Institute, New Orleans, LA.

Fairbrother, G., Stuber, J., & Galea, S. (2003). *Do single parents need extra assistance following a traumatic event?* Unpublished manuscript.

Fairbrother, G., Stuber, J., Galea, S., Fleischman, A. R., & Pfefferbaum, B. (2003). Posttraumatic stress reactions in New York City children after the September 11, 2001, terrorist attacks. *Ambulatory Pediatrics, 3,* 304-311.

Garbarino, J., & Kostelny, K. (1996). The effects of political violence on Palestinian children's behavior problems: A risk accumulation model. *Child Development, 67,* 33-45.

Garbarino, J., Kostelny, K., & Dubrow, N. (1991). *No place to be a child: Growing up in a war zone.* Toronto: Lexington Books.

Gorman-Smith, D., & Tolan, P. (1998). The role of exposure to community violence and developmental problems among inner city youth. *Development and Psychopathology, 10,* 101-116.

Gurwitch, R. H., Pfefferbaum, B., & Leftwich, M. J. T. (2002). The impact of terrorism on children: Considerations for a new era. In S. N. Gold & J. Faust (Eds.), *Trauma practice in the wake of September 11, 2001* (pp. 101-124). Binghamton, NY: The Haworth Press, Inc.

Gurwitch, R. H., Sitterle, K. S., Young, B. H., & Pfefferbaum, B. (2002). Helping children in the aftermath of terrorism. In A. M. La Greca, W. K. Silverman, E. M. Vernberg, & M. C. Roberts (Eds.), *Helping children cope with disasters: Integrating research and practice* (pp. 327-357). Washington, DC: American Psychological Association.

Hoven, C. W. (2002, June 10). *Testimony regarding unmet mental health needs of New York City public school children as a result of the September 11th attacks on the World Trade Center.* U.S. Senate Health, Education, Labor and Pensions (HELP) Committee Hearing.

Klein, T. K., DeVoe, E. R., & Miranda, C. (2003, April). The impact of the WTC attacks on young children. In L. R. Sherrod (Chair), *Reactions of children and youth to the World Trade Center disaster.* Symposium conducted at Biennial Meeting of the Society for Research on Child Development, Tampa, FL.

Koplewicz, H.S., Vogel, J. M., Solanto, M. V., Morrissey, R. F., Alonso, C. M., Abikoff, H., et al. (2002). Child and parent response to the 1993 World Trade Center bombing. *Journal of Traumatic Stress, 15*(1), 77-85.

Miller, K. E. (1996). The effects of state terrorism and exile on indigenous Guatemalan refugee children: A mental health assessment and an analysis of children's narratives. *Child Development, 67,* 89-106.

Pfefferbaum, B., Nixon, S. J., Krug, R. S., Tivis, R. D., Moore, V. L., & Brown, J. M. et al. (1999). Clinical needs assessment of middle and high school students following the 1995 Oklahoma City bombing. *American Journal of Psychiatry, 156,* 1069-1074.

Pfefferbaum, B., Nixon, S. J., Tucker, P. M., Tivis, R. D., Moore, V. L., & Gurwitch, R. H. et al. (1999). Posttraumatic stress responses in bereaved children after the Oklahoma City bombing. *Journal of the American Academy of Child and Adolescent Psychiatry, 38*(11), 1372-1379.

Pfefferbaum, B., North, C. S., Doughty, D. E., Fullerton, C. S., Gurwitch, R. H., & Kyula, J. (2003). Posttraumatic stress and functional impairment in Kenyan children following the 1998 American Embassy bombing. *American Journal of Orthopsychiatry, 73,* 133-140.

Pfefferbaum, B., Seale, T. W., McDonald, N. B., Brandt, E. N., Jr., Rainwater, S. M., & Maynard, B. T. et al. (2000). Posttraumatic stress two years after the Oklahoma City bombing in youths geographically distant from the explosion. *Psychiatry*, *63*(4), 358-370.

Phillips, D., Scheibelhut, L., & Prince, S. (2003, April). Children's responses to the terrorist attacks of September 11th: An exploratory study. In J. Lawrence Aber & D. Phillips (Chairs), *The aftermath of September 11th, 2001: Developmental effects and policy implications.* Symposium conducted at the Biennial Meetings of the Society for Research in Child Development, Tampa, FL.

Punamäki, R. L. (1996). Can ideological commitment protect children's psychological well-being in situations of political violence? *Child Development, 67*, 55-69.

Pynoos, R. S., Goenjian, A., & Steinberg, A. M. (1998). A public mental health approach to the post-disaster treatment of children and adolescents. *Child and Adolescent Clinics of North America, 7*, 195-210.

Pynoos, R. S., Steinberg, A. M., & Piacentini, J. C. (1999). A developmental psychopathology model of childhood traumatic stress and intersection with anxiety disorders. *Biological Psychiatry, 46*, 1542-1554.

Rutter, M. (1987). Psychosocial resilience and protective mechanisms. *American Journal of Orthopsychiatry, 57*(3), 316-331.

Schlenger, W. E., Caddell, J. M., Ebert, L., Jordan, B. K., Rourke, K. M., & Wilson, D. et al. (2002). Psychological reactions to the terrorist attacks: Findings from the National Study of Americans' Reactions to September 11. *Journal of the American Medical Association, 288*(5), 581-588.

Schuster, M. A., Stein, B. D., Jaycox, L. H., Collins, R. L., Marshall, G. N., & Elliott, M. N. et al. (2001). A National Survey of Stress Reactions after the September 11, 2001, terrorist attacks. *The New England Journal of Medicine, 345*(20), 1507-1512.

Slone, M., Adiri, M., & Arian, A. (1998). Adverse political events and psychological adjustment: Two cross-cultural studies. *Journal of the American Academy of Child and Adolescent Psychiatry, 37*(10), 1058-1069.

Slone, M., & Hallis, D. (1999). The impact of political life events on children's psychological adjustment. *Anxiety, Stress, and Coping, 12*, 1-21.

Stuber, J., Fairbrother, G., Galea, S., Pfefferbaum, B., Wilson-Genderson, M., & Vlahov, D. (2002). Determinants of counseling for children in Manhattan after the September 11 attacks. *Psychiatric Services, 53*, 815-822.

Stuber, J., Galea, S., Pfefferbaum, B., Vandivere, S., Moore, K., & Fairbrother, G. (in press). Behavior problems in New York City's children after the September 11, 2001, terrorist attacks. *American Journal of Orthopsychiatry.*

Zero to Three/National Center for Clinical Infant Programs. (1994). *Diagnostic classification: 0-3. Diagnostic classification of mental health and developmental disorders of infancy and early childhood.* Arlington, VA: National Center for Clinical Infant Programs.

Voice:
I Don't Want to Go to Any More Funerals
of Eight Year Olds

The planes smashed into the World Trade Center barely 72 hours after I had returned home from two months of covering the Israeli-Palestinian agony. I was *The New York Times* bureau chief in Jerusalem for four years in the first half of the 1990s. Those were years of hope for a genuine peace between those two peoples, or years of self-delusion; take your pick. Your choice will no doubt be guided by your politics.

Back then, I saw mainly the hope. Like many, I had thought that the Oslo agreements provided the psychological breakthrough for both Israelis and Palestinians. Each side now truly accepted the inevitability of the other's existence and the validity of its national aspirations. Sure, important details remained to be worked out; there would be difficult days ahead. And even then, optimism was sorely tested by Palestinian suicide bombings, a relatively new and singularly ugly phenomenon at the time. I covered half a dozen or more bombings before I left the Middle East in 1995. But I accepted the proposition advanced by the Israeli government that these atrocities were part of the

Address correspondence to: Clyde Haberman, 229 West 43rd Street, New York, NY 10036 USA (E-mail: haberman@nytimes.com).

[Haworth co-indexing entry note]: "Voice: I Don't Want to Go to Any More Funerals of Eight Year Olds." Haberman, Clyde. Co-published simultaneously in *Journal of Aggression, Maltreatment & Trauma* (The Haworth Maltreatment & Trauma Press, an imprint of The Haworth Press, Inc.) Vol. 9, No. 3/4, 2004; and: *The Trauma of Terrorism: Sharing Knowledge and Shared Care, An International Handbook* (ed: Yael Danieli, Danny Brom, and Joe Sills) The Haworth Maltreatment & Trauma Press, an imprint of The Haworth Press, Inc., 2005.

peace process's growing pains. They would end. Humanitarian issues aside, they made no political sense. Good faith would prevail.

I was wrong, of course. It didn't help that so were many others. By the time I went back to Jerusalem for a two-month stint in the summer of 2001, the situation seemed hopeless. Bombings continued at a shocking pace. Palestinians had their own pain, trapped in a virtual lockdown in their villages. What depressed me most, perhaps, was that each side had lost all compassion for the other. Palestinians didn't want to hear about Israelis' legitimate security fears. Israelis didn't want to hear about Palestinians' legitimate despair over the wretchedness of their lives.

At the end of my stay, I wrote a long essay comparing present moods and realities with what existed in 1995. I began by talking about Israeli Jerusalemites listening for the ambulance sirens. The first siren may mean nothing. But then comes a second siren, then a third and a fourth. And then everyone knows that terrorists have struck again. So they reach for cell phones. But often they cannot get through because everyone else is doing the same thing, jamming the system. So they wait for excruciating minutes or hours wondering if their wives or husbands or children chose this wrong time to stop at that wrong café. This article ran on the front page of *The New York Times on* September 9, 2001.

Two days later, much of it proved distressingly prescient. It was our turn in New York to listen for the sirens, to reach for the cell phones that didn't work, to wait fearfully and wonder where loved ones were when the terrorists turned airplanes into missiles. Israel's daily reality, it seemed, had arrived on our shores. That was my theme on September 11 as I resumed my regular New York column.

"Do you get it now?" I wrote.

It was a refrain that I repeated and weaved throughout that column. Do you get what it is like to live with terror as Israelis do? In fact, however, I myself didn't get it, not precisely. Despite the horror of 9/11, New Yorkers do not live with the grinding reality of daily life in Israel. Yes, we suffered great pain that September morning. Perhaps there is more to come. But we do not really know what it is like to have no idea if the bus or subway train will blow up, or if the coffee shop will suddenly explode, or if taking the kids out for a pizza may mean losing them forever. In conversations, I have often said that we will be more like Jerusalem when a bomb goes off at a diner in Jackson Heights, a neighborhood in the borough of Queens with no special symbolic or economic significance.

That summer, I discovered that I was not immune to fear. I had not felt it when I was the regular correspondent in Jerusalem. But in 2001, I tended to stay away from outdoor cafes, for they seemed vulnerable to attack. One evening when Jerusalem was on high terrorist alert, I felt skittish enough to insist on a rear table at a restaurant. I figured that if a terrorist blew himself up, he would probably do it near the entrance. Don't misunderstand, back in 1994 when the suicide attacks began, I also took reasonable precautions. I insisted that no one in my family ride buses, which were frequent targets. When in a crowd, I was aware of who stood near me. But there was no fear factor. Covering terrorism was essentially safe for journalists. With rare exceptions, we were not at the scene when a bomb went off. We recreate events after the fact. And after a while, a depressingly familiar routine set in.

During the Rabin-Peres years, the stories would start out by saying how many people were killed and describing the terrible scene. That was quickly followed by a government disclaimer that the extremists would not knock the peace process off course. Cold as this might sound, the stories developed a dreary sameness.

The Sharon government's reaction, obviously, is different. It has struck back, and hard, almost every time. But even that response acquired a predictability of its own. An occupational hazard for those who cover terrorism is that a numbness of sorts can take hold.

Up to a point. There is no such numbness at the funerals of terror's victims. I went to so many of them. It was at graveside that the anguish of terrorism truly struck home. I felt it keenly in August 2001, after 15 people perished in the bombing of a Jerusalem pizzeria. Five of them were from a single family: mother, father, and three children. Looking at their bodies lined up, I realized that there are limits to even a journalist's endurance for emotional pain. Mine had been reached. Standing there, I decided that I didn't want to go to any more funerals of 8-year-olds. Since then, I haven't.

The Immediate Psychological Consequences of Terror Attacks in Children

Esti Galili-Weisstub
Fortu Benarroch

SUMMARY. Two hundred and sixty young terror victims were evaluated in the Emergency Room (ER) of a general hospital immediately after several terrorist attacks in Jerusalem. The developmental perspective is presented through descriptions of the psychological presentation in different ages. Less than 20% of the victims presented with a pathological acute stress reaction. Detailed examples of the clinical reactions are included. Issues of the intrapsychic difficulties stemming from the traumatic experience are raised. Finally, the role of the parent in the formulation and intensity of the child's psychological reaction is discussed.

KEYWORDS. Children, adolescents, immediate reaction, psychological reaction, terror, trauma

Address correspondence to: Esti Galili-Weisstub, MD, Child & Adolescent Psychiatry, Hadassah University Hospital, Kiryat Hadassah P.O.B. 12000, Jerusalem, Israel 91120 (E-mail: galili@hadassah.org.il).

[Haworth co-indexing entry note]: "The Immediate Psychological Consequences of Terror Attacks in Children." Galili-Weisstub, Esti, and Fortu Benarroch. Co-published simultaneously in *Journal of Aggression, Maltreatment & Trauma* (The Haworth Maltreatment & Trauma Press, an imprint of The Haworth Press, Inc.) Vol. 9, No. 3/4, 2004; and: *The Trauma of Terrorism: Sharing Knowledge and Shared Care, An International Handbook* (ed: Yael Danieli, Danny Brom, and Joe Sills) The Haworth Maltreatment & Trauma Press, an imprint of The Haworth Press, Inc., 2005.

In recent years, much effort has been invested in prospective clinical research projects on children and adolescents exposed to trauma. Most focused on the intermediate and long-term consequences. The majority of the clinical presentations of Post Traumatic Stress Disorder (PTSD) were collected from victims who have sought professional help weeks, months, and sometimes years after the traumatic event. There are still only a limited number of descriptions of the immediate clinical presentation of acute stress, particularly in children and adolescents exposed to severe acute trauma (Cohen, 2003; Daviss, Racusin, Fleischer, Mooney, Ford, & McHugo, 2000; Fein, Kassam-Adams, Vu, & Datner, 2001; March, 2003; Milgram, Toubiana, Klingman, Raviv, & Godstein, 1998; Vila, Porche, & Mouren-Simeoni, 1999; Winston et al., 2002).

Victims of acute trauma may be seen minutes after the trauma, at the scene of the traumatic event or in the emergency rooms (ERs) of general hospitals. Immediate psychiatric evaluation, including detailed clinical description and psychological assessment, provides the starting point for understanding the resolution of trauma in most cases and the evolution of PTSD or other posttraumatic psychiatric sequelae in others. Early clinical evaluation also provides the basis for developing tools for early detection of minors at risk for developing a significant clinical disorder. Detailed data collected immediately after the traumatic event are a necessary baseline for determining immediate intervention and evaluating their contribution to diminishing or even preventing the development of Acute Stress Disorder (ASD) and PTSD in children and adolescents.

The clinical description of immediate emotional and physiological reactions to trauma should include the perspective of the trauma itself. Was the trauma acute or chronic? Natural or human made? Was the minor alone? Was the caretaker hurt? What did the child actually witness? And what are the chronological age, gender, cultural background, and cognitive, emotional, and social developmental stage of the child?

During the last three years, due to the escalation of violence in the Middle East, we have seen over 260 minors evacuated to the ER of two general hospitals (in Jerusalem) directly from a terror event. They were exposed to violent terrorist acts: suicide bombers exploding in buses or shopping areas, terrorists shooting at cars or pedestrians, and explosives going off unexpectedly on the street, in cafeterias, and in open fields. The threat of terrorism has become an ongoing part of children's lives in the Middle East. As time passed, we met children involved in more than one event. We have thus been dealing not with a simple reaction to a single-event trauma but with a more complex situation of "acute on chronic" trauma (Shalev et al., 2002).

We saw the victims in an ER setting. They were examined and treated immediately following evacuation from the terror scene. All victims were evaluated regardless of whether they had any specific physical or emotional complaints. The majority of minors (73%) suffered from minimal physical injury, and were released from the ER within hours after the event. The psychological/psychiatric evaluation and intervention were conducted by senior child and adolescent psychiatrists, who are experienced in the field of emotional trauma in children.

It is important to note that the professionals live and work in the same social context of ongoing terrorist threat as the victims. In addition, during the last three years there seems to have been a change in the social attitude toward and acceptance of emotional reaction to the trauma of terrorism. An increasing number of young victims and their parents feel freer to express their immediate terrifying experience and are less concerned with "stigma" when they seek support and guidance. Most of the victims (80%) were adolescents (ages 12 to 18 years old). They were usually with other peers at the scene. Most of the children (ages 3 months to 11 years) were with their parents and other family members when the attacks took place. A small number had lost a parent or an immediate family member at that same event. The total number of males and females was almost equal: 53% boys and 47% girls.

ACUTE STRESS REACTION: DEFINING THE NORMAL RANGE

Most of the terror victims (82%) we saw did not present with significant clinical symptoms that we would consider "pathologically" acute stress reaction. They were fully oriented, could give a clear description of the event, had appropriate affect for the situation, and understood the meaning of what had occurred.

It is a difficult and debatable question where the line crosses between normal and pathological immediate stress reaction. Although it seems that the subjectivity of the clinician plays a central part, it is still a valuable demarcation to make if one of the aims is to assess the risk of development of a disorder in the aftermath.

Considering the horrifying experience that the 260 terror victims we observed were exposed to, we regarded sadness (sometimes accompanied by crying), anxiety, some excitement, and restlessness to be normal non-pathological reactions. The guidelines were: intact cognition, reasonable emotional control, and a downward trend in measures of physiological hyperarousal (heart rate, blood pressure and other physical symptoms of anxiety) (Shalev, 2000). By intact cognition, we mean, for example, normal orientation and clear memory of the traumatic event. Reasonable emotional control is demonstrated by a capacity for self regulation (Cohen, 2003; March, 2003; Shalev et al., 2002); for example, a boy who was crying but nevertheless could cooperate and engage in conversation.

We describe our observations of immediate psychological reactions of child victims of terrorist attacks, in two parallel conceptual frameworks:

1. The phenomenological description as included in the definition of ASD. The main rationale for this approach is that although the validity of ASD as an entity in children remains controversial (Cohen, 2003; March, 2003; Pfefferbaum, 1997), studies of children exposed to trauma have shown a correlation between the score in measures of ASD-like signs and symptoms taken close to the trauma and the later development of PTSD (Daviss et al., 2000; Fein et al., 2001; Milgram, 1998; Vila et al., 1999; Winston et al., 2002).
2. The intrapsychic description of the affects and thought contents, in order to understand the inner subjective experience of the trauma, in search of themes that should be considered in future therapeutic interventions.

DEVELOPMENTAL ASPECTS IN THE CLINICAL PRESENTATION IMMEDIATELY AFTER EXPOSURE TO TERROR

Infants and Toddlers. Evaluating children who are a few months to 2 years old is complex. In general, the child's concept of and reactions to the traumatic event are affected significantly by the reactions of the caretaker (Scheeringa & Zeanah, 2001). When accompanied by their parents, one can directly observe the parents' or caretaker emotional reaction and their ability to attend to the baby's needs, be it through contact, verbal soothing, or feeding. At the same time, one gathers a clinical impression of the child's emotional state. Some babies react to their parents stress by becoming reticent, very quiet, sometimes falling asleep. Most babies react with restlessness. They cry, are hard to soothe, and may take a while before they are settled and able to eat. Babies who are apart from their parents experience acute separation. It may be of short duration, or the first stage of orphanhood.

The infants and young children we have seen in the ER were involved in a terrorist event as part of their family. In a few instances, they were in a car that was shot at and both parents were killed. Sometimes siblings were injured or killed as well. Usually within minutes of their arrival at the ER, they were held and looked after by older brothers/sisters or by grandparents. The majority of the cases did not exhibit apparent stress or anxiety symptoms. Even in the state of shock from the sudden tragedy, close family members were able to mobilize empathy, tenderness, and caring for the young ones.

Preschool-Age Children. Preschoolers are capable of verbal interaction and description of their experience. Again, the presence of a close family member or a familiar person seemed to affect the child in a positive manner. Some described the event in their own words; others were playing (free play). On the whole, we have not encountered any acute emotional reaction in preschool terrorist victims.

Although we have not seen any posttraumatic dissociative reactions in very young children (4-5 years old) even if they were involved in extremely violent terrorist attacks, we did observe obvious dissociative states in children from the same age group who witnessed severe domestic violence. It remains unclear whether the difference stems from the more emotionally conflictual experience of domestic violence (e.g., father murdering mother), or from the fact that the number of very young terror victims we have seen is relatively small.

Some of the very young children who experienced terrorist trauma later developed PTSD with a significant separation anxiety component. In these cases, at least one parent had PTSD as well. It was apparent that when these young children were observed in the ER, they were still protected from the immediate impact of the event. In the long run, they are exposed to the damage and loss caused by the incident. The development of the disorder may thus occur months after the event.

School Age Children. Similar to younger children, school age children (6-11 years old) are usually accompanied by close family/friends; however, they are more independent, and it is not unusual for them to spend the time immediately after the trauma trying to locate family members who were on the site of the explosion/attack with them. They present with a spectrum of emotional reactions. Some are sad and subdued, communicative when approached, with no apparent problem in their cognitive perception of the event. Others are anxious about parents, siblings, or themselves, focusing their concern on very small cuts or minor therapeutic interventions. The communication with school age children is verbal and directive. One can usually conduct a full psychiatric evaluation with their cooperation very shortly after arrival at the ER.

Adolescents. Adolescents present a different clinical picture. Most have been at the event with friends. Their traumatic experience happened usually in a social rather than a family context. Some might refuse (at first) to involve their parents. They are occupied with cellular phones locating other friends who were at the site with them. Often they seem unaware or unconcerned about their injury, yet some behave like the younger children (e.g., over focusing on superficial wounds). Most express obvious acute stress reaction with signs of emotional shock, anxiety, and sadness. They are clearly upset by what they witnessed and readily describe the event and the horrific scenes.

IMMEDIATE PATHOLOGICAL REACTIONS

Eighteen percent of the minors exhibited what we termed an extreme acute stress reaction. Among the clinical phenomena were dissociative states, conversion reactions, intense anxiety, and psychosis.

Dissociative Reactions. Very few studies describe the rate of dissociation in children and adolescents immediately after a traumatic event. Most studies question the victims about their feelings when the event took place days or longer after the trauma. Terr (1979) stressed that none of the children interviewed after the Chowchilla kidnapping exhibited memory lapses, emotional numbing, or blurring of consciousness. Like others, she gathered the information from the children in retrospect. Fein, Kassam-Adams, Vu, and Datner (2001) described 81 young violence victims (8-24 years old) who were evaluated immediately after the assault. Seventy-eight percent of the victims reported peritraumatic dissociative symptoms, and 41% reported post traumatic dissociative symptoms.

Our sample of young terror victims reported mild to moderate peritraumatic dissociation. The most common experiences were feeling that during the event time passed very slowly or extremely fast, and as if it were not real, as if they were in a movie. By the time they were evaluated in the ER, only 10% of the minors observed by us presented with acute dissociative reaction.

Since there is no clear-cut demarcation for what defines the clinical term of dissociative reaction in each of the studies, the understanding of the difference in these observations (Terr's, Fein's and ours) remains a challenge. The following illustrates what we defined as an acute dissociative reaction:

> G, a 16-year-old boy, took a bus in the afternoon with his older brother. It was full and they were separated. G went in and his brother stayed close to the entrance. The explosion was horrifying; an extremely loud blast, and the whole bus seemed to go up in the air. There were corpses, blood, body parts all over, and tremendous confusion and fear. The ambulances arrived almost instantaneously and G was rushed into the hospital within ten-fifteen minutes after the explosion. He was covered with blood and the nurses asked him to take off his clothes and change into a hospital gown. He cooperated without hesitation and was walking around the ER, wearing dark tight underwear, his back exposed, talking cheerfully and intensely (like one would after a rollercoaster ride). When questioned about the event, he gave a very clear and coherent description. He did not complain about pain (his arm was significantly wounded and required several stitches). He did not express any concern about his brother and, when family members asked about his brother, he answered that he is not worried because as he escaped the burning bus he saw his

brother and he was fine (which contradicted independent reports that he saw his brother's corpse, and was thus a partial dissociative amnesia with secondary compensatory confabulation). During the four hours G was in the ER, his mood remained elated and his conduct was clearly inappropriate for the situation. His brother was killed in the explosion. G himself needed to be hospitalized for several days for treatment of the injury in his arm.

Conversion Reaction. Conversion reaction has been observed among a small number of children and adolescents, the most common symptom in this category being aphonia.

T skipped school that day. It was her 14th birthday, and she went downtown on her own. T had significant learning difficulties. Socially, she did not feel accepted by her peers in the religious school she attended. The explosion, a suicide bomber, caught her on the way to a friend's house. In the ER, T looked very frightened. There was no apparent physical injury. She gestured that she was unable to speak. With patient and empathic contact, she managed to whisper a word or two at a time. The older of two, she had not met her father until she was 12. Her parents never married. Her father was an Arab, her mother Jewish, and that became a clear emotional struggle under the present circumstances. The terror attack caught T in the midst of a deep identity conflict complicated by academic and social difficulties.

Acute Psychotic Reactions. Only one of all the victims we have seen presented with an acute psychotic reaction. She was almost 18, a school dropout, who left home and abused drugs. L was extremely restless, crying and shouting. She described different events in detail, and it took a while for the treating team to realize that those events did not actually take place. There were rapid mood swings mostly between anger and sadness, and a clear lack of awareness and appropriate judgment.

THE INTRAPSYCHIC DESCRIPTIVE PERSPECTIVE

It is important to pay attention to fantasies and concepts born in the immediate emotional reaction to the trauma since they may become the basis for intrusive post-traumatic thoughts, repetitive dreams, or play reenactments (Terr, 1979). Feelings expressed in the immediate reaction are also important since they may serve as a clue for understanding main themes that arise in cases of unresolved trauma (Pynoos et al., 1987; Pynoos & Nader, 1989; Terr, 1979). Some will be reality-based, such as anger, loss, and helplessness; others will be misconceptions (distortions or misattributions) such as guilt, time distortion, or changes in self-image. The following examples illustrate some of these themes.

Magical Thinking or Omens. Magical thinking or omens refer to psychic efforts to make sense of the trauma. One of the psychological phenomena Terr (1979) related to in her pioneering contribution to understanding the emotional reaction to acute trauma in young children is "the ego's repeated attempt to gain retrospective mastery or control through the discovery of 'omens'" (p. 563). In the group that she described, the trauma went on for a long time (days) and this 'omen' phenomenon took place at the event itself. The trauma that the children and adolescents we observed were exposed to was mostly of short duration (seconds-minutes), and the 'omen' phenomenon, both positive and negative, was observed in the ER.

> D and her sister S attend the same high school. D, the older, is disorganized and tends to be late. S is ambitious and responsible. In the mornings, they would often get into arguments while preparing to leave the house and go to school. More than once, S went ahead and took a bus to school, leaving D behind to miss the first class. Thursday morning, as usual, D wasn't getting out of the house. S kept urging her sister to move, but for some unclear reason did not go ahead that morning. As they finally ran and arrived at the bus stop, they saw number 7 leave. Seconds later the bus exploded. S felt strongly that her sister had saved her life and that some unknown guiding force prevented her from going on her own and getting on that bus that morning.

> E was with his mother and siblings on a bus that exploded on the way back from the Wailing Wall. His retrospective narrative of the events was filled with negative omens: When he and his family were waiting for the bus, his mother remembered that she needed something from the house and they let the first bus pass. When they finally got on the next bus, they met on the way passengers of the first bus who had to get off it due to some mechanical problem. E was thinking to himself "this is not a good day, too many problems." As they continued to the Wailing Wall in the crowded bus, he couldn't help thinking: "this is a perfect opportunity for a suicide bomber."

> S did not describe any pre-event thoughts. She just noted that her out-of-routine behavior that morning saved her life. E, on the other hand, did experience pre-event, semi-prophetic thoughts but did not act upon them. Both S, a secular 17-year-old girl, and E, a 12-year-old religious boy, experienced what could be described as magical thinking. In both cases, it seems clear that there was a psychological effort to process the

experience in a manner that would offer some defense against a severe feeling of helplessness.

In some instances, magical thoughts can be haunting, especially if they are connected to significant and not easily resolved guilt.

> B was 13. The school year had begun and his parents decided that in order to overcome his separation anxiety symptoms, he had to be encouraged to take a bus home from school on his own. B accomplished that once, but on the second day of school he felt extremely anxious and wanted his parents to come and pick him up. His mother refused. B begged his father, who came reluctantly to drive him home. On the way home, they stopped for a falafel and a suicide bomber exploded at the food stand. The boy was injured and his father died at the site. B's guilt was overwhelming. There was nothing abnormal in his mental status, only extreme sadness and a feeling of total responsibility for his father's death.

The same guilt reaction can occur in situations that are less clear than the above. We recommend asking questions about the circumstances prior to the traumatic event, aiming to learn about the subjective experience of the child and the amount of responsibility s/he might feel.

THE ROLE OF THE PARENTS

The connection between the parents' emotional status, their reaction to the trauma, and the child's perception of the event and later development of PTSD is well established (Cohen, 2003; March, 2003; Pfefferbaum, 1997; Scheeringa & Zeanah, 2001). It has been observed in different types of trauma, and in events where only the children were involved and the parent was not even present.

> Fourteen-year-old V ran from the exploding bus so fast that she hardly saw a thing. She was taken immediately to the ER and, lying on a bed waiting for a physical evaluation, was relatively calm. As part of his job, her father, a policeman, arrived at the terror scene. Knowing his daughter was on that bus, unable to reach her on her mobile phone, he was horrified to see a covered body wearing his daughter's shoes. Even though he was notified within minutes that she was safe and uninjured, he could not overcome his emotional shock. He hurried to the hospital, rushed to her bed, and there and then the event took on different meaning and power for V herself. Her father was shaken and broken. It was only

through his subjective perception of the event that the life-threatening element of the daughter's subjective experience became significant.

A and D, two adolescent girls, were sitting on the hospital bed waiting for their mother. They were taken to the ER from the explosion site. They were emotionally shaken but had no physical injury. Their mental status was intact. Mrs. C's arrival was heard in the whole ER area. She was shouting, pulling her hair, and scratching her face. As she approached, both started crying loudly, and the older started shaking all over. They became uncommunicative. Only physical separation between the girls and the mother allowed a gradual calming down.

A was driving his 5-year-old son and his 10-year-old daughter to school. The explosion happened a few cars ahead of them, and the front glass of the car shattered. At first, A thought they were being shot at. He shoved the children under the car seat, went out carefully, and evaluated the scene. When he realized that they were in no immediate danger, he instructed them to stay in the car, protecting them from seeing the many casualties. Only upon arriving at the ER did he let down his control. He was flooded by feelings of fear and helplessness and could not stay in the same room with his children. The young boy remained quiet, mainly concerned about the blood on his sister's face. The girl was terrified by the need to clean her forehead from broken glass, but readily connected and was calmed by the psychiatrist. Their traumatic exposure was "censored" by their father, thus preventing a much worse experience.

It is interesting to note that all but two of the minors cooperated with our intervention. One was a sixteen-year-old runaway who was terrified that social services would place her in a foster family. The other was a fourteen-year-old Palestinian who was injured when a bomb exploded in a cafeteria where he worked. He was worried about being accused of involvement with the placing of the bomb and of being interrogated.

CONCLUSIONS AND DIRECTIONS FOR FUTURE RESEARCH

Space limitations do not permit the description of the therapeutic intervention in the ER, nor the follow-up data of this group months and years after the terrorist trauma. We consider it important to stress that while the issue of group debriefing is still very controversial in the literature on adult victims of trauma, there are almost no empirical data on children (Cohen, 2003; Vila et al., 1999). A very careful approach is therefore mandatory. We also believe that it is potentially harmful to intervene in the immediate circumstance in a group setting. It might aggravate the exposure at a very critical point in the encoding and processing of the experience (Cohen, 2003; March, 2003). The exception to this is a natural group, such as family members or peers.

Although we do not rule it out completely, in our sample we did not need to use pharmacological means to overcome psychiatric symptomatology in the ER. A direct, supportive intervention allowed for significant clinical improvement in all cases. The duration of the interventions varied from 15 minutes to two hours.

In order to evaluate the objectivity of our clinical observations, and broaden the understanding of the significance of immediate psychological reaction to trauma, we are conducting a multi-center clinical study, which includes a standard evaluation, therapeutic intervention, and short questionnaires to be completed in the ER.

REFERENCES

Cohen, J. A. (2003). Treating acute post traumatic reactions in children and adolescents. *Biological Psychiatry, 53*, 827-833.

Daviss, W. B., Racusin, R., Fleischer, A., Mooney, D., Ford, J. D., & McHugo, J. D. (2000). Acute stress disorder symptomatology during hospitalization for pediatric injury. *Journal of the American Academy of Child and Adolescent Psychiatry, 39*, 569-575.

Fein, J. A., Kassam-Adams, N., Vu, T., & Datner, E. M. (2001). Emergency department evaluation of acute stress disorder symptoms in violently injured youths. *Annals of Emergency Medicine, 38*(4), 391-396.

March, J. S. (2003). Acute stress disorder in youth: A multivariate prediction model. *Biological Psychiatry, 53*, 809-816.

Milgram, N. A., Toubiana, Y. H., Klingman, A., Raviv, A., & Godstein, I. (1998). Situational exposure and personal loss in children's acute and chronic stress reactions to a school bus disaster. *Journal of Traumatic Stress, 1*, 339-352.

Pfefferbaum, B. (1997). Posttraumatic stress disorder in children: A review of the last ten years. *Journal of the American Academy of Child and Adolescent Psychiatry, 36*, 1503-1511.

Pynoos, R. S., Frederick, C. J., Nader, K., Arroyo, W., Steinberg, A., & Eth, S. et al. (1987). Life threat and posttraumatic stress in school-age children. *Archives of General Psychiatry, 44*, 1057-1063.

Pynoos, R. S., & Nader, K. (1989). Children's memory and proximity to violence. *Journal of the American Academy of Child and Adolescent Psychiatry, 28*, 236-241.

Scheeringa, M. S., & Zeanah, C. H. (2001). A relational perspective on PTSD in early childhood. *Journal of Traumatic Stress, 14*(4), 799-815.

Shalev, A., Adessky, R., Boker, R., Benhat, Y., Bar-Gay, N., & Hadar, H. et al. (2002). Clinical interventions during repeated stressful events. *Sihot-Dialogue, Israel Journal of Psychotherapy, 17*(1), 8-19.

Shalev, A. Y. (2000). *Psycho-biological perspectives on early reactions to traumatic events.* Unpublished manuscript, Hebrew University at Jerusalem, Israel.

Terr, L. C. (1979). Children of Chowchilla: A study of psychic trauma. *Psychoanalytic Study of the Child, 34,* 547-623.

Vila, G., Porche, L. M., & Mouren-Simeoni, M. C. (1999). An 18-month longitudinal study of posttraumatic disorders in children who were taken hostage in their school. *Psychosomatic Medicine, 61,* 746-754.

Winston, F. K., Kassam-Adams, N., Vivarelli-O'Neil, C., Ford, J., Newman, E., & Baxt, C. et al. (2002). Acute stress disorder symptoms in children and their parents after pediatric traffic injury. *Pediatrics, 109*(6), e90.

Post-Traumatic Distress in Israeli Adolescents Exposed to Ongoing Terrorism: Selected Findings from School-Based Screenings in Jerusalem and Nearby Settlements

Ruth Pat-Horenczyk

SUMMARY. This article examines the impact of exposure of ongoing terrorism on post-traumatic stress disorder (PTSD) symptoms, functional impairment, somatization, and depression among Israeli adolescents in the context of the Al Aqsa Intifada. An in-school screening of 1,010 adolescents was conducted in Jerusalem and nearby settlements

Address correspondence to: Ruth Pat-Horenczyk, PhD, Israel Center for the Treatment of Psychotrauma, Herzog Hospital, P.O. Box 3900, Jerusalem 91035, Israel (E-mail: rpat@herzoghospital.org).

This project was funded by UJA Federation of New York. Special appreciation to colleagues Claude Chemtob, PhD, Robert Abramovitz, MD, and Shelley Horwitz from the UJA Federation of New York, who assisted in the development of the study instruments; to Naomi Baum, PhD, Osnat Doppelt, MA, and Ayala Daie, MA, of the Israel Center for the Treatment of Psychotrauma, who took part in data collection and analysis; and to the school staff and students who participated in the project. The author would like to thank Prof. Arlene F. Tucker-Levin for the encouragement and her illuminating comments.

[Haworth co-indexing entry note]: "Post-Traumatic Distress in Israeli Adolescents Exposed to Ongoing Terrorism: Selected Findings from School-Based Screenings in Jerusalem and Nearby Settlements." Pat-Horenczyk, Ruth. Co-published simultaneously in *Journal of Aggression, Maltreatment & Trauma* (The Haworth Maltreatment & Trauma Press, an imprint of The Haworth Press, Inc.) Vol. 9, No. 3/4, 2004; and: *The Trauma of Terrorism: Sharing Knowledge and Shared Care, An International Handbook* (ed: Yael Danieli, Danny Brom, and Joe Sills) The Haworth Maltreatment & Trauma Press, an imprint of The Haworth Press, Inc., 2005.

that were subjected to intensive terrorist attacks. The screening procedure proved effective in identifying posttraumatic distress and triaging
students for school-based treatments. The relationship between level of
exposure and gender and the psychological sequelae, the differences between adolescents in Jerusalem and the settlements, and the role of spirituality and community are discussed.

KEYWORDS. Screening, PTSD, trauma, terrorism, adolescents, post-traumatic stress disorder

*T., a 14-year-old boy, lives in a Jerusalem neighborhood. Asked about
his personal experiences during the Al Aqsa Intifada, he replied that
nothing happened to him. Later, it emerged that his mother was driving
her car when the bus next to her exploded; his father was on his way to
lunch at a pizzeria that was bombed just a few minutes before he arrived;
his cousin's boyfriend was killed in a suicide bombing in the city center;
and a rocket fell in the courtyard of his junior high school. For months,
T.'s neighborhood was repeatedly targeted by sharpshooters and rocket
launchers. Living near a main road that leads to a major hospital, he
constantly hears the sirens of the ambulances rushing past. T. "knows"
that he is next.* (T. was a participant in a school-based treatment group
for adolescents screened for PTSD.)

Ongoing terrorism poses complex questions about normal and pathological
development in children and adolescents. What does it mean to grow up and mature in the shadow of ongoing terrorism? How does terrorism affect developmental stages, coping mechanisms, and resilience? How does it affect childrens'
and adolescents' *Weltanschauung*, perception of the future, and perception of
themselves? What are the risk factors and, most importantly, what can be done
to prevent, identify, and treat post-traumatic distress in youngsters exposed to
ongoing terrorism?

Israel provides an *in vivo* empirical laboratory for exploring these questions.
For more than three years, since the outbreak of the current wave of violence,
known as the Al Aqsa Intifada, in September 2000, Israelis have been living in a
state of "routine emergency," constantly aware that suicide bombers can ex-

plode at any time and that knife and gun attacks can occur anywhere. The basic beliefs in the existence of "a safe place" and "safety rules" have been shaken.

There is growing interest in exploring the long-term impact of war and terrorism on children (Joshi & O'Donnell, 2003; Shaw, 2003). Literature on the effects of terrorist attacks, mostly from the United States, has focused almost exclusively on single events, such as the 1993 World Trade Center attack (Koplewicz et al., 2002); the Oklahoma city bombing (Pfefferbaum et al., 2003); and September 11 (Hoven, Duarte, Lucas, Mandell, Wu, & Rosen, 2002). Several Israeli studies focus on the effect of the war (Klingman, Sagi, & Raviv, 1993). However, only a handful of studies have focused recently on the psychological effects of ongoing terrorism on Israeli children and adolescents (Gurvitch, Sitterle, Young, & Pfefferbaum, 2002), and on the emotional effect of the Al Aqsa Intifada on Palestinian children (Thabet, Abed, & Vostanis, 2003). The reality of ongoing terrorism calls for more investigation to clarify the unique effects of multiple exposures to unpredictable threats to life.

The recently redefined diagnosis of post-traumatic stress disorder in children and adolescents in the DSM IV-TR (American Psychiatric Association, 2000) includes: exposure to a traumatic event; subjective experience of fear, helplessness, and horror; and symptoms in each of three clusters (re-experiencing, avoidance, and hyper-arousal). Each of these must be present for at least one month and severe enough to cause functional impairment in school performance or interpersonal domains. It is unclear how the new requirements affect the incidence of PTSD diagnoses in youths and adolescents. Furthermore, Perry and Azad (1999) have shown that in most prevalence studies the number of children who do not meet the criteria for a full diagnosis yet suffer from significant symptoms is twice the number of children who are given the full diagnosis.

Studies of PTSD among youth are characterized by striking variability in the estimates of its prevalence, ranging from 0% to 100% (Saigh, Yasik, Sack, & Koplewicz, 1999). This amazing variability in the literature may be explained, at least in part, by differences in the type and intensity of the precipitating stressors, substantial differences in the duration between stress exposure and assessment of PTSD distress, sampling techniques, variability in the methods of the assessment of PTSD, and the contrasting sets of diagnostic developed since 1980. In contrast to adults, diagnosis of children and adolescents is complicated by developmentally specific and age-related behaviors and divergent clinical presentations (Lonigan, Phillips, & Richey, 2003).

RISK FACTORS

Age. Due to their dependence on caregivers, fluid developmental schemata, incomplete biological development, and immature concepts of themselves and their surroundings, children may be particularly vulnerable to trauma and suffer higher rates of PTSD symptoms than adults (Perrin, Smith, & Yule, 2000). Children may be particularly vulnerable when both they and their parents face ongoing terrorism and its resultant stress, since the parents may then be less available and unable to utilize the parent-child relationship as a buffer against stress reactions. The evidence regarding the vulnerability of younger children is inconclusive. Reviewing data from 177 articles published between 1981 and 2001, Norris, Friedman, Watson, and Byrne (2002) found that school-age children tend to be the most affected. In contrast, there is evidence that older children are more vulnerable to the psychological effect of trauma than younger children (Green et al., 1991).

Gender. In their review, Saigh et al. (1999) found seven studies indicating greater prevalence of PTSD among females, while 13 reported no significant differences. Adolescent girls were found to be two to six times as likely as adolescent boys to develop PTSD (Breslau & Kessler, 2001; Giaconia, Reinherz, Silverman, Pakiz, Frost, & Cohen, 1995). Girls who meet the full PTSD criteria show evidence of other psychopathology as well as poorer school performance (Lipschitz, 2000).

Exposure and Response. Exposure to an extremely distressing event is usually not sufficient to induce PTSD (Saigh et al., 1999), nor is the impact of major national trauma limited to those with direct experience. Thus, simple objective measures of exposure cannot predict degree of response (Cohen-Silver, Holman, McIntosh, Poulin, & Gil-Rivas, 2002). The relationship between exposure and the development of PTSD-related symptoms is mediated by factors such as proximity; extent and severity of exposure including degree of life threat (Anthony, Lonigan, & Heath, 1999); direct and indirect exposure (Pfefferbaum et al., 2003; Schlenger et al., 2002); duration of exposure (Pynoos et al., 1987); and the level of identification with the victims (Raviv, Sadeh, Raviv, Silberstein, & Diver, 2000).

SCREENING AND TREATMENT

Most of the studies reviewed by Chemtob, Nakashima, and Hamada (2002) conclude that psychological treatment, both group and individual, is helpful in the reduction of posttraumatic symptoms in children. Assessing the effectiveness of a school-based, trauma- and grief-focused group psychotherapy protocol, Saltzman, Pynoos, Layne, Steinberg, and Aisenberg (2001) found that group participation was associated with improvement in post-traumatic stress, grief symptoms, and academic performance.

However, the avoidance and numbing symptoms, combined with the natural tendency of adolescents to strive for independence and deny or minimize problems in all areas of their lives, may negatively affect treatment-seeking (Pfefferbaum et al., 2003). Teachers and parents are often unable to identify posttraumatic stress symptoms in adolescents and rarely refer them to treatment services, and children may minimize or deny symptoms for fear of overtaxing their already over-burdened parents (Chemtob et al., 2002). Hoven et al. (2002) found that 2/3 of children with PTSD and impaired functioning in New York City following September 11th have not sought any form of treatment. Similarly, Pfefferbaum et al. (2003) found that only 5% of those diagnosed with PTSD after the Oklahoma bombing sought counseling. There is thus a need for universal screening of at-risk groups after major traumatic incidents and for more attention to those who may be suffering silently.

School-Based Interventions

School settings encourage normalcy and minimize stigma (Pfefferbaum et al., 2003), and therefore provide natural, accessible sites for universal screening, identification of children in need of post-traumatic intervention, and service delivery. Furthermore, many stress symptoms are likely to emerge in classroom settings. Finally, some believe (Chemtob et al., 2002) that schools have an obligation to establish mechanisms to identify and counsel children with disaster-related symptoms. School-based screening is thus the best method for effective identification of symptomatic children and youth.

SCHOOL-BASED INTERVENTION IN THE JERUSALEM AREA

Context

The Jerusalem Screening Project was developed to examine the effects of direct and indirect exposure to terrorism on PTSD and functional impairment among adolescents living in highly exposed areas and to provide school-based intervention for affected students. The integrative school-based program is aimed at addressing the needs of the entire school population and tailoring the comprehensive and modular program according to the unique needs of each school. This program included building resilience among school staff and students, empowering parents, direct screening of posttraumatic symptoms and functional impairment in students, and providing school-based group interventions for students identified with posttraumatic related distress (for a detailed description of the project of building resilience in schools, see Baum, this volume).

Project Description

Three junior and senior high schools in a Jerusalem neighborhood and nearby settlements in the Etzion Bloc participated in the project during June 2002 (for an in-depth description of the Jerusalem area screening project, see Pat-Horenczyk et al., 2003). These schools were selected because Jerusalem has suffered from more terrorist attacks than any other city in Israel, and the children in the Etzion Bloc settlements were also exposed to high levels of security stress and threats of terrorism. There were 695 students from Jerusalem and 315 students from the Etzion Bloc in grades 7-12, ranging in age from 12 to 18 years old ($M = 15.1$, $SD = 1.77$). No differences were found in age and gender between Jerusalem and Etzion Bloc students. The participants completed a battery of self-report questionnaires: (a) demographic data; (b) The Israeli Trauma Exposure Questionnaire (Pat-Horenczyk, Chemtob, Abramovitz, Baum, Daie, & Brom, 2002), developed specifically for the Israeli setting, which assesses exposure to terrorism. The exposure items were then collapsed into three aggregate levels of exposure: Personal exposure (someone close who was injured or killed in such an attack),[1] Indirect exposure (having been near the site of a terrorist attack, having been there before/after an attack, or having planned to be at the site of an attack), or No exposure (no exposure to a terrorist attack, either directly or indirectly, except for media coverage). (c) The UCLA PTSD Reaction Index-Adolescent Version (Rodriguez, Steinberg, & Pynoos, 1999), which assesses the frequency of posttraumatic stress symptoms. The questionnaire was translated, adapted to the Israeli context, and used previously by Lavi (2002). (d) The Brief BDI is an abbreviated self-report measure of depressive symptoms (Beck, Rial, & Rickles, 1974). (e) A self-report somatization scale for somatic complaints, and (f) the Functional Impairment Questionnaire (Lucas et al., 2001), which assesses reported changes in functioning in four domains (e.g., academic functioning, social and family relationships, and after school activities). Upon receiving permission from the Ministry of Education and informed consent from the parents, the teachers provided the students with a brief explanation of the purpose of the screening and administered the questionnaires in the classes, a procedure that took up to 30 minutes. Each questionnaire received a code number, according to which the data were analyzed. The list of names and codes remained in the school. The school counselors met with the students who were identified with PTSD-related distress and used a semi-structured interview to confirm the current status of posttraumatic distress and functional impairment. In appropriate cases, the parents were then consulted regarding possible referral to school-based interventions.

SELECTED RESULTS FROM THE SCREENING
FOR POSTTRAUMATIC DISTRESS IN JERUSALEM
AND THE ETZION BLOC SETTLEMENTS

Exposure to Ongoing Terrorism

The results of the screening of the 1,010 students who participated in the project, in both Jerusalem and the Etzion Bloc settlements, showed that 41.7% of the adolescents ($n = 421$) reported "Personal Exposure" (i.e., were actually present at a terrorist attack, whether injured or not, or know someone who was injured or killed at such an event). An additional 20.5% ($n = 207$) reported "Indirect Exposure" (being or having intended to be near the site of the terrorist attack, or being at the site before or after the attack); and only 37.8% ($n = 382$) reported "No Exposure" (i.e., they knew of the attacks only through media coverage).

Boys and girls did not differ in their level of exposure to terrorism. However, a significant difference was found between adolescents living in Jerusalem and in the West Bank settlements. The latter were more "personally exposed" to terrorist attacks (61.3% in the settlements vs. 32.8% in Jerusalem) whereas "indirect exposure" to terrorism was higher in Jerusalem (22.3% in Jerusalem vs. 16.5% in settlements).

PTSD Diagnosis and Symptoms

Although two-thirds of the students who took part in the screening project (67%) reported high levels of fear, helplessness, and horror, the full diagnosis of Posttraumatic Stress Disorder according to DSMIV-TR[2] was found in only 5.1% ($n = 52$) of them. Higher rates of full PTSD diagnosis, as well as posttraumatic-related symptoms, were found among those adolescents who were "personally" or "indirectly" exposed to terrorism as compared to those who reported "no exposure." These findings suggest that exposure is indeed a risk factor for developing Posttraumatic Stress Disorder and are consistent with previous findings reported by Pynoos et al. (1987).

It is noteworthy that six students, comprising 2.1% of those students reporting "no exposure," had developed symptoms that meet the PTSD diagnosis. This subgroup, although subjectively defined as "not exposed" to terrorism, comprises 11.5% of those adolescents who meet all the criteria for PTSD diagnosis. We thus suggest that the PTSD of those adolescents reporting "no exposure" to terrorist attacks may be attributed, at least in part, to the intense exposure to media coverage of the ongoing terrorist attacks in Israel (see Ahern, Galea, Resnick, & Vlahov, this volume). Another etiological explanation that cannot be ruled out is non-terror-related prior trauma, which underscores the need to assess prior exposure to trauma as a component of a comprehensive PTSD screening.

More girls than boys report high levels of subjective fear, helplessness, and horror as responses to terrorism (71.1% vs. 57.7%). Gender differences were also found in the rate of PTSD diagnosis in the different levels of exposure to terrorism, suggesting a differential impact of exposure on the rate of post-traumatic stress in boys and girls. Among those students who reported exposure to terrorism (whether personally or indirectly), more girls than boys fulfilled all criteria for PTSD, whereas no such gender differences were found among those adolescents who indicated "no exposure." This differential sensitivity to exposure raises important questions regarding the vulnerability of the genders to terrorism-related trauma, loss, and bereavement.

In spite of greater exposure to terrorism among adolescents living in the settlements, lower rates of full PTSD were found than in the adolescents living in Jerusalem (6.3% vs. 2.5%, respectively). The same pattern was found for the intensity of posttraumatic symptoms; in other words, all clusters of posttraumatic symptoms reported by adolescents in Jerusalem were more severe than those of their counterparts in the settlements.

Depression, Somatic Symptoms, and Functional Impairment

Examining the impact of exposure level on functional impairment, somatic complaints, and depression showed a greater prevalence of reported distress among youngsters with higher degree of exposure to terrorism. More adolescents exposed to terrorism, whether "personally" or "indirectly," than "non-exposed" youth reported functional impairment (23.3% and 25.1% vs. 11.8%, respectively), somatic complaints (33.5% and 26.6% vs. 21.5%, respectively) and severe or very severe depression (16.6% and 15.0% vs. 10.2%, respectively). Furthermore, the intensity of functional impairment and somatic complaints were more pervasive among those students who were exposed to terrorism.

Girls tended to report more somatic complaints and to rate them as more severe than boys, whereas boys reported more functional impairment than girls. Adolescents in Jerusalem complained more of somatic symptoms than adolescents in the settlements, but did not differ in the level of functional impairment or depression.

Co-Morbidity of PTSD. As previously indicated, adolescents suffering from PTSD are more at risk for co-morbidity with other distress symptoms and functional difficulties than those who do not qualify for this diagnosis. Our findings showed consistently that the adolescents diagnosed with PTSD reported *greater* severity of posttraumatic related symptoms, *higher* levels of depression, *more* functional impairment, and *more* somatization symptoms than the general student population. Co-morbidity of emotional distress with PTSD was found in both genders and occurred in Jerusalem and the settlements at a similar rate.

CONCLUSIONS AND IMPLICATIONS

The findings of the Jerusalem Screening Project reveal that DSMIV-TR's stringent criteria yielded 5.1% full PTSD diagnosis among adolescents exposed to ongoing terrorism. As predicted by Breslau and Kessler (2001), and in contrast to literature surveys of subjective stress, the inclusion of functional impairment as a necessary criterion for the diagnosis of PTSD resulted in a relatively low rate of clinical diagnosis. Consistent with prior reports, students with full PTSD exhibited higher co-morbidity.

Intensity of exposure proved to be a significant factor for posttraumatic symptoms. It is noteworthy, however, that within the group of students identified with full PTSD, more than 11% indicated neither personal nor indirect exposure. As Pfefferbaum et al. (2003) suggest, indirect exposure can hinder the identification of problems in children and adolescents and thus limit their referral to treatment services. School-based screening is therefore the method of choice for early detection of PTSD in youngsters, whether they have been directly or indirectly exposed to traumatic events.

Diagnosis on the basis of self-report scales, rather than on the basis of a clinical interview such as CAPS-C (Nader et al., 1996), necessarily raises questions concerning clinical validity. However, self-report instruments about thoughts and feelings have been shown to be very effective and are the consensus method for screening adolescents (Chemtob et al., 2002). It has also been shown that questionnaire information about mental health has good validity compared with structured clinical interviews for children and adolescents, such as the diagnostic schedule for children or the National Institute of Mental Health's diagnostic interview for children (Reijneveld, Crone, Verhulst, & Verloove-Vanhorick, 2003).

Several findings require further investigation. The relatively low prevalence of PTSD, despite the unremitting exposure to ongoing and unpredictable terrorist attacks, reflects the resilience of Israeli youth. The even lower subjective distress among youth living in the settlements, despite their higher exposure, suggests a possible relationship between exposure level and mediating factors, such as community cohesiveness and support, faith, religion, and ideology. The presence of a differential "dose effect" of exposure for girls and boys (that is, the fact that a higher level of exposure resulted in increased PTSD in girls but not in boys) is also intriguing.

Comprehensive school-based programs, which integrate screening, secondary prevention, and school-based treatments, have the potential to directly and effectively reach a large community at risk for PTSD-related distress. The screening for PTSD-related distress has led us to the development of clinical solutions for implementation within the school system, based on the premise that programs for adolescents must be provided in a non-stigmatizing and non-clinical manner by school staff within the school setting. Two treatment modules were developed to address the needs of students identified by the screening battery. The first treatment protocol (Pat-Horenczyk & Kaplansky, 2003a), which consists of six sessions, is geared to students with moderate amounts of distress. The second treatment module (Pat-Horenczyk & Kaplansky, 2003b), which consists of 12 sessions, is suitable for students suffering from full PTSD symptoms. School-based mental health professionals are currently being trained to run this intervention program in schools. This training will empower the school staff to deal with the ongoing stressful situation and prepare the school system for developing long-term resources using internal personnel. By working with in-place educational staff, we are laying the foundations for creating and maintaining resilience in the entire educational system.

NOTES

1. Loss or injury of significant others for adolescents may carry major adverse consequences, sometimes no less than, or even worse than direct exposure to traumatic events or being injured themselves.
2. DSM diagnosis of PTSD was determined based on: exposure questionnaire–for criteria A1, A2; Reaction Index–for criteria B, C and D; Functional impairment questionnaire–for criteria F and duration.

REFERENCES

Ahern, J., Galea, S., Resnick, H., & Vlahov, D. (2004). Television watching and mental health in the general population of New York City after September 11. *Journal of Aggression, Maltreatment, & Trauma, 9*(1/2/3/4), 109-124.

American Psychiatric Association. (2000). *Diagnostic and statistical manual of mental disorders* (4th ed., text rev.). Washington, DC: Author.

Anthony, J. L., Lonigan, C. J., & Heath, S. (1999). Construct validity of posttraumatic stress disorder in children exposed to disaster: A confirmatory analysis of alternative models. *Journal of Abnormal Psychology, 108*, 326-336.

Baum, N. L. (2004). Building resilience: A school-based intervention for children exposed to ongoing trauma and stress. *Journal of Aggression, Maltreatment, & Trauma, 10*(1/2/3/4), 487-498.

Beck A. T., Rial W. Y., & Rickles, K. (1974). Short form of depression inventory: Cross validation. *Psychological Reports, 34*, 1184-1186.

Breslau, N., & Kessler, R. C. (2001). The stressors criterion in DSM-IV posttraumatic stress disorder: An empirical investigation, *Biological Psychiatry, 50*, 699-704.

Chemtob, C. M., Nakashima, J. P., & Hamada, R. S. (2002). Psychosocial intervention for post disaster trauma symptoms in elementary school children. *Archives of Pediatric and Adolescent Medicine, 156*, 211-216.

Cohen-Silver, R., Holman, A., McIntosh, D. N., Poulin, M., & Gil-Rivas, V. (2002). National longitudinal study of psychological responses to September 11. *Journal of the American Medical Association, 288*(10), 1235-1244.

Giaconia, R. M., Reinherz, H. Z., Silverman, A. B., Pakiz, B., Frost, A. K., & Cohen, E. (1995). Traumas and posttraumatic stress disorder in a community population of older adolescents. *Journal of the American Academy of Child and Adolescent Psychiatry, 34*, 275-280.

Green, B. L. Korol, M., Grace, M. C., Vary, M. G., Leonard A. C., Gleaser, G. C. et al. (1991). Children and disaster: Age, gender and parental effects on PTSD symptoms. *Journal of the American Academy of Child and Adolescents Psychiatry, 30*, 945-951.

Gurvitch, R. H., Sitterle, K. A., Young, B. H., & Pfefferbaum, B. (2002). The aftermath of terrorism. In A. M. Le Greca, W. K.Silverman, E. M. Verenberg, & M. Roberts (Eds.), *Helping children cope with disasters and terrorism* (pp. 327-358). Washington DC: American Psychological Association.

Hoven, C. W., Duarte, C. S. Lucas, C. P., Mandell, D. J., Wu, P., & Rosen, C. (2002). *Effects of the World Trade Center attack on NYC public school students: Initial report of the New York Board of Education.* New York: Applied Research and Consulting, LLC & Columbia University Mailman School of Public Health & New York State Psychiatric Institute.

Joshi, P. T., & O'Donnell, D. A. (2003). Consequences of child exposure to war and terrorism. *Clinical Child and Family Psychology Review, 6*(4), 275-292.

Klingman, A., Sagi, A., & Raviv, A. (1993). The effect of war on Israeli children. In L. A. Leavitt & N. A. Fox (Eds.), *The psychological effects on war and violence on children* (pp. 75-92) Hillsdale, NJ: Lawrence Erlbaum.

Koplewicz, H. S., Vogel, J. M., Solanto, M. V., Morrissey, R. G., Alonso, C. M., & Gallagher, R. et al. (2002). Child and parent response to the 1993 World Trade Center bombing. *Journal of Traumatic Stress, 15*(1), 77-85.

Lavi, T. (2002, June). *Both sides of the fence: Psychological adjustment of Palestinians and Israeli children exposed to the Intifada.* Paper presented at the First Bi-national Conference on Treating Traumatized Children and Adolescents, Schneider Medical Center, Petach Tikva.

Lipschitz, D. S. (2000). Clinical and functional correlates of posttraumatic stress disorder in urban adolescent girls at a primary care clinic. *Journal of the American Academy of Child and Adolescent Psychiatry, 39*(9), 1104-1111.

Lonigan, C. J., Phillips, B. M., & Richey, J. A. (2003). Posttraumatic stress disorder in children: Diagnosis, assessment, and associated features. *Child and Adolescent Psychiatric Clinics of North America, 12*, 171-194.

Lucas, C. P., Zhang, H., Fisher, P. W., Shaffer, D., Regier, D. A., & Narrow, W. E. et al. (2001). The DISC Predictive Scales (DPS): Efficiently screening for diagnoses. *Journal of the American Academy of Child and Adolescent Psychiatry, 40*, 443-449.

Nader, K., Kriegler, J. A., Blake, D. D., Pynoos, R. S., Newman, E., & Weather F. W (1996). *Clinician Administered PTSD Scale, Child and Adolescent Version.* White River Junction, VT: National Center for PTSD.

Norris, F. H., Friedman, M. J., Watson, P. J., & Byrne, C. M. (2002). 60,000 disaster victims speak: Part I. An empirical review of the empirical literature, 1981-2001. *Psychiatry, 65,* 207-239.

Pat-Horenczyk, R., Abramovitz, R., Brom, D., Doppelt O., Daie, A., & Horowitz, S. et al. (2003). *Progress report: Screening for PTSD in adolescents in the Jerusalem area.* Jerusalem: Israel Center for the Treatment of Psychotrauma.

Pat-Horenczyk, R., Chemtob, C. M., Abramovitz, R., Baum, N., Daie A., & Brom, D. (2002). *The Israeli Trauma Exposure and Functional Impairment.* Unpublished instrument.

Pat-Horenczyk, R., & Kaplinsky, N. (2003a). *School-based treatment protocol for coping with persistent stressful situations: A counseling group for adolescents-counselor's guide (adolescent version).* Unpublished manuscript.

Pat-Horenczyk, R., & Kaplinsky, N. (2003b). *School-based treatment protocol for posttraumatic related distress (adolescent version).* Unpublished manuscript.

Perrin, S., Smith, P., & Yule, W. (2000). Practitioner review: The assessment and treatment of post-traumatic stress disorder in children and adolescents. *Journal of Child Psychology and Psychiatry, 41*(3), 277-289.

Perry, B. D., & Azad, I. (1999). Post-traumatic stress disorders in children and adolescents, *Current Opinions in Pediatrics, 11*(4), 121-132.

Pfefferbaum, B., Sconzo, G. M., Flynn, B. W., Kearns, L. J., Doughty, D. E., & Gurwitch, R. H. et al. (2003). Case findings and mental health services for children in the aftermath of the Oklahoma City bombing. *The Journal of Behavioral Health Services & Research, 30*(2), 215-227.

Pynoos, R. S., Frederick, C., Nader, K., Arroyo, W., Steinberg, A., & Eth, S. et al. (1987). Life threat and posttraumatic stress in school-age children. *Archives of General Psychiatry, 44*(12), 1057-1063.

Raviv, A. M., Sadeh, A., Raviv, A., Silberstein, O., & Diver, O. (2000). Young Israelis reactions to national trauma: The Rabin assassination and terror attacks. *Political Psychology, 21,* 299-322.

Reijneveld, S. A., Crone, M. R., Verhulst, F. C., & Verloove-Vanhorick, S. P. (2003). The effect of a severe disaster on the mental health of adolescents: A controlled study. *The Lancet, 362,* 691-694.

Rodriguez, N., Steinberg, A., & Pynoos, R. S. (1999). *UCLA PTSD index for DSM IV.* Unpublished instrument, UCLA Trauma Psychiatry Services.

Saigh, P. A., Yasik, A. E., Sack, W. H., & Koplewicz, H. S. (1999). Child-adolescent posttraumatic stress disorder: Prevalence, risk, factors, and co-morbidity. In P. A. Saigh & J. D. Bremner (Eds.), *Posttraumatic stress disorder: A comprehensive text* (pp. 18-43). New York: Allyn and Bacon.

Saltzman, W. R., Pynoos, R. S., Layne, C. M., Steinberg, A. M., & Aisenberg, E. (2001). Trauma-and grief-focused intervention for adolescents exposed to community violence: Results of a school-based screening and group treatment protocol. *Group Dynamics, 5*(4), 291-303.

Schlenger, W. E., Caddell, J. M., Ebert, L., Jordan, B. K., Rourke, K. M., & Wilson, D. et al. (2002). Psychological reactions to terrorist attacks: Findings from the national study of Americans' reactions to September 11, *Journal of the American Medical Association, 288*(5), 581-588.

Shaw, J. A. (2003). Children exposed to war/terrorism. *Clinical Child and Family Psychology Review, 6*(4), 237-246.

Thabet, A. M., Abed, Y., & Vostanis, P. (2003). Emotional problems in Palestinian children living in a war zone: A cross-sectional study. *The Lancet, 359*, 1801-1804.

Voice:
Koby's Death

Sherri Mandell

Koby's death is a murder that is shocking in its raw pain and its unmediated cruelty. Two Jewish boys, my son, Koby Mandell, and his friend, Yosef Ish-Ran, were attacked in a cave by Arab terrorists, and bludgeoned to death with stones the size of bowling balls. I can't think about a murderer pummeling my thirteen-year-old-boy to death with rocks. I don't know how to cope with the pain and the evil. I imagine my son afraid, crying out, and dying alone, in horror and agony. The boys' blood was wiped all over the cave. The murderers have not been caught.

Since Koby's murder, I am unable to read the paper or listen to the news because what I hear is pain. The television broadcasts, the articles in the press . . . none of them got it right. Each article had a mistake or two. They said nothing about what was important to us, the way that you had left the house that morning, laughing and happy. The fear when we waited for your return and the way my friend Shira told me that you were dead; intercepting the police, she told me later, so that she could tell me with love.

When I watch the attack on the World Trade Center, all I think about are the mothers. I feel like a voyeur and can no longer listen, because I know that behind the news are families that are suffering. I know that suffering is a knife that keeps digging into the most tender areas, and then pierces even deeper.

Address correspondence to: Sherri Mandell, Tekoa, Gush Etzion, Israel.

Excerpted from *The Blessing of a Broken Heart* by Sherri Mandell (The Toby Press, 2003). Printed with permission.

[Haworth co-indexing entry note]: "Voice: Koby's Death." Mandell, Sherri. Co-published simultaneously in *Journal of Aggression, Maltreatment & Trauma* (The Haworth Maltreatment & Trauma Press, an imprint of The Haworth Press, Inc.) Vol. 9, No. 3/4, 2004; and: *The Trauma of Terrorism: Sharing Knowledge and Shared Care, An International Handbook* (ed: Yael Danieli, Danny Brom, and Joe Sills) The Haworth Maltreatment & Trauma Press, an imprint of The Haworth Press, Inc., 2005.

At 7:00 a.m.on May 8, 2001, I listened to the radio as I made Koby two sa-lami sandwiches. I didn't kiss him goodbye because Yosef was there so I just went upstairs to finish getting ready. That was the last time I saw my son.

At 8:00 a.m., I left to go swimming with a friend about twenty minutes away. Then, I got to town and edited a manuscript for my friend, Aryih, a mur-der mystery. As I edited, I thought, "What does Aryih know about murder? What do I know about murder? How can I edit a murder scene?" Later, I had a meeting with the editor of Hadassah magazine, where we discussed article as-signments for the coming year. Mine was to write an article on miracles.

I got home a little before 6:00 p.m. Then, at about 8:30 p.m., my ten-year-old daughter, Eliana, returned from youth group activities. I hoped that she had seen Koby, but she told me that she hadn't seen him. I put the two smaller children to sleep and then I began to really worry.

I call Koby's friends and Yosef's mother, Rena. She says that she thinks they might have gone to the demonstration in Jerusalem calling for more protection for our roads and settlements. Then at ten o'clock at night I begin to dial madly. I call Koby's friends in Efrat and Jerusalem. I call Rena four times, who assures me that they're at the demonstration. Then, suddenly, it's eleven o'clock and Koby isn't home. I call the police. They check the hitchhiking posts.

Then Shlomo, Koby's friend, comes over and tells us that Koby and Yosef had said they were going to the wadi, a dry riverbed that cuts through a magnifi-cent rugged canyon nearby. They must have gotten lost, I think. He's stuck somewhere in there, it's happened to other kids before. He'll come home and I'll yell at him, and we'll go on. I truly think I'll suffer nothing more than lost sleep.

All night there are neighbors in my house. They say, "Welcome to the teen years. He's your oldest. We've all been through this." I believe them. One's fourteen-year-old daughter had been missing until three o'clock one morning. One's eight-year-old son had been lost in the cave. "They don't think like we do," Orly tells me. That is the hope I cling to. I imagine them, stuck on some ledge in the cave, unable to go up or down, to rise or fall. Or they are on a bus to Eilat, on a whim. It's a foolish act, but it makes sense, they are living in a war zone. They've been through eight months of the Intifada, of drive-by shootings every day. People could crack and just run away, do things that weren't like them. They could.

Shoshana sits knitting in my living room and says, "Go see if you can feel him somewhere, feel his being." It's already four o'clock in the morning. Seth and I walk to the entrance of the wadi. I don't feel him. But when the sun rises and they're still not home, it hits me. They need to come home now. I remem-ber something about missing children, if they aren't found the first day, chances are they won't be found alive. I plead with God and with Koby, "Come back now! Come back now!" I remember giving birth and how the midwife, worried after listening to Koby's heartbeat, said, "Push this baby out! Push this baby out!" I say Come home now! Come home now! with the same kind of urgency. I can will him to come home. My friend Shira walks into the house and I see the fire of fear in her eyes. I know that there's pain there, more pain than I am willing to admit, to let enter my heart. Now I know that I am being too optimistic.

I say, "I'm going in the backyard." I think I can protect myself, as if bad news can only come to the front door. Then Shira comes out to me a short while later. She looks at me, takes my hand in hers, and says, "They found them. They're dead."

I say, "No he's not. Koby is not dead. He's not dead. He's not dead." There is one thing I know, I do not want to live in a world where Koby is dead, even worse, where Koby is murdered.

Friends tell me I fainted. I remember lying on the dirt in my backyard. Just lying there. I remember holding my husband, holding him and crying. I remember people talking to us about telling the other kids. Seth went up to tell them.

Now people ask me, "How are you?" The question is one from my former world. Now, it is one that I cannot answer. I have lost the ability to be in a world where I answer okay. There is no okay. Nothing will ever again be okay. I can never again take anything for granted, that the sun will rise, that my husband will return from work. I carry the weight of my son's death everywhere I go, even into my dreams. Jewish tradition says that each person is a world. I have lost a whole world.

In the Shadow of Terror:
Changes in World Assumptions
in Israeli Youth

Zahava Solomon
Avital Laufer

SUMMARY. This study examined the effects of terror on world assumptions in Israeli youth. The sample comprised 2,999 adolescents aged 13-16 who were exposed to different levels of terror. Relations of objective and subjective exposure to terror, life events, ideological, religious commitment, and social support with world assumptions were assessed. Results show that personal and social resources made a more substantial contribution to the explained variance of world assumptions than exposure to terror. Implications of the associations between religious and ideological commitment and social support with world assumptions are discussed.

address:

Address correspondence to: Zahava Solomon, PhD, Adler Research Center, Tel-Aviv University, Tel Aviv 69978, Israel (E-mail: Solomon@post.tau.ac.il).

This study was supported by the Adler Center, Tel Aviv University.

[Haworth co-indexing entry note]: "In the Shadow of Terror: Changes in World Assumptions in Israeli Youth." Solomon, Zahava, and Avital Laufer. Co-published simultaneously in *Journal of Aggression, Maltreatment & Trauma* (The Haworth Maltreatment & Trauma Press, an imprint of The Haworth Press, Inc.) Vol. 9, No. 3/4, 2004; and: *The Trauma of Terrorism: Sharing Knowledge and Shared Care, An International Handbook* (ed: Yael Danieli, Danny Brom, and Joe Sills) The Haworth Maltreatment & Trauma Press, an imprint of The Haworth Press, Inc., 2005.

KEYWORDS. Terror, world assumptions, adolescents, religion

Intifada El Aqsa, the Palestinian uprising that commenced in 2000 with no end in sight, is being fought in densely populated areas. Both Palestinian and Israeli children are thus inevitably exposed to terror. No place in Israel is safe, but some areas are at higher risk than others. The settlements in the disputed territories have often been attacked and settlers, including children, killed or wounded in their homes. Several other areas of Israel within the internationally accepted borders have also been repeatedly hit by terror. Hundreds of Israeli children and adults have been killed and wounded, mostly by suicide bombers in crowded public places.

Prolonged and repeated exposure to political violence has often been implicated in numerous psychological problems and may affect many aspects of the survivor's life, including cognitions (e.g., Ehlers & Clark, 2000). Among the cognitive changes that have been ascribed to exposure to trauma are changes in the individual's world assumptions (WAS). Several theoreticians (e.g., Janoff-Bulman, 1989) argue that some perceptions or world assumptions protect us from fully appreciating our vulnerability and that exposure to catastrophes unsettles or even shatters the illusion of safety, and forces people to examine and revise their assumptions and often replace them with new and less positive ones.

Janoff-Bulman (1989) developed a conceptual model of the relevant world assumptions and an instrument to measure them. This model maintains that there are three primary categories of perception of the world: (a) Benevolence of the World, (b) Meaningfulness of the World, and (c) Worthiness of the Self. Each consists of several assumptions.

Benevolence of the World (BW) concerns the degree to which one views the impersonal world and people positively or negatively. The more positive one's assumptions are in this category, the more one expects good things, rather than bad, to happen and the more one views people as basically good, kind, helpful and caring.

Meaningfulness of the World (MN) concerns the way in which outcomes are distributed. Three dimensions are at issue: justice, controllability, and randomness. The assumption that the world is just entails the belief that people get what they deserve and deserve what they get. The assumptions that outcomes are controllable represents the belief that people can directly control their world through their own behavior and minimize their vulnerability by engaging in the "proper" behaviors (e.g., caution, foresight). The assumption that outcomes are random entails the belief that they occur by chance and that there is little that one can do to sway their course. These three assumptions are not mutually exclusive. People are inclined to hold all three of them to different degrees.

Worthiness of the Self (SW) involves three assumptions about the self and the world. These pertain to one's self-worth, self-controllability, and luck. Self-worth entails the degree to which individuals perceive themselves as good, decent, and moral persons. Self-controllability portrays the degree to which they view themselves as engaging in the "right" behaviors (e.g., precautionary, appropriate) to minimize their vulnerability to negative outcomes. Luck entails the belief that they are somehow protected from ill fortune, though they cannot point to anything in their character or behavior to account for this protection. The more one views oneself as a moral individual, who engages in the right behaviors, and as a lucky person, the greater one's sense of worthiness and, presumably, the less one's vulnerability to negative events.

These compelling theoretical formulations were assessed in several studies in adults (e.g., Magwaza, 1999; Solomon, Iancu, & Tyano, 1997) but, as far as we know, never in children and young adolescents. The present study aims to fill this gap in the literature and assess the relationship between exposure to political and world assumptions in Israeli youth.

The noxious effects of traumatic stress are often modified or attenuated by personal and social attributes. Among the most prominent socio-cultural variables that have been identified as stress buffers are ideology, religion and social support. Several studies have shown that adult and youth with higher religious or ideological commitment may be less vulnerable to the harmful effects of stress (e.g., Kostelny & Garbarino, 1994). Religious or ideological beliefs may give meaning to traumatic experiences and suffering and hence attenuate the noxious effects (Bettelheim, 1961; McIntosh, Silver, & Wortman, 1993). In addition, the protective role of social support derived from family members or belonging to a larger social group has been repeatedly documented. Studies found that social support buffers the detrimental effects of stress and is implicated in enhanced psychological adjustment among children and youth exposed to political violence (Punamaki, Qouta, & El-Saraaj, 2001).

The present study aims to assess (a) the relationship of past life events, recent life events and exposure to terror to world assumptions; and (b) the unique and combined contribution of several recognized stress buffers: ideological commitment, religious commitment and social support to world assumptions of Israeli youth in the aftermath of a wave of terror attacks.

METHOD

Participants and Methodology

The sample is comprised of 2,999 adolescents from grades 7-9 from four zones: (a) Areas within the international border, not exposed to terror incidents; (b) Areas within the green line that were exposed to terror; (c) Areas in the disputed territories which had low levels of terrorist incidents; and (d) Zones in the territories with repeated exposure to terrorist incidents. In each zone, we randomly chose one secular and one religious high school. The questionnaires were filled out in the classes in the presence of a research assistant.

The participants included 42.2% boys and 57.8% girls. 35.5% of the participants were in grade 7, 36.5% in grade 8, 26.9% in grade 9, and 1% in grade 10. Of all the participants, 0.7% were ultra-orthodox, 39.0% were religious, 27.4% were traditional, and 32.9% were secular. When defining their economic situation, 0.6% of the students classified their status as very low, 4.3% as low, 70.4% as similar to their friends, and 20.4% as above that of their friends, and 4.3% as very high.

Measures

Sociodemographic, Life Events, and Social Support. We asked the youth about gender, religious observance, political stance, economic status, and parents' education and occupation. In addition, the questionnaire asked the participants to list any lifetime and recent life events (e.g., death or severe illness).

Exposure to Terror. Exposure to terror was assessed via Lavi's exposure questionnaire (Lavi & Solomon, 2004). In its present form, the questionnaire lists seventeen terror-related traumatic events (e.g., a relative was shot at in a terror attack). Factor analysis has revealed four zones of exposure that matched the four sampled areas. Therefore, for further analysis it was decided to include only the exposure of the child (i.e., the total number of terror incidents which the respondent endorsed).

World Assumptions Scale. The World Assumptions Scale (WAS; Janoff-Bulman, 1989) self-report scale examines subjects' cognitive schemes. Three global indices including benevolence of the world (BW), meaningfulness of the world (MN), and worthiness of the self (SW) are calculated by summing responses across the items with higher scores indicating higher beliefs in this assumption. The questionnaire was translated into Hebrew using back translation. For the Hebrew version, an $\alpha = 0.78$ for BW was achieved and for SW, $\alpha = 0.77$ for MN was achieved.

Ideological Commitment. This questionnaire was devised for this study to assesses ideological commitment regardless of the context of the political view. It is comprised of 3 factors: (a) practical commitment (e.g., I am willing to participate in demonstrations) (α = .87); (b) ideological conviction (α = .68); and (c) intolerance of other political views (α = .72). A global score, which is the average number, was calculated and three levels of ideological commitment were defined as low (between 1-2), medium (2-4), and high (4 and above).

The Revised Religious Orientation Scale. The revised Religious Orientation Scales (Gorsuch & McPherson, 1989) was used to assess intrinsic and extrinsic religious orientations. The questionnaire was translated into Hebrew using back translation. Factor analysis yielded three factors that were different from the original factors obtained for Christian subjects: (a) Religion as a lifestyle, which reflects the extent to which a person runs his life according to religious values (α = .90). (b) Religion as a social aspect (e.g., I attend the synagogue because I enjoy meeting people) (α = .78). (c) Religion as defining identity (α = .69). In addition, an average score was computed and three levels (low, medium and high) of religious commitment were defined.

Social Support. Social support was assessed via the Support Persons Scale (Mailgram & Toubiana, 1996); the original questionnaire was in Hebrew. Factor analysis for this study yielded three groups of supporters: (a) family (α = .75); (b) professional (e.g., teacher, counselor) (α = .78), and (c) friends (only 1 item). Level of support was divided into low (below 2.5) and high (2.5 and above).

Neighborhood Cohesion Instrument. The Neighborhood Cohesion Instrument (NCI; Buckner, 1988 in Seidman et al., 1995) was used to assess cohesion and sense of connectedness to one's community. This scale has reportedly good psychometric properties. The questionnaire was translated from English to Hebrew using back translation. Subjects were divided into 2 groups: those reporting low sense of connectedness (below 2.5) and high level of connectedness (2.5 and above).

RESULTS

The relationships between number of negative life events and the three indices of WAS were examined via a one-way analysis of variance. Results reveal a significant difference among the groups only in BW, $F(2,2029) = 5.87$, $p < 0.01$. Scheffe's test indicated that children who had experienced three or more life events in the course of their life held more negative views of the world than children who experienced two or less negative events. With regard to recent life events, results show that children who had experienced two life events in the last year endorsed more negative BW and SW than children who did not experience stressful life events in the previous year, $F(3,2029) = 6.81$, $p < 0.001$ for BW; $F(3,2002) = 3.80$, $p < 0.05$ for SW.

In terms of exposure to terror incidents, a one-way analysis of variance was performed. Exposure was divided into 5 levels ranging from 0 (no exposure) to 4 (6 or more terror events). Contrary to expectation, results indicate that children who were exposed to 6 or more terror events perceive the world as more meaningful and benevolent than children who were exposed to 3 or less terror events, $F(4,2026) = 16.66$, $p < 0.001$ for BW; $F(4,1967) = 12.93$, $p < 0.001$ for MN.

We also examined the relationships between WAS and ideological and religious commitment and social support. One-way analysis of variance reveals that there are significant differences in all three indices of WAS according to level of reported ideological commitment, $F(2,2029) = 27.31$, $p < 0.001$ for BW; $F(2,1970) = 27.69$, $p < 0.001$ for MN; $F(2,2002) = 22.64$, $p < 0.001$ for SW. Results of the Scheffe test revealed that children who are less ideologically committed report more negative BW, MN, and SW than children who are more ideologically committed.

With regard to religious commitment, one-way analysis of variance reveals significant differences in all indices of WAS, $F(2,2029) = 14.03$, $p < 0.001$ for BW; $F(2,1970) = 18.75$, $p < 0.001$ for MN; $F(2,2002) = 3.60$, $p < 0.05$ for SW. The Scheffe test shows that children who report low religious commitment perceive the world more negatively than children characterized by high religious commitment.

A series of two-tailed t-tests was conducted to assess the relationships between the measures of social support and the WAS indices. Results reveal that children who tend to report that there is someone with whom they can share their feelings in the aftermath of terror perceive the world and people as more benevolent and also endorse higher SW than children who have no one to turn to, $t(1892) = -5.46$, $p < 0.001$ for BW; $t(447.05) = -6.50$, $p < 0.001$ for SW. Similarly, children who turn to their family to share their feelings in the aftermath of terror also view the world and themselves more positively $[t(1142.52) = -4.99$, $p < 0.001$ for BW] $[t(1166.20) = -6.91$, $p < 0.001$ for SW]. In the same vein, children who share feelings connected with terror with their friends see the world as more benevolent and meaningful and themselves as more worthy, $t(2028) = -6.71$, $p < 0.001$ for BW; $t(1969) = -3.45$, $p < 0.01$ for MN; $t(1298.63) = -5.05$, $p < 0.001$ for SW. With regard to feeling connected with their community, children who reported a stronger sense of connectedness held more positive world assumptions as indicated in all three

WAS indices than children who endorsed a weaker sense of connectedness, $t(2028) = -9.35$, $p < 0.001$ for BW; $t(1385.21) = -2.93$, $p < 0.01$ for MN; $t(2001) = -7.05$, $p < 0.001$ for SW.

To assess the unique and cumulative contributions of the independent variables to WAS we conducted a series of stepwise linear regressions for the three WAS scores. In the first step of the regression, sociodemographics and life events were entered. In the second step, exposure to terror was entered. The third step comprised religious and ideological commitment, and the fourth the social support measures (see Table 1).

The regression model for BW explained 27.9% of the variance. The most significant contribution was made by the social support and religious and ideological commitment (R^2 change of 12.2% for social support, and 9.8% for ideology and religious commitment). Youth who tended to perceive the world and people as benevolent reported less fear in the aftermath of terror; were willing to act on behalf of their ideology; endorsed intrinsic religious commitment; and received support from their family and friends.

A similar regression was computed for MN (see Table 1). The model explained 15.35% of the variance. The most significant contribution was made by religious and ideological commitment (R^2 change of 10.7%). Youth who endorse high intrinsic religious commitment, who are intolerant of other political views, and who are self reliant and do not seek social support from family endorse more MN.

Finally, a stepwise linear regression was performed for SW. The model explains 26.6% of the variance. The major contribution was made by the social support variables (R^2 change of 24.2%). Children who report more general support report more enhanced sense of self worth.

DISCUSSION

This study assessed the effects of stress and trauma on world assumptions. Janoff-Bulman (1992) used the term "traumatic life events," and the consequent studies included a large variety of events. Her choice to use the term "traumatic life events" seems to have left room for other works that examined both traumatic and stressful events. These studies show conflicting results with some studies supporting the theory (e.g., Magwaza, 1999; Solomon et al., 1997) while others do not (e.g., McDermut, Haaga, & Kirk, 2000; Overcash, Calhoun, Cann, & Tedeschi, 1996). The literature is instructive in suggesting that a more refined conceptualization of traumatic life events is needed. Studies show that the effects of traumatic versus stressful events are more detrimental for world assumptions in adults (e.g., Magwaza, 1999). Repeated

TABLE 1. Stepwise Linear Regression Models for WAS

	BW		MN		SW	
	β	R² chng.	β	R² chng.	B	R² chng.
Step 1		3.7		.3		−.5
[1]Gender	−.07		.05		.01	
Grade	.18 ***		.06		.02	
Life events	−.01		−.04		−.00	
Current life events	−.04		.01		−.02	
Step 2		2.2		.9		−.3
Gender	−.12 **		.03		.04	
Grade	.13 **		.02		.04	
Life events	−.03		−.06		−.00	
Current life events	−.03		.02		−.03	
Fear of terror	−.06		.01		.03	
[2]Int.Exposure–religious	−.16 ***		−.11 **		.07	
Step 3		9.8		10.7		2.4
Gender	−.08 *		.05		.05	
Grade	.09 *		−.00		.02	
Life events	−.03		−.05		−.00	
Current life events	−.02		.04		−.01	
Fear of terror	−.06		−.01		.02	
[2]Int.Exposure–religious	−.12 **		−.07		.13 ***	
Practical commitment	.18 **		−.03		.13 *	
Ideological conviction	−.11 *		−.06		−.02	
Intolerance of other views	−.06		.15 **		.02	
Relig. as a lifestyle	.24 ***		.24 ***		.09 *	
Relig. as social aspect	−.14 **		−.13 **		−.05	
Relig. as defining identity	.05		.10 *		.05	
Step 4		12.2		3.4		24.2
Gender	.00		.09 *		.10 *	
Grade	.04		−.04		−.04	
Life events	−.04		−.05		.00	
Current life events	−.01		.05		−.02	
Fear of terror	−.10 **		−.03		−.03	
[2]Int.Exposure–religious	−.10 **		−.06		.14 **	
Practical commitment	.13 **		−.04		.05	
Ideological conviction	−.12 *		−.07		−.01	
Intolerance of other views	−.06		.15 **		.03	
Relig. as a lifestyle	.19 ***		.23 ***		.00	
Relig. as social aspect	−.12 **		−.11 *		−.02	
Relig. as defining identity	.03		.08		.02	
Community support	.07		.01		.10 **	
Family support	.18 **		−.13 **		.26 ***	
Friend support	.21 ***		−.01		.20 ***	
Professional support	.03		−.01		.12 *	
Adj. R²		27.9		15.3		26.6

$p < .05$ $p < .01$ $p < .001$
[1](0 = girls 1 = boys)
[2]Due to the higher exposure of religious youth to terror attacks, exposure to terror was included in the model as an interaction with religiosity.

terror attacks that are maliciously committed are therefore expected to affect negatively cognitive schemes in youth. The results of this study reveal a complex picture. Whereas life events were associated with negative world assumptions, exposure to terror was not. Contrary to expectation, youth who were exposed to more terror-related events endorsed more positive perceptions of BW and MN.

What can account for this surprising finding? It seems that the children who were exposed to life events came from all sectors of Israeli society, but the children who were exposed to the highest levels of terror constitute a unique group. They live in remote secluded settlements in the occupied territories and are characterized by both high religious and ideological commitments. Furthermore, these small, close-knit settlements provide their youth with a highly cohesive and supportive environment.

These findings raise the need to assess not only the characteristics of the traumatic event, but also to examine the personal attributes of survivors and their social world. When we examined the association between personal attributes, we found that youth with strong religious and ideological commitment and social support reported more positive perceptions as reflected in all three indices of world assumptions: BW, MN, and SW.

The role played by these personal attributes became even more salient when we examined the results of the multiple regressions. Analysis showed that in all three world assumptions indices, the contribution of both types of life events and terror was marginal. On the other hand, the contribution of religious and ideological commitment and social support was most significant. This suggests that as far as adolescents are concerned the social milieu has a more powerful effect on the interpretation and meaning of their experiences and thus also on their WAS than the events themselves.

This finding compels the reexamination of Janoff–Bulmann's (1992) assumptions. She had maintained that in working through the traumatic experience one has to change or accommodate one's basic assumptions and thus give them a new meaning. Not all researchers agree with this contention. Some claim that the assimilation can be done through other avenues, including religious schema (e.g., Overcash et al., 1996). Religion constitutes a cognitive schema that may help a person interpret the world and guide behavior (Koenig, 1995). The Jewish religion entails explicit guidance for coping with trauma and loss by stating: "Naked came I out of my mother's womb, and naked shall I return: the Lord gave, and the Lord hath taken away; blessed be the name of the Lord" (Job 1: 21; King James Version) and provides meaning to suffering. Religion thus portrays trauma and suffering as integral parts of life rather than as external events that challenge one's cognitive assumptions. Overcash et al. (1996) write: "religious beliefs may be more resilient than empirical assumptions about the world, perhaps because religious beliefs are less subject to empirical disconfirmation" (p. 462). They found that traumatic events did not challenge or shatter existing schema but rather strengthened it.

At the same time, religion is a multifaceted concept. While intrinsic religious orientation (i.e., observance of commandments) was positively related to WAS, extrinsic religious orientation (i.e., religion as a social obligation) was negatively associated with WAS. Intrinsic orientation implies that religion is the goal itself, whereas extrinsic orientation assumes that religion is a means for some other aim (e.g., social status, security) (Allport & Ross, 1967). Previous studies have also linked intrinsic religious orientation with well-being and mental health and extrinsic orientation with high levels of anxiety, and low self-esteem. (Bergin, Masters, & Richards, 1987; Pargament et al., 1992). We therefore speculate that when facing adversity individuals with intrinsic religious orientation will be helped by their religious schema whereas those who hold extrinsic religious orientation will not be served and protected by the religious prism and their WAS will be challenged.

Our findings also supported the protective role of ideology that had been found in several studies (Kostelny & Garbarino, 1994; Punamaki et al., 2001). Bettelheim (1961), for example, who survived the Holocaust, observed that inmates who were religious or held a strong ideological conviction fared better than other prisoners. He argued that their enhanced coping stemmed from their ability to ascribe meaning to their suffering. In Janoff-Bulman's (1992) terms, inmates who did not have the psychological protection of religion and ideology had to undergo the painful process of rebuilding the cognitive schema, which in turn was reflected in their intense suffering.

Terror Management Theory (Becker, 1971) holds that the major aim of culture is to protect people from death-related paralyzing anxiety. Humanity created culture and within it structures such as religion and ideology to provide a sense of order and stability that help make sense of human experiences. Culture also plays a role in protecting self esteem by linking the individual to a larger structure that will endure after his or her death. Studies found that when death anxiety is aroused, people tend to reaffirm their connections with cultural structures which in turn help them keep their anxiety at bay (e.g., Greenberg et al., 1990; Sowards et al., 1991).

Our findings show that the use of ideology and religion made a major contribution to WB and MN but only a marginal contribution to SW. It seems that while religion and ideology assist in meaning making they do not help maintain SW.

Social support made the most significant contribution to SW. Israeli youth who received support from numerous sources reported an enhanced self worth. This finding is consistent with a considerable body of research that suggests that self esteem in adolescents stems mostly from ties with and input from their social network (Cotterell, 1992; Gecas & Seff, 1990).

The results of this study suggest that the impact of traumatic events requires not only the consideration of various aspects of world assumptions but also the characteristics of both the person and the social environment. Results show different patterns among the three world assumptions. Meaningfulness of the World seems to stem from existing cultural assumptions; Benevolence of the World is affected by both culture and the adolescent's social world; and Self Worthiness is most affected by the adolescent's social network. It thus seems that these three world assumptions should not be viewed as one entity but rather as basic schemes reflecting different aspects of a person's life.

REFERENCES

Becker, E. (1971). *The birth and death of meaning.* New York: Free Press.

Bergin, A. E., Master, K. S., & Richards, P. S. (1987). Religiousness and mental health reconsidered: A study of an intrinsically religious sample. *Journal of Counseling Psychology, 34,* 197-204.

Bettelheim, B. (1961). *The informed heart.* New York: Free Press.

Cotterell, J. L. (1992). The relation of attachments and supports to adolescent well-being and school adjustment. *Journal of Adolescent Research, 7,* 28-42.

Ehlers, A., & Clark, D. M. (2000). A cognitive model of posttraumatic stress disorder. *Behavior Research and Therapy, 38,* 319-345.

Gecas, V., & Seff, M. A. (1990). Families and adolescents: 1980's decade review. *Journal of Marriage and the Family, 52,* 941-958.

Gorsuch, R. L., & McPherson, S. E. (1989). Intrinsic/extrinsic measurement: I/E–Revised and single-item scales. *Journal for the Scientific Study of Religion, 28*(3), 348-354.

Greenberg, J., Solomon, S., Veeder, M., Pyszczynski, T., Rosenblatt, A., & Kirkland, S. et al. (1990). Evidence for terror management theory II: The effects of mortality salience on reaction to those who threaten or bolster the cultural worldview. *Journal of Personality and Social Psychology, 58,* 308-318.

Janoff-Bulman, R. (1989). Assumptive worlds and the stress of traumatic events: Applications of the schema construct. *Social Cognition, 7,* 113-136.

Janoff-Bulman, R. (1992). *Shattered assumptions.* New York: The Free Press.

Koenig, H. G. (1995). Religion as cognitive schema. *The International Journal for the Psychology of Religion, 5,* 31-37.

Kostelny, K., & Garbarino, J. (1994). Coping with the consequences of living in danger: The case of Palestinian children and youth. *International Journal of Behavioral Development, 17,* 595-611.

Lavi, T., & Solomon, Z. (2004). *The psychological effects of terror on Palestinian youth.* Manuscript in progress.

Magwaza, A. S. (1999). Assumptive world of traumatized South African adults. *The Journal of Social Psychology, 139,* 622-630.

McDermut, J. F., Haaga, D. A. F., & Kirk, L. (2000). An evaluation of stress symptoms associated with academic sexual harassment. *Journal of Traumatic Stress, 13,* 397-411.

McIntosh, D. M., Silver, R. C., & Wortman, C. B. (1993). Religion's role in adjustment to negative life events: Coping with the loss of a child. *Journal of Personality and Social Psychology, 65,* 812-821.

Milgran, N., & Toubiana, Y. H. (1996). Children's selective coping after a bus disaster: Confronting behavior and perceived support. *Journal of Traumatic Stress, 9*(4), 687-702.

Overcash, W. S., Calhoun, L. G., Cann, A., & Tedeschi, R. G. (1996). Coping with crises: An examination of the impact of traumatic events on religious beliefs. *The Journal of Genetic Psychology, 157,* 455-464.

Pargament, K. I., Olsen, H., Reilly, B., Falgout, K., Ending, D. S., & Van Haitsma, K. (1992). God help me (II): The relationship of religious orientations to religious coping with negative life events. *Journal for the Scientific Study of Religion, 31*(4), 504-513.

Punamaeki, R. L., Quota, S., & El-Samir, E. (2001). Resiliency factors psychological adjustment after political violence among Palestinian children. *International Journal of Behavioral Development, 25,* 256-267.

Seidman, E., LaRue, A., Aber, J. L., Mitchell, C., Feinman, J., & Yoshikawa, H. et al. (1995). Development and validation of adolescent-perceived microsystem scales: Social support, daily hassles and involvement. *American Journal of Community Psychology, 23,* 355-388.

Solomon, Z., Iancu, I., & Tyano, S. (1997). World assumptions following disaster. *Journal of Applied Social Psychology, 27,* 1785-1798.

Sowards, B. A., Moniz, A. J., & Harris, M. J. (1991). Self esteem and bolstering: Testing major assumptions of terror management theory. *Representative Research in Social Psychology, 19,* 95-106.

SECTION III
THE IMPACT OF TERRORISM
ON INDIVIDUALS, GROUPS
AND SOCIETY

Terrorism's Toll on Civil Liberties

Nadine Strossen

SUMMARY. The toll that terrorism takes on civil liberties has become clear in the United States in the aftermath of the 9/11 attacks. Horrendous as those attacks were, they were hardly unique in the fear that they spurred on the part of the politicians and the public, resulting in a counterattack on civil liberties in the name of preventing terrorism. The cost to civil liberties is thus imposed not directly by terrorism itself, but rather by unjustified policies that are labeled "counter-terrorist." In that sense, this chapter would more aptly be entitled, "Counter-Terrorism's Toll on Civil Liberties."

Address correspondence to: Nadine Strossen, JD, 57 Worth Street A903, New York, NY 10013 USA.

The author would like to thank, for research and administrative assistance with preparing this chapter, the following NYLS students: David Rankin, Matthew Rench, Jennifer Meyer, and Jennifer Amore.

[Haworth co-indexing entry note]: "Terrorism's Toll on Civil Liberties." Strossen, Nadine. Co-published simultaneously in *Journal of Aggression, Maltreatment & Trauma* (The Haworth Maltreatment & Trauma Press, an imprint of The Haworth Press, Inc.) Vol. 9, No. 3/4, 2004; and: *The Trauma of Terrorism: Sharing Knowledge and Shared Care, An International Handbook* (ed: Yael Danieli, Danny Brom, and Joe Sills) The Haworth Maltreatment & Trauma Press, an imprint of The Haworth Press, Inc., 2005.

KEYWORDS. Civil liberties, security measures, USA PATRIOT Act, minority groups

THE SCAPEGOATING OF CIVIL LIBERTIES

In the post-9/11 situation, as in the past, the many cutbacks on civil liberties have not in fact increased protection from terrorism. Ironically, too many purported "counterterrorism" measures actually advance the very goals of the terrorists themselves: they sabotage the ideals of liberty, equality and justice that the terrorists attacked, and they simultaneously divert the government from more constructive counterterrorism policies in favor of the high-profile, politically appealing tactic of scapegoating civil liberties. Real freedom is traded for the illusion of security.

This point was stressed by the celebrated FBI whistleblower, longtime agent Coleen Rowley, in a letter she wrote to FBI Director Robert Mueller in February 2003, criticizing the government's post-9/11 dragnet detention and incarceration of many Muslim immigrants from the Middle East and South Asia. "After 9-11," she wrote, "[FBI] headquarters encouraged more and more detentions for . . . essentially PR [public relations] purposes. Field offices were required to report daily the number of detentions in order to supply grist for statements on our progress in fighting terrorism" (Rowley, 2003).

The foregoing typical pattern of sacrificing real rights for the semblance of safety no doubt reflects common psychological reactions to danger, as well as common political reactions. In the wake of terrorist attacks, members of the public are understandably afraid and, in a democracy, they want their government to take action to protect them. Politicians understandably want to "do something," or to be perceived as doing something, to allay their constituents' concerns.

The cheapest "quick fix" for any societal problem, including terrorist threats to national security, is to enhance government power and cut back on civil liberties. Such approaches initially require minimal resource expenditures and hence no new taxes. They tend not to engender much opposition, since there is not a large lobby for the rather abstract concept of civil liberties, especially when the issue is posed as a choice between national security and personal safety versus civil liberties. As polls in the 9/11 aftermath confirmed, most Americans were willing, if not eager, to trade in their freedoms in order to gain increased security or even the mere appearance of increased security.

Additionally, even more Americans were willing to trade in the freedoms of *other* people–for example, immigrants, or members of certain ethnic or religious minorities–in order to enhance their *own* security. Therefore, not surprisingly, as in all national security crises, the disproportionate targets of post-9/11 civil liberties violations are indeed members of minority groups. This phenomenon was also confirmed by Agent Rowley when she complained to FBI Director Robert Mueller that FBI field offices were subjected to "undue pressure" from FBI Headquarters after 9/11 "to detain or round up" suspects, "particularly those of Arabic origin" (Rowley, 2003).

It may well be rational to be willing to give up some freedom in return for some security, as proponents of government security measures maintain. But surely it is also rational to be *un*willing to give up some freedom *without* gaining security in return, or if the same security gain could be achieved without giving up as much freedom. Moreover, while proponents of government security measures rightly note that life and safety are prerequisites for enjoying liberty, it is also true that liberty is a prerequisite for enjoying life and safety. Even the chief author of the PATRIOT Act, former Assistant U.S. Attorney General Viet Dinh, has cited "the boy in the bubble" as exemplifying the kind of completely safe, but completely unfree, life that would be antithetical in America. For all of these reasons, the goals of protecting civil liberties and preventing terrorism are not unalterably opposed–as too many officials and citizens assume–but rather are mutually reinforcing.

My own personal background confirms the positive interrelationship between security and freedom. My father was born in Germany in 1922 as what the Nazis called a "Jew of the second degree," since one of his parents was Jewish. For that "crime," he was imprisoned and almost died in the forced labor camp at Buchenwald. He was liberated by American armed forces and came to this country as a refugee after the war. For the rest of his life, he continued to feel, and to convey to me, his undying gratitude toward the U.S. military personnel who gave him freedom in the most literal sense.

Moreover, the U.S. forces freed him just one day before he had been scheduled to undergo forced sterilization. Therefore, I literally owe my life to the U.S. military! And I continue to depend on the U.S. military–as well as intelligence and law enforcement officials–to protect my life and our cherished American way of life. But what many of us most cherish about that way of life is precisely its dedication to the ideals of "liberty and justice for all." As the U.S. Supreme Court said, in striking down a Cold War era security measure that undermined constitutional rights, "It would indeed be ironic if, in the name of national defense, we would sanction the subversion of . . . those liberties . . . which make[s] the defense of the Nation worthwhile" (*U.S. v. Robel*, 1967, pp. 258, 264).

THE COSTS TO THE CIVIL LIBERTIES OF EVERYONE IN THE U.S.

Following the predictable patterns described above, it was not surprising that, promptly after the 9/11 attacks, the government proposed a new law that gave it sweeping new powers of surveillance, detention, and prosecution. The law was based on the assumption that the cause of the terrorist attacks was that the government did not already have enough power to obtain information about terrorist plots. This was not supported by any evidence.

In the two years since the PATRIOT Act was passed, Congress has investigated the causes of the attacks and concluded that most of the intelligence failures had nothing to do with lack of government power to gather information, but rather resulted from the government's failure to effectively analyze and act on the massive amounts of information it already possessed through its already great surveillance powers. Moreover, many of the government's intrusive new surveillance powers can be exercised not only against suspected terrorists but also against law-abiding citizens who are not suspected of any crime at all. Therefore, these measures are the worst of both worlds: they do demonstrably violate the freedoms of everyone in the U.S., but they do not demonstrably enhance national security.

Under one section of the PATRIOT Act, government agents may obtain any records about anyone from any entity that holds them, so long as the government "specif[ies]" that the records are sought in connection with a terrorism investigation (USA PATRIOT Act, 2001, Section 215). On that basis, even our most personal records can be turned over by banks, hospitals, Internet Service Providers, libraries, universities, and any other of the multiple entities that maintain personal information about us. This enormous new power not only violates fundamental privacy rights, but it also endangers freedom of speech, since many of us may well be deterred from such activities as borrowing certain library books, or visiting certain Websites, knowing that the government can be looking over our shoulders as we read.

The same chilling effect on free speech and other First Amendment rights follows from another expansive post-9/11 surveillance power: the Attorney General's guidelines, issued in May 2002, which allow government agents to infiltrate secretly any gatherings, including political meetings and religious worship services, even without any suspicion whatsoever that any participants are engaging in illegal activities. This was precisely the kind of political spying that targeted Martin Luther King and many other pro-civil rights and anti-Vietnam War activists a generation ago, prompting Congressional hearings and investigative guidelines that prohibited surveillance without at least some suspicion of criminal activity. In the 9/11 aftermath, Attorney General John Ashcroft unilaterally rolled back those protections and again unleashed government power to spy on Americans merely because of their political and religious beliefs.

While the government's increased surveillance powers can be used against anyone, including American citizens, since 9/11 many publicized government investigative programs have singled out Muslim immigrants from the Middle East and South Asia. Therefore, individuals in these groups reasonably fear that they are the prime targets of clandestine surveillance measures. Immigrants and Muslims have said that they are no longer attending meetings or religious services for fear that they will be subject to government surveillance and harassment. Even if they "have nothing to hide" in terms of any wrongdoing, they understandably still do not want government officials to spy surreptitiously on their political and religious expressions and beliefs.

It is becoming increasingly difficult to maintain some sphere of personal privacy that the government may not invade even with no specific justification. "Thanks" to rapidly developing information-gathering technology, including the linking of computerized databases, we are approaching the dystopia depicted in George Orwell's classic novel *1984*. One's freedom of action certainly can be limited by the fear of facing a terrorist attack, but it may also be limited by the fear, or indeed, knowledge, that "Big Brother is watching."

THE DISPROPORTIONATELY HIGH COSTS TO THE CIVIL LIBERTIES OF CERTAIN MINORITY GROUPS

While precious rights of everyone in the U.S. have been forfeited in the domestic "War on Terrorism," the rights of some people have been hit especially hard, namely, young Muslim men from certain countries in the Middle East (including Israel) and South Asia. Thousands have been interrogated and hundreds have been incarcerated, in secret, based only on national origin and religion. In a scathing report issued in June 2003, the Justice Department's own Inspector General concluded that these "indiscriminate and haphazard" arrests and detentions led to the prolonged incarceration of hundreds of individuals who had no ties whatsoever to terrorism (Department of Justice, 2003). Worse yet, many were held incommunicado without access to lawyers or family members and in inhumane conditions.

These current discriminatory practices replicate the errors of the past, when the U.S. government repeatedly has demonized particular immigrant groups as alleged national security threats based on no individualized suspicion but rather on ethnic prejudices. While the post-9/11 incarcerations involved "only" hundreds of innocent immigrants–as opposed to the 120,000 innocent Japanese-Americans who were incarcerated during World War II–the very same principles are at stake. The well-respected legal journalist Stuart Taylor wrote: "Despite the unprecedented secrecy imposed by Attorney General John Ashcroft, evidence has mounted that [since September 11, 2001] his Justice Department has put hundreds of harmless Muslim men from abroad behind bars for far too long, treated many of them worse than convicted criminals, and arguably violated their constitutional rights–all without finding enough evidence to charge a single one . . . with a terrorist crime" (Taylor, 2002, p. 52).

Disproportionate sacrifices of the rights of "the usual suspects," members of targeted minority groups, create a false sense on the part of the majority of our citizenry that only "other people's rights are at stake." The lesson the American Civil Liberties Union has been trying to teach in the current climate is that it is not only wrong to demonize Muslim men from certain countries, but also that everyone else has a direct personal stake in righting this wrong. This fundamental concept was memorably captured by Stephen Rohde, a civil liberties lawyer in Los Angeles, who composed a post-9/11 variation on the famous 1937 prose poem by the Reverend Martin Niemoller about Nazi Germany. Stephen Rohde's (2001) moving words follow:

> First they came for the Muslims, and I didn't speak up because I wasn't a Muslim.

> Then they came for the immigrants, detaining them indefinitely solely upon the certification of the Attorney General, and I didn't speak up because I wasn't an immigrant.

> Then they came to eavesdrop on suspects consulting with their attorneys, and I didn't speak up because I wasn't a suspect.

> Then they came to prosecute non-citizens before secret military commissions, and I didn't speak up because I wasn't a non-citizen.

> Then they came to enter homes and offices for unannounced "sneak and peek" searches, and I didn't speak up because I had nothing to hide.

Then they came to reinstate Cointelpro and resume the infiltration and surveillance of domestic religious and political groups, and I didn't speak up because I no longer participated in any groups.

Then they came to arrest American citizens and hold them indefinitely without any charges and without access to lawyers, and I didn't speak up because I would never be arrested.

Then they came to institute TIPS, the Terrorism Information and Prevention System, recruiting citizens to spy on other citizens, and I didn't speak up because I was afraid.

Then they came to institute Total Information Awareness, collecting private data on every man, woman and child in America, and I didn't speak up because I couldn't do anything about it.

Then they came for immigrants and students from selective countries luring them under the requirement of "special registration" as a ruse to seize them and detain them, and I didn't speak up because I was not required to register.

Then they came for anyone who objected to government policy because it only aided the terrorists and gave ammunition to America's enemies and I didn't speak up . . . because I didn't speak up.

Then they came for me and by that time no one was left to speak up.

THE THREAT TO FREE EXCHANGE OF INFORMATION

As the Rohde/Niemoller piece underscores, a critical right, especially in the counter-terrorism context, is the right "to speak up" against government abuses. Great costs to civil liberties, in the current security crisis as well as others, result from the government's efforts to stifle dissent. This specific type of rights violation is particularly pernicious since it hampers efforts to counter all other rights violations. Since 9/11, the U.S. government has sought to suppress criticism in many ways, both indirectly, by suggesting that dissent is unpatriotic, and directly, by illegally arresting individuals who are simply seeking to exercise their right to peaceful protest. These crackdowns on fundamental First Amendment freedoms violate not only the core individual right of self-expression, but also an essential tenet of democratic self-government: that "We the People" must be free to criticize the policies that our elected representatives adopt in our name.

An early effort to discourage criticism of the government's anti-terrorism policies occurred only weeks after the terrorist attacks, with the government's heavy-handed promotion of its draconian new, so-called "anti-terrorism" law. I use the term "so-called" to underscore that most of the law's intrusive new powers apply to people who are suspected of non-terrorist crimes, and some even apply to people who are suspected of no wrongdoing at all. The law's title, the "USA PATRIOT" Act, signifies that anyone who dares to dissent from this law, or to criticize it, is not patriotic, or at least will face politically powerful charges of lack of patriotism.

The message that true patriots willingly give up freedom and hand over power to the government during national security crises was asserted even more explicitly by U.S. Attorney General John Ashcroft in testimony before the U.S. Senate Judiciary Committee in December, 2001. He charged that anyone who raised what he derided as "phantoms of lost liberty" would "only aid terrorists" and "give ammunition to America's enemies."[1] This charge was especially harsh, since it closely echoed the U.S. Constitution's definition of treason.[2]

Following historic patterns, since 9/11 both federal and local officials have employed a variety of tactics not only to discourage individuals from expressing critical opinions but also to make it difficult for government leaders and the general public to hear those opinions even when they are expressed. For example, in cities throughout the U.S., peaceful demonstrators against the war in Iraq have been subjected to various forms of official mistreatment, from physical abuse, to false arrest, to interrogations about their political and religious beliefs. Moreover, when President Bush or other top Administration officials make public appearances, the Secret Service has consistently restricted members of the public who seek to criticize Administration policies to locations that are far away not only from the officials at whom the messages are aimed, but also from the TV cameras that are covering the officials' appearances (American Civil Liberties Union, 2003). This policy not only violates the cherished First Amendment rights of the would-be protestors themselves, but it also violates the First Amendment rights of everyone in this country, since we are deprived of information about the range and strength of perspectives on these critically important issues that so profoundly affect us all.

In addition to preventing or discouraging citizens from conveying critical viewpoints to their elected officials post-9/11, the government also has completely silenced many communications that should be taking place in the other direction–from the government to the citizenry. The government has thrown an unprecedented shroud of secrecy over essential aspects of its counter-terrorism policies in ways that are not justified by security concerns. This makes it impossible for "We the People" to assess what our government is doing in our name. For example, the Bush Administration has consistently refused to provide even statistical information about how it is deploying the intrusive new surveillance powers it gained under the Patriot Act. The government has pursued blanket policies of secret arrests, secret incarcerations, secret deportation hearings, and secret deportations without justifying the need for such secrecy in any particular instance. In lawsuits brought by the ACLU and our allies to challenge these sweeping secrecy policies, judges have denounced the policies as "odious to a democracy" (*American Civil Liberties Union v. County of Hudson*, 2002). In one widely quoted pronouncement, federal appellate Judge Damon Keith decried the secret deportation policy by declaring, "Democracies die behind closed doors" (*Detroit Free Press v. Ashcroft*, 2002, p. 683).

THE COSTS TO THE CONSTITUTIONAL SYSTEM OF CHECKS AND BALANCES

In addition to undermining democratic self-government through suppressing the free flow of information and ideas between government officials and citizens, the current counter-terrorism policies have also eroded another essential pillar of our democracy: the system of checks and balances designed to prevent any single branch of government from amassing excessive power and abusing individual rights. A pervasive pattern running through many post-9/11 policies, as well as many prior anti-terrorism policies, is the consolidation of power in the executive branch of government, thus substantially diminishing the powers of both other branches of the federal government, the Congress and the courts.

The Administration has circumscribed Congress's powers in several ways. First, it has exerted enormous pressure on members of Congress to rush through laws that it asserts to be essential to the anti-terrorist arsenal, such as the PATRIOT Act, with only minimal deliberations, in derogation of standard legislative processes. The executive branch prevailed upon Congress to pass this lengthy, complex Act in record time, even before most members of Congress had had time to read it. Second, the executive branch has thwarted Congress's attempts to exercise its important oversight responsibilities to ensure that government officials are exercising their pervasive new powers in ways that do not abuse individual rights. Administration officials have stonewalled Congress's requests for information and documents, provoking harsh criticism even from some Republican members of Congress. Third, the executive branch has unilaterally implemented many rights–restricting anti-terrorism policies on its own without even consulting with Congress, let alone seeking Congressional authorization.

The Administration has resisted Congress' effective participation in counter-terrorism policymaking with a "trust us" argument: trust us to know what is best for the American people. Politicians and members of the public might well find such an argument appealing in one significant sense because of an understandable desire to be able to trust our national leaders at times of crisis. Whatever the psychological realities that encourage many individuals to accept the government's self-described beneficence on the basis of trust or faith, political and historical realities demonstrate that the "trust us" approach is a thin reed on which to rest either liberty or democracy. The great former U.S. Supreme Court Justice Louis Brandeis eloquently explained this, in a much-quoted opinion: "Experience should teach us to be most on our guard to protect liberty when the government's purposes are beneficent. . . . The greatest dangers to liberty lurk in insidious encroachment by men of zeal, well-meaning but without understanding" (*Olmstead v. United States*, 1928, pp. 438, 479). Justice Brandeis's insight is in fact hard-wired into the U.S. constitutional system of checks and balances.

Even more dangerous to civil liberties and democracy than the Administration's attempts to reduce, and in some instances, even to eliminate Congress's role in shaping anti-terrorism policies is the Administration's consistent erosion of the checking powers of the third branch of our federal government, the federal courts. The framers of the U.S. Constitution deliberately provided some distance between the federal courts and the electorate in order to maximize judicial independence. Since federal judges are appointed rather than elected, and since they have lifetime tenure, they are well positioned to serve as the ultimate safety net for the rights of individuals and members of minority groups when elected officials are not as likely to protect these rights. This role of the federal courts is especially important in times of national security crisis, when elected officials are particularly susceptible to political pressures–as illustrated, for example, by the very few votes against the Patriot Act, despite its many cutbacks on fundamental freedoms and despite the lack of any showing that these new powers would even be effective in countering terrorism, let alone necessary to do so.

To counter this tendency of politicians to succumb to political and popular pressures, especially during times of crisis, it is in those very times that the courts must most rigorously review government actions to ensure that they do not unjustifiably sacrifice the rights of individuals or minority groups. This point was stressed by the Chief Justice in Israel, a country that certainly has had more than its share of terrorist attacks. Aharon Barak, President of the Israeli Supreme Court, said: "The real test of [judicial] independence and impartiality comes in situations of war and terrorism. . . . Precisely in these times, we judges must hold fast to fundamental principles and values; we must embrace our supreme responsibility to protect democracy and the constitution" (Lewis, 2003, p. A-17).

In short, vigorous judicial review is more important than ever in the context of counter-terrorism efforts. Unfortunately, since 9/11 too many anti-terrorism policies have moved in exactly the opposite direction to cut back or even eliminate the courts' time-honored power to check executive branch over-reaching and to protect individual rights. Judges no longer may exercise meaningful review over secret seizures of personal records from any entity that holds them, secret searches and seizures of items in homes and offices, interception of communications between attorneys and their clients, and the holding of certain hearings in secret.

The most dramatic Administration post-9/11 assertion of unilateral power, with the exclusion of meaningful judicial review, concerns "enemy combatants." I put that term in quotes, since it is not a legal term of art and the Administration has not defined it, other than to describe one American citizen whom it labeled an "enemy combatant" as being "a bad guy" ("Dirty Bombs," 2002). The President has claimed the power to pronounce anyone, including an American citizen who is arrested in the U.S., to be an "enemy combatant." Moreover, once the Administration has tarred someone with that stigmatizing label, it also asserts the power to imprison him or her indefinitely, incommunicado, without charge, without trial, and without access to a lawyer or anyone else. The Administration has further claimed that the courts are powerless to review the "enemy combatant" designation and its draconian consequences so long as it produces "some evidence," no matter how conclusory or questionable, in support. Such unfettered, unchecked government power is antithetical to both personal liberty and democratic government. That conclusion is confirmed by a sadly apt comment that Winston Churchill made in 1943:

> The power of the executive to cast a man into prison without formulating any Charge . . . and to deny him the judgment of his peers, is in the highest degree odious, and the foundation of all totalitarian governments, whether Nazi or Communist. (The United Kingdom Parliament Joint Committee on Human Rights, 2003, February)

CONCLUSION

The costs to civil liberties resulting from U.S. post-9/11 counter-terrorism efforts reflect consistent patterns that we see whenever any government seeks to protect national security against serious threats. As we have learned from past experience, too many sacrifices of civil liberties prove in retrospect to be not only unprincipled, but also unpractical. This is especially true when the victims are members of minority groups who are targeted because of who they are, not what they have done. By demonizing innocent people, we deflect attention from guilty ones. As President George W. Bush declared, in his first words to a shattered nation on that dreadful date of September 11, 2001, the terrorists attacked the U.S. because it is "the brightest beacon for freedom and opportunity in the world," and he vowed that "No one will keep that light from shining" (Bush, 2001). Accordingly, if our own counter-terrorism policies dim the very light of liberty that the terrorists targeted, that would be the greatest cost of all, not only to civil liberties, but also to our struggle against terrorism.

NOTES

1. This is a close paraphrase of Attorney General John Ashcroft's testimony before the Senate Judiciary Committee on December 6, 2001, in which he said that the government's civil libertarian critics would "only aid terrorists" and "give ammunition to America's enemies."

2. U.S. Constitution, Article III, Section 3: "Treason against the United States, shall consist . . . in adhering to their Enemies, giving them Aid and Comfort."

REFERENCES

American Civil Liberties Union. (2003). *Freedom under fire: Dissent in post 9/11 America*. New York: Author.

American Civil Liberties Union v. County of Hudson. (2002, March 27). No. HUD-L-463-02. Hudson City: New Jersey Superior Court.

Ashcroft, J. (2001, December 6). *DOJ oversight: Preserving freedoms while defending against terrorism*. Hearing before the Senate Committee on the Judiciary, 107th Congress.

Bush, G.W. (2001, September). *Statement in his Address to the nation*. Washington, DC. Copy of the transcript available at www.whitehouse.gov

Department of Justice. (2003, June). *Report on the September 11 detainees: A review of the treatment of aliens held on immigration charges in connection with the investigation of the September 11 attacks*. Washington, DC: Government Publishing Office.

Detroit Free Press v. Ashcroft, 303 F.3d 681, 683 (6th Cir. 2002).

Dirty bombs and civil rights. (2002, June 12). *The New York Times*, p. A-28.

Lewis, A. (2003, February 24). Marbury v. Madison v. Ashcroft. *The New York Times*, p. A-17.

Olmstead v. United States, 277 U.S. 438, 479 (dissenting opinion) (1928).

Rohde, S. (2001). *Then they came for me*. (Inspired by the Rev. Martin Neimoller, 1937). Unpublished manuscript.

Rowley, C. (2003, February 26). *Rowley Letter to FBI Director.* Published March 6, 2003. Retrieved from: http://www.startribune.com/stories/484/3738192.html

Taylor, S. Jr. (2002, June 3). Stop locking up Muslims. *Legal Times*, p. 52.

The United Kingdom Parliament Joint Committee on Human Rights. (2003, February). *Continuance in force of Sections 21 to 23 of the Anti-Terrorism, Crime and Security Act 2001.* Fifth report.

U.S. v. Robel, 389 U.S., 258-264 (1967).

USA PATRIOT Act. Business Records Provision. 50 USC § 1861 (2003)(b)(2).

The Theater of Terror:
The Psychology of Terrorism
and the Mass Media

Gabriel Weimann

SUMMARY. Modern terrorists became aware of the new opportunities for exerting mass psychological impact using the latest means of mass communications. Academic observers remarked increasingly on the theater-like nature of terrorist operations. According to this notion, modern terrorism can be understood in terms of the production requirements of theatrical engagements. Several terrorist organizations realized the potentials of media-oriented terror, in terms of effectively reaching huge audiences. This article examines the strategies and tactics of this new pattern of media-oriented terrorism and their impact on the audiences who, through the media's mediation, join the widening circles of victims of terrorism.

Address correspondence to: Gabriel Weimann, PhD, United States Institute of Peace, 1200 17th Street NW, Washington, DC 20036 USA (E-mail: weimann@soc.haifa.ac.il).

[Haworth co-indexing entry note]: "The Theater of Terror: The Psychology of Terrorism and the Mass Media." Weimann, Gabriel. Co-published simultaneously in *Journal of Aggression, Maltreatment & Trauma* (The Haworth Maltreatment & Trauma Press, an imprint of The Haworth Press, Inc.) Vol. 9, No. 3/4, 2004 and: *The Trauma of Terrorism: Sharing Knowledge and Shared Care, An International Handbook* (ed: Yael Danieli, Danny Brom, and Joe Sills) The Haworth Maltreatment & Trauma Press, an imprint of The Haworth Press, Inc., 2005.

379

KEYWORDS. Terrorism, media, psychology, propaganda, Internet, suicide

Historically, the term terrorism has entailed a mass psychological aspect. Specifically, the word "terror" comes from the Latin word "terrere," which means "to frighten" or "to scare." The first use of large-scale terrorism was during the "popular" phase of the French Revolution. For example, in September 1793 the "Reign of Terror" was officially declared and activated, causing the execution of 17,000 people. Executions were conducted before large audiences and were accompanied by sensational publicity thus spreading the intended fear.

The emergence of media-oriented terrorism led several communication and terrorism scholars to re-conceptualize modern terrorism within the framework of symbolic communication theory (Jenkins 1975; Weimann, 1983, 1986; Weimann & Winn, 1994). According to this theory, terrorism as a symbolic act can be analyzed much like other forms of communication, consisting of four basic components: (a) transmitter (the terrorist), (b) intended recipient (target), (c) message (bombing, ambush) and (d) feedback (reaction of target audience). Karber (1971) has pointed out that "the terrorist's message of violence necessitates a victim, whether personal or institutional, but the target or intended recipient of the communication may not be the victim" (p. 529). On the other hand, Weimann and Winn (1994) adopted the theater of terror metaphor to examine modern terrorism as an attempt to communicate messages through the use of orchestrated violence.

The growing use and manipulation of modern modes of communication by terrorist organizations have led governments and several media organizations to consider certain steps in response. These included limiting terrorists' access to the conventional mass media, reducing and censoring news coverage of terrorist acts and their perpetrators, and minimizing the terrorists' capacity for manipulating the media (Weimann, 1999). However, the new media technologies allow terrorist organizations to transmit messages more easily and freely than through other means of communication, as well as to exerting a mass psychological impact.

The networks of computer-mediated communication (CMC), or the Internet, are ideal for terrorists-as-communicators. This is a decentralized medium, it cannot be subjected to control or restriction, it is not censored, and it allows access to anyone who wants it (Tzfati & Weimann, 1999, 2002). This article examines the psychological importance of the mass media in modern terrorism, the media tactics of terrorists, and the challenges they present to media organizations and governments.

THE THEATER OF TERROR

From its early days, terror has entailed a mass psychological aspect. Contemporary terrorists have become exposed to new opportunities for exerting mass psychological impacts as a result of technological advances in communications and transportation. The most significant change was the emergence and widespread diffusion of television broadcasting. Paralleling the growth in technology-driven opportunities for terrorist action were efforts by terrorists themselves to hone their communications skills. As one of the terrorists who orchestrated the attack on the Israeli athletes during the 1972 Munich Olympic Games testified:

> We recognized that sport is the modern religion of the Western world. We knew that the people in England and America would switch their television sets from any program about the plight of the Palestinians if there was a sporting event on another channel. So, we decided to use their Olympics, the most sacred ceremony of this religion, to make the world pay attention to us. We offered up human sacrifices to your gods of sport and television. And they answered our prayers. From Munich onwards, nobody could ignore the Palestinians or their cause. (Dobson & Paine, 1977, p. 15)

During the 1970s, academic observers remarked increasingly on the theatrical proficiency with which terrorists conducted their operations. As Jenkins (1975) concluded in his analysis of international terrorism:

> Terrorist attacks are often carefully choreographed to attract the attention of the electronic media and the international press. Taking and holding hostages increases the drama. The hostages themselves often mean nothing to the terrorists. Terrorism is aimed at the people watching, not at the actual victims. Terrorism is a theater. (p. 4)

Modern terrorism can be understood in terms of the production requirements of theatrical engagements. Terrorists pay attention to script preparation, cast selection, sets, props, role playing, and minute-by-minute stage management. Just like compelling stage plays or ballet performances, the media orientation in terrorism requires full attention to detail in order to be effective.

Several terrorist organizations realized the potentials of media-oriented terror, in terms of effectively reaching huge audiences. Our study (reported in Weimann & Winn, 1994) examined 6,714 incidents of international terrorism from the late 1960s to the early 1990s. The analysis revealed a significant increase in terrorist acts that victimize Western nations (though most perpetrators are non-Western) and are directed to attract the attention of the Western publics. No wonder that Bell (1976) argued: "It has become more alluring for the frantic few to appear on the world stage of television than remain obscure guerrillas of the bush" (p. 89). Terrorist theory was gradually realizing the potential of the mass media. Acts of terrorism were more and more perceived as means of persuasion and psychological warfare, when the victim is described as being "the skin on a drum beaten to achieve a calculated impact on a wider audience" (Schmid & de Graaf, 1982, p. 14).

THE STRATEGY OF MEDIA-ORIENTED TERRORISM

One of the most influential theorists of modern terrorism was the Brazilian Carlos Marighela, whose *Minimanual of the Urban Guerrilla* became a sourcebook for many terrorist movements all over the world. In his publications, Marighela (1971a) outlined the various uses that can be made of the media:

> To kidnap figures known for their artistic, sporting, or other activities who have not expressed any political views may possibly provide a form of propaganda favorable to the revolutionaries. . . . Modern mass media, simply by announcing what the revolutionaries are doing, are important instruments of the propaganda. The war of nerves, or the psychological war, is a fighting technique based on the direct or indirect use of the mass media. . . . (pp. 87-90)

Marighela (1971b) continued by outlining additional uses of the media in acts of terrorism stating:

> The coordination of urban guerrilla action, including each armed action, is the principal way of making propaganda. These actions, carried out with specific and determined objectives, inevitably become propaganda material for the mass communication system. Bank assaults, ambushes, desertion and diverting of arms, the rescue of prisoners, executions, kidnapping, sabotage, terrorism, and the war of nerves, are all cases in point. Airplanes diverted in flight, ships and trains assaulted and seized by guerrillas, can also be solely for propaganda effects. (p. 103)

The emergence of media-oriented terrorism led several communication and terrorism scholars to reconceptualize modern terrorism within the framework of a symbolic communication theory. Karber (1971) suggested a new model of analysis: "As a symbolic act, terrorism can be analyzed much like other media of communication" (p. 529). Dowling (1986) suggested applying the concept of "rhetoric genre" to modern terrorism, arguing that "terrorists engage in recurrent rhetorical forms that force the media to provide the access without which terrorism could not fulfill its objectives" (p. 14). Some terrorist events become what Bell (1976) has called "terrorist spectaculars" that can be best analyzed by the "media event" conceptualization (p. 50; for a comparative analysis of media events and terrorist spectaculars, see Weimann, 1987).

The growing importance attributed to publicity and mass media by terrorist organizations was revealed both in the diffusion of media-oriented terrorism (Brosius & Weimann, 1991; Weimann & Brosius, 1989, 1991; Weimann & Winn, 1994) as well as in the tactics of modern terrorists who have become more media-minded.

THE TACTICS OF MEDIA-ORIENTED TERRORISM

To study media tactics of terrorists, we analyzed terrorist literature from pamphlets, personal diaries, and press interviews. We conducted interviews with terrorists, some jailed and some free, in various countries. We analyzed the place of the mass media in the strategy of modern terrorism and found convincing evidence of the importance terrorists attribute to the media in their plans and tactics (Weimann & Winn, 1994).

Terrorists see the media as a powerful tool in their psychological warfare. They believe that fear and panic can be spread by the coverage of terrorist attacks. They also look at the media as instruments of propaganda, targeting various audiences as they can create awareness (on a global scale) of the problems and issues motivating them. They can use terrorist attacks to promote their cause on the media agenda and thus on the public agenda, they can turn to their own people seeking legitimacy, support, and funding and even recruit new members. The mass media are a valuable instrument in terrorist strategy, and consequently in terrorist tactics too.

It is clear that media-wise terrorists plan their actions with the media as a major consideration. They select targets, location and timing, according to media preferences, trying to satisfy the media criteria for newsworthiness, media timetables and deadlines, and media access. They prepare visual aids for the media, like video clips of their actions, taped interviews and declarations of the perpetrators, films, PRs or VNRs (Press Releases and Video News Releases). Hizbollah's attacks on Israeli targets were always taped, leading some analysts to suggest that every terror unit consists of at least four members: (a) the perpetrator, (b) a cameraman, (c) a soundman, and (d) a producer. Modern terrorists feed the media, directly and indirectly, with their propaganda material, often disguised as news items. They also monitor the coverage, examin-

ing closely the reporting of various media organizations. The pressure of terrorists on journalists takes many forms, from open and friendly hosting to
direct threats, blackmailing and even killings of journalists. The lynch-style
execution of two Israeli soldiers as well as the execution of Palestinians suspected of collaboration with Israel were taped but not broadcast or printed by
news organizations as a result of a massive campaign of threats by Palestinian
terrorists. Finally, terrorist organizations operate their own media, from television channels (Al-Manar of the Hizbollah), news agencies, newspapers and
magazines, radio channels, video and audio cassettes, and recently, terrorist
websites on the Internet.

SUICIDE TERRORISM
AND THE COMMUNICATIONS PERSPECTIVE

Suicide terrorism is a relatively new production in the Theater of Terror but
it certainly follows some of the patterns and formats suggested by scriptwriters
like Marighela and his followers. Nevertheless, this new production presents
new challenges, not only from the security and military perspectives but also
from the mass media perspective.

Suicide attacks are one of the most effective weapons of psychological warfare. As such, the importance of the media in this type of terrorism is crucial,
as illustrated by several examples from recent Israeli experiences:

Pre-Planning. These attacks are planned carefully with the media in mind.
The events are not only very dramatic, very photographic, and emotionally
powerful, they also satisfy the requirements of the Theater of Terror. Locations and timing are carefully chosen to carry symbolic meanings (i.e., the attacks on the centers of major cities, on restaurants and discotheques, during
Jewish holidays such as the Passover meal or Purim, the Jewish carnival, killing people at parties, at weddings and during their daily routine).

Feeding. The terrorists continuously feed the media. Before the attack they
warn about suicide bombings, send tapes of volunteers preparing for their mission, and distribute pictures and tapes of former attacks; after the attack they
release tapes of the terrorist reading his last testament, usually with all the necessary props (i.e., flags, Koran, weapons, photos, symbols, and the statement
written for him by one of the "script writers"). Other mass media actions will
include taking responsibility, sending relatives of the dead terrorist to interviews, showing continuously the footage of the attack and its devastating results on television or on video cassettes and their websites. Indeed, terrorist
websites carry pages devoted to suicide terrorists, including their names, pic-

tures, personal background, actions, and praises of their heroism and holy sacrifice.

Monitoring. Terrorists use the media to follow and monitor the success of their actions, as illustrated by a recent example. Israeli officials arrested Marwan Barguti, the leader of the Palestinian Tanzim, and are prosecuting him for causing the death of hundreds of Israelis. The indictment included the following: On March 5, 2002, the suicide terrorist Ibrahim Hassouna attacked a restaurant in Tel Aviv with an M-16 machinegun and hand grenades, killing two policemen and wounding many of the restaurant's guests. Security officers shot and killed him. Nasser Avis and Ahmed Barguti, the personal aides of Marwan Barguti, who is accused of planning this assault, had recruited Hassouna. At 3 o'clock that night, Ahmed Barguti phoned Marwan Barguti to tell him that the act had been committed. He asked Barguti to watch the live broadcasting from the scene of the attack, on Israeli television. Barguti answered that he was already watching the coverage, and even told Ahmed not to claim responsibility yet and to consult him before the Tanzim formally assumed responsibility.

Suicide terrorism introduces new challenges but not only from the military and security perspective. It also challenges the media, the journalists, the policies of media organizations, and their daily routines in covering and reporting events.

MEDIA CHALLENGES IN THE THEATER OF TERROR

The recent attacks in Israel have not only exposed some basic dilemmas and problems of covering such events; they have also promoted an open and often very bitter and vocal debate, one which in turn has promoted studies, experiments, and attempts to find guideless, red lines and agreements between the media and the administrations and among the media themselves. To highlight only some of these dilemmas: (a) Breaking news: what is the threshold for breaking normal broadcasting? How should such terrible events be reported? And who decides? (b) How live should live coverage be? The lessons of direct feed, straight from the terrorist scene, have sparked a debate about the impact of such violent and disturbing images, identification of victims on television before informing the relatives, inaccurate reports on the number of victims, and the spread of panic. (c) Drawing red lines: what are the red lines of such coverage, who should draw them, how can they be implemented by all media organizations? What sanctions should be used against those who cross the lines? (d) Commercial channels: when the normal routines are broken commercial channels stop broadcasting advertisements and commercials; when should commercials be stopped? For how long? Who decides? Who will compensate the broadcasters for their losses?

Journalists face tough dilemmas in their everyday work but terrorist acts present even tougher choices, such as the conflicting roles of a citizen and a journalist, the clash between care for the victims and the duty to report, photograph and tape. Journalists know the news value of terrorism but they are also aware of their being the carriers of the fear, the threat, and the messages.

THE NEW ARENA: TERRORISM IN CYBERSPACE

The same advantages the Internet and advanced communication technology bring to the general public and to business (i.e., speed, easy access and global linkage) help international terrorist groups organize their deadly and disruptive activities. Paradoxically, the very decentralized structure that the American security services created out of fear of a Soviet nuclear attack now serves the interests of the greatest foe to the West's security services since the end of the Cold War, namely, international terror. The nature of the network, its international character and chaotic structure, the simple access, and the anonymity all furnish terrorist organizations with an ideal arena for action.

The story of cyberspace presence of terrorist groups has barely begun to be told. In 1998, nearly half of the 30 organizations designated as Foreign Terrorist Organizations under the U.S. Antiterrorism and Effective Death Penalty Act of 1996 (AEDPA) maintained websites; by the end of 1999, nearly all terrorist groups had established their presence on the net. These websites, whatever other language versions they might be available in, are invariably in English and pose complex and hitherto unexplored questions about the constituencies that find cyberspace hospitable for the fulfillment of their political goals. Two studies reveal the growing attraction of the Internet to modern terrorists. Tzfati and Weimann (1999, 2002) applied a systematic content analysis to a sample of terrorist sites, and repeated this analysis after three years (see Table 1).

What Is the Content of Terrorist Sites? They usually include information about the history of the organization and biographies of its leaders, founders, heroes, commanders, or revered personalities, information on the political and ideological aims of the organization, and up-to-date news. Most of the sites give a detailed historical review of the social and political background, a selective description of the organization's notable activities in the past, and its aims. Almost all the terror sites detail their goals in one way or another. The most common presentation of aims is through direct criticism of their enemies or rivals. The terrorist sites do not concentrate only on information concerning their organizations; direct attack on the enemy is the most common strategy of the Internet terrorists. By contrast, almost all sites avoid presenting and detail-

TABLE 1. Who Are the Terrorists on the Web? A List of Terrorist Groups Currently Using Websites[1]

1. Hamas (the Islamic Resistance Movement)
2. The Lebanese Hizbollah (Party of God)
3. The Egyptian Al-Gama'a al Islamiyya (Islamic Group, IG)
4. The Popular Front for the Liberation of Palestine (PLFP)
5. The Palestinian Islamic Jihad
6. The Peruvian Tupak-Amaru (MRTA)
7. 'The Shining Path' (Sendero Luminoso)
8. The Kahane Lives movement
9. The Basque ETA movement
10. The Irish Republican Army (IRA)
11. The Japanese Supreme Truth (Aum Shinrikyo)
12. The Colombian National Liberation Army (ELN-Colombia)
13. The Liberation Tigers of Tamil Eelam (LTTE)
14. The Armed Revolutionary Forces of Colombia (FARC)
15. The Popular Democratic Liberation Front Party in Turkey (DHKP/C)
16. The Kurdish Workers' Party (PKK)
17. The Zapatista National Liberation Army (ELNZ)
18. The Japanese Red Army (JRA)
19. The Islamic Movement of Uzbekistan (IMU)
20. The People's Mujahedin of Iran (PMOI–Mujahedin-e Khalq)

All these organizations not only pursue the peaceful act of establishing Internet sites, but also engage in actual violence (some of them with a long record that includes killings, kidnapping, assaults, and bombings).

ing their violent activities. While avoiding the violent aspects of their activities, the Internet terrorists, regardless of their nature, motives, or location, usually stress two issues: freedom of expression and political prisoners. The terrorists appear to aim at Western audiences, who are sensitive to the norms of freedom of expression and human rights and thus emphasize the issues that provoke sympathy in democratic societies.

What Is the Rhetoric of Terrorist Sites? Tzfati and Weimann (2002) found four rhetorical structures frequently used on the terrorist sites, all used to justify the use of violence. The first one is the "no choice" motive. Violence is presented as a necessity foisted upon the weak as the only means with which to deal with an oppressive enemy. A second rhetorical structure related to the legitimacy of the use of violence is the demonizing and de-legitimization of the enemy. The members of the movement or organization are presented as freedom fighters, forced against their will to use violence because a ruthless enemy is crushing the rights and dignity of their people or group. The enemy of the movement or the organization is the real terrorist, many sites insist, and "our violence is dwarfed in comparison with his aggression" is a routine slogan. Terrorist rhetoric tries to shift the responsibility to the opponent, displaying his brutality, his inhumanity, and his immorality. The violence of the 'freedom' and 'liberation' movements is dwarfed beside the cruelty of the opponent. The third rhetorical tactic is to emphasize weakness. The organizations attempt to substantiate the claim that terror is the weapon of the weak. As noted earlier, despite the ever-present vocabulary of 'the armed struggle' or 'resistance,' the terror sites avoid mentioning or noting how they victimize others. Finally, in the fourth method, the actions of the authorities against the terror groups are heavily stressed, usually with words such as 'slaughter,' 'murder,' 'genocide,' and the like. The organization is constantly being persecuted, its leaders are subject to assassination attempts and its supporters massacred, its freedom of expression is curtailed, and its adherents are arrested. This tactic, which portrays the organization as small, weak, and hunted down by a power or a strong state, turns the terrorists into the underdog.

Whom Do the Internet Terrorists Target with Their Sites? Are they appealing to potential supporters, to their enemies (i.e., the public who are part of the opposing socio-political community in the conflict), or are they targeting international public opinion? An analysis of their contents indicates an attempt to approach all three audiences. Reaching out to supporters is evinced from the fact that the sites offer appropriate items for sale, including printed shirts, badges, flags, and video and audiocassettes. The slogans at these sites also appeal strongly to the supporter public. Of course, the sites in local languages target these audiences more directly. These sites include much more detailed information about recent activities of the organizations and about internal politics (i.e., the relationship between local groups). But an important target audience, in addition to supporters of the organizations, is the international 'bystander' public and surfers who are not involved in the conflict. This is evident from the presentation of basic information about the organization and the extensive historical background material (with which the supporter public is presumably familiar). Similarly, the sites make use of English in addition to the local language of the organization's supporters. Judging from the content of many of the sites, one might also infer that journalists constitute another bystander target audience. Press releases by the organizations are often placed on the websites. The detailed background information might also be useful for international reporters. One of Hizbollah's sites specifically addresses journalists and invites them to interact with the organization's press office via e-mail. Approaches to the 'enemy' audiences are not as clearly apparent from the content of many sites. However, in some sites the desire to reach this audience is evident in the efforts to demoralize the enemy or to create feelings of guilt. The organizations try to utilize the websites to change public opinion in their enemies' states, to weaken public support for the governing regime, to stimulate public debate, and of course to demoralize the enemy. A good example is the following declaration by a Hizbollah leader: "By means of the Internet

Hizbollah has succeeded in entering the homes of Israelis, creating an important psychological breakthrough" (Rapoport, 1998, p. 16).

CONCLUSION

The emergence of media-oriented terrorism presents a tough challenge to democratic societies and their liberal values. The threat is not limited to media manipulation and psychological warfare launched by terrorists; it also includes the danger of restrictions imposed on the freedom of the press and freedom of expression by those who try to fight terrorism. One should consider that the fear that terrorism generates can be, and in the past has been, manipulated by politicians to pass questionable legislation, undermining individual rights and liberties, that otherwise wouldn't stand a chance of being accepted by the public. After the September 11 attack in New York and Washington, the U.S. House of Representatives approved an anti-terrorism bill that gave law enforcement officials expanded surveillance powers to monitor Internet behavior and e-mail. The tool they use to conduct that investigation is the controversial e-mail surveillance system, Carnivore. This is one example of the hidden threat of modern terrorism, which causes an infringement on basic democratic and liberal values (see also Strossen, this volume). The challenge facing democratic societies by modern media-wise terrorism should lead to collaboration among the mass media, the administration and the academic community. Only by reaching self-imposed restrictions and guidelines, based on empirical findings, can we attempt to find optimal ways of maximizing security while minimizing the damages to the free flow of information and civil rights. This requires an open debate, bargaining and negotiation among the administration, security officials and representatives of the mass media, a process that should be directed and navigated by scholars and researchers who come from the disciplines of communication, psychology, terrorism and civil rights.

REFERENCES

Bell, J. B. (1978). Terrorist script and live-action spectaculars. *Columbia Journalism Review, 17*(1), 47-50.

Brosius, H. B., & Weimann, G. (1991). The contagiousness of mass-mediated terrorism. *European Journal of Communication, 6*, 63-75.

Dobson, C., & Paine, R. (1977). *The Carlos complex: A pattern of violence*. London: Hodder and Stoughton.

Dowling, R. E. (1986). Terrorism and the media: A rhetorical genre. *Journal of Communication, 56*(1), 12-24.

Jenkins, B. (1975). *International terrorism.* Los Angeles: Crescent Publication.

Karber, P. (1971). Urban terrorism: Baseline data and a conceptual framework. *Social Science Quarterly, 52*, 527-33.

Marighela, C. (1971a). *For the liberation of Brazil.* Harmondsworth: Pelican.

Marighela, C. (1971b). Minimanual of the urban guerrilla. In J. Mallin (Ed.), *Terror and the urban guerrilla* (in Appendix). Coral Gables, FL: University of Miami Press.

Rapoport, A. (1998, December 16). Hizbollah On-line, Yediot Aharonot, p. 16.

Schmid, A., & de Graaf, J. (1982). *Violence as communication.* Beverly Hills: Sage.

Strossen, N. (2004). Terrorism's toll on civil liberties. *Journal of Aggression, Maltreatment, & Trauma, 9*(1/2/3/4), 365-377.

Tzfati, Y., & Weimann, G. (1999). Terror on the Internet. *Politika, 4*, 45-64.

Tzfati, Y., & Weimann, G. (2002). www.terrorism.com: Terror on the Internet. *Studies in Conflict and Terrorism, 25*(5), 317-332.

Weimann, G. (1983). The theater of terror: Effects of press coverage. *Journal of Communication, 33*, 38-45.

Weimann, G. (1986). Mass mediated theater of terror: Must the show go on? In P. Bruck (Ed.), *The news media and terrorism* (pp. 1-22). Ottawa: Carleton University Press.

Weimann, G. (1987). Media events: The case of international terrorism. *Journal of Broadcasting and Electronic Media, 31*(1), 21-39.

Weimann, G. (1999). The theater of terror as a challenge to democracy. In R. Cohen-Almagor (Ed.), *Basic issues in Israeli democracy* (pp. 247-264). Tel Aviv: Sifriat Poalim.

Weimann, G., & Brosius, H. B. (1989). The predictability of international terrorism: A time-series analysis. *Terrorism, 11*(6), 491-502.

Weimann, G., & Brosius, H. B. (1991). The newsworthiness of international terrorism. *Communication Research, 18*(3), 333-354.

Weimann, G., & Winn, C. (1994). *The theater of terror: Mass media and international terrorism.* New York: Longman.

Guide:
Media Guidelines:
From the "Trauma Vortex"
to the "Healing Vortex"

Gina Ross

The media can play a leadership role in helping to reduce individual and national traumatic reactivity by understanding the intrinsic connection between violence and trauma. They can begin by assessing the impact of tragedy, violence and terror on their own perceptions and how it affects their reporting of events. The goal is to lessen the results of traumatic reactivity on themselves, the public, and politics.

A nation hit by terrorist attacks may well keep its initial reaction of panic, fear, helplessness and impulsivity. But it can also take the path of awareness and use this opportunity for transformation. By helping to inform a nation of healthy coping mechanisms and healing, we can strengthen resiliency and take the critical time to address root causes that could lead to mediation and the hopeful extinguishing of terrorism. *To address trauma at mass levels, we need mass information and the help of mass media* (Ross, 2003).

The media are an asset for helping people deal with fear and terror. They can be the perfect vehicle to introduce a common and shorthand language that

Address correspondence to: Gina Ross, MFCT, 269 South Lorraine Boulevard, Los Angeles, CA 90004 USA (E-mail: ginaross@aol.com).

[Haworth co-indexing entry note]: "Guide: Media Guidelines: From the 'Trauma Vortex' to the 'Healing Vortex'." Ross, Gina. Co-published simultaneously in *Journal of Aggression, Maltreatment & Trauma* (The Haworth Maltreatment & Trauma Press, an imprint of The Haworth Press, Inc.) Vol. 9, No. 3/4, 2004; and: *The Trauma of Terrorism: Sharing Knowledge and Shared Care, An International Handbook* (ed: Yael Danieli, Danny Brom, and Joe Sills) The Haworth Maltreatment & Trauma Press, an imprint of The Haworth Press, Inc., 2005.

can help recovery from collective traumatic events, stem recurring cycles of violence and begin cycles facilitating peace. The media's use of metaphoric language such as the *"trauma vortex and healing vortex"* (Levine, 1997, pp.197-199) can help develop this common language and transform destructive energies into creative and constructive movements.

Unresolved trauma sits stagnant in the body. A bio-psychological event that deregulates the nervous system, it affects biological, emotional, mental and social balance, hindering the innate ability for self-regulation (Levine, 1997; Van der Kolk, 1996). At the individual level, the "trauma vortex" metaphor helps illustrate trauma's dynamic nature and how it rivets attention and pulls towards repetition, creating a downward spiral. At the collective level, the metaphor illustrates trauma's contagiousness and magnetic pull and its capacity to destroy people and projects (Ross, 2003). Action or language generating fear, rage, hopelessness, victimization, and violence fuels the "trauma vortex" (Ross, 2003).

The good news: also contagious, the "healing vortex" illustrates an opposite and upward spiraling effect, and refers to mankind's ability to cope and heal. It generates a language supporting trust, self-control, hope, creative problem solving, and the cultivation of healing (Ross, 2003; Staub, 1989). It requires developing sufficient internal, external and collective resources, whichever helps us feel better (Ross, 2003).

THE ROLE OF THE MEDIA

Overexposure to the details of death, destruction, and hatred is destabilizing, terrifying and enraging to the public (Ross, 2003). Adding healing aspects to coverage, such as how people cope and care, the media can help reassure and promote hope and meaning. Media activities designed to help the public shift "from the trauma vortex into the healing vortex" are simple and come under the following categories:

Protecting the Public from Secondhand Trauma

1. Frontline media professionals monitor their own levels of traumatic stress, learning how to release safely and discharge traumatic energies.
2. Asking the following guiding questions:
   Have we balanced the coverage of the trauma vortex with coverage of the healing vortex? Is caring for the victims obvious (Cote & Simpson, 2000)? Has secondhand trauma determined the pull for repeated trauma-driven coverage? Are ratings indicators of public opinion or simply indicators of secondhand trauma-driven attention?

3. Warning viewers of upcoming disturbing sounds/images. Children and sensitive viewers are vulnerable to traumatic images on television.
4. Recognizing the impact of language (i.e., predictions of doom) on a public in shock (Ross, 2003).
5. Encouraging viewers to watch the news in small doses. They need to be informed, but also "resourced" in between viewing (Ross, 2003).
6. Avoiding excessive use of gory details (Cote & Simpson, 2000).
7. Avoiding repetitive showing of the same traumatic images. Repetition drives traumatic images deeper, putting people at risk for flashbacks and panic (Thoman, 1993).
8. Heavy focus on negative news reinforces fears and desires for revenge.
9. Being aware that non-governmental organizations (NGOs) and U.N. personnel, who are also vulnerable to secondhand trauma, may not be "impartial witnesses." They may be pulled into the traumatic narrative of the people they are helping (Ross, 2003).

Informing and Encouraging the Public

1. Normalizing initial traumatic responses and cautioning about the characteristics of unresolved trauma, including that trauma impairs the ability to think clearly.
2. Providing information on cutting-edge coping and healing methods and working in tandem with trauma expertise.
3. Informing the public of all available help during and after tragic events.
4. Running videos on emotional first aid.
5. Inserting images inspiring trust: acts of kindness and compassion and stories of courage and perseverance.
6. Continued reporting of individual and group recovery (i.e., vigils, healing rituals) helps communities overcome feelings of helplessness or dread and recuperate hope (Cote & Simpson, 2000).

The media's leadership in handling trauma can lead the way for other sectors that have the potential to amplify unwittingly the "trauma vortex" or promote the "healing vortex." Whether regarding the microcosm of an individual, or the macrocosm of a people, trauma awareness and healing by mental health and medical professionals, schools, justice systems, clergies, diplomats, NGOs, political leaders, and militaries can help the world counter terrorism.

REFERENCES

Cote, W., & Simpson, R. (2000). *Covering violence: A guide to ethical reporting about victims and trauma.* New York: Columbia University Press.

Levine, P. (1997). *Waking the tiger: Healing trauma.* Berkeley, CA: North Atlantic Books.

Ross, G. (2003). *Beyond the trauma vortex: The media's role in healing fear, terror and violence.* Berkeley, CA: North Atlantic Books.

Staub, E. (1989). The roots of evil: The psychological and cultural origins of genocide. Cambridge, UK: Cambridge University Press.

Thoman, E. (1993). *Beyond blame: Media literacy as violence prevention.* Center for Media Literacy, 62.

Van der Kolk, B. A. (1996). *The body keeps the score: Approaches to the psychobiology of posttraumatic stress disorder.* New York: Guilford.

Voice:
Wrong Place at the Wrong Time

Chris Cramer

"We supply the ink . . . others supply the blood."

I forget who said it, but it has real resonance and takes on real meaning for journalists when we experience terrorism close up and personal. My awakening came on a dull April morning in 1980 when, fresh back from an assignment for BBC News in Zimbabwe, I found myself, bad tempered and tired, waiting in a downstairs office inside the Iranian Embassy in Knightsbridge, London.

I was sweating on an entry visa to visit Tehran to cover the capture of American hostages by Iranian dissidents in that troubled country. Phone calls and faxes to the embassy had gone unanswered so, ever the arrogant journalist, I had arranged to bang the tables in frustration at the London embassy itself, and hopefully, walk away with my passport stamped. It wasn't to be.

With exquisite irony, urban terrorism confronted me, not overseas but in my own country, at the embassy itself, when six armed gunmen smashed and shot their way into the London building and rounded up me and two dozen or so other hapless souls. I have one burning memory of that experience, and it stays with me more than two decades later. A diminutive Arab boy, headscarf

Address correspondence to: Chris Cramer, Managing Director, CNN International ONE, CNN Center 6SW636A, Atlanta, GA 30303 USA (E-mail: chris.cramer@cnn.com).

[Haworth co-indexing entry note]: "Voice: Wrong Place at the Wrong Time." Cramer, Chris. Co-published simultaneously in *Journal of Aggression, Maltreatment & Trauma* (The Haworth Maltreatment & Trauma Press, an imprint of The Haworth Press, Inc.) Vol. 9, No. 3/4, 2004; and: *The Trauma of Terrorism: Sharing Knowledge and Shared Care, An International Handbook* (ed: Yael Danieli, Danny Brom, and Joe Sills) The Haworth Maltreatment & Trauma Press, an imprint of The Haworth Press, Inc., 2005.

wrapped tightly around his head, a machine pistol clutched tightly in his tiny hand, and a bright green hand grenade in the other. I say "boy" because he was barely 20, scared half as much as me, bright flashing eyes and a nervous habit of jumping to the left and then to the right, like a crab disturbed on a beach. Something even more frightening occurred next. His fingers snatched out the safety pin of the hand grenade and pushed it toward me, and then he smiled with his eyes and replaced it again.

Terrorism for me was the collapse of my own self-esteem, a slow, terrifying realization that a child with a gun and explosives could overpower me physically, and more seriously, mentally. Your emotions shut down when you are at the mercy of a terrorist. You seek to shrink into the carpet and out of sight. Out of sight and hopefully out of mind.

And then, in my case, your journalistic instincts fire up and you slip into type. "I work for the BBC," I said "Can I help you get your message and your demands to the authorities on the outside? Maybe telex the outside world? Maybe interview your leader?" At this distance of time, it seems pathetic. And yet, when confronted by the modern day terrorist, it is perhaps all you can do to reassert your dignity, a small clutch at a straw before you slip under the water.

My captors allowed me to do my job and telex their demands to the British police and government of Margaret Thatcher. They let me set up phone calls to the BBC to interview them and set out their list of ridiculous instructions: freedom for their fellow fighters in Iran, political representation, free passage to a country of their choice. Their list was endless and destined to fail, though it came with a threat to kill all of us, all the hostages, if their demands were not met.

Despite this and in a moment of singular stupidity, I decided to try and pass vital details about the terrorists and their weaponry to the authorities. I hadn't realized that the terrorist leader, Salim, understood more English than he spoke and during a telephone call to my colleagues at the BBC, he exploded in anger, screaming and jabbing me with his pistol.

I realized then that journalists are not a protected species. We have no guardian angel hovering over us to protect the free flow of information that we believe in so deeply. We are just human beings, as fragile as the rest of the population. That night, I decided that escape from the embassy was the only defense for me. A minor stomach ailment, a legacy from my recent trip to Africa, was going to be my passport out of the building and out of this particular horror. For the next 12 hours, I willed myself into a state of anxiety and illness and the following morning, at a little after 11 AM, I was carried, writhing in pain, to the front door of the embassy and bundled out onto the street outside.

"Walk straight ahead," said the terrorists. "If you look behind you, or turn left or turn right, we will kill you."

I did their bidding. I walked in a crouch across the road and past the parked cars in the street outside, eventually ducking down behind one of them and waiting until two plain clothed police officers picked me up and carried me to a waiting ambulance.

The Iranian Embassy Siege in London lasted another four days, and after one hostage was brutally murdered, was ended when Prime Minister Thatcher sent in soldiers from Britain's Special Air Service (SAS), motto "Who Dares Wins," to smash the siege and rescue the remaining hostages. A second hostage was shot in the final seconds of the siege, and all but one of the terrorists was killed by the SAS.

The after-effects of that brief encounter with terrorism stayed with me for at least a decade. It changed my professional ambitions to be a war correspondent and haunted me privately for longer than I thought possible. It also made me a better person and a better journalist. Once you have experienced terrorism for what it is, for the horror it is designed to bring, it changes the way you report on it. It makes you ultra sensitive to the victims.

If you look, albeit briefly, into your own open grave and have the fortune to walk away, you capture a new enthusiasm for life. It is never again possible to be a cynic.

Cultural Issues in Terrorism
and in Response to Terrorism

Kathleen Nader
Yael Danieli

SUMMARY. Among the multiple causes of terrorism is a clash of cultures. Trauma and the destruction of culture may create fertile ground for violent cultures and future terrorists. Cultural differences are important elements in the prevention, assessment, and treatment of post-terrorism psychological sequelae. Cultural and spiritual practices have been used or adapted to reduce anxiety, enhance recovery, and provide supplemental interventions. Learning within a community and engaging community and religious leaders, community members, and the individual patient in order to be guided by the specific needs of a group or an individual is essential to effective interventions following terrorism.

address: *<docdelivery@haworthpress.com>* *Website:*

KEYWORDS. Culture, terrorism, coping, violence, religion, spiritual, gender, individual, collective, regression, suicide bombers, shame, stigma, rituals

---

Address correspondence to: Kathleen Nader, DSW, Two Suns, 2809 Rathlin Drive, Suite 102, Cedar Park, TX 78613 USA (E-mail: knader@twosuns.org).

[Haworth co-indexing entry note]: "Cultural Issues in Terrorism and in Response to Terrorism." Nader, Kathleen, and Yael Danieli. Co-published simultaneously in *Journal of Aggression, Maltreatment & Trauma* (The Haworth Maltreatment & Trauma Press, an imprint of The Haworth Press, Inc.) Vol. 9, No. 3/4, 2004; and: *The Trauma of Terrorism: Sharing Knowledge and Shared Care, An International Handbook* (ed: Yael Danieli, Danny Brom, and Joe Sills) The Haworth Maltreatment & Trauma Press, an imprint of The Haworth Press, Inc., 2005.

Cultural, religious, and ethnic differences are important elements in the prevention, assessment, and treatment of post-terrorism psychological sequelae. Cultural issues may contribute to the emergence of terrorism, reactions to terrorism, and recovery from terrorism. Culture, thus, can function as an instigator, buffer, healer, and transmitter of trauma (Danieli, 1998, 2003; also see Introduction, this volume).

CULTURAL ISSUES IN THE EMERGENCE OF TERRORISM

Clash of Cultures

> It is my hypothesis that the fundamental source of conflict in this new world will not be primarily ideological or primarily economic. The great divisions among humankind and the dominating source of conflict will be cultural. . . . The fault lines between civilizations will be the battle lines of the future. . . . Civilizations are differentiated from each other by history, language, culture, tradition, and, most important, religion. The people of different civilizations have different views on the relations between God and man, the individual and the group, the citizen and the state, parents and children, husband and wife, as well as differing views of the relative importance of rights and responsibilities, liberty and authority, equality and hierarchy. These differences are the product of centuries. (Huntington, 1993, pp. 22-24)

Cultural issues have played an important part in the hatred and violence that led to September 11 and to other acts of terrorism. Although the causes of war-analogous conditions such as terrorism are multiple (e.g., reactions against inequality or perceived tyrannical bullying; the struggle for power and resources; issues of exclusion or abandonment), they often include a clash of cultures or factions (Canada & the World Backgrounder, 2003; Huntington, 1993, 2001; Picco, this volume). For example, the war between the former Yugoslavian republics included a clash among the predominantly Orthodox Serbs, Macedonians, and Montenegrins, the predominantly Roman Catholic Croats and Slovenes, and the increasing number of Bosnian Muslims (Mooren & Kleber, 1999). Much of the current threat of terrorism is that of Islamic factions against the West. In 2001, the United States was the target of 63% of international terrorist attacks (Canada & the World Backgrounder, 2003). Huntington (1993) outlined the following as perceptions pertinent to this terrorism: inequality between the West and the world of Islam; America as a bully, backing corrupt regimes; America as a decadent society (obsessed with materialism, the glorification of violence and sex) that puts the needs of the rich above those of others and flaunts a belief in its superiority; and that Islam is convinced of its cultural superiority and is obsessed with the inferiority of its power. Others have suggested that the combination of factors contributing to the culture clash includes the faulty wielding of power and the use of the traumatized and humiliated by terrorist groups (Scheff, 1997; Volkan, 2001; see The Construction of a Violent Culture below).

Polls show that Arab Middle Easterners value American technology, education, democracy, and the potential for advancement but abhor its Middle Eastern policies and its morality (e.g., dating practices, premarital birth control, women living alone, explicit movies, the divorce rate, acceptance of homosexuality; Canada & the World Backgrounder, 2003; Inglehart & Norris, 2003; Meleis, 2003). Inglehart and Norris (2003) suggest that the cultural fault line is primarily about gender equality and sexual liberation. According to Meleis (2003), if asked, Middle Eastern men would describe a fear that, under American influence, their women would adopt Western values that separate them from established cultural, family, and, religious values (e.g., their daughters would lose their virginity, their wives would dominate them).

The Destruction of Culture

The destruction of culture (as a consequence of colonization, oppression, war, or terrorism) itself has traumatic effects (Danieli, 1998; Kinzie, Bohnlein, & Sack, 1998; Kupelian, Kalayjian, & Kassabian, 1998; see also Duran, Duran, Brave Heart, & Yellow Horse-Davis, 1998). The devastation of cultural identity with an accelerated loss of language, customs, and values, personal and economic status, and individual and collective power may result in intense responses of helplessness and estrangement (Nagata, 1998). Kinzie et al. (1998) suggest that trauma-related accelerated de-acculturation has resulted in, among other things, the breaking down of social values, which has a major consequence for the traumatized and succeeding generations.

Lira (2001) has delineated the use of predominant ideological arguments that lead to social division and polarization and then make one group the target of violence, thereby enhancing the power of another group. The target group or subculture is defined in some negative way (e.g., as outsiders, enemies, subversives, criminals, terrorists, infidels, evil, non-religious; see Cromer, this volume) that makes their actions unacceptable and strips their members of their humanity. Violence toward the identified group then appears to be legitimate (Lira, 2001; Scheff, 1997; Volkan, 2001), and the victimizers characterize themselves as defenders, saviors, or heroes rather than perpetrators. These techniques have been used in the partial or attempted destruction of cultures during genocides (e.g., the Nazi Holocaust, Bosnia, Rwanda) and by terrorists (e.g., Al Qaeda; see Picco, this volume).

The Construction of a Violent Culture

Similar to war-like conditions, ongoing terrorism can create a culture of death, terror, and violence that remains a part of a national psyche and of the psyches of the people themselves (Awwad, 1999; Bar-On, 1999; Lira, 2001; Nader, 2003, 2004). For example, according to Lira, political repression and violence in Chilean society resulted in a "culture of death and terror," a rigid social framework, sociopolitical polarization, constrained and ruptured sense of everyday life, weakened personal autonomy and self-confidence, and the devaluation of human life.

Techniques that neutralize the norms that oppose crime/violence provide a cultural foundation for violence (described by Alvarez, 1997 and Sykes & Matza, 1957 in Scheff, 1997). The techniques include: (a) Denial of responsibility (e.g., "only carrying out orders"; "sanctioned by God"); (b) Denial of injury (e.g., euphemisms such as "ethnic cleansing"); (c) Blaming the victim (e.g., the victim brought it on himself); (d) Condemning the condemners (e.g., suggesting that the countries denouncing these actions are guilty of worse crimes such as mistreatment of native inhabitants of their lands/colonies or of specific races); (e) Appeal to higher loyalties (e.g., patriotic, religious); and (f) Denial of humanity (e.g., the Nazi portrayal of Jews, Serbs' portrayal of Bosnians).

Post-trauma cultures are often characterized by hatred and rage. Scheff (1997) suggests that hatred and rage are products of unacknowledged emotions (e.g., those generated [or exacerbated] by alienation and by cultural scripts for demonizing purported enemies). For example, when feelings of rejection or inadequacy are unacknowledged, the subsequent rage and aggression may mask shame. This composite of shame and anger becomes rage, "the motor of violence." Scheff concludes that any steps that decrease mass alienation (e.g., providing post-disaster assistance, desired reconstruction, genuine regret/sorrow/shame for directly or indirectly inflicting harm) lessen pressure toward conflict.

Volkan (2001) suggests that large-group regression (i.e., a return to some of the fears, wishes, expectations, and defense mechanisms from an earlier stage of development) follows massive traumas, humiliation, or the impositions of a regressed, paranoid leader. This regression includes attempts to repair, maintain, or protect the large-group identity and to separate it from "the enemy's" identity. A strong leader and his cohorts may reinforce the group's symptoms and either encourages its members to remain regressed or to progress. A regressed society imposes rigid obligations that must be obeyed at all times while permitting what would normally be considered antisocial or antihuman behaviors. The world is perceived as a place of lurking dangers. Fears and other internal demons (e.g., rage) are projected onto "the enemy" or other. "They" (the demonized others) are all bad; "we" (their own ethnic/cultural group) are all good. "They" are associated with things foul, made less human, and ultimately dehumanized, thus making their killing or torture justified (Volkan, 2001). Chosen historical traumas are reactivated by new collective traumas, folklore (e.g., myths, songs) and rituals are created, and at the same time parts of history may be erased in order to confirm these beliefs and to fuel aggression or a sense of victimhood (Klain, 1998; Volkan, 2001).

Post-trauma group regression, with its real or fantasized humiliation or victimization, forms a fertile ground for the creation of suicide bombers and other terrorists (Scheff, 1997; Volkan, 2001). Volkan (2001) defines the two essentials for creating suicide bombers: a youth whose personal identity is already disturbed and who is seeking an outside source to stabilize this disturbed inner world, and a training method that forces a large-group identity to fill the damaged or subjugated individual identity. Youth who have endured concrete traumas (i.e., actual humiliation such as loss of a parent, beating, or torture by an enemy; e.g., in the Gaza strip, Afghanistan) are the best candidates to become suicide bombers/killers, because there is a natural match between their developmentally normative search for identity and autonomy, and the struggle for autonomy of the group. Their education is most easily accomplished when a religious element of group identity provides a solution for a personal sense of shame, humiliation, or helplessness. Sanctioned by God, they may feel a sense of omnipotence in carrying out their acts of destruction. The killings are ritualized and made psychologically easy (Volkan, 2001).

CULTURAL ISSUES IN THE AFTERMATH OF TERRORISM

After terrorist acts as well as after other traumatic experiences, understanding culture is integral to understanding the predicaments of trauma survivors and their families, whether or not their cultural identity played a role in their victimization and perhaps more so if it did. Many clinicians consider it essential to use culturally appropriate therapies incorporating elements of traditional culture into the healing process (Duran et al., 1998; Weine, Danieli, Silove, Van Ommeren, Fairbank, & Saul, 2002). Particularly following war or other conflict, a central challenge is to transform the destructive use of culture into a healing one. In countries recovering from war, combining culturally-sensitive therapies leading to the restoration of traditional skills and values with a program of national reconciliation offers hope to the remnants of indigenous people, as well as to former warring parties.

Numerous cultural issues are important to post-terrorism interventions. The importance of reading and learning about the cultural group to unearth an individual's cultural story cannot be overemphasized. We must know what to look for, what and how to ask, and how our own cultural lenses and biases motivate us to organize our thinking, anchor our lives, blind us to the unfamiliar and unrecognizable (Laird, 1998; Weine et al., 2002), and impede our ability to help.

Spiritual and Religious Beliefs as Coping Strategies

Every individual in a particular culture or subculture learns to use culturally specific coping strategies to promote health and development and to deal with stress (Shiang, 2000). For example, after 9/11 the New York Asian community used cleansing (e.g., to clear away the evil) and other protection practices to reduce anxiety. Some religions (e.g., Buddhist, Hindu) provide an answer (e.g., karma) for the question asked frequently following tragedy: Why (me, him, her, us)? Some faiths (e.g., Jewish, Muslim, Christian) assign practices to ward off future suffering, to make amends, or to overcome guilt (New Advent, 2001; Shu`aib, 2001; Strassfeld, 1985). Prescribed rituals assist us through life's transitions, difficulties, social interactions, group bonding, and separations. They have been used therapeutically following terrorism and other violent experiences (Johnson, Feldman, Lubin, & Southwick, 1995). At the same time, infusing a large-group identity and altering religious rituals have been used to create terrorists from youth seeking a method of coping with a damaged identity.

Religious or spiritual beliefs may influence or dictate responses to crisis (e.g., culpability, view of therapy, coping strategies, needed rituals; Bibb & Casimir, 1996; McGoldrick, 1996). In a crisis, beliefs may either function as a source of comfort and as anchors or may promote a sense of hopelessness and helplessness (Hines, 1998; Tully, 1999). Medical studies have confirmed that faith, prayer, and rituals have strengthened health and healing presumably by triggering emotions that influence the immune and cardiovascular systems (Walsh, 1998; see also Davidowitz-Farkas & Hutchinson-Hall, this volume). Congruence between beliefs and practices may generate an overall sense of well-being and wholeness; incongruence may induce shame or guilt (Walsh, 1998).

Religion has been an important part of the recovery process following war or terrorism. Church/temple/mosque attendance has often increased. Religious beliefs and practices have been frequently used to reconstruct a meaningful narrative following traumatic experiences (Ogden, Kaminer,Van Kradenburg, Seedat, &

Stein, 2000). The injustice and senselessness of trauma/terrorism and suffering belong in the spiritual dimension as well. Traumatic events have precipitated the questioning of long-held spiritual beliefs and a quest for something new that can be sustaining (Peterson, 2002; Walsh, 1998). Spiritual distress can impede coping and the sense that life has meaning. Spiritual renewal can be found in a variety of ways (e.g., rituals, nature, beauty, spiritual teachings and places, music or dance, love, and transporting imaginations; Tully, 1999; Walsh, 1998).

Rituals

Ninety-five percent of the respondents to Danieli's surveys of the 9/11 anniversaries mentioned the importance of public and private rituals (in Spratt, 2002). To be therapeutic, rituals must help manage stressful emotions (e.g., grief, anger, shock) and provide symbolic enactments that may serve as metaphors for transformation (e.g., of feelings, of injured relationships, of disturbed social connection). Johnson et al. (1995) suggest that the ritual situations must contain rather than suppress emotions, permit more individual expression, designate specific times for spontaneous comments or actions, and allow for greater arousal of the disturbing experience toward greater catharsis.

Funerals, the need to have or view a deceased body, and grieving vary across and within cultures. Whether funerals are somber and silent or loud, celebratory or mournful, or distracting or focused on the death varies by culture (Mooren & Kleber, 1999; Peddle, Monteiro, Guluma, & Macaulay, 1999; Tully, 1999). Following the September 11 terrorist attacks, many bodies were never found. In their place, dust from the World Trade Center location, donated blood, or body parts have served as concrete representations or for burial (Yee, 2003).

Providing Mental Health Interventions

Although "Western" societies tend to be individualistic rather than collectivistic, many American subcultures include interdependence as an essential value (e.g., African American, Chinese American; Boyd-Franklin & Franklin, 1998; Watson, 1998). At the center of individualistic societies is the relatively isolated nuclear family (Falicov, 1998). In contrast, in interdependence-based cultures (e.g., Asian Indian; Japanese), the nuclear family is embedded in an extended network. The marital tie is not elevated above other ties. Lifelong parent-child bonds insure continuity with the family of origin. The "familial self" (as opposed to the "individual self") entails connectedness; emotional involvement, empathy with and receptivity to the family of origin; and strong identification with the honor and reputation of the extended family over attachments to outsiders (Falicov, 1998). Most psychological theories were developed in Western Europe and White North America and consider individual self-worth as primary. Concepts such as individual destiny, responsibility, legitimacy, and even human rights, as well as self, assertiveness, and fulfillment are central to most related therapies (Waldegrave, 1998). In contrast, questions of self-exposure and self-assertion are confusing or even alienating for people who come from communal or extended family cultures, where questions about the self can be considered intrusive and rude (Waldegrave, 1998).

In some cultures, expressing mental health problems is associated with shame or stigma (Kinzie, 1993; Shiang, 2000). They may express emotional problems through somatic complaints, as complaining of physical symptoms allows the elicitation of support without the implied stigmatization (Shiang, 2000). The taboo against having mental problems may be greater for males in some cultures (e.g., Hispanic, Arabic). The length of time (weeks, months, or years) it takes for a person to reveal the extent of personal traumatic reactions varies by culture as well (Kinzie, 1993).

Many of New York's approximately 800,000 Asian residents came to the United States from the war zones of Vietnam, Laos, and North Korea in order to feel safe (Kinzie, this volume). In addition, their livelihood was affected by the 9/11 destruction as well as by the subsequent SARS scare. The latter exacerbated their isolation and escalated their fears (Hall, Norwood, Fullerton, Gifford, & Ursano, this volume). A quick phone survey in English completed one month after 9/11 (Yee, 2003) suggested that, although Asians were in closer proximity to the terrorist attacks and more exposed, they had the least anxiety, followed by Blacks and then Latinos. Yee (2003) believes that the real truth is that Asian people were not willing to discuss their anxiety on the phone or with someone who was not speaking their language. They would have been more willing to discuss their symptoms in person, with individuals speaking their own language who would make them feel comfortable. Deeply conscious of the associated stigmatization, they do not verbalize their discomfort and avoid seeking assistance. Even Asian clinicians are reluctant to admit to mental health problems in their own family members. Folk remedies (e.g., placing garlic around the room to dispel evil) and prescribed actions (e.g., marrying a mentally ill offspring to someone healthy to counteract the bad karma) are used instead.

To address this resistance, Yee (2003) and his colleagues recruited well-respected community members (e.g., pastors and pastors' wives among Koreans, respected members of the Buddhist Temple, the garment factory union, ex-restaurant workers, and teachers) rather than clinicians to engage in outreach and trained them to use some simple counseling techniques (providing a supportive presence, advocacy, breathing techniques, re-engagement in normal activities including pleasurable ones).

Articles and voices in this volume (e.g., see Davidowitz-Farkas & Hutchinson-Hall, Engdahl, Bar-on, Solomon, Somasundaram, and Thielman) contain numerous additional examples of culture-bound effects of terrorism and culture-sensitive interventions.

CONCLUSIONS

The causes of terrorism are multiple. Terrorism often develops on the basis of a clash of cultures with fault lines along civilizations with varying histories, values, religious heritages, and gender-related issues. Traumatic in itself, the actual or feared destruction of culture may create fertile ground for violent cultures and the education of future terrorists.

Cultural, religious, and ethnic differences are important elements in the prevention, assessment, and treatment of post-terrorism psychological sequelae. Cultural and spiritual practices have been used or adapted to reduce anxiety, enhance recovery, and provide supplemental interventions. A deep appreciation of an individual's and family's culture, historical roots, beliefs, and views of mental health and healing requires an ongoing commitment to building knowledge. Learning within a community, engaging community and religious leaders as well as its members, and the individual patient in order to be guided by the specific needs of the group or an individual is essential to effective interventions following terrorism.

REFERENCES

Awwad, E. (1999). Between trauma and recovery: Some perspectives on Palestinian's vulnerability and adaptation. In K. Nader, N. Dubrow, & B. Stamm (Eds.), *Honoring differences: Cultural issues in the treatment of traumatic stress* (pp. 234-256). Philadelphia: Taylor & Francis.

Bar-On, D. (1999). Israeli society between the culture of death and the culture of life. In K. Nader, N. Dubrow, & B. Stamm (Eds.), *Honoring differences: Cultural issues in the treatment of traumatic stress* (pp. 211-233). Philadelphia: Taylor & Francis.

Bibb, A., & Casimir, G. J. (1996). Haitian families. In M. McGoldrick, J. Giordano, & J. Pearce (Eds.), *Ethnicity and family therapy* (pp. 86-111). New York: Guilford Press.

Boyd-Franklin, N., & Franklin, A. J. (1998). African American couples in therapy. In M. McGoldrick (Ed.), *Re-visioning family therapy* (pp. 268-281). New York: Guilford.

Canada & the World Backgrounder. (2003). Clash of civilizations? *Canada & the World Backgrounder, 68*(5), 17-21.

Cromer, G. (2004). A terrorist tale. *Journal of Aggression, Maltreatment & Trauma, 9*(1/2/3/4), 45-55.

Danieli, Y. (Ed.) (1998). *An international handbook of multigenerational legacies of trauma.* New York: Plenum Press.

Danieli, Y., Engdahl, B., & Schlenger, W. E. (2003). The psychological aftermath of terrorism. In F. M. Moghaddam & A. J. Marsella (Eds.), *Understanding terrorism: Psychological roots, consequences, and interventions* (pp. 223-246). Washington, DC: American Psychological Association.

Danieli, Y., Brom, D., & Sills, J.B. (Eds.). (2004). Introduction. *Journal of Aggression, Maltreatment & Trauma, 9*(1/2/3/4), 1-17.

Davidowitz-Farkas, Z., & Hutchinson-Hall, J. (2004). Religious care in coping with terrorism. *Journal of Aggression, Maltreatment & Trauma, 10*(1/2/3/4), 565-576.

Duran, E., Duran, B., Brave Heart, M., & Yellow Horse-Davis, S. (1998). Healing the American Indian soul wound. In Y. Danieli (Ed.), *An international handbook of multigenerational legacies of trauma* (pp. 341-354). New York: Plenum Press.

Engdahl, B. (2004). Integrating international findings on the impact of terrorism. *Journal of Aggression, Maltreatment & Trauma, 9*(1/2/3/4), 265-276.

Falicov, C. J. (1998). The cultural meaning of family triangles. In M. McGoldrick (Ed.), *Re-visioning family therapy* (pp. 37-49). New York: Guilford.

Hall, M. J., Norwood, A. E., Fullerton, C. S., Gifford, R., & Ursano, R. J. (2004). The psychological burden of bioterrorism. *Journal of Aggression, Maltreatment & Trauma, 9*(1/2/3/4), 293-305.

Hines, P. M. (1998). Climbing up the rough side of the mountain: Hope, culture, and therapy. In M. McGoldrick (Ed.), *Re-visioning family therapy* (pp. 78-89). New York: Guilford.

Huntington, S. P. (1993). The clash of civilizations? *Foreign Affairs, 72*(3), 22-50.

Huntington, S. P. (2001, December 17). The age of Muslim wars. *Newsweek, 138*(25), 42-48.

Inglehart, R., & Norris, P. (2003). The true clash of civilizations. *Foreign Policy, 135,* 62-66.

Johnson, D., Feldman, S., Lubin, H., & Southwick, S. (1995). The therapeutic use of ritual and ceremony in the treatment of post-traumatic stress disorder. *Journal of Traumatic Stress, 8*(2), 283-298.

Kinzie, J. D. (1993). Posttraumatic effects and their treatment among southeast Asian refugees. In J. Wilson & B. Raphael (Eds.), *The international handbook of traumatic stress syndromes* (pp. 311-319). New York: Plenum Press.

Kinzie, J. D. (2004). Some of the effects of terrorism on refugees. *Journal of Aggression, Maltreatment, & Trauma, 9*(1/2/3/4), 411-420.

Kinzie, J. D., Bohnlein, J., & Sack, W. H. (1998). The effects of massive trauma on Cambodian parents and children. In Y. Danieli (Ed.), *An international handbook of multigenerational legacies of trauma* (pp. 211-221). New York: Plenum Press.

Klain, E. (1998). Intergenerational aspects of the conflict of the former Yugoslavia. In Y. Danieli (Ed.), *An international handbook of multigenerational legacies of trauma* (pp. 279-296). New York: Plenum Press.

Kupelian, D., Kalayjian, A., & Kassabian, A. (1998). The Turkish genocide of the Armenians: Continuing effects on survivors and their families eight decades after massive trauma. In Y. Danieli (Ed.), *An international handbook of multigenerational legacies of trauma* (pp. 191-210). New York: Plenum Press.

Laird, J. (1998). Theorizing culture: Narrative ideas and practice principles. In M. McGoldrick (Ed.), *Re-visioning family therapy* (pp. 20-36). New York: Guilford.

Lira, E. (2001). Violence, fear, and impunity: Reflections on subjective and political obstacles for peace. *Peace and Conflict: Journal of Peace Psychology, 7*(2), 109-118.

McGoldrick, M. (1996). Irish families. In M. McGoldrick, J. Giordano, & J. Pearce (Eds.), *Ethnicity and family therapy* (pp. 310-339). New York: Guilford Press.

Meleis, A. (2003). Reflections on September 11, 2001. *Health Care for Women International, 24*, 1-4.

Mooren, G. & Kleber, R. (1999). War, trauma, and society: Consequences of the disintegration of former Yugoslavia. In K. Nader, N. Dubrow, & B. Stamm (Eds.), *Honoring differences: Cultural issues in the treatment of traumatic stress* (pp. 76-97). Philadelphia: Taylor and Francis.

Nader, K. (2003). *Assessing trauma in children and adolescents.* Manuscript submitted for publication.

Nader, K. (2004). Treating traumatized children and adolescents: Treatment issues, modality, timing, and method. In N. B. Webb (Ed.), *Mass trauma, stress, and loss: Helping families cope* (pp. 50-74). New York: Guilford Press.

Nagata, D. (1998). Intergenerational effects of the Japanese American internment. In Y. Danieli (Ed.), *An International Handbook of Multigenerational Legacies of Trauma* (pp. 125-140). New York: Plenum Press.

New Advent. (2001). The sacrament of penance. *The New Catholic Encyclopedia* [on-line]. Available: http://www.newadvent.org/cathen/11618c.htm

Ogden, C., Kaminer, D., Van Kradenburg, J., Seedat, S., & Stein, D. J. (2000). Narrative themes in responses to trauma in a religious community. *Central African Journal of Medicine, 46*(7), 178-184.

Pardess, E. (2004). Training and mobilizing volunteers for emergency response and long-term support. *Journal of Aggression, Maltreatment & Trauma, 10*(1/2/3/4), 609-620.

Peddle, N., Monteiro, C., Guluma V., & Macaulay, T. (1999). Trauma, loss, and resilience in Africa: A psychosocial community based approach to culturally sensitive healing. In K. Nader, N. Dubrow, & B. Stamm, (Eds.), *Honoring differences: Cultural issues in the treatment of traumatic stress* (pp. 121-149). Philadelphia: Taylor and Francis.

Peterson, C. (2002, August). Character strengths before and after September 11. In R. G. Tedeschi (Chair), *Posttraumatic growth in the aftermath of terrorism.* Symposium conducted at the meeting of the American Psychological Association, Chicago, Illinois, USA.

Picco, G. (2004). Tactical and strategic terrorism. *Journal of Aggression, Maltreatment, & Trauma, 9*(1/2/3/4), 71-78.

Scheff, T. (1997). *Deconstructing rage* [on-line]. Retrieved September 17, 2003 from http://www.soc.ucsb.edu/faculty/scheff/7.html

Shiang, J. (2000). Considering cultural beliefs and behaviors in the study of suicide. In R. Maris, S. Canetto, J. McIntosh, & M. Silverman (Eds.), *Review of suicidology* (pp. 226-241). New York: Guilford.

Shu`aib, T. B. (2001). *Essentials of Ramadan, The Fasting Month, Da`awah Enterprises International, Los Angeles, California, USA.* [on-line]. Available: http://www.usc.edu/dept/MSA/fundamentals/pillars/fasting/tajuddin/fast_8.htm l#HEADING7

Solomon, Z. (2004). Overview of recent Israeli data on the consequences of terror. *Journal of Aggression, Maltreatment & Trauma, 9*(1/2/3/4), 353-364.

Somasundaram, D. (2004). Short- and long-term effects on the victims of terror in Sri Lanka. *Journal of Aggression, Maltreatment & Trauma, 9*(1/2/3/4), 215-228.

Spratt, M. (2002, August 28). *9/11 media may comfort, terrify.* Retrieved August 28, 2002 from www.dartcenter.org

Strassfeld, M. (1985). *The Jewish Holidays.* New York: Harper & Row.

Thielman, S. B. (2004). The effects on Kenyan employees of the attacks on the American embassies in East Africa. *Journal of Aggression, Maltreatment & Trauma, 9*(1/2/3/4), 233-240.

Tully, M. (1999). Lifting our voices: African American cultural responses to trauma and loss. In K. Nader, N. Dubrow, & B. Stamm, (Eds.), *Honoring differences: Cultural issues in the treatment of traumatic stress* (pp. 23-48). Philadelphia: Taylor and Francis.

Volkan, V. D. (2001). September 11 and societal regression. *Mind and Human Interaction, 12,* 196-216.

Waldegrave, C. (1998). The challenges of culture to psychology and postmodern thinking. In M. McGoldrick (Ed.), *Re-visioning family therapy* (pp. 404-413). New York: Guilford.

Walsh, F. (1998). Beliefs, spirituality, and transcendence: Keys to family resilience. In M. McGoldrick (Ed.), *Re-visioning family therapy* (pp. 62-77). New York: Guilford.

Watson, M. F. (1998). African American sibling relationships. In M. McGoldrick (Ed.), *Re-visioning family therapy* (pp. 282-294). New York: Guilford.

Weine, S., Danieli, Y., Silove, D., Van Ommeren, M., Fairbank J. A., & Saul, J. (2002). Guidelines for international training in mental health and psychosocial interventions for trauma exposed populations in clinical and community settings. *Psychiatry, 65*(2), 156-164.

Yee, P. (2003, August 6). *New York's Asian population following the terrorist attacks of 9/11.* An unpublished interview reported to Kathleen Nader. Peter Yee is the Assistant Executive Director of Hamilton Madison House and the President of the New York Coalition for Asian American Mental Health.

Some of the Effects of Terrorism on Refugees

J. David Kinzie

SUMMARY. Highly traumatized people are vulnerable to exacerbation of symptoms when confronted with stressful situations. The extensive TV coverage of the 9/11 attacks provided such a stressful stimulus. Many patients from Vietnam, Cambodia, Laos, Somalia, and Bosnia had severe reactions. Nightmares and flashbacks occurred most among Somalis, who felt less safe; depressive symptoms increased most among Bosnians. Encouraging patients to turn off the TV was very therapeutic. The Patriot Act severely affected refugee immigration to the United States, leaving many families separated and increasing suspicions of discrimination among Muslim refugees. Terrorism's effects are pervasive and destructive. Some countermeasures may have similar unintended consequences.

Address correspondence to: J. David Kinzie, MD, Oregon Health & Science University, 3181 SW Sam Jackson Park Road, Portland, OR 97239 USA (E-mail: kinziej@ohsu.edu).

The author appreciates the very helpful assistance of Crystal Riley in preparing this manuscript.

[Haworth co-indexing entry note]: "Some of the Effects of Terrorism on Refugees." Kinzie, J. David. Co-published simultaneously in *Journal of Aggression, Maltreatment & Trauma* (The Haworth Maltreatment & Trauma Press, an imprint of The Haworth Press, Inc.) Vol. 9, No. 3/4, 2004; and: *The Trauma of Terrorism: Sharing Knowledge and Shared Care, An International Handbook* (ed: Yael Danieli, Danny Brom, and Joe Sills) The Haworth Maltreatment & Trauma Press, an imprint of The Haworth Press, Inc., 2005.

KEYWORDS. Terrorism, refugees, PTSD, counter terrorism, 9/11, media

Terrorism, with its indiscriminate destruction of human life, has profound effects on its victims, their families and the community. With almost instantaneous TV coverage throughout the world, the vicarious effects of terrorism can be experienced by almost everyone. This is true for refugees who have often directly experienced the atrocities of wars, forced migration, and resettlement. This article reports the effects on traumatized refugees in the United States of viewing military and terrorist activities, particularly with regards to the September 11, 2001 terrorist attacks. It also describes the effects on these refugees of some of the counter-terrorism measures taken by the United States government.

Lindeman (1944) observed back in 1944 that current stresses could clearly reactivate memories of prior losses and traumatic events. Initial reactivation, either physiological or psychological, based on exposure to cues that symbolize an aspect of the traumatic event is included in the diagnostic criteria of Posttraumatic Stress Disorder (PTSD) (American Psychiatric Association, 2000). Several studies report that exposure and subsequent traumatic events serve as a reminder of past trauma. Solomon, Garb, Bleich, and Grupper (1987) report that combat-related reactivated PTSD can take several forms and is a complex phenomenon. Traumatized former POWs were found to be vulnerable to the detrimental effects of life events (Solomon, 1995). Post-disaster negative life events have been found to increase incidence and severity of PTSD (Maes, Mylle, Delmerse, & Janca, 2001). In a study of the Gulf War Scud Missile survivors, the threat of additional Iraqi missile attacks was found to have a detrimental effect on a previously exposed population (Toren, Wolmer, Weizman, Magel-Vandi, & Laor, 2002).

In our study exposing Cambodian refugee patients to traumatic video scenes, we found a general nonspecific arousal (by self-reports and heart rate increases) compared to normal volunteers and Vietnam veterans (Kinzie et al., 1998). This study, as well as previously reported studies, indicated that reactivation is not only a response to cues that represent or symbolize a traumatic event, but can occur as a response to negative, threatening, or disturbing life events. In our experience, events associated with fear or loss can bring back the whole posttraumatic syndrome.

A study from Israel, a country where there is ongoing terrorism, found that 16.4% of the population was directly exposed to terrorism and 37.3% had a family member or friend exposed (Bleich, Gelkopf, & Solomon, 2003). Nevertheless, the rate of PTSD was rather moderate (9.17%). This was thought to be related to accurate information about loved ones and social support, which are often lacking for refugees. A recent study of Asian and Middle Eastern immigrants in Oklahoma City found PTSD symptoms associated with the bombing on April 19, 1995. Most had experienced prior trauma in their homelands and this prior trauma was associated with the bombing symptoms (Trautman et al., 2002). This result is very similar to the one we reported below.

The Intercultural Psychiatric Program at Oregon Health & Science University has treated refugees for the past 25 years, beginning with those fleeing from the effects of the Vietnam War and the Pol Pot regime in Cambodia. More recently, we have treated victims from wars and civil violence in Bosnia and Somalia. A consistent clinical finding for many patients with PTSD is reactivation of posttraumatic stress symptoms in response to current stresses, such as an accident, surgery, an assault, or even viewing a violent TV show (Berthold, 1999; Kinzie, 1988). Our patients describe increased symptoms from TV viewing of the war in Bosnia, the first Gulf war, the war in Afghanistan, and the most recent Iraqi war. Their most severe reaction, however, was due to the terrorist destruction of the World Trade Center on September 11, 2001. A summary of that study follows; for a full description, see Kinzie, Boehnlein, Riley, and Sparr (2002).

THE EFFECT OF 9/11 TELEVISION VIEWING ON TRAUMATIZED REFUGEES

In our clinical work with refugees it became apparent that the rather constant television exposure to the events of 9/11 had profound and disturbing effects, including recurrent nightmares, intrusive memories, depressed mood, and a sense of not being safe in America, a place where most had found safety and security. Added to this was further insecurity and vulnerability experienced by the two Muslim groups, the Bosnians and Somalis, who felt singled out by their appearance and religious background. Because of this, we decided to do a clinical study to assess the changes and symptoms of five ethnic groups in response to viewing the events of 9/11 and to describe the sense of personal vulnerability experienced by these groups. The groups studied were as follows:

1. Vietnamese, the largest patient population, who endured the Vietnam War.
2. Laotians, who had suffered the effects of the Indochinese war in Laos.
3. Cambodians, a group severely traumatized by the 4 years of extreme cruelty from 1975-1979 of the Pol Pot regime.

4. Bosnians, who came to the United States shortly after experiencing brutal conflict, including the Serbian-controlled concentration camps, that
occurred in former Yugoslavia from 1992-1993. Bosnians are Muslims,
although less traditional and strict than the Somalis.

5. Somalis, who endured a civil war with tribal conflict since 1991, resulting in general lawlessness, looting, mass starvation and indiscriminate
killing. Those refugees who came to the United States had lived for several years in refugee camps, primarily in Kenya. They were the most recent arrivals, having been in the United States usually less than 3 years;
all were strict Muslims and most of the women wore traditional Islamic
clothing.

Method

We developed a simple analogue questionnaire on a 10-point scale, with 10
being the highest (worst) and 0 being no or least effect. The Visual Analogue
Scale could be used cross-culturally without any specific language requirements. The patients were then asked to judge how much the 9/11 events affected them, based on how much their nightmares, flashbacks, and depression
changed. In addition, they were asked how safe they felt after 9/11 compared
with before. The questionnaire also included an open-ended question about
their major feelings since 9/11. The sample is a sample of convenience of
those who came to the clinic within two months of 9/11 and were able to complete the interview required for the questions. Overall, 177 patients participated: 74 Vietnamese, 43 Cambodians, 17 Laotians, 26 Bosnians, and 17
Somalis. They represented between 29% and 54% of their respective patient
population. Being patients in a general psychiatric clinic, they had a wide
range of diagnoses. The individual groups ranged from 100% PTSD and often
with another comorbid disorder among the Somalis, to 64% PTSD among the
Laotians.

Results

Virtually all (95%) reported seeing the TV images of the 9/11 disaster, and
92% said that it affected them. Table 1 summarizes the data from patients with
PTSD, indicating that a large effect was reported from almost every group.
The largest single effect (meaning extremely or nearly so) came from the Somalis and the Bosnians. The greatest change in nightmares as well as flashbacks occurred within the Somalis. Depression changed most in the Bosnians.
Table 2 shows respondents' change of perception after 9/11. Clearly, the Somalis felt the most change, from feeling safe to currently feeling only mildly to
moderately safe. As shown in Table 3, patients with depression alone (al-

though a smaller number) had a comparable effect to those with PTSD. The schizophrenic patients were the least affected, which was true for all ethnic groups. Each ethnic group's rating of post 9/11 feelings of safety can be found in Table 4.

Clearly, the traumatized refugees showed a strong reaction to 9/11, and the strongest reaction tended to be among patients with PTSD from Bosnia and Somalia. These two had experienced the most recent war atrocities, which were also widely covered by television. Their reactions seemed to be related to their Muslim religious background. The Cambodians had a more muted response, which could be related to the relative remoteness of their experiences in both time and place. It may also be that this response is due both to a sense of fatalism and acceptance at the core of Buddhism. Patients with PTSD and depression had the largest reaction; however, patients with schizophrenia, even schizophrenia with PTSD, reacted the least of all diagnostic categories in regard to ethnicity. The isolation of emotions in schizophrenia perhaps explains this phenomenon. Fear was the most common open-ended response to questions about feelings and was the response given in 73% of Bosnians and 47% of Somalis. Uncertainty was the most common response among Laotians (53%); however, no single reaction stood out among Vietnamese and Cambodians.

Television coverage of this highly graphic and disturbing event had serious psychiatric consequences for our refugees that needed to be addressed in treatment. A practical suggestion was to encourage patients to turn off their TV sets. Clinically, most patients reverted to their pre-9/11 levels in 2 to 3 months, and although they reacted dramatically to the events, the effects were not prolonged.

THE EFFECTS ON REFUGEES OF POST 9/11 U.S. MEASURES

The reactions to the events of 9/11 have been multiple, confusing, and with probable unintended consequences for refugees. The refugee patients, in addition to their personal reactions, were universally appalled that some people could kill over 3,000 innocent victims. The greatest outrage seemed to be expressed by the Muslim community, who saw this act as a violation of Islamic beliefs and feared a terrible reflection on all Muslims. Most had adopted America as a tolerant place of safety and felt stunned that others would attack a benevolent sanctuary. The response of the local community ranged from support towards the refugees, including Muslims, to clear hostility, especially to the traditionally dressed women, who felt shunned and were occasionally told

TABLE 1. Patients with Posttraumatic Stress Disorder (N = 129)

1. How much did 9/11 affect you?										
Not at all			Mildly		Moderately		Very		Extreme effect	
0	1	2	3	4	5	6	7	8	9	10

2. Since 9/11 how much did your nightmares change?
3. Since 9/11 how much did your flashbacks change?
4. Since 9/11 how much did your depression change?

Ethnicity	Effect[a]	Nightmare Changes[b]	Flashback Changes[c]	Depression Changes[d]
Vietnamese (*n* = 42)	7.33	6.13	4.65	6.09
Cambodian (*n* = 37)	6.65	2.57	5.05	3.92
Somali (*n* = 37)	9.00	6.94	8.00	6.24
Laotian (*n* = 10)	7.10	2.40	3.50	6.20
Bosnian (*n* = 18)	9.22	4.56	6.50	8.56

Note. ANOVA test of significance: [a]F = 5.414; significance = .000; [b]F = 9.274; significance = .000; [c]F = 4.303; significance = .003; [d]F =10.384; significance = .000

TABLE 2. Changes in Feeling Safe

Not safe at all			Mildly safe		Moderately safe		Very		Extremely safe	
0	1	2	3	4	5	6	7	8	9	10

Ethnicity	How safe before 9/11 M (SD)	How safe now M (SD)	Change[a] M (SD)
Vietnamese (*n* = 73)	7.92 (2.66)	3.74 (2.62)	4.19 (2.85)
Cambodian (*n* = 46)	9.52 (1.21)	6.54 (2.39)	2.98 (2.93)
Somali (*n* = 17)	9.89 (.46)	3.58 (2.85)	6.32 (2.79)
Laotian (*n* = 17)	8.00 (1.17)	3.99 (2.22)	4.01 (2.59)
Bosnian (*n* = 27)	8.93 (2.09)	4.59 (3.35)	4.33 (3.10)

Note. [a]ANOVA: F = 5.17; significance = .001

to dress "like Americans." There were some hate crimes in the area involving vandalism to local mosques.

Changes in the government procedures of new applications for refugee status had a more far-reaching effect. Seventy thousand refugees were approved for admission in the year 2003, but only 28,455 were actually admitted into the United States. The biggest drop was from the 22,000 ceiling of admissions from Africa to the actual number of 10,717 who were admitted. Of the 15,000 approved in 2002 from the Near East and South Asia, only 3,554 were admitted (U.S. State Department, 2003).

TABLE 3. Results Based on Diagnosis (All Ethnicities)

Diagnosis	Effect[a]	Change in Depression[b]	Change in Feeling Safe[c]
PTSD ($n = 124$)	7.60	5.24	4.24
Depression ($n = 27$)	7.44	5.84	4.24
Schizophrenia ($n = 17$)	5.41	3.94	3.00
Other ($n = 80$)	6.00	4.00	3.12

Note. ANOVA: [a]$F = 4.048$, significance $= .008$; [b]$F = 2.857$, significance $= .039$; [c]NS

TABLE 4. Post 9-11 Feeling of Safety in Percentage

		Not Safe (0-3)	Moderately Safe (4-7)	Very Safe (8-11)
Vietnamese	($n = 73$)	51	34	15
Cambodian	($n = 47$)	6	57	36
Somali	($n = 18$)	56	28	17
Laotian	($n = 18$)	50	44	6
Bosnian	($n = 24$)	42	29	29

These were the results of the State Department's implementation of additional overseas security checks for refugees entering the United States following the events of 9/11. These procedures included security checks on applicants for refugee status prior to interviews with INS offices, the requirement that photographs of refugees be taken at the on-site overseas processing location, and the return of already approved cases to an INS anti-fraud and security review. These caused the flow of refugees to the United States to slow dramatically and at times to stop altogether. Not only did this mean that there was a total decrease in new refugees to the United States, but it also meant that many refugee families were kept in limbo while their family members were stranded abroad, unable to join them, and with no indication of when family reunification would occur. This affected Africans and Middle Easterners the most.

The Patriot Act and the creation of the Department of Homeland Security following 9/11 combined several services for the purposes of sharing information on immigration, criminal activity, fraud, and of course, security risk. These have had multiple effects on refugees and immigrants. Muslim men were singled out for particular scrutiny. As reported by the BBC on June 10,

2003, 82,000 Arab and Muslim adult males obeyed a government request that they register with the Immigration Service on the grounds that they came from 25 mainly Muslim countries said to harbor terrorists. Having cooperated with the anti-terrorism measures, more than 13,000 have been or are facing deportation. Only 11 of those who registered, among the tens of thousands screened, were found to have links with terrorism. Immigration deportation processes have been mostly based on lapses in immigration status. These aggressive techniques have stirred passions in the community and left many refugees bewildered.

Even before the PATRIOT Act, soon after 9/11, many refugees felt unsafe in their new home; the Somalis particularly felt discriminated against. Table 4 indicates the feeling of safety that was present in the months following 9/11. Clearly, all groups except Cambodians felt much less safe after 9/11. Fifty-six percent of Somalis felt not safe at all. Only 17% of them felt very safe (as did 15% of Vietnamese and 6% of Laotians).

Our study confirms that post-9/11 anti-immigrant policies have made many refugees, particularly Muslims, feel unwelcome in the United States.

Case Example

This patient is a 45-year-old Somali mother of seven children. Both she and her children were separated from her husband in the process of fleeing from the tragic events in Somalia. She eventually received refugee status in Kenya and came to the United States with her children 3 years ago. She found out that her husband had made his way to Egypt and had started the process of applying for refugee status so that he could join her. The events of 9/11 changed all that. Although he was approved prior to 9/11, the on-site processing locations in Africa periodically closed down. In addition, there were increased background checks requiring fingerprints and photographs, which had to be processed in the United States. For more than 2 years, he has been waiting to join his family without any clear indication of when, or if, that will be possible.

CONCLUSION

This article addresses the effects of terrorism on refugees in the United States, including television viewing of the World Trade Center bombing and reactions to the U.S. Government' s post-9/11 policies on refugees. Refugees have suffered in their countries of origin through civil wars, ethnic cleansing, starvation, death of family members, and random acts of violence, looting and rape in the aftermath of total societal disintegration. Some of these atrocities, especially in ethnic conflicts, included indiscriminate violence against civilian populations, which likely meets some definition of terrorism (Wessells, 2003). Although some refugees in the United States are victims of terrorism, that term is inadequate to describe the multiple losses (forced migration, dislocation, and resettlement experiences) that they have experienced prior to arriving in the United States.

Undoubtedly some refugee camps, especially those of long duration, breed hopelessness in which terrorists can be recruited (Taylor & Louis, 2003). However, it is inaccurate and prejudicial to feel and act toward some refugees in the United States as if they were terrorists. The Oklahoma City and World Trade Center bombings were not committed by people who came to America as refugees. On the contrary, from the author's experience evaluating and treating over 1,000 refugees in 25 years, refugees have been grateful for this country's security and generosity. Indeed, most have contributed greatly to the strength and diversity of our society. As the United States seeks ways to strengthen its security, this author urges us to remember the commitment to openness, tolerance and civil rights on which this great society is based.

REFERENCES

American Psychiatric Association. (2000). *Diagnostic and statistical manual of mental disorders* (4th ed., text rev.). Washington, DC: Author.

Berthold, S. M. (1999). The effects of exposure to community violence on Khmer refugee adolescents. *Journal of Traumatic Stress, 12*, 455-471.

Bleich, A., Gelkopf, M., & Solomon, Z. (2003). Exposure to terrorism, stress-related mental health symptoms and coping behaviors among a nationally representative sample in Israel. *Journal of the American Medical Association, 290*, 612-620.

Kinzie, J. D. (1988). The psychiatric effects of massive trauma on Cambodian refugees. In J. P. Wilson, Z. Harel, & B. Kahana (Eds.), *Human adaptation to extreme stress* (pp. 305-317). New York: Plenum Press.

Kinzie, J. D., Boehnlein, J. K., Riley, C., & Sparr, L. (2002). The effects of September 11 on traumatized refugees: Reactivation of posttraumatic stress disorder. *Journal of Nervous and Mental Diseases, 190*, 437-441.

Kinzie, J. D., Denney, D., Riley, C., Boehnlein, J., McFarland, B., & Leung, P. (1998). A cross-cultural study of reactivation of posttraumatic stress disorder symptoms. *Journal of Nervous and Mental Diseases, 186*, 670-676.

Lindeman, E. (1944). Symptomatology and management of acute grief. *American Journal of Psychiatry, 101*, 141-148.

Maes, M., Mylle, J., Delmerse, L., & Janca, A. (2001). Pre- and post-disaster negative life events in relation to the incidence and severity of posttraumatic stress disorder. *Psychiatry Research, 105*, 1-12.

Solomon, Z. (1995). The effect of prior stressful experience on coping with war trauma and captivity. *Psychological Medicine, 25*, 1289-1294.

Solomon, Z., Garb, R., Bleich, A., & Grupper, D. (1987). Reactivation of combat-related posttraumatic stress disorder. *American Journal of Psychiatry, 144*, 51-55.

Taylor, D. M., & Louis, W. (2003). Terrorism and the quest for identity. In F. M. Moghaddam, & A. J. Marsella (Eds.), *Understanding terrorism* (pp. 169-185). Washington, DC: American Psychological Association.

Toren, P., Wolmer, L., Weizman, R., Magel-Vandi, O., & Laor, N. (2002). Retraumatization of Israel civilians during a reactivation of the Gulf War threat. *Journal of Nervous and Mental Diseases, 190*, 43-45.

Trautman, R., Tucker, P., Pfefferbaum, B., Lensgraf, S. J., Doughty, D. E., & Buks, A. et al. (2002). Effects of prior trauma and age on posttraumatic stress symptoms in Asian and Middle Eastern immigrants after terrorism in the community. *Community Mental Health Journal, 38*, 459-474.

U.S. State Department. (2003, November). Refugees and migration. *U.S. Refugee Admissions Program News, Bureau of Population, 1*(2).

Wessells, M. G. (2003). Terrorism and the mental health and well-being of refugees and displaced people. In F. M. Moghaddam, & A. J. Marsella (Eds.), *Understanding Terrorism* (pp. 247-263). Washington, DC: American Psychological Association.

Voice:
The Effects of Terror on Ethiopian Israelis: What I Have Left

Micha Feldmann

ANDALAU'S STORY

Andalau (Elad) Wasa, 26, was severely injured in a suicide bombing in the shuk (open air market) in Netanya on May 19, 2002. After 10 days in a coma in the Intensive Care Unit, he awoke to find that he was paralyzed from the hips down. Andalu uses a wheelchair and lives in a rented apartment in Netanya. This is Andalau's story.

When I arrived in Israel via Sudan, I was a small boy, but I remember that it was very strange to see white people all around me. But I soon got used to it, I learned the language and I adjusted pretty well. In school I had Ethiopian as well as white friends. You can say that despite the difference in color, I felt I belonged, I felt I had returned home, just like the village elders had promised in their stories.

Address correspondence to: Micha Feldman, SELAH, Israel Crisis Management Center (ICMC), 15 Chevrat Shas Street, Neve Tzedek, Tel Aviv 65156, Israel (E-mail: icmc@selah.org.il).

The voices of Ethiopian Isarelis are from interviews conducted by Micha Feldmann of SELAH, the Israel Crisis Management Center for this volume.

[Haworth co-indexing entry note]: "Voice: The Effects of Terror on Ethiopian Israelis: What I Have Left." Feldmann, Micha. Co-published simultaneously in *Journal of Aggression, Maltreatment & Trauma* (The Haworth Maltreatment & Trauma Press, an imprint of The Haworth Press, Inc.) Vol. 9, No. 3/4, 2004; and: *The Trauma of Terrorism: Sharing Knowledge and Shared Care, An International Handbook* (ed: Yael Danieli, Danny Brom, and Joe Sills) The Haworth Maltreatment & Trauma Press, an imprint of The Haworth Press, Inc., 2005.

When I came home from boarding school on holidays, I would work in the Netanya shuk so I would have a few shekels in my pocket. My parents did not have money to give me. Over time, my boss's family became my family and till today they treat me like one of their own.

In the army, I also felt a part of things. My fellow soldiers accepted me like everyone else and till today I am in touch with friends from the army. I took advantage of every vacation to work in the shuk and when I finished the army, it was only natural that I would go back to my job. I was not cut out for studying. I liked carrying sacks and crates and arranging vegetables in the stand.

On the day of the bombing, we were very busy, so I went to eat lunch late. As usual, I went to my boss's sister's restaurant. When I finished eating, she offered me a glass of tea, but I was in a hurry to get back to work. If I had drunk that tea, what happened to me would not have happened. A few minutes after I arrived back at work, the bomb exploded.

After 10 days, I woke up in the hospital. I did not feel my legs. The doctors explained that I would never be able to walk again. Everyone tried to encourage me, but I did not want to hear anyone, I did not want to talk to anyone. For two months I did not speak, not even to my mother. As an Ethiopian, I knew that for my parents there is no greater pain than having their son not talk to them. But I simply could not. At night and even during the day, I dreamt I was walking, but when I awoke, I would find myself in the same position.

After two months, I woke up one morning and said to myself: "I'm alive. I got my life as a gift. It is true that God took my legs but he left me my hands and most importantly, my head works. With what I have left, I will do something." I do not know what caused this but since then, I put every ounce of my energy into moving forward. I'm learning to walk with the help of a special implement and I began studying in order to finish my matriculation exams. I play basketball and work out. I believe that one day I will be able to do everything. Everything is dependent on my will.

Despite what happened to me, I still feel like I belong here. This is my country, my home, I have nowhere to run to. And more than that, here, in my land, when what happened to me happens to someone, you discover that you are not forgotten, that the country and the people take care of you, that there are many people around you who believe in you and help you. For me, that is first and foremost my family who stood by me even when I was not speaking to them. I also have many friends, like the SELAH volunteers, who do not leave my side. This gives me the strength to go on. God gives and God takes away.

VADA'S STORY

Vada (Varda) Hyela's daughter, Orit, was killed in a bus bombing on June 18, 2002. Orit studied and worked in a program for newly religious girls in Jerusalem. That morning, she took a bus from her home in Gilo to her job in the center of town. Just before the Pat Junction, a suicide bomber exploded himself in the middle of the bus, causing the death of many young people who were on their way to school and to work. This is Vada's story.

Twenty years ago, we began walking to Sudan on the way to Jerusalem. My grandparents always told us that Ethiopia was not our country, that our country was Jerusalem. Because everyone started to go, we believed the time had come. We did not know how we would go, we did not know how we would arrive, we just believed that time had come. Even the elders said: "We do not know how we will get there. The distance to Jerusalem is bigger than the distance between the earth and the sky." We sold what we could and left. We were happy because we were about to arrive in Jerusalem. But we also cried because we left people behind.

The journey was very difficult. We were thirsty, hungry, and tired. Little ones died. But the older people said, "Do not cry for them. God knows . . . God will guide us." Some people wanted to go back but we heard that those who returned were put in jail. We were also very afraid, and many times people wept from fear. Even though I was sick, I carried Orit on my back. After a month, we arrived in Sudan.

We were in a refugee camp in Sudan for nine months. Many died there. We lived in a big tent on the sand. I put plants on the sand so that my children would not sleep on the ground. I made sure they stayed healthy. I slept on the sand myself, it did not bother me. My husband did not help me with the children. He had taken another wife when I got sick.

When we arrived in Israel, we were welcomed nicely and taken care of. We were sent to an absorption center in Mevasseret Tzion. Everyone in my house was sick. My grandson was very sick. I tried to help him but my hands shook. Three months after we arrived, my grandson died. After that, they separated us and sent my daughter to another place. I worried about her because she was also sick.

When I arrived in Israel, I was not happy inside because my husband and I did not get along. I had pains all over my body. But I was happy for my children, especially for Orit. All my children were nice, healthy, and diligent. But none of them was like Orit. When she was four or five, she taught me how to use the telephone. In exchange, she would ask for a sweet. She would make me laugh. Everyone praised her. People always said, "How cute she is." I would take second-hand clothes for my kids but for Orit, I bought everything new. Guests, and we always had guests, would be amazed at her intelligence. She would go everywhere with me, her hand in mine. Everyone spoiled her. I always walked to school with her and would walk to meet her on her way home. When it came to my children, nothing was difficult. It was not hard for me to cook for them, it wasn't hard for me to clean. I liked taking care of them.

I feel that Israel is my home and that feeling has not changed after what happened to Orit. People ask how they can help me. It would have been better if I had nothing and my daughter was alive. The terrorist did not come to kill my daughter, he wanted to kill Jews. It just happened to be my daughter. It hurts me that she died without having children.

How can I be angry at the State? Like everyone, I prayed to come to Jerusalem. Many families suffer when their children are murdered. My daughter's death is not connected to the State of Israel, it's connected only to God. God gives and God takes away. I do not know when I will go, only He knows.

SECTION IV
PSYCHOLOGICAL FIRST AID, ACUTE AND LONG-TERM TREATMENT FOLLOWING TERRORIST ATTACKS

Mental Health Interventions in a General Hospital Following Terrorist Attacks: The Israeli Experience

Ilan Kutz
Avi Bleich

SUMMARY. Over three years of repeated terrorist attacks in Israel have shown that the victims suffering from acute stress syndromes constitute the bulk of the casualties. The large number of psychological victims presents an immediate problem of hospital surge capacity. The need for alleviating acute suffering and preventing chronic, disabling posttraumatic syndromes requires organizational and clinical skills. The

Address correspondence to: Ilan Kutz, MD, Director, Psychiatric Services, Meir General Hospital, Kfar Saba 44281, Israel (E-mail: ikutz@netvision.net.il).

[Haworth co-indexing entry note]: "Mental Health Interventions in a General Hospital Following Terrorist Attacks: The Israeli Experience." Kutz, Ilan, and Avi Bleich. Co-published simultaneously in *Journal of Aggression, Maltreatment & Trauma* (The Haworth Maltreatment & Trauma Press, an imprint of The Haworth Press, Inc.) Vol. 10, No. 1/2, 2005; and: *The Trauma of Terrorism: Sharing Knowledge and Shared Care, An International Handbook* (ed: Yael Danieli, Danny Brom, and Joe Sills) The Haworth Maltreatment & Trauma Press, an imprint of The Haworth Press, Inc., 2005.

article reviews deployment and intervention protocols for the treatment of victims and affected staff members in a general hospital setting. *ticle copies available for a fee from The Haworth Document Delivery Service:*

KEYWORDS. Acute stress, hospital preparedness, EMDR, hypnosis, CBT, group debriefing, staff support

While the world is busy with the probability of a terror attack with chemical or biological weapons with a potential for mass destruction, the Oklahoma City bombing, and particularly the Twin Towers attack on September 11, have shown that under certain deployment conditions conventional devices can be as deadly as non-conventional ones. However, even less spectacular events, particularly when repeated, can achieve the prime aim of terrorist organizations: to instill fear and disrupt the fabric of normal life. In Israel, the past few years have painfully shown that while all forms of conventional terror are fatal, suicide bombings are the most lethal forms because of the difficulty of stopping the intended bombers from fulfilling their mission and because of the carnage that follows (see Table 1).

Statistics following terror attacks in Israel show that the number of those responding with acute psychological stress responses far outweighs those with physical injuries and may be as high as 10:1 or even higher. During a mega-attack by a conventional weapon or non-conventional terrorism, this ratio is expected to be much higher and produce mass psychogenic or sociogenic illness (Bartholomew & Wessely, 2002) with all the hallmarks of a contagious epidemic. Masses of terrorized people may jam the emergency wards of general hospitals, thwart efforts to render adequate help, and overload health facilities and other public services. Hence, advance planning and well-rehearsed deployment of trained mental health teams are paramount to ensuring the continuation of effective care.

Based on our accumulated experience with terror attacks in Israel, we present the psychiatric aspects of terror attacks with particular emphasis on general hospital preparedness and on intervention in the immediate phase.

CLINICAL SYNDROMES FOLLOWING TERROR ATTACKS

Clinically, one can roughly distinguish two symptom groupings: one related to threat and anxiety and the other to loss and depression (see Table 2). Sadly, mixed pictures are all too common.

TABLE 1. Casualties Since 09.30.00 Updated 10.12.03

Casualties	Civilians	Security Forces	Total Number of Israeli Casualties
Injured	**4259**	**1750**	**6009**
Killed	**632**	**266**	**898**

Details of Security Forces and Israeli Civilians Killed

Type of Attack	Israeli Civilians	Security Forces	Total
Rocks	2	0	2
Stabbing	6	0	6
Running Over	1	7	8
Lynching	17	2	19
Shooting	92	101	193
Drive-by Shooting	28	9	37
Shootings at Vehicle from an Ambush	59	11	70
Shootings at Towns and Villages	15	6	21
Shootings at Military Installations	0	26	26
Bombings	24	36	60
Suicide Bombing	372	40	412
Car-bomb	15	23	38
Mortar Bombs	0	1	1
Other	1	4	5
Total	632	266	898

Acute Stress Reaction, Acute Stress Disorder and Post-Traumatic Stress Disorder: Time Frames and Clinical Relevance. The diagnoses of acute stress reaction (ASR) and acute stress disorder (ASD) differ in their time frame. The time frame in ASR was first defined in the ICD-10 (World Health Organization, 1993, pp. 98-99) as: "Criterion D. If the stressor is transient or can be relieved, the symptoms must begin to diminish after not more than 8 hours. If exposure to the stressor continues, the symptoms must begin to diminish after not more than 48 hours." The ASD diagnosis, which first appeared in the DSM-IV in 1994, begins when the ASR ends: "Criterion G. The disturbance lasts for a minimum of 2 days and a maximum of 4 weeks, and occurs within 4 weeks of the traumatic event" (American Psychiatric Association [APA], 2000, pp. 429-432). Post-traumatic stress disorder (PTSD), according to the DSM-IV-TR (APA, 2000), continues where the ASD ends: 1 month or more after the traumatic event (see Table 3).

TABLE 2. Clinical Syndromes Following Terrorist Attacks

Anxiety-related syndromes
• Acute stress reaction
• Acute stress disorder
• Post-traumatic stress disorder
• Mass psychogenic illness (mass hysteria)
Loss-related syndromes
• Traumatic grief reaction
• Depressive reaction

TABLE 3. Timetable of Stress Responses

ASR (ICD 10):	First 8 hours (up to 48 hours)
ASD (DSM IV):	2 days to 4 weeks
Acute PTSD:	1-3 months
Delayed-onset PTSD:	Symptoms appearing at least 6 months after the stressor

Further distinction can be found in the clinical picture itself. While the ASR definition describes a more undifferentiated picture of distress, one that Yitzhaki, Solomon, and Kotler (1991) describe as polymorphous and shifting symptoms, the ASD definition already distinguishes between several distinct clusters of symptoms (arousal, dissociation, re-experiencing, and avoidance) that are more akin to PTSD.

Although certain researchers (Brewin, Andrews, & Rose, 2003; Harvey & Bryant, 2002) have questioned the clinical relevance of ASD, our experience with thousands of terror victims indicates that the concepts of ASR and ASD, though in need of some refinement, are conceptually helpful as well as clinically practical. Applying them early on contributes to the early detection of those at risk and to the effectiveness of intervention decision-making.

CORE PRINCIPLES FOR MANAGING AND TREATING STRESS DISORDERS IN GENERAL HOSPITAL SETTINGS

Objectives of mental health interventions in a general hospital include:

1. To reduce distress and restore functioning of all victims by ameliorating symptoms of ASR.
2. To identify those at risk for ASD in the hope of preventing subsequent PTSD. The likelihood of developing a chronic disorder like PTSD is

much higher in those diagnosed as suffering from ASD and is estimated to be 30-80% (Harvey & Bryant, 1998; Koren, Arnon, & Klein, 1999; North et al., 1999).

3. To intervene as soon as possible. ASR and ASD represent acute dysregulation of the physiology and psychology of affected individuals that within hours or days should begin correcting itself (Shalev, 2002). These psycho-physiologic considerations together with ample clinical observations suggest that the early period presents a window of opportunity for intervening and preventing prolonged syndromes. While only one controlled study documents the importance of timing of clinical intervention with ASR and ASD victims (Campfield & Hills, 2001), its conclusions, as well as the many non-controlled intervention attempts, dictate the following working hypothesis: *the sooner victims can be approached, diagnosed and treated, the better the long-term prognosis.* Sustained symptoms of PTSD suggest a more permanent form of psycho-physiologic dysregulation (Yehuda, 2002) that is notoriously harder to treat.

WAVES OF ARRIVAL
OF PSYCHOLOGICALLY AFFECTED INDIVIDUALS
TO THE EMERGENCY DEPARTMENT

Reports from all medical centers in Israel confirm that, invariably, whenever a large number of people are present at a terror attack site, three waves of victims arrive at the general hospital emergency department (ED).

The First Wave. Arriving within minutes to a few hours includes most of those suffering from acute distress who have been directly evacuated from the terror scene. Their selection is not conducted by professionals but by lay people and ambulance service personnel who are instructed to bring in all those who seem affected. Most of these people will be suffering from ASR.

The Second Wave. These individuals trickle in four to eight hours after the attack. They were not identified at the scene of the attack, had run away from the scene and later developed symptoms, or were identified by others as suffering from physical or psychological distress. They will also display symptoms of ASR.

The Third Wave. These are the people who arrive one to seven days after the attack. They had gone home, unaware of their psychological reaction or hoping that their initial reaction would subside. When they realize that their symptoms have not ameliorated or may have even exacerbated with time, they call or come to the ED or their local doctor's office. These individuals may be suffering from ASR or already from the more pronounced and sustained symptoms of ASD.

In addition to the clinical pictures of ASR and ASD, some individuals–either victims arriving from the scene, or family members who have come to locate their relatives–may respond with acute grief reaction due to the loss of loved ones.

MENTAL HEALTH TEAM DEPLOYMENT CONSIDERATIONS IN THE GENERAL HOSPITAL

Certain organizational steps are essential to ensure adequate treatment for large numbers of psychologically impacted survivors who arrive at the general hospital following a terror attack.

Deploying the Acute Stress Intervention Site (ASIS). As a cardinal principle for managing the many victims of the first wave, all victims with ASR initially have to go through the main ED for a physical checkup, usually involving ear or eye examination, X-ray or at times computed tomography scans. However, once their physical condition has been cleared, it is preferable to reposition them outside the ED. Numerous terror attacks have demonstrated that the ED is not a suitable location for mental health intervention; there is no therapeutic space to assess seriously and intervene, the presence of many ASR victims adds to the mayhem that impedes the life-saving intervention for the physically injured, and the exposure to gruesome scenes in the ED may increase the psychological distress of those already affected by ASR.

The ASIS is a pre-designated space isolated from the turmoil of the ED. It is staffed by a mental health team, including psychiatrists, psychologists, social workers and nurses. Clerks monitor the checking in and out, and security personnel block the perimeter from unrelated intruders. The ASIS includes several treatment rooms for group and individual interventions and a common corridor space for select family members and patients awaiting intervention or release. Snack food and drinks are available at all times, offered by a designated volunteer team. Phone connections are available for locating and contacting family members.

All psychologically affected individuals who arrive at the ED are evaluated at the ASIS, including those who upon arrival to the ED seem fairly calm and relatively composed. Experience has shown repeatedly that the early cursory psychiatric examination in the ED, performed by a psychiatrist, is not sufficient to capture a developing clinical picture of ASR. Such an evaluation may be misleading. An additional, more elaborate evaluation at a later time and under different settings is necessary.

Deploying the Information and Communication Center. This center is also physically removed both from the ED and from the ASIS. It is primarily staffed by social workers and administrators and assists and orients concerned family members and friends who call by phone or arrive at the hospital inquiring about their loved ones. A mental health worker may be added to assist if a crisis develops. Experience has shown that families appreciate the effort made on their behalf, even when information is not immediately available. On the other hand, unmet needs of family members may be a source of disruption and unnecessary painful clashes.

NON-SPECIFIC INTERVENTION PRINCIPLES FOR ASR FOLLOWING TERRORIST ATTACKS

During the very immediate care for survivors, whether in the vicinity of the terror attack, during evacuation, or initially within the hospital's ED, the survivors may still be disoriented and suffering from additional stressors such as pain, uncertainty, lack of clarity about further threat, fear for loved ones, and disconnection from their familiar support system. In this acute phase, when the victims are still in the midst of experiencing the event, all steps are aimed at providing a sense of physical and psychological safety by offering physical comfort, support and reassurance. Mental health professionals, non-mental health professionals, and trained volunteers can provide such non-specific functions after adequate basic training. The higher the number of casualties, the more likely is the need for early interventions by non-professionals. This may be particularly true for a mega-terror attack, when the numbers of survivors with ASR can flood the hospital gates.

The general principles for intervention by non-professionals, adopted by the Israel Ministry of Health (2002), are:

a. Establish personal contact with the survivors and provide words of comfort or supportive touch.
b. Encourage survivors to verbalize their experiences.
c. Provide orienting information about what happened and what is about to happen in the hospital.
d. Ensure physical needs such as hydration, food, and rest when appropriate.
e. Enable contact with any significant other as soon as possible through phone or personal contact.

PROFESSIONAL INTERVENTIONS FOR ACUTE STRESS SYNDROMES

Group Interventions for ASR in the ASIS. Once the ASR survivors have been cleared to move to the ASIS, group intervention can proceed as soon as a sufficient number of people (optimal 5-12) have assembled. Each group is led by two experienced mental health workers. The participants may be of mixed gender and age (adolescents and adults). Younger children have their own site. The group intervention usually occurs 1-3 hours after the initial cursory evaluation in the ED and provides a more prolonged and interactive monitoring opportunity.

The economic benefits of group intervention are obvious. The average group intervention time is 45 minutes so that several groups can be handled sequentially by the same team if needed. Thus, a team of two professionals can "process" 30-45 people within 3 hours. Since parallel groups can be held simultaneously by different teams of group leaders–holding three or four groups at a time is not unusual–the number of survivors that can be observed and treated within the first few hours is considerable. As Everly (2000) and Terr (1992) point out, when a massive number of casualties is present, larger group formats can be deployed.

This formation of groups helps structure the work at the ASIS and reduces the mayhem that is always a potential problem when dealing with a large number of survivors and their families. In our experience, group work has considerable clinical advantages. The group encounter we describe is by no means identical to Mitchell's Critical Incident Stress Debriefing (CISD, 1983) that has recently been heatedly debated (Arendt & Elklit, 2001; Bisson, 2003; Van Emmerik, Kamphuis, Hulsbosch, & Emmelkamp, 2002), though it contains some useful elements of that method in a briefer and less structured way, while relying more on recognized group dynamics. The immediate objectives are to restore orientation in time and space, turn chaos into order, and provide a safe place and a sense of control.

GROUP MECHANISMS INVOLVED
IN ACHIEVING THESE OBJECTIVES

Shared Fate. The group is a unique community of individuals with a shared recent fate. The awareness that other people were "there" reduces the sense of isolation.

Mutual Support and Human Contact. Whether helping others or being helped by them, the repeated process of mutual containment and support enhances coping and fosters the sense of autonomy and safety.

Construction of a Narrative. The ability to create a coherent narrative of events allows the structuring of time and space and helps differentiate the past from the present. Putting experience into words enhances the sense of control. The initial perceived meaning of the narrative, particularly its negative aspects of shame or guilt, can be reframed by the group and facilitators.

Repeated Exposure. By retelling the event rather than by re-experiencing it through flashbacks alone, the tendency to apply avoidance is challenged and a sense of control is regained.

"Heart-Storming." The process of sharing and reconstruction often involves emotional upheaval or abreaction. Group support helps each member to express emotions seething under the surface and contains expression of these emotions.

Roles of the group leaders include:

1. *Allow the group process to proceed* with minimal interruption, while facilitating and guiding the flow.
2. *Provide a locus for positive transference.*
3. *Provide information and context* by pointing out, for example, that ASR is a normal, expected reaction to an abnormal, unexpected event.
4. *Prepare group members for possible future symptoms,* stressing in general their subsiding course while alerting them to risk of intensification.
5. *Identify those at risk* in the group whose condition has not improved after the intervention.
6. *Serve as an address for further queries and guidance.*

At the termination of the group intervention, those who are identified as low risk for ASD are provided with oral instructions as well as information cards detailing how to contact the general hospital trauma unit or other support centers in case of continuing symptoms. Group members whose condition has not improved either continue to be treated individually or are scheduled for further individual evaluation and treatment on the following day (see below).

GROUP TREATMENT FOR HOSPITAL STAFF

Although staff members exposed to the aftermath of a terror event are not in the same extreme state of disorganization and stress as those directly impacted by terror, they may need some form of intervention, particularly if the event was gruesome, resulted in tragic consequences, or if the staffs have been exposed to multiple frequent events. This may be true for the ED teams, nursing staffs on the surgery floor, the social and mental health teams, and others. We found that a proactive approach is superior to passive response to an emergency outbreak on one of the wards. Forming a "defusing group" for teams who took part in an emotionally intense event in the very first few days may be of great benefit (see also Danieli, 2002). The mechanisms that operate in such groups are very similar to those described above for the traumatized patients in the ASIS.

INDIVIDUAL INTERVENTIONS WITH ASD

While some of these interventions may be attempted in the ASIS, most are carried out on an outpatient basis in the days following the terrorist event. The treatment population includes scheduled patients, non-scheduled victims who report worsening of their symptoms, third-wave victims who report in for the first time, and all injured patients who had been hospitalized in the surgical wards. Accordingly, the staff of the surgical wards is trained in identifying symptoms of ASD.

More important than the treatment modalities listed below is the comprehensive approach to the victim. *Involving the family* is necessary at times for understanding the patient's background, maintaining support, and improving compliance with intervention programs. *Staying with the survivor* is another crucial principle. Our experience has repeatedly shown that willingness to assume proactive responsibility for the survivor in the first few weeks and providing frequent interventions when needed ensures continuity of care and maximizes the chances for recovery. Sending or referring away, more frequently than not, results in the patient's dropping out of the system in this crucial therapeutic period.

Eye Movement Desensitization and Reprocessing (EMDR; Shapiro, 1995) is primarily used for patients with established PTSD symptoms. Although its efficacy for PTSD seems promising (Davidson & Parker, 2001; Heber, Kellner, & Yehuda, 2002; Shepherd, Stein, & Milne, 2000), its mechanisms of intervention remain unknown and in need of further study. We have found EMDR to be impressively effective in alleviating intrusive ASD symptoms (Kutz, 2003). In this acute phase, a single, brief EMDR session can markedly alleviate or eliminate the recurring intrusions in over 50 percent of the victims.

Cognitive Behavior Therapy, a psycho-educational intervention, combines prolonged exposure to disturbing images using principles of re-adjusting thoughts, beliefs and perceptions to modify the emotions and techniques of anxiety control. This method has been increasingly recognized as an effective technique for treating PTSD (Bryant, Sackville, Dang, Moulds, & Guthrie, 1999; Ehlers & Clark, 2003) and reported as an effective treatment for ASD following assault (Foa, Hearst-Ikeda & Perry, 1995).

Hypnosis with Cognitive Behavioral Elements: Converging evidence suggests that acute stress and PTSD are associated with higher levels of hypnotizability (Bryant, Guthrie, & Moulds, 2001; Bryant, Guthrie, Moulds, Nixon, & Felmingham, 2003). Specifically designed to treat symptoms of ASD, such interventions combine elements of hypnotic technique with cognitive and behavior elements such as exposure and desensitization. It has recently been shown that hypnosis and CBT are overall more effective than CBT alone in treating PTSD (Bryant, Moulds, Guthrie, Dang, & Nixon, 2003).

Psychopharmacology of ASR and ASD: The effect of medications in the area of acute trauma is largely an uncharted territory. While anecdotal reports abound, more systematic data are lacking (Morgan, Krystal, & Southwick, 2003). Our clinical experience indicates that selective serotonin re-uptake inhibitors (SSRIs), which help alleviate symptoms of PTSD, may be even more effective in ASD (with or without accompanying depression, which has already been found to be a risk factor for subsequent PTSD; Shalev et al., 1998). Trials with beta-blockers (Pitman et al., 2002) and other candidate drugs are underway. In the meantime, symptomatic support for severe restlessness or troubling insomnia can be achieved by a judicious use of benzodiazepines for brief intermittent periods (Lavie, 2001).

CONCLUSION AND RECOMMENDATIONS

Adopting these organizational principles and clinical skills may enhance the effective approach to managing, treating, and preventing long-term consequences of psychic trauma. However, if terrorist events are overwhelming and exceed the surge capacity of the hospital, other deployment strategies may be needed that require relocating the emergency sites and altering of some of the triage principles (Shemer & Shapira, 2001).

REFERENCES

American Psychiatric Association. (2000). *DSM-IV-TR diagnostic and statistical manual of mental disorders.* Washington, DC: Author

Arendt, M., & Elklit, A. (2001). Effectiveness of psychological debriefing. *Acta Psychiatrica Scandinavica, 104,* 423.

Bartholomew, R. E., & Wessely, S. (2002). Protean nature of mass sociogenic illness: From possessed nuns to chemical and biological terrorism fears. *British Journal of Psychiatry, 180,* 300-306.

Bisson, J. I. (2003). Single-session early psychological interventions following traumatic event. *Clinical Psychology Review, 23*(3), 481-499.

Brewin, C. R., Andrews, B., & Rose, S. (2003). Diagnostic overlap between acute stress disorder and PTSD in victims of violent crime. *American Journal of Psychiatry, 160*(4), 783-786.

Bryant, R. A., Sackville, T., Dang, S. T., Moulds, M., & Guthrie, R. (1999). Treating acute stress disorder: An evaluation of cognitive behavior therapy and supportive counseling techniques. *American Journal of Psychiatry, 156,* 1780-1786.

Bryant, R. A., Guthrie, R. M., & Moulds, M. L. (2001). Hypnotizability in acute stress disorder. *American Journal of Psychiatry, 158*(4), 600-604.

Bryant, R. A., Guthrie, R. M., Moulds, M. L., Nixon, R. D., & Felmingham, K. (2003). Hypnotizability and posttraumatic stress disorder: A prospective study. *International Journal of Clinical and Experimental Hypnosis, 51*(4), 382-389.

Bryant R. A., Moulds, M. L., Guthrie, R. M., Dang, S. T., & Nixon, R. D. (2003). Imaginal exposure alone and imaginal exposure with cognitive restructuring in treatment of posttraumatic stress disorder. *Journal of Consulting and Clinical Psychology, 71*(4), 706-712.

Campfield, K. M., & Hills, A. M. (2001). Effect of timing of critical incident stress debriefing (CISD) on posttraumatic symptoms. *Journal of Traumatic Stress, 14*(2), 327-340.

Danieli, Y. (Ed.). (2002). *Sharing the front line and the back hills: International protectors and providers, peacekeepers, humanitarian aid workers and the media in the midst of crisis.* New York: Baywood Publishing Company, Inc.

Davidson, P. R., & Parker, K. C. (2001). Eye movement desensitization and reprocessing (EMDR): A meta-analysis. *Journal of Consulting and Clinical Psychology, 69,* 305-316.

Ehlers, A., & Clark, D. (2003). Early psychological interventions for adult survivors of trauma: A review. *Biological Psychiatry, 1, 53*(9), 817-826.

Everly, G. S. (2000). Crisis management briefings (CMB): Large group crisis intervention in response to terrorism, disasters, and violence. *International Journal of Emergency Mental Health, 2*(1), 53-57.

Foa, E. B., Hearst-Ikeda, D., & Perry, K. J. (1995). Evaluation of a brief cognitive-behavioral program for the prevention of chronic PTSD in recent assault victims. *Journal of Consulting and Clinical Psychology, 63,* 948-955.

Harvey, A. G., & Bryant, R. A. (1998). The relationship between acute stress disorder and posttraumatic stress disorder: A prospective evaluation of motor vehicle accident survivors. *Journal of Consulting and Clinical Psychology, 66*(3), 507-512.

Harvey, A. G., & Bryant, R. A. (2002). Acute stress disorder: A synthesis and critique. *Psychological Bulletin, 128*(6), 886-902.

Heber, R., Kellner, M., & Yehuda, R. (2002). Salivary cortisol levels and the cortisol response to dexamethasone before and after EMDR: A case report. *Journal of Clinical Psychology, 58*(12), 1521-30.

Israel Ministry of Health. (2002). *A position paper of the National Council for Mental Health: Guidelines for the assessment and professional intervention with terror victims in the hospital and community.* (Hebrew). Jerusalem: Ministry of Health Publication.

Koren, D., Arnon, I., & Klein, E. (1999). Acute stress response and posttraumatic stress disorder in traffic accident victims: A one-year prospective, follow-up study. *American Journal of Psychiatry, 156*(3), 349-351.

Kutz, I. (2003). *The use of EMDR in acute stress disorder following terrorist attacks and motor vehicle accidents: An uncontrolled study of 65 victims.* Unpublished manuscript.

Lavie, P. (2001). Sleep disturbances in the wake of traumatic events. *New England Journal of Medicine, 345*(25), 1825-1832.

Mitchell, J. T. (1983). When disaster strikes: The critical incident stress debriefing process. *Journal of Emergency Medical Services, 8*, 36-39.

Morgan, C. A., Krystal, J. H., & Southwick, S. M. (2003). Toward early pharmacological posttraumatic stress intervention. *Biological Psychiatry, 53*(9), 834-843.

North, C. S., Nixon, S. J., Shariat, S., Mallonee, S., McMillen J. C., Spitznagel, E. L. et al. (1999). Psychiatric disorders among survivors of the Oklahoma City bombing. *Journal of the American Medical Association, 282*, 755-762.

Pitman, R. K., Sanders, K. M., Zusman, R. M., Healy, A. R., Cheema, F., Lasko, N. B. et al. (2002). Pilot study of secondary prevention of posttraumatic stress disorder with propranolol. *Biological Psychiatry, 51*(2), 189-192.

Shalev, A. Y., Freedman. S., Peri, T., Brandesm D., Sahar, T., Orr, S. P. et al. (1998). Prospective study of posttraumatic stress disorder and depression following trauma. *American Journal of Psychiatry, 155*, 630-637.

Shalev, A. Y. (2002). Acute stress reactions in adults. *Biological Psychiatry, 51*, 532-543.

Shapiro, F. (1995). *Eye movement desensitization and reprocessing: Basic principles, protocols and procedures.* New York: The Guilford Press.

Shemer, J., & Shapira, S. C. (2001). Terror and medicine–the challenge. *Israeli Medical Association Journal, 3*, 799-802.

Shepherd, J., Stein, K., & Milne, R. (2000). Eye movement desensitization and reprocessing in the treatment of post-traumatic stress disorder: A review of an emerging therapy. *Psychological Medicine, 30*, 863-871.

Terr, L. C. (1992). Mini-marathon groups: Psychological "first aid" following disasters. *Bulletin of the Menninger Clinic, 56*(1), 76-86.

Van Emmerik, A. A., Kamphuis, J. H., Hulsbosch, A. M., & Emmelkamp, P. M. (2002). Single session debriefing after psychological trauma: A meta-analysis. *Lancet, 360*, 766

World Health Organization (1993). International Statistical Classification of Diseases and Related Health Problems. Geneva: Author.

Yehuda, R. (2002). Post-traumatic stress disorder. *New England Journal of Medicine, 346*(2), 108-114.

Yitzhaki, T., Solomon, Z., & Kotler, M. (1991). The clinical picture of acute combat stress reaction among Israeli soldiers in the 1982 Lebanon war. *Military Medicine, 156*, 193-197.

Voice: When News Comes Close

Tali Arad

September 2000 will be remembered in collective memory as the month of the beginning of the Al Aksa Intifada. In my own memory as a young journalist on a local newspaper in Jerusalem, September will be remembered as the beginning of reporting on the most difficult terrorist attacks during the last four years.

In July of the same year I began working at the newspaper, my life's dream was fulfilled. Since I can remember I have wanted to be a journalist, to be in the field in places where important things happen, to bring interesting and important news to the public, and perhaps even to help a person or two through the profession I chose. Looking back on this period, I never imagined that an integral part of my work would be at the attack sites, to speak with the wounded, to cover funerals, and to interview families who, less than 24 hours earlier had lost their dearest children, including a son, a daughter, a father, a mother, a friend, and a husband. In a few attacks, whole families were erased by the flick of the terrorist's hand on the activation mechanism of the explosive belt he was wearing on his body. Three years of attacks passed by. Every attack and its people, every attack and the human story in it. With the time passing and the number of attacks increasing, the paper asked me to bring new angles, to look for other human stories, those stories that have not yet been told. A family that lost two children in two different attacks, a person who was

Address correspondence to: Tali Arad, 20 Davidson Street, Neve Granot, Jerusalem 93706, Israel (Email: taltol500@yahoo.com).

[Haworth co-indexing entry note]: "Voice: When News Comes Close." Arad, Tali. Co-published simultaneously in *Journal of Aggression, Maltreatment & Trauma* (The Haworth Maltreatment & Trauma Press, an imprint of The Haworth Press, Inc.) Vol.10, No. 1/2, 2005; and: *The Trauma of Terrorism: Sharing Knowledge and Shared Care, An International Handbook* (ed: Yael Danieli, Danny Brom, and Joe Sills) The Haworth Maltreatment & Trauma Press, an imprint of The Haworth Press, Inc., 2005.

present in more than one attack. What should we do? There are many attacks and there is a lot of work, and the reader, they said, is thirsty for information. In the tireless journalistic coverage I forgot myself.

My breaking point as a journalist and as a human being was Saturday night, March 9, 2002, the attack in Café Moment. The headlines cried that, "eleven killed and dozens injured." That evening I went out on a date with a man with whom I had just started a relationship. Three days earlier, after a wedding of a mutual friend, we continued the night with a glass of beer in Café Moment, which we both thought of as our "second home." That Saturday we decided to meet at another café, Cafit, where two days earlier, one of the waiters there caught a suicide bomber in the middle of the café, and thus prevented another murderous attack. On my way to the date, I called a friend, also a journalist, and, as usual for us, we joked on the number of (intelligence) warnings in Jerusalem. When I told her that I was on the way to Cafit, she said that I was crazy, "only yesterday they caught a terrorist there, maybe you should go to another place, for example, Moment. It is safe there. It is near the prime minister's house." I dismissed her feeling and said, "whatever has to happen will happen and I will not stop my life. If something happens, you know where my parents live." I said this so she would be able to take a photograph to the paper if need be, if I die in an attack. This was a part of the black humor we developed.

We had barely ordered and were served our beer when a police car passed, and another one. I understood that something had happened. My 24-hour-a-day beeper did not signal a special event. My partner got up for a minute and I asked the hostess what had happened. She told me of the attack at Moment. I immediately gathered my things and ran to the car. My date wanted to join me. I explained to him that this is an unpleasant experience and that it will be best if he goes home. He insisted. I drove frantically to the café. On the way, I tried to reach all the emergency services, the Magen David Adom (Red Star of David ambulance services), the spokespersons for the hospitals and the police, to get an update. I did not succeed in reaching anyone. Police cars, ambulances, and fire trucks passed us in both directions. I got as close as possible with my car, stopped, and ran to the café. The police had already cordoned the place off with plastic tapes. They did not let journalists in. I crossed the police line anyhow, but a large policeman returned me to my place. Suddenly, I heard someone call my name. It was the journalist friend with whom I had just spoken by phone. She broke up crying and said out loud what we all felt, "I can't anymore. How many more attacks will we cover?" I hugged her and when I realized that it did not help I did what seemed right at the moment, I slapped her and told her that we will cover this attack together, each for her own medium. This helped. As matter of routine we looked for eyewitnesses, and when I found some I called her to come and hear them. I stayed near the café all night despite my stated role that I have to be in hospitals to interview the injured. I could not leave the place. I felt that my home was destroyed, that I must make sure that none of my close friends was hit. When communication became possible, I received dozens of messages from concerned friends who know that I loved to frequent this cafe and, like them, I left messages for dozens of my friends whom I knew also loved to come to this typical Jerusalem café. At some point I returned my date to his own car and drove to Hadassa Hospital to interview the injured. I moved around all night among hospitals, looking for special stories. I found them only the next day. All the wounded I spoke to said, "they destroyed our home."

Suddenly, the attacks came near the place that I and my friends frequented. We became a part of it. I became a part of it. I forbade my parents from doing their shopping at the "Mahane Yehuda" market in town, I warned them to answer the cell phone when there was an attack. And where am I in this whole craziness? Work? Live? Or living in an insane world and somehow succeeding in looking at it all from the side and writing about it? Maybe!

The attacks continue, and the emotional exhaustion with them. Politics, as strange as it may seem, do not interest me. As a journalist I try to be objective. As a human being I understand that both sides, Jews and Arabs, hurt. But all I want is to be a good journalist, to bring stories that will make people think and might even help a person or two.

Today, every ambulance that passes near my house makes me jump. I wait quietly to hear whether another one or more will pass. I check the beeper to see when the "First announcement. An explosion was heard . . . " will appear. Physically I am ready to go. My car always has enough gasoline. The jeans and the blouse are always at an arms length to enable me to leave as fast as possible. Emotionally, I do not want to be ready. I want quiet.

Treating Survivors of Terrorism While Adversity Continues

Rhonda S. Adessky

Sara A. Freedman

SUMMARY. The current situation in Israel of continuous terrorist attacks poses unique challenges to the treatment of Posttraumatic Stress Disorder (PTSD). This article addresses issues that arise when treating survivors of ongoing terrorism. These include: (a) Is PTSD treatable during ongoing adversity? (b) When should treatment be offered? (c) Is avoidance maladaptive or adaptive? (d) How does one deal with re-exposure? (e) How to define the end of treatment? and (f) What are the effects on the therapist when conducting treatment during ongoing adversity? Case studies are provided to illustrate these issues when treating clients with PTSD during ongoing terror.

www.HaworthPress.com>

Address correspondence to: Rhonda S. Adessky, PhD, Center for The Treatment of Traumatic Stress and Anxiety Disorders, Hadassah University Hospital, Department of Psychiatry, POB 12000, Jerusalem, Israel (E-mail: rhondaadessky@hotmail.com).

[Haworth co-indexing entry note]: "Treating Survivors of Terrorism While Adversity Continues." Adessky, Rhonda S., and Sara A. Freedman. Co-published simultaneously in *Journal of Aggression, Maltreatment & Trauma* (The Haworth Maltreatment & Trauma Press, an imprint of The Haworth Press, Inc.) Vol. 10, No. 1/2, 2005; and: *The Trauma of Terrorism: Sharing Knowledge and Shared Care, An International Handbook* (ed: Yael Danieli, Danny Brom, and Joe Sills) The Haworth Maltreatment & Trauma Press, an imprint of The Haworth Press, Inc., 2005.

KEYWORDS. Trauma, terror, cognitive behavior treatment, re-exposure, avoidance, coping

The current situation in Israel of ongoing terror attacks poses unique challenges to the treatment of Posttraumatic Stress Disorder (PTSD). Since September 2000, there have been 20,530 terrorist attacks in Israel and her territories (Israel Defense Force, 2003), with 6,139 civilian and security forces injured and 920 killed. The number of witnesses to each attack and the number of people exposed to graphic images of the scene through the media are manifold. By definition, terrorism is random. Thus, terrorist attacks do not occur daily, at any particular time, or in any particular place. While the threat of terror attacks is continuous with no defined end, people in Israel are continuously being re-exposed to multiple discrete traumatic events that occur randomly. How are people living under such conditions affected?

Taken at face value, one would hypothesize that continuous re-exposure to traumatic events, particularly those of the same nature, places individuals at higher risk for developing PTSD. Ehlers and Clark (2000) argue that PTSD becomes persistent when individuals process the trauma in a way that leads to a sense of serious current threat. This sense arises as a consequence of: (a) excessively negative appraisal of the trauma and/or its sequelae and (b) a disturbance of autobiographical memory characterized by poor elaboration and contextualization, strong associative memory, and strong perceptual priming. In Israeli reality, however, negative appraisal of the trauma such as "nowhere is safe" and "the next disaster will strike soon" may actually be reality-based rather than excessive. Moreover, autobiographical memories are continuously being primed and associated with each new attack. Foa and Kozak (1986) theorize that following a trauma, individuals develop fear structures that incorporate all features of the traumatic event and generalize to associated features. Fear structures are accessed and strengthened when information compatible with the original trauma is presented. Thus, continuous exposure to trauma may strengthen fear structures and place people at higher risk for the development of PTSD.

This article addresses the following issues arising from prolonged adversity as they affect psychological interventions for adults with diagnosable PTSD as a result of exposure to terrorist attacks: (a) Is PTSD treatable while terrorism is ongoing? (b) When is the most opportune time to offer treatment? (c) Is avoidance maladaptive or adaptive? (d) Re-exposure to terror attacks, (e) Coping with re-exposure, (f) Defining the end of treatment, and (g) Therapist effects when conducting treatment during ongoing adversity.

IS PTSD TREATABLE WHILE TERRORISM CONTINUES?

Although terrorism has debilitating effects, PTSD resulting from terror attacks is treatable during ongoing adversity. The questions then are how is PTSD treated while terrorism continues and what challenges arise while treating PTSD during ongoing adversity? At the Center for the Treatment of Traumatic Stress and Anxiety Disorders, we successfully use Cognitive Behavior Therapy, an empirically validated treatment approach for PTSD (Foa, Keane, & Friedman, 2000). We have found that 75% of our clients exhibit a 65% reduction in symptoms and a return to a relatively normal life. The work is best illustrated through the following case example:

> B, a 25-year-old woman, was eating lunch when a terrorist entered the restaurant and blew himself up. She was only slightly wounded; however, several people were killed and scores were seriously injured in the attack. Knowing only basic first aid, B recalled helping the wounded as best she could. She witnessed horrific images of charred human remains, pools of blood, pieces of flesh, and decapitated bodies.

B presented for treatment three months after the event, stating that she had not been herself since the attack. Even the slightest reminder of things she saw, smelled, heard, or felt in the attack caused flashbacks, avoidance, or both and controlled her life. For instance, at a dinner party a guest dropped a bottle on the table, causing a loud crash that brought back the image of the attack in the restaurant in a terrible flashback. As a result, she began avoiding eating with others. The smell of burning flesh and sight of raw meat triggered horrific images in her mind, causing her to avoid restaurants, supermarkets, and social gatherings at homes of friends where these things could be found. A puddle of water caused by rain reminded her of the pools of blood on the floor of the restaurant and prevented her from going out in inclement weather.

At intake, B was assessed using structured clinical interviews and self-report questionnaires. She was experiencing flashbacks, nightmares, sleep disturbance, and hyper-arousal; avoidance of thinking about, or activities that reminded her of, the event; emotional numbness, detachment, and difficulty concentrating. She also endorsed symptoms of depression including depressed mood, lack of interest or pleasure, loss of appetite, psychomotor retardation, and feelings of guilt and worthlessness. As can be seen in Table 1, her scores on the Posttraumatic Stress Scale (Foa, Riggs, Dancu, & Rothbaum, 1993) were 46, and on the Beck Depression Inventory (Beck, 1988) 40, indicating significant symptoms of PTSD and depression. Her therapy, lasting 11 sessions, was challenging but successful. Because of the difficulty of the im-

TABLE 1. Summary Scores on Self-Report Measures

Date (session)	Posttraumatic Stress Scale-Self Report (PSS-SR)	Beck Depression Inventory (BDI)	Subjective Units of Distress (SUDS)
2/28/2003 intake	46	40	
3/11/2003 (1)	46	35	
3/25/2003 (3)	33	28	100-60
4/8/2003 (5)	27	22	80-40
4/29/2003 (7)	29	21	60-35
5/11/2003 (9)	22	19	40-20
6/1/2003 (11)	17	15	20-10
7/1/2003 (1 month follow up)	13	10	

ages she witnessed and her distress when she reviewed them, she needed a great deal of encouragement to continue with imaginal exposure. In retelling the story, she often felt nauseous and cried a great deal. Nonetheless, she managed to habituate to the images, and her Subjective Units of Distress began to decrease significantly by the third session (see Table 1). Through in vivo exposure, B learned to habituate to the smells of burnt meat, foods she had been eating when the bomb exploded, images of body parts from anatomy text books, public places, loud noises, and eating in restaurants and at friends' homes. As can be seen in Table 1, B exhibited marked decrease in symptoms but was clearly experiencing some. Her quality of life improved drastically.

WHEN TO OFFER TREATMENT?

The question of when is the most opportune time to treat patients suffering from PTSD, particularly when similar traumata are occurring, is paramount. Until recently, it was generally assumed that early intervention, such as psychological debriefing or critical incidence stress debriefing immediately following a traumatic event, is useful in preventing chronic problems (Everly & Mitchell, 1999). However, recent reviews (Raphael & Ursano, 2001; Rose, Bisson, & Wessely, 2001) of the results of controlled studies failed to confirm its efficacy, and some studies reported adverse long-term effects (Mayou, Ehlers, & Hobbs, 2000).

Moreover, research indicates that the presence of PTSD symptoms within a few days of a traumatic event is typical and disappears rapidly (Shalev, Freedman, Peri, Brandes, & Shahar, 1997; Shalev et al., 1998). In addition, patients presenting with symptoms one month post-trauma had fully recovered five months later. These data suggest that recovery from PTSD symptoms may occur in many individuals without intervention. However, for those who do not recover, chronic PTSD has set in with all the potentially accompanying disruptions, including unemployment, family distress, and depression.

Thus, timing of intervention remains a difficult dilemma: on the one hand, when resources are limited, we do not want to offer treatment to those who may recover on their own. On the other, we do not want to wait until chronic PTSD has become entrenched or the occurrence of additional attacks strengthens beliefs that maintain PTSD, cause excessive fears, and avoidance. It is difficult to predict who will develop PTSD (Shalev et al., 1997). However, research has indicated that people suffering from Acute Stress Disorder following a traumatic event may be at higher risk for developing PTSD (Bryant, Harvey, Dang, Sackville, & Basten, 1998). Thus in defining an early intervention treatment group, assessing levels of acute stress symptoms and targeting those individuals with significant symptoms for treatment appears to be the most efficient approach.

Several studies suggest that cognitive behavioral interventions within the first month of the trauma offer promising results in preventing the onset of chronic PTSD (Bisson, Shepard, Joy, Probert, & Newcomb, 2004; Bryant, Sackville, Dang, Moulds, & Guthrie, 1999; Foa, Hearst-Ikeda, & Perry, 1995). In view of the repeated exposure to terror attacks and our concern that this may place people at even greater risk for developing PTSD, we are currently administering CBT treatment within a month of the trauma to survivors who present to the Emergency Department following an attack and who exhibit high levels of acute stress symptoms within the first two weeks following the trauma. Preliminary results appear promising.

MALADAPTIVE AND ADAPTIVE AVOIDANCE

According to the cognitive model of PTSD, avoidance is not only a defining symptom of PTSD but also a factor in maintaining the disorder (Ehlers & Clark, 2000). In a situation of ongoing terror, however, avoidance may actually be helpful in maintaining health. If encouraged, does it also maintain PTSD as suggested by PTSD researchers? To address this issue, we have come up with the concepts of "adaptive avoidance" and "maladaptive avoidance." Adaptive or healthy avoidance is considered avoidance of places or situations that increase the risk for direct exposure to terrorism, such as city center, buses, and cafes. This type of avoidance has become the norm for the general population. However, we encourage clients to return to their previous level of activity as much as possible. For example, a client who survived an attack on a bus agreed to ride the bus but disembarked as it drove down the street where the attack had taken place, left the bus, walked down side streets, and got back on the bus several blocks past the site of the attack. During ongoing terror, we deem this as appropriate avoidance. However, if such behavior were to continue once the terrorist attacks cease, this avoidance would be seen as maladaptive and would require attention. Thus, appropriate avoidance is encouraged, whereas excessive avoidance and unrealistic or overgeneralization of danger are discouraged.

In situations where returning to the site of the attack is potentially dangerous, as when several attacks were carried out in the same area and it was not essential for the client to return to the area (e.g., open-air market for shopping rather than going to a neighborhood store), we use modified avoidance. Clients do not return to the site but use maps and photos in lieu of returning to the actual site of the attack. This enables the client, for whom any reminder of the site is difficult, to have partial exposure, which aids in processing the fears and memories and decreases the type of avoidance that maintains PTSD. Some of the "avoidance solutions" are adaptive in the current situation of prolonged adversity and will require modification if and when the daily terror ceases.

RE-EXPOSURE TO TERROR ATTACKS

The issue of re-exposure to terror attacks and its impact on treatment is of extreme significance. Unfortunately, we have seen clients who have been re-exposed to terrorist attacks during the period in which they are in therapy and also weeks or months after therapy has ended. Experiencing a second or third attack can be particularly detrimental to the person and the therapy process. Both direct exposure as well as indirect exposure, such as seeing images of another attack on television or hearing about others wounded or killed in an attack, elicit horrific memories in victims of terrorism. Re-exposure may also reinforce beliefs such as "the world is an unsafe place" or "bad things keep happening to me" that maintain PTSD (Ehlers & Clark, 2000).

Our initial intervention when a patient is re-exposed to an additional attack while in treatment is to offer support, identify resources, and implement effective coping mechanisms. In the subsequent therapy session, patients are able to discuss their fears, memories, and experiences of the initial attack. However, processing the original traumatic event remains a necessary goal to help them change their fear structures and habituate to the fear of the trauma memories. Focus on the original trauma resumes within one or two sessions. If additional processing of the second attack is necessary, extra sessions are devoted to it.

We have also found that re-exposure to a similar attack may not always be detrimental in the long run. For example, R, an 18-year-old who was in treatment following an attack in a café, decided that it was extremely important for him to return to cafes so as to resume his previous social life. During his 'homework assignment,' the café next to his was blown up. R was not injured but witnessed horrific images. He learned in the second attack that his reaction of fear and helplessness in the first attack was typical for everyone. This enabled him to change his maladaptive appraisal "I am not normal for having such a reaction" that, in turn, was maintaining his PTSD. Similarly, A, a client who had witnessed a shooting near her home and avoided returning to live in her home for fear of another attack in her neighborhood, was treated successfully for her PTSD. Two weeks after she completed treatment and was back living in her home, a shooting attack occurred in a house next door. Her greatest fear came true and, despite experiencing extremely high levels of anxiety immediately following the attack, her anxiety decreased and she was able to cope. These examples illustrate the importance of assessing idiosyncratic fears that maintain PTSD and the fact that re-exposure may not have only negative outcomes. Despite initial increase in symptoms immediately following re-exposure to terror attacks, we find that anxiety levels decrease within a few hours to a few days and clients resume their previous level of functioning.

COPING WITH RE-EXPOSURE

We expect that all of our clients will be, at a minimum, indirectly exposed to subsequent terrorist attacks. Methods for coping with future attacks are thus a crucial aspect of treatment. In the treatment of other traumatic events like sexual assault and car accidents, patients are taught to avoid potential risks for re-exposure (e.g., reckless driving with car accidents or dark secluded places with sexual assault). Defining risk when dealing with terror, which by definition is random and intended to create the sense that danger exists everywhere, is much more challenging. Random terrorist acts create the sense that every public venue is a potential risk for direct exposure and every media broadcast or conversation is a potential for indirect exposure. Moreover, given that some terrorist incidents have even occurred in private homes and bombs have exploded in residential neighborhoods, some people have developed schemas that no place, including home, is safe. A colleague who lives across the street from a café that was bombed in Jerusalem was sitting in his living room when the thunderous bomb exploded, causing his building to shake and windows to shatter. Within seconds, shocked and wounded survivors, covered in blood and human flesh, ran into his home seeking shelter and safety. Describing his experience, he stated poignantly that, unlike the Persian Gulf Crisis, which was referred to as the "living room war" because CNN's live 24-hour coverage of the military events brought the war into America's living rooms, the Al-Aksa Intifada has literally brought war into Israeli living rooms.

How do terror attack survivors cope with the possibility of re-exposure? Cognitive reappraisal of risk is used in therapy to help clients cope with the possibility of being in a future attack. Despite a 300% increase in number of terror attacks between 1999 and 2000, the risk of being killed in an attack is still relatively small. Cognitive reappraisal helps decrease the anxiety caused by cognitive distortions such as overestimation of danger and emotional reasoning. For example, clients are helped to see that their fear of riding buses after being in an attack on a bus does not increase the likelihood that an attack will occur. Thus, it is important to note that the pathology of PTSD is the catastrophic perception of danger and not the avoidance behavior. Those with PTSD irrationally believe that they will be in another attack. While this does happen in some cases, therapy can be used to appraise realistically the danger and weigh the costs and benefits of excessive avoidance and worry.

An additional coping mechanism is to help clients plan and prepare in advance what they would do in the event of a future attack, which allows for some sense of control. Moreover, clients are taught that re-occurrence of symptoms is normal in the event of future attacks and is to be expected so they are not distressed by their reactions.

Recent Israeli research (Gidron, Gal, & Zahavi, 1999) has supported the hypothesis put forth by Lazarus and Folkman (1984) that the use of emotion-focused coping (calming-distraction) would be most helpful in situations of uncontrollable stress. Following re-exposure, clients are encouraged to use relaxation techniques, to disengage from media coverage, and to engage in pleasurable but safe activities (e.g., watching movies at home rather than in a public theatre or meeting friends at home rather than at a café). Clients are encouraged to call their therapists when feeling distressed, particularly in the event of an additional attack. In addition, after all major terrorist attacks, therapists call their clients to provide support. They help to normalize the fear and the temporary increase in their PTSD symptoms.

DEFINING THE END OF TREATMENT

Treating victims of terrorism during ongoing adversity raises the question of defining the end of treatment or a return to health. Unlike many interventions for PTSD that assume the end-point of treatment is a return to normal daily functioning (Foa, Keane, & Friedman, 2000), the goals of treatment during continuous terrorism are to help patients process effectively their discrete traumatic event and teach them to cope with direct and indirect future terror attacks. We expect a significant reduction in most symptoms but assume that certain symptoms will continue and a change in daily functioning may persist. Symptoms such as increased arousal, some avoidance of public places, and hypervigilance are to be expected. These symptoms have indeed become typical in the general population. Recent studies in Israel have found that most people (77%) endorse experiencing at least one symptom of traumatic stress (Bleich, Gelkopf, & Solomon, 2003). Shalev et al. (2003) collected data in 2001 on a civilian community exposed to continuous and repeated terrorist attacks. Twenty-five percent of the community met the diagnosis of PTSD, whereas the remaining 75% tended to express some post-traumatic symptoms. Few people expressing symptoms, however, reported significant distress and functional impairment or sought treatment. The prevalence of post-traumatic stress symptoms is not surprising given the significant rise in number of terror attacks in the last few years in Israel. The population at large is constantly warned to remain vigilant for potential suicide bombers and suspicious objects. Hypervigilance in the public domain is considered adaptive and helpful rather than pathological. In the current situation of ongoing adversity, having "symptoms" can in fact be considered a good thing. We can no longer use the definition of lack of symptoms as a measure of treatment success or good health. Thus, the end of treatment is defined as when a patient attains relief from the severity of symptoms that are interfering with his or her life, processes effectively the traumatic event, and does not overestimate the level of danger.

THERAPIST EFFECTS WHEN CONDUCTING TREATMENT DURING ONGOING ADVERSITY

Therapists who treat terror survivors are equally indirectly and occasionally even directly exposed to horrific events. They may know someone injured or killed in the attack their client is describing. Such personal involvement makes the therapy much more challenging for the therapist. Therapists who themselves have experienced an attack or were close to a relative or friend who was involved in an attack may find it difficult to listen to their patients' experiences without becoming too emotional and over-identified with their patients. Such therapists are always given the choice to not treat terror attack patients. If they do continue with the therapy, they are given additional supervision and support by the treatment team. Therapists are discouraged from treating too many trauma survivors at one time to prevent burn-out. Listening to horrific stories, gruesome details, and tremendous grief and despair can be very difficult. Therapists remain motivated and fresh by seeing the tremendous results of a client emerging from the shattered life s/he initially presented with to a fully functioning, recovered survivor, able to resume his/her previous level of functioning.

Therapists' personal beliefs and attitudes may also influence their treatment of their clients. For instance, therapists who do not ride buses or frequent public places may be more reluctant to encourage their clients to engage in such activities than therapists who themselves are less fearful or avoidant. While it is always up to the client to decide what he or she is willing to avoid, therapists' personal choices may indirectly impact the client's choices.

Working with trauma survivors increases the awareness in some therapists of personal impact of terrorism. Despite denying exaggerated avoidance, it increases their hypervigilance in situations like riding buses or choosing seats in cafes, which they did not experience prior to working at the center (even after the beginning of the terrorist attacks). We view this change in behavior as a normal consequence of working with terror survivors, similarly to those in therapists working with motor vehicle accident survivors who drive more cautiously. Extensive support and intensive supervision to therapists treating survivors of terrorist attacks are essential.

CONCLUSION

This article focused on issues arising when treating trauma survivors in an ongoing terrorist situation. Trends suggest that Israelis are relatively resilient to developing PTSD despite years of ongoing random terror attacks. Given the existing dangers, the increase in symptoms is seen as normal (for cultural issues that may apply, see, for example, chapters by Nader & Danieli, Kinzie, Lahad, and Solomon & Berger, this volume). The majority of those who do develop PTSD respond well to cognitive behavioral interventions. Challenges include re-experiencing and avoidance behaviors, which occur for the entire population and are addressed by cognitive therapy, proactive coping and therapeutic support. Though patients respond well to treatment offered 3-12 months after the trauma, the effectiveness of early intervention (i.e., within 3-4 weeks post trauma) is currently being investigated. The current paper is based on descriptive data and a limited number of case histories. Additional research that includes control groups such as a waitlist or different types of therapy is essential.

REFERENCES

Beck, A. T. (1988). *Beck Depression Inventory*. New York: Psychological Corporation.

Bisson, J. I., Shepard, J. T., Joy, D., Probert, R., & Newcomb, R. G. (2004). Early cognitive behavioral therapy for posttraumatic stress symptoms after physical injury. *British Journal of Psychiatry, 184,* 63-69.

Bleich, A., Gelkopf, M., & Solomon, Z. (2003). Exposure to terrorism, stress-related mental health symptoms, and coping behaviors among a nationally representative sample in Israel. *Journal of the American Medical Association, 290,* 612-620.

Bryant, R. A., Harvey, A. G., Dang, S. T., Sackville, T., & Basten, C. (1998). Treatment of acute stress disorder: A comparison of cognitive behavioural therapy and supportive counselling. *Journal of Consulting and Clinical Psychology, 66,* 862-866.

Bryant, R. A., Sackville, T., Dang, S. T., Moulds, M., & Guthrie, R. (1999). Treating acute stress disorder: An evaluation of cognitive behavior therapy and supportive counseling techniques. *American Journal of Psychiatry, 156,* 1780-1786.

Ehlers, A., & Clark, D. M. (2000). A cognitive model of posttraumatic stress disorder. *Behaviour Research and Therapy, 38,* 319-345.

Everly, G. S., & Mitchell, J. T. (1999). *Critical Incident Stress Management (CISM): A new era and standard of care in crisis intervention* (2nd ed.). Ellicott City, MD: Chevron.

Foa, E. B., Hearst-Ikeda, D. E., & Perry, K. J. (1995). Evaluation of a brief cognitive-behavioral program for the prevention of chronic PTSD in recent assault victims. *Journal of Consulting and Clinical Psychology, 63,* 948-955.

Foa, E. B., Keane, T. M., & Friedman, M. J. (Eds.). (2000). *Effective treatments for PTSD: Practice guidelines from the International Society for Traumatic Stress Studies.* New York: Guilford Press.

Foa, E. B., & Kozak, M. J. (1986). Emotional processing of fear: Exposure to corrective information. *Psychological Bulletin, 99,* 20-35.

Foa, E. B., Riggs, D. S., Dancu, C. V., & Rothbaum, B. O. (1993). Reliability and validity of a brief instrument for assessing posttraumatic stress disorder. *Journal of Traumatic Stress, 6,* 459-473.

Gidron, Y., Gal, R., & Zahavi, S. (1999). Bus commuters' coping strategies and anxiety from terrorism: An example of the Israeli experience. *Journal of Traumatic Stress, 12,* 185-192.

Israel Defense Force. (2003). *Statistics*. [On-Line]. Available from, http://www.idf.il/english/statistics

Kinzie, J. D. (2004). Some of the effects of terrorism on refugees. *Journal of Aggression, Maltreatment, & Trauma, 9*(1/2/3/4), 411-420.

Lahad, M. (2004). Terrorism: The community perspective. *Journal of Aggression, Maltreatment, & Trauma, 10*(1/2/3/4), 667-679.

Lazarus, R. S., & Folkman, S. (1984). *Stress, appraisal and coping.* New York: Springer Publishing Company.

Mayou, R. A., Ehlers, A., & Hobbs, M. (2000). Psychological debriefing for road traffic accident victims: Three-year follow-up of a randomised controlled trial. *British Journal of Psychiatry, 176,* 589-593.

Nader, K., & Danieli, Y. (2004). Cultural issues in terrorism and in response to terrorism. *Journal of Aggression, Maltreatment, & Trauma, 9*(1/2/3/4), 399-410.

Raphael, B., & Ursano, R. J. (2001). Psychological debriefing. In Y. Danieli (Ed.), *Sharing the front line and the back hills: International protectors and providers: Peacekeepers, humanitarian aid workers and the media in the midst of crisis.* (pp. 343-352). Amityville, NY: Baywood Publishing Co, Inc.

Rose, S., Bisson, J., & Wessely, S. (2001). Psychological debriefing for preventing posttraumatic stress disorder (PTSD). (Cochrane Review). In *The Cochrane Library, 2,* Oxford: Update Software.

Shalev, A. Y., Adessky, R., Boker, R., Bargai, N., Cooper, R., Freedman, S. et al. (2003). Clinical interventions for survivors of prolonged adversities. In R. Ursano, C. S. Fullerton, & A. E. Norwood (Eds.), *Terrorism and disaster* (pp.162-188). Cambridge, UK: Cambridge University Press.

Shalev, A. Y., Freedman, Peri, D., S., Brandes, T., & Sahar, T. (1997). Predicting PTSD in civilian trauma survivors: Prospective evaluation of self report and clinician administered instruments. *British Journal of Psychiatry, 170,* 558-564.

Shalev, A. Y., Freedman, S., Peri, T., Brandes, D., Sahar, T., Orr, S. P. et al. (1998). Prospective study of posttraumatic stress disorder and depression following trauma. *American Journal of Psychiatry, 155,* 630-637.

Solomon, Z. (2004). In the shadow of terror: Changes in world assumptions in Israeli youth. *Journal of Aggression, Maltreatment, & Trauma, 9*(1/2/3/4), 353-364.

The Treatment of Children Impacted by the World Trade Center Attack

Sandra J. Kaplan
David Pelcovitz
Victor Fornari

SUMMARY. This article presents, from a developmental perspective, the authors' experiences treating children and families who were traumatized by and who lost relatives in the World Trade Center attack. The treatments took place within the Trauma Treatment Development Center, National Child Traumatic Stress Network (NCTSN) of the Division of Child and Adolescent Psychiatry, North Shore University Hospital, Manhasset, New York, of the North Shore-Long Island Jewish Health System. Case vignettes address treatments for toddlers, preschool, and school-age children and adolescents. Family, individual cognitive-behavioral, school, social, and parenting treatment strategies utilized are discussed.

Address correspondence to: Sandra J. Kaplan, MD, Vice-Chairman of the Department of Psychiatry, North Shore University Hospital, 400 Community Drive, Manhasset, NY 11030 USA (E-mail: sandrak@nshs.edu).

[Haworth co-indexing entry note]: "The Treatment of Children Impacted by the World Trade Center Attack." Kaplan, Sandra J., David Pelcovitz, and Victor Fornari. Co-published simultaneously in *Journal of Aggression, Maltreatment & Trauma* (The Haworth Maltreatment & Trauma Press, an imprint of The Haworth Press, Inc.) Vol. 10, No. 1/2, 2005; and: *The Trauma of Terrorism: Sharing Knowledge and Shared Care, An International Handbook* (ed: Yael Danieli, Danny Brom, and Joe Sills) The Haworth Maltreatment & Trauma Press, an imprint of The Haworth Press, Inc., 2005.

KEYWORDS. Child, 9/11 impact, mental health interventions

The events of 9/11 profoundly impacted the New York City and Washington, DC metropolitan areas and Shanksville, Pennsylvania. Children and families sustained particularly intense trauma. Coping strategies were challenged. For many, their lives will always be remembered as before and after 9/11.

Traumatized children, adolescents, and adults in the New York City area had a variety of reactions to the World Trade Center (WTC) attack. Some became numb; many thought calmly about what needed to be done; others were frantic and panic-stricken. The prolonged search and rescue fueled enormous anxiety, and parents sought ways to minimize the traumatic impact on children. Those who sustained losses found themselves immersed in the complexities of traumatic losses. Emotions were intense, and resilience was striking. The outpouring of volunteerism was dramatic; many reacted with selflessness and generosity.

This article presents, from a developmental perspective, the authors' experiences treating children and families who were traumatized by, and who lost relatives in, the WTC disaster. The treatments took place within the Trauma Treatment Development Center, a Center of the National Child Traumatic Stress Network (NCTSN),[1] of the Division of Child and Adolescent Psychiatry, North Shore University Hospital, North Shore-Long Island Jewish Health System. The Center is located in Manhasset, New York in Long Island's Nassau County, near the border of the New York City Borough of Queens.

The North Shore-Long Island Jewish Health System includes the tertiary care North Shore University Hospital. The System comprises 18 hospitals including two tertiary care hospitals, four nursing homes, a home health care agency, and a network of primary and specialty care ambulatory sites serving 5,400,000 residents, including 1,426,655 children under 18 years of age in the Counties of Nassau, Suffolk, Queens, and Richmond (Staten Island) of the New York City Metropolitan Area. The System is affiliated with the New York University and Albert Einstein Schools of Medicine.

Areas served by the Center and the Health System were severely impacted by the WTC attacks. As of August 16, 2002, 2,726 death certificates related to the attacks had been filed. Of these, 1,169 (43%) of the decedents were residents of New York City and 593 (22%) resided elsewhere in New York State (Centers for Disease Control and Prevention, 2002). Three hundred ninety-seven decedents, comprising 14.5% of the total number of WTC decedents, resided in the suburban Long Island Counties of Nassau and Suffolk. The Queens and Richmond Counties of New York City, where the Health System is also located, were, respectively, the locations of the residences of 257 (9.5%) and of 189

(6%) of decedents (*Newsday*, 2004). Thus, the Health System serves the areas of the residence of 30.1% of WTC attack decedents' families.

Between September 11, 2001 and September 30, 2002, the System's Trauma Treatment Development Center focused primarily on assisting the WTC disaster child mental health response for Long Island and New York City. These activities included the provision of public education for parents and other community members; training for mental health professionals; and psycho-education for teachers, psychologists, social workers, public and parochial school administrators, nurses, clergy and religious congregations, and emergency medical services (EMS) personnel. Crisis counseling was provided for personnel of the schools of students and/or staff whose relatives died in the WTC attacks.

Both Center- and field-based child and family mental health services were provided for family members of victims, which consisted of psycho-education, crisis counseling, and psychotherapy. Field-based services were provided to families belonging to religious groups who lost family members in the attacks.

The Center participated in Project Liberty's production of videotapes for the Catholic community on helping children, parents, and educators to understand 9/11-related child traumatic stress and associated mental health intervention (Project Liberty Catholic Charities, 2002). The Center also participated in the New York State Office of Mental Health Child and Adolescent Trauma Treatment and Services (CATS) Consortium[2] for implementing evidence-based interventions for children and adolescents impacted by the WTC disaster.

The developmental levels of children and adolescents guide all of our interventions. The youngest victims were infants and toddlers, without the necessary language to benefit from traditional therapy. For them, recommendations were often based on the continuation of pre-disaster routines to the extent possible. Preschoolers and young school age children required age-appropriate verbal explanations, including describing the death of a loved one at a time when the concept of death might not be fully understood. Preadolescents and adolescents required more sophisticated descriptions, even though traumatized adults found themselves without words to describe these unspeakable facts and with challenged coping abilities.

The following case vignettes, organized according to the involved child's developmental level, illustrate some of our therapeutic interventions for children and families.

THE TODDLER AGE CHILD (AGES 1.5-3)

A single, female New York City Police Officer who had only been on the Force for two years lost several colleagues and became overwhelmed after the attack. She was close to her brother, his wife, and their 2 1/2-year-old son. Prior to 9/11, she had spent at least one day a week with her nephew. She had no prior history of depression, but became tearful and sad six weeks following 9/11. Encouraged by her family to seek treatment, she initially felt that there was nothing wrong. Following the attack, however, she had withdrawn from her nephew and rarely saw him. The child became increasing clingy when he did see his aunt and had tantrums following their visits.

During her evaluation, she spoke of her nephew's questions about 9/11. "How does one begin to explain this to him?" Her style had been not to discuss feelings. Now she said: "Why do I need to talk about this so much?" Validating and normalizing these reactions and focusing on her during her 12 weekly treatment sessions were important. She also agreed to begin anti-depressant medication, which reduced her anxiety, elevated her mood, and allowed her to resume more of her routines, including her weekly time with her nephew. However, she continues to have a sense of foreboding and impending doom and to feel that a terrorist attack is imminent. Her vigilance remains high.

THE PRESCHOOL CHILD (AGES 3-5)

The concrete thinking style of preschoolers makes it more likely that they will view traumatic events through a prism that might distort such experiences by blaming themselves or viewing traumatizing events as punishment for their actions or thoughts. Death is often viewed as reversible and magical thinking may predominate. Preschoolers often respond to trauma with global, disorganized behavior and affect. Regression, irritability, and clinginess are common. Research suggests that the level of a preschooler's dysfunction is highly correlated with levels of parental distress. The following vignette illustrates a typical preschool reaction to the events of 9/11.

Five-year-old twins, who lost their father in the WTC attack, were not responding to maternal reassurance in the weeks 9/11. Three weeks after the attack, as her mother was putting her to sleep, one of the twins asked: "Mommy, why do people hate twins?"

Another preschooler, Marcus,[3] was five when his father, Mr. B., a New York City policeman, was killed in the WTC. The older of two children, Marcus has a sister who was then two. Mrs. B. was too overwhelmed by grief to care for her children in the month immediately following the attacks, and Marcus and his sister went to live with their maternal aunt and uncle. They and other members of the extended family provided a protective shield around him. This cushioned some of the pain from his father's death and his mother's unavailability.

Sessions with Marcus' mother, aunt, and uncle, as well as weekly play therapy sessions for him, began five weeks after Mr. B's death. The treatment goals included facilitating the return of Marcus and his sister to their home, providing guidance to Mrs. B. on helping her son and daughter grieve for their father and their former lives, and to cope with the drastic change in her ability to care for them. Many of the treatment strategies described below can be found in Lieberman, Compton, Van Horn, and Ghosh-Ippen (2003).

Family Interventions

The initial treatment focus was on supporting Marcus's emotional connection with his new primary caregivers, his aunt and uncle, and on helping him to reconnect with his mother. Mrs. B. was encouraged to work towards having her children return home. As noted by Lieberman and her colleagues (2003), returning to predictable routines is a cornerstone of healing for the bereaved preschooler.

Mrs. B. was also referred for individual therapy and to a group for 9/11 widows. Within a month, she was able to have her children return to her full-time care. The aunt and uncle were encouraged to remain involved in Marcus' life. They continue to provide concrete and emotional supports for him.

School and Peer Interventions

Marcus's mother was asked to read him a book written for preschool children that discusses a young child whose pet mouse dies (Harris, 2001). The book focuses on the permanence of death and the validity of experiencing angry and sad feelings afterward. Marcus begged her to take him to school with the book and to read it to his classmates, explaining, "They don't understand." After she did so, Marcus expressed relief that his friends now "understood" what it means to have a father die and his mood at school improved. Several weeks later, the therapist was asked by Marcus's teacher and Mrs. B. for advice on ways to respond when Marcus engaged in traumatic play marked by repetitively building large towers and then toppling them. As the year progressed, with the teacher's and Mrs. B's encouragement, these reenactments gave way to play reflecting less helplessness.

Dealing with Traumatic Loss Reminders

Although Mr. B's body had not been recovered, efforts were made to help Marcus preserve his father's memory in a reassuring way. A memorial service was held that included burying a reproduction of Marcus's favorite picture of his father and him on a trip to Disneyland and pictures drawn by him depicting playing ball with his father. This ritual helped Marcus to have happy memories of his father when he visited his father's grave rather than traumatizing memories of his death. Recalling and reinforcing comforting memories proved to be soothing for Marcus both during his graveside visits and when coping with daily loss reminders.

THE SCHOOL AGE CHILD (AGES 6-11)

School-age survivors of trauma often do not show trauma-specific symptoms. They frequently respond with somatic concerns, sleep difficulties, and school problems. While they may appear resilient, there might be a sleeper effect with subsequent onset of symptoms. A "family practice" treatment model of encouraging parents to bring even well-adjusted school age trauma survivors for follow-ups as they enter new developmental stages may be advisable.

Family and School Interventions

The Jones family resided in Battery Park City near Ground Zero and included children who attended school and parents who worked near the WTC. Living in Manhattan, walking to work instead of commuting, and walking together to the children's school had made their life style 'just what they wanted,' that is, until 9/11. That morning, after the children were dropped off at school, the couple waved each other goodbye. One went to the dentist; the other went to the office at the WTC. Then there was panic. Cell phones did not work. Both parents rushed to the school, and together the family walked up the West Side Highway while the first Tower burned. The second plane came so low overhead that they thought it might hit them. They watched it hit the second Tower and thought that they would die. They proceeded uptown to a friend's apartment, trying not to look back; they arrived terrified and exhausted, like refugees fleeing war. They thought about losing their apartment and their belongings. A few days later, they moved to the maternal grandparents' Long Island home.

Therapy addressed the disaster's social/community implications for this family. A cognitive-behavioral approach was used to help clarify the reality of their circumstances, mindful that none of them was physically injured or lost. Uprooted, but grateful to be alive, the children were registered in school in the grandparents' community. There was a gradual rebuilding of family life as they adapted to their new environment. Consultation with their new school facilitated the transition for the children. They spoke of their sense of loss of both their previous lives and their home. They all suffered repeated intrusive visualizations of the planes hitting the Towers, of people jumping and of bodies falling from the buildings, and of smoke and ashes. These images were conjured up without warning, and their stress was compounded by fears of another terrorist attack and warnings of impending danger. Trains, subways, bridges, and tunnels all seemed unsafe. The children longed for their friends and their belongings. Two years after the events, the family has begun to feel at home in the new community and has chosen not to return to their city home. The mother obtained a job on Long Island and the father commutes by ferry. The children remain in counseling together to address their anxieties and fears.

Cognitive-Behavioral, Family, and Traumatic Loss Reminder Interventions

Joseph, age 11, was referred for treatment by his mother six months after his father died in the WTC attacks. The youngest of three children, Joseph had resisted help earlier because he "already felt different enough" from his friends without facing the additional perceived stigma of psychotherapy. His family had already received much support from their friends and community. He perceived a loss of privacy stemming from his mother's friends spending time in his family's home and felt a strong need to find space for himself to grieve privately.

Joseph experienced intense anger at his 5th grade teacher, a man who Joseph perceived as cold and non-supportive. Conflict existed between Joseph and his teacher regarding Joseph's frequent failure, after his father's death, to complete homework assignments. In the first treatment session, Joseph acknowledged that his father had often helped him with science and math homework, the two subjects in which Joseph was most frequently missing assignments.

As weekly sessions progressed, Joseph shared his feelings of loss, anger, and sadness. He had enjoyed a warm and close relationship with his father. He expressed sadness, often triggered by loss reminders including music or visiting places previously enjoyed by them and his father, family celebrations, like weddings, and birthday parties. Individual sessions focused on a balance between giving Joseph an opportunity to express feelings of grief and loss, sharpening his awareness of activities that triggered sadness, and developing plans for anticipated loss/trauma reminders and a toolbox of coping strategies for responding to these difficult situations.

Cognitive-Behavioral Interventions. Joseph was helped to understand his feelings of sadness and anger and to anticipate and cope with such intense feelings. This gradually led to greater feelings of control. These interventions included helping him plan his first birthday party without his father. He invited his closest friends and family and related comforting feelings of his father be-

ing there "in spirit." By September 11, 2002, Joseph became increasingly confident and successful by using coping skills including relaxation exercises and
calming self-talk before, during, and after situations that evoked intense feelings.

Social Interventions. While his mother and older siblings appreciated the
support of their family, friends, and community, Joseph felt "crowded," overwhelmed, and embarrassed by his loss of privacy since his father's death. Joseph's uncle was close to him before 9/11 and was recruited as a gatekeeper to
enable Joseph greater control over his time. They discussed a schedule that reserved specific weekday and weekend times when neighbors and extended
family would be asked to allow private time for the nuclear family. Joseph was
also invited to use his uncle's home as a refuge if he felt overwhelmed by visitors' presence. Joseph was taught interpersonal skills to identify and recruit
specific types of social supports (Layne et al., 2001). During therapy, he became skilled in identifying his needs and in recruiting extended family for
problem solving and emotional support.

School Consultation. A school consultation relationship was established.
The teacher shared that his "coldness" to Joseph came from intense feelings of
distress about Joseph's loss. As a child of concentration camp survivors, he
was raised in an environment hypersensitive to loss, while also conveying that
discussing feelings about death and loss was forbidden. With support, the
teacher became increasingly warm and was viewed more positively by Joseph.

Traumatic Loss Reminders. Joseph identified his loss reminders, which included music that he and his father listened to, and his science and math homework. Among coping strategies that worked best for Joseph in dealing with
these triggers were distracting himself by going on walks or playing basketball
with friends and reframing his perspective by focusing on positive changes
that took place after 9/11, including increased closeness and supportiveness
among his family members. Joseph became more adept at anticipating loss reminders, and planning and implementing effective coping strategies.

Commemoration. In an early session, Joseph expressed a desire to have
something of his own to remind him of his father. This request led to the creation of a book that helped Joseph preserve positive memories of his father. He
and his mother assembled pictures and memorabilia of vacations, birthday
parties, and graduations. Joseph became increasingly able to articulate mixed
feelings of sadness and comfort afforded him by these memories.

THE ADOLESCENT (AGES 12-18)

Research has documented that adolescence is a particularly vulnerable time
regarding the impact of trauma, a developmental period when a strong need

for independence emerges and a stable sense of identity is being formed. Rape victims and combat veterans have been reported to have increased risk for PTSD if they experience trauma during adolescence (Van der Kolk, 1985).

Treatment for a Teenager with Pre-Disaster Vulnerability

Mabel, an excellent high school student, attended school near Ground Zero and stared out of its windows and watched the Towers fall. She reported panic, disbelief, and shock. Flashbacks and nightmares prevented her from returning to school. Already preoccupied with her weight and feeling fat prior to 9/11, her weight plummeted. "They won't make me go to school if I'm too thin!" she declared. Her vivid nightmares included loved ones dying in her lap. "There is no way I can go back to that school!" she declared. Individual counseling, nutritional support, and the threat of a medical hospitalization contributed to weight restoration. Family intervention focused on reassurance and support. A cognitive-behavioral approach was taken to clarify thoughts, maintain a realistic perspective, and instill a sense of calm. Consultation with Mabel's school and family led to the assurance that she would not have to return to that school. Having sufficient credits, she decided to graduate early from high school, allowing the flexibility of beginning college in another city. Unfortunately, her younger brother developed symptoms of panic and their father suffered a heart attack. Both children were increasingly anxious about safety. Interventions continue to reduce her brother's anxiety and to support her transition to college life.

Family-Focused Treatment

The Vincent family included four children (all adolescent and college age) who lost their father in the WTC. Their initial reactions were shock, disbelief, and hopes of a miraculous return by him. When the children accepted their father's loss, they and their mother came together to therapy to seek how to proceed without the father's remains to begin to have closure. His remains were subsequently located and a funeral burial was organized. Over subsequent weeks and months, there were six calls announcing that more remains were identified. Mrs. Vincent decided not to inform the children about these calls, wondering "What might it mean to them to have repeated funerals? What images of the remains might such events conjure?" She decided to cremate subsequent remains and have the ashes interred at the gravesite without repeated funeral proceedings. Other families of WTC decedents chose different ways to deal with the delayed finding of relatives' remains, according to their religious and cultural beliefs.

The reactions of the children to their father's death was different. Two appeared ready to accept and move on; one was in disbelief; one was numb. Over time, each accepted the reality in his or her own way. The mother has attempted to model for the children that life goes on. They reacted differently to her efforts, some with relief and others with resentment. Of the four children, one is significantly depressed and has continued treatment. Another, also depressed, questioned the necessity of therapy.

Interventions began with a family meeting soon after 9/11. Most family members had never had contact with mental health providers. The therapist met with combinations of the children and mother utilizing a supportive approach. Antidepressant medication was prescribed for the mother and proved helpful. The youngest of the four children was prescribed a psycho-stimulant to treat his previously diagnosed but untreated Attention-Deficit/Hyperactivity Disorder.

Cognitive-Behavioral and Family-Focused Therapy

Sheila, an 18-year-old Long Island High School senior, lost her father in the WTC attacks. Her father's co-workers said that they were on a floor low enough for him to have escaped but that he stayed behind to ensure that all of his colleagues, including an elderly asthmatic man, were safe. As he escorted this associate down the steps of the North Tower, it collapsed. Sheila began treatment the summer after her father's death because of her uncertainty over attending college in California as she had planned. Her younger sister, Anna, entering high school, begged her to stay home. Anna had been very dependent on her father for schoolwork help. She expressed fear that she could not succeed in high school without Sheila's emotional and academic support. Anna viewed her mother as being too fragile since the loss of her husband to provide her with the help she felt was needed. These themes emerged during her weekly individual psychotherapy sessions:

Traumatic Reminders. Sheila reported difficulty managing traumatic loss reminders that followed the death of her father. Although she did not have a full constellation of Post Traumatic Stress Disorder symptoms, she had frequent flashbacks of Towers collapsing. She avoided radio, television, and newspapers because she found it impossible to cope with media coverage related to the 9/11 attacks. Some of her friends began avoiding her after an initial outpouring of support. The cognitive behavioral and social coping strategies described by Layne and colleagues (2000) for use with adolescents were employed. A combination of coping self-statements, use of journals and approaches to recruit social support were utilized, during and after her exposure to traumatic reminders.

Family Issues. Several sessions were held jointly with Sheila's mother and sister. Their goals were to help Sheila find a more adaptive balance between feeling overburdened by perceived responsibilities for them while finding a realistic role for her to facilitate the family's response to the tragedy. Werner (1993) found that "required helpfulness" can be a protective factor for children following adversity. Sheila's mother and sister helped her to feel that it was her decision whether to stay in New York for another year. Once Sheila felt empowered to decide based on a realistic appraisal of how much her family needed her, rather than from guilt stemming from feeling burdened unfairly by family demands, she decided to defer going to California for one year. Sheila, now attending college in California, reports that she did the right thing by remaining with her family when she feels her presence was critical to her mother's and sister's recoveries.

Ambivalence. Early in treatment, Sheila reluctantly acknowledged having mixed feelings about the nature of her father's death. She was proud of his heroism but angry that he chose to rescue a "stranger" instead of choosing life with his family. After several months of treatment, Sheila shared, for the first time, an incident that involved her and her father during the Saturday before his death. She had then wanted to borrow his car to go to a party with her friends. He refused, citing concerns about alcohol and drug use by members of the crowd planning to attend the party. A screaming match ensued and she had a fleeting thought wishing that he would "drop dead." She felt guilty and ashamed about having harbored such thoughts.

During therapy, she discussed feelings about this incident and her relationship with her father in the context of normal parent-adolescent struggles that would have resolved had her father lived. In keeping with the guidelines of Cohen and Mannarino (2001), Sheila was encouraged to have imaginary conversations with her father, which reminded her that their relationship had always been strong enough to weather even the most stormy fights.

CONCLUSION

The above clinical vignettes are only a few examples of the reactions elicited by the events of 9/11. Working with families with children requires clinicians to be mindful of the children's ranges of reactions and needs for treatments appropriate for their developmental levels. Monitoring of the impact on clinicians is also crucial. Vicarious traumatization is anticipated, but clinicians working in teams can minimize it. When disasters affect communities, as do war and terrorism, clinician responders are also impacted.

NOTES

1. Project Liberty, New York State Office of Mental Health and the U.S. Center for Mental Health Services (CMHS), Substance Abuse and Mental Health Services Administration (SAMSHA).
2. Child and Adolescent Trauma Treatment and Services Consortium (CATS), sponsored by the New York State Office of Mental Health.
3. All names have been changed to protect the identity of the individuals and families.

REFERENCES

Centers for Disease Control and Prevention. (2002, September 11). Deaths in World Trade Center terrorist attacks–New York City 2001. *Morbidity & Mortality Weekly Report, 51*(Special Issue), 16-18.

Cohen, J., & Mannarino, A. (2001). *Cognitive behavioral therapy for traumatic bereavement in children.* Pittsburgh, PA: Center for Traumatic Stress in Children and Adolescent, Allegheny General Hospital.

Harris, R. (2001). *Goodbye mousie.* New York: Simon & Schuster.

Layne, C., Saltzman, W., & Pynoos, R. (2000). *School-based trauma/grief group psychotherapy program.* Los Angeles: Department of Psychiatry, University of California, Los Angeles.

Layne, C. M., Pynoos, R. S., Saltzman, W. R., Arslanagic, B., Savjak, N., Popovic, T. et al. (2001). Trauma/grief-focused group psychotherapy: School-based postwar intervention with traumatized Bosnian adolescents. *Group Dynamics: Theory, Research and Practice, 5,* 277-290.

Lieberman, A., Compton, N., Van Horn, P., & Ghosh-Ippen, C. (2003). *Losing a parent to death in the early years: Guidelines for treating traumatic bereavement in infancy and early childhood.* Washington, DC: Zero to Three.

Newsday. (2004, January 15). Remembering the lost. Retrieved January 15, 2004 from, cf1.newsday.infi.net/911/victimsearchframe.cfm.

Project Liberty Catholic Charities (Producer). (2002). *Putting the pieces together remembering 9/11* [Educational video]. (Available from Catholic Charities, 90 Cherry Lane, Hicksville, NY 11801.)

Van der Kolk, B. (1985). Adolescent vulnerability to PTSD. *Psychiatry, 48,* 365-370.

Werner, E. (1993). Risk, resilience and recovery: Perspectives from the Kauaii Longitudinal Study. *Development and Psychopathology, 54,* 503-515.

Terror, Trauma, and Bereavement: Implications for Theory and Therapy

Ruth Malkinson
Simon Shimshon Rubin
Eliezer Witztum

SUMMARY. How is interpersonal loss incurred in a terror event similar and different from loss under non-terror conditions? Because terror and bereavement are located in the individual's experience of the event, this has important implications for assessment and intervention. In the Two-Track Model of Bereavement (TTMoB), the relationship between life threat, symptomatic response, and the ongoing relationship to the deceased allow therapy to target difficulties in functioning as well as relationship to the deceased. Two case vignettes are presented to ground the discussion.

KEYWORDS. Bereavement, loss, traumatic grief, Two-Track Model of Bereavement, assumptive world

---

Address correspondence to: Ruth Malkinson, PhD, Bob Shapell School of Social Work, Tel Aviv University, Ramat Aviv, Tel Aviv 69978, Israel (E-mail: malkins@agri.huji.ac.il)

[Haworth co-indexing entry note]: "Terror, Trauma, and Bereavement: Implications for Theory and Therapy." Malkinson, Ruth, Simon Shimshon Rubin, and Eliezer Witztum. Co-published simultaneously in *Journal of Aggression, Maltreatment & Trauma* (The Haworth Maltreatment & Trauma Press, an imprint of The Haworth Press, Inc.) Vol. 10, No. 1/2, 2005; and: *The Trauma of Terrorism: Sharing Knowledge and Shared Care, An International Handbook* (ed: Yael Danieli, Danny Brom, and Joe Sills) The Haworth Maltreatment & Trauma Press, an imprint of The Haworth Press, Inc., 2005.

Persons exposed to a terrorist attack are potentially exposed also to a significant dislocation and change in their life course. It is common to experience the physical attack as one that assaults the sense of safety, predictability, and continuity of self and environment that are important to the experience of security. People exposed to terror attacks are challenged to reorganize and reorient their lives. While the loss of a loved one is assuredly their disappearance from the "real" world of interpersonal interaction, it is less clear to what extent their death will be accompanied by a diminution of their presence in the internal world of the bereaved (Rubin, Malkinson, & Witztum, 2000). The bereaved are challenged to reorganize and reorient their lives.

And yet, for all their similarities, there are numerous ways in which terror and bereavement are radically different types of life events with significantly different phenomenology and impact. Not surprisingly, someone can bear the brunt of interpersonal loss and be involved in a terror event simultaneously. We seek to provide a conceptual framework to clarify appraisal and intervention in cases of the combination of these events.

Is interpersonal loss incurred under terrorism always different from loss under non-terror conditions? What are some of the clinical implications of the interaction of terror and loss?

The terms "trauma" and "bereavement" are often joined together. The frequent use of the terms in combination has resulted in a category of loss considered to be "traumatic bereavement" or "traumatic grief" (Prigerson & Jacobs, 2001). Despite the prominent and increasing usage of these terms, there remains a degree of ambiguity (Shear & Smith, 2002; Silverman, Johnson, & Prigerson, 2001; Stroebe, Schut, & Finkenauer, 2001). Part of the tension stems from the competing trauma and bereavement perspectives that vie for primacy in the hybrid. Each field may highlight its terminology and perspective so as to emphasize why the phenomena are best grouped under either the loss matrix or the trauma and stress rubric (Brom & Kleber, 2000). We advance the argument for a multi-faceted approach to the phenomena of traumatic bereavement. While this is particularly relevant to bereavement occurring under conditions of terror, it has general relevance as well.

Regardless of the conceptual framework, both terror and bereavement are located in the individual's experience of the event. This is true both when the bereaved individual was physically exposed to the terror threat as well as when s/he was not present. The individual who was not present, yet experienced the loss of a loved one, has special needs that overlap with those of individuals exposed to terrorism but who were not bereaved or injured. One could say that the experience of terror and bereavement is located in the interaction of the two in a relatively elastic function, and there are patterns rather than clear-cut "rules." Despite the complexity of the interaction, we believe that there are major sequelae of trauma, traumatic bereavement, and terror.

The range of symptomatic response to trauma is broad. It may take on the characteristic of stress disorders, such as Acute Stress Disorder or Post Traumatic Stress Disorder (PTSD), or it may present with any symptomatic picture. Almost any psychological responses are possible outcomes in the aftermath of trauma and traumatic bereavement.

There are many advantages to maintaining a focus on the response to both loss and trauma in ways that encompass the significance of how bereaved persons manage their lives following loss. In the Two-Track Model of Bereavement (TTMoB; Rubin, 1999), attending to a multidimensional view of psychosocial functioning and its derivatives is balanced by a parallel focus on the emotional, cognitive and psychological relationship to the deceased (Rubin, Malkinson, & Witztum, 2000, 2003). Expanding and clarifying these twin tracks of (a) Functioning, which comprises an array of symptoms, including the symptom picture of distress, various other mental and physical types of upset, and numerous features of disruption in integration with the worlds of relationships, and meaning matrixes, and (b) Relationship to the deceased, which includes numerous features of the way the deceased and the relationship to him or her is conceptualized and experienced, are key to evaluating, researching, and intervening at the juxtaposition of terror, trauma and bereavement.

The TTMoB is particularly useful in assessing the magnitude of the traumatic experience as well as the loss components of the experience. We present two case vignettes, then our view that trauma (including terror attacks) and bereavement overlap so that they are best treated as mixed rather than either separate or independent phenomena. A further analysis of the cases will clarify clinical implications.

VIGNETTE 1: SPOUSAL BEREAVEMENT: DIRECT EXPOSURE

Dave M. was seated next to his wife Noa on the bus when a suicide bomber boarded and almost immediately activated her explosive device. The last thing he remembered before the blast was a stylish, pregnant Arab woman who looked too well bred to be traveling by public transportation. In the explosion, a flurry of ball bearings, nuts, and bolts tore through the first part of the bus and the people grouped there. Noa was killed instantly, while Dave himself was lightly wounded. He remembers the screams of the victims, the horrible smell of burning, the hands pulling him away from his dead wife to safety, and the smoke that was everywhere. Moments later, Dave immediately returned to the bus for his wife, but all he found was a severed hand that he thought was hers.

Noa had already been carried out and her body covered with makeshift articles of clothing. Despite profuse bleeding from a head wound, Dave resisted being transferred to the hospital, insisting he had to remain with his wife's body since, if the hand was hers, it should be taken to the morgue at Abu Kabir and eventually buried with her. Later, he was told by the social worker at the hospital that the hand was not his wife's and that she would be buried as completely as possible. A month after the funeral, which he barely remembers, Dave was hypertense, experienced flashbacks of pictures before and after the bus bombing, and ruminated whether he should have taken the hand out of the bus with him to have made sure that it was not Noa's. He missed his wife terribly, was sleeping and eating poorly, was unable to concentrate at work or at home, and had contemplated suicide but thought that it would be too hard for his young adult children to bear at this time. He was referred for individual treatment by the National Insurance Rehabilitation Division.

In his case, the exposure to terror and the traumatic bereavement occurred simultaneously. The multiple sources of "trauma" include the particular horrific images that Dave was exposed to. The next case of spousal bereavement in a terrorist attack occurred at a distance, but still with devastating effect.

VIGNETTE 2: SPOUSAL BEREAVEMENT: INDIRECT EXPOSURE

Susan Y. lost her chemist husband Zack in a terror attack. Zack had gone out drinking with his friends and did not return. Susan had called the police, who belittled her concern and told her to call back if he remained missing for another day. Her friends also minimized her concern, saying that Zack was probably on a "binge" with his friends. Susan was upset by their response and remained very anxious and uneasy. Two days later, Zack's body was found, bound and burned in the shell of his still smoldering car. Dental records confirmed his identity. The police ruled it a terrorist attack, and Susan felt her concerns had been vindicated and that her friends had totally let her down. In the following weeks, anxiety, depression, insomnia, and restlessness continued to interfere with her life. After attempting to deal with "this" herself, she approached her family physician, who prescribed medication. This did not help, and after several months she requested therapy to help her cope with her sadness and anxiety.

These two cases of spousal bereavement illustrate how traumatic bereavement may manifest itself under conditions of terrorism. What can be so disruptive and traumatizing in these losses is best understood as some combination of the attack upon self, other, and worldview that accompanies both losses.

BEREAVEMENT AND TRAUMA AS THE LOSS OF COHERENCE, CONTINUITY AND CAPABILITY

Loss and exposure to terrorism are two classes of events that disrupt life patterns and functioning and require major responses by the individual to restore homeostasis. Grouping loss as well as other dislocations of self as predictors for depression and anxiety takes into account the multiple ways in which individuals are vulnerable to psychological dislocation produced by a variety of stress factors. One recent example, emerging from a study of twins, examined the relationship of depression and anxiety resulting from a variety of life crises and/or psychological threats to the self system (Kendler, Hetlema, Butera, Gardner, & Prescott, 2003). The fact that numerous events can produce seemingly similar response patterns and disorders has led to theoretical and clinical confusion. In particular, the unique aspects of bereavement have often been overlooked by the focus on the shared elements of life crises and shared symptomatology.

In the wake of exposure to events of overwhelming magnitude, the individual must cope with attacks upon mostly deeply held (and often unarticulated) beliefs about the self, the outside world, and about one's relationship to the forces that shape our lives. Janoff-Bulman's work on shattered assumptions (1992) is relevant for terror, trauma, and bereavement. She suggests that exposure to certain life events of great psychological magnitude attacks basic assumptions about the benevolence of the world, meaningfulness, and self-worth. Establishing new beliefs and changed beliefs is a task for the individual in adapting to this new world reality. This is one of the tasks of adaptation to a world that has changed forever (Kauffman, 2002). At a national level, Pearl Harbor in 1941 was a defining moment of change for a U.S. generation, as was the Yom Kippur war in 1973 for Israel, and the events of September 11, 2001 for most of the Western world.

Several relevant examples of the interface between bereavement and terrorism emerged from the New York World Trade Center (WTC) experience. On the basis of survey of adult response to the 9/11 attack and its aftermath, Galea et al. (2002) reported on the occurrence of PTSD and major depressive disorder in the short-term aftermath. They found that gender, ethnicity, physical proximity to the event, and personal experience of loss of a relative or friend were among the predictors of diagnosable disorder. Being involved in such an attack turned out to be not only a function of physical proximity, but also of psychological proximity and involvement via the conduit of important relationships. In other words, having a relative involved in the terrorist attack yielded a number of symptomatic behaviors characteristic of exposure and proximity to the terrorist event.

Similar findings emerged from the preliminary report prepared in 2002 by Hoven and colleagues (Hoven et al., 2002) for the New York City Board of Education examining how the emotional health of New York City schoolchildren was affected by the September 11 attack. In that report, the exposure of a family member to the attack was a better predictor of PTSD than was personal physical exposure or proximity of the child him or herself. In another study (DeLisi et al., 2003), 1,009 adults were interviewed in Manhattan about themselves before and after September 11. Results revealed that over half had some emotional sequelae three to six months after the event, and only a small portion of those with severe responses was seeking treatment.

In Israel, Karniel-Lauer (2003) compared individuals injured in terror attacks with those who lost relatives in such attacks. The population consisted of 180 subjects in three groups: the first included subjects that were injured in terror attacks; the second, subjects that lost a meaningful figure in a terrorist attack; the third (control) group had socio-demographic characteristics similar to those in the other two groups. Each group consisted of 60 subjects. Each subject was interviewed individually and filled out a questionnaire that included demographic data, exposure to the event, world assumptions, damage to self-perception, traumatic grief, and symptoms of the post-traumatic stress disorder.

The findings indicate that terrorist attacks should be viewed as events with particular pathogenic potential for both the injured and the bereaved (51.5% of the subjects developed PTSD, and 20% of the subjects developed a grief response). However, the rate of PTSD among the injured was higher than among bereaved subjects. The two world assumptions, the "benevolent world" and the "self-worth," changed after the traumatic event; whereas the group of victims regarded the world as less benevolent, the bereaved group related lower self-value to themselves. The findings confirmed a risk for both, but with important differences in their response patterns. On matters of viewing the world and the self, the traumatic event affected both groups. But whereas the injured tended to experience change in their view of the world, the bereaved tended to experience change in self-perception.

A related area to meaning has to do with the self-experience of the individual. Here, too, is an underlying commonality to terror, trauma and loss that is only partially related to the extent of behavioral change following exposure and response to these life experiences. Studies revealed that these life experiences change the individual. Significant individual change was reported in the case of bereavement, infant loss, loss of sons due to military causes (Malkinson & Bar-Tur, 2000; Rubin, 1992; Rubin & Malkinson, 2001) and road accidents (Shalev, 1999). These changes to the integration and organization of self are common to both bereavement and non-bereavement trauma

(Neimeyer, Keesee, & Fortner, 2000). The change in the view of self and world is a fundamental similarity between trauma and bereavement. There is a greater sense of vulnerability, and many other features that involve recognizing that things can no longer be seen as they once were (Janoff-Bulman, 1992).

BEREAVEMENT AND TRAUMA
AND THE TWO-TRACK MODEL OF BEREAVEMENT

In every loss, the necessity of reorganizing the relationship to the now deceased loved one is a task of great complexity. This forces us to reorganize our mental schemata and emotional response to the memories of their presence and their impact, their absence, and the nature of their intertwining with our lives. Loss under particularly traumatic circumstances compounds the recovery process. Witnessing the death of a loved one is traumatic in many cases (illness, accident, violent deaths). In the WTC disaster, with family and friends witnessing this openly on TV, they swayed between despair and hope. When the terrible reality dawned, they were left with the finality of the loss with no bodies to mourn for (Rubin, Malkinson, & Witztum, 2003). The general approach to assessment and intervention at the trauma-bereavement interface should remain sensitive to both foci of the disruptive life experience. There are a range of bereavements that are particularly traumatic. Examples of these may be: the loss of a child suddenly and without warning; loss occurring under conditions of massive violence with the bereaved not present (homicide or terrorism); or loss occurring at the same time that the bereaved is exposed to immediate life threat (such as escaping from a violent event while one's beloved is struck down). In all of these cases the approach to the assessment of the trauma and the bereavement are fundamentally the same. In all, a parallel assessment of the ongoing reorganization of the internal psychological relationship to the deceased, and the manner in which a multidimensional set of tasks of life function are affected, is warranted. The particular profile of the response to these losses, along the two-pronged demarcation provided by the TTMoB, assists in the measurement of, and potential intervention following, many kinds of bereavement.

The two cases presented illustrate the application and the clinical decisions faced by the dual focus of this bereavement model.

CASE ILLUSTRATIONS

The major elements characterizing trauma include intrusive re-experiencing of the trauma and/or its avoidance, anxiety, and depression. The major elements of loss and bereavement include preoccupation with, reliving and yearning for the lost person, profound sad and painful feelings following the loss, and anxiety. These reactions can coexist, and this is the variation of traumatic loss, depending on the circumstances of the death and the response of the bereaved (Rubin, Malkinson, & Witztum, 2003).

> Dave M. was exposed to a terrorist attack in which he lost his wife. From the perspective of the TTMoB, there are numerous indicators of response on Track One: the post traumatic symptoms of hyper vigilance, problems with concentration, flashbacks of the trauma, insomnia, loss of appetite and suicidal ideation. Indicators of Track Two appeared later and were characterized by memories that were not focused on the trauma but related to mutual experiences with his wife.

> Susan Y. experienced a traumatic loss that involved a terrorist event without personal exposure to the event and an interpersonal loss. In telling the details of her husband's traumatic death, she repeatedly mentioned the longstanding reservations she had about that specific group who were his childhood friends. He was very attached to them and they used to spend time drinking together, which she detested. She said she always felt uncomfortable in their company and had tried many times to convince her husband to stop meeting them. Therefore, when he invited her to join him, she refused to go, as she had done previously. She said she felt guilty for failing to convince him not to go, a thought that she was obsessed with. Her family physician prescribed medication to alleviate symptoms of anxiety and insomnia, which Susan stopped taking after a while.

What should be the foci of intervention in Susan's case? We can see why the severity of her depression and anxiety symptoms may, in the physician's opinion, justify medication, but we also know that a rapid relief of symptoms could be counterproductive to Susan's experiencing the pain of loss and guilt feelings she has been encountering.

From the TTMoB perspective, Susan's story has elements of both the Functioning Track (anxiety, insomnia and depression) and the Relationship Track (conflict and guilt feelings), so both will need to be addressed in the course of therapy. It seems that magnitudes of elements of the trauma are more pronounced and therefore should receive priority at the initial phase of therapy.

In Susan's situation, not only were the violent circumstances of the death sufficient to meet criteria for major overwhelming trauma, but there were other features as well. The sudden, unexpected nature of the death, the anxiety of the waiting period, and the mutilation of the body were also traumatagenic. Finally, the absence of social support for her husband added additional sources of trauma, disruption, and difficulty to this loss. Working with Track Two on Case 2 will revolve around relationship issues, especially those of guilt and responsibility as experienced by Susan. These issues require special interventions for acute and chronic grief (Daie & Witztum, 1991; Malkinson, 2001; Witztum & Roman, 2000).

These two cases demonstrate aspects of what we are suggesting: that the interface of traumatic bereavement is more adequately addressed as a broad and inclusive concept. In that way, the multiple aspects of what can be so disruptive and traumatizing in loss are better clarified by considering the additive and complementary contributions of various factors in the loss process.

CONCLUDING REMARKS

Ultimately, what is traumatic in "bereavement as the result of terrorism" leads to a multiple and cumulative view of trauma and bereavement, with direct implications for assessment, research, and intervention. For both the clinicians and researchers among us, it is useful to stress the following points:

1. Bereavement accompanying exposure to terrorism and similar external trauma that threatens life is a particular kind of traumatic bereavement. Much of the literature on trauma stems from non-bereavement related events that directly place the individual at risk for harm, injury, and death. A death occurring at the same time as a life threat is common in terrorist attacks. This is bereavement occurring under conditions of trauma.
2. While not all bereavement occurs under conditions of terror, any bereavement can be experienced as traumatic. We know that the loss of a loved one and responding to that loss, which are by definition at the heart of bereavement, make up a painful and disruptive process. Bereavement is traumatic in the sense that it overwhelms. There is always a "wound" (trauma), which reflects the attack on self, world, and relationship to a specific other, but its impact varies.
3. Traumatic bereavement originates at the interface of the individual and the event. The more severe the so-called "objective" traumatic proportions of the type of bereavement, the more likely one is to have complications in the "traumatic bereavement."
4. There are types of loss that are more likely to result in complications due to circumstances even though they may not meet external criteria for "traumatic proportions." This does not reflect on how painful or dislocating they may be.

The empirical and clinical materials described in this chapter lend support to the importance of multi-dimensional assessment in cases of traumatic grief following terrorism in order to determine intervention strategies suited for the individual case. The Two-Track Model of Bereavement provides a framework for addressing the relationship between terrorism, traumatic response and interpersonal loss. Appropriate therapy will match its focus to the relative significance of each of these features.

REFERENCES

Brom, D., & Kleber, R. (2000). On coping with trauma and coping with grief: Similarities and differences. In R. Malkinson, S. Rubin, & E. Witztum (Eds.), *Traumatic and nontraumatic loss and bereavement: Clinical theory and practice* (pp. 41-66). Madison, CT: Psychosocial Press.

Daie, N., & Witztum, E. (1991). Short-term strategic treatment in traumatic conversion reactions. *American Journal of Psychotherapy, 55*, 335-347.

DeLisi, L. E., Maurizio, A., Yost, M., Papparozzi, C. F., Fulchino, C., Katz, G. et al. (2003). A survey of New Yorkers after the Sept. 11, 2001, terrorist attacks. *American Journal of Psychiatry, 160*, 780-783.

Galea, S., Ahern, J., Resnick, H., Kilpatrick, D., Bucyvalas, M., Gold, J. et al. (2002). Psychological sequelae of the September 11 terrorist attacks in New York City. *New England Journal of Medicine, 346*(13), 982-987.

Hoven, C. W., Duarte, C. S. Lucas, C. P., Mandell, D. J., Wu, P., & Rosen, C. (2002). *Effects of the World Trade Center attack on NYC public school students: Initial report of the New York Board of Education.* New York: Applied Research and Consulting, LLC & Columbia University Mailman School of Public Health & New York State Psychiatric Institute.

Janoff-Bulman, R. (1992). *Shattered assumptions: Towards a new psychology of trauma.* New York: The Free Press.

Karniel- Lauer, E. (2003). *Post traumatic stress disorder and grief response: Their interrelationship, and the contribution of damage to "world assumption" and "self perception."* Unpublished doctoral dissertation, Tel Aviv University, Tel Aviv, Israel.

Kauffman, J. (Ed.). (2002). *Loss of the assumptive world: A theory of traumatic loss.* New York: Brunner-Rutledge.

Kendler, K. S., Hetlema, J. M., Butera, F., Gardner, C. O., & Prescott, C. A. (2003). Life event dimensions of loss, humiliation, entrapment, and danger in the prediction of onset of major depression and generalized anxiety. *Archives of General Psychiatry, 60*, 789-796.

Malkinson, R., & Bar-Tur, L. (2000). The aging of grief: Parents' grieving of Israeli soldiers. *Journal of Personal & Interpersonal Loss, 5*(2-3), 247-262.

Malkinson, R. (2001). Cognitive-behavioral therapy of grief: A review and application. *Research on Social Work Practice, 11*(6), 671-698.

Niemeyer, R., Keesee, N. J. & Fortner, B. V. (2000). Loss and meaning reconstruction: Propositions and procedures. In R. Malkinson, S. Rubin, & E. Witztum (Eds.), *Traumatic and nontraumatic loss and bereavement: Clinical theory and practice* (pp. 173-196). Madison, CT: Psychosocial Press.

Prigerson, H., & Jacobs, S. (2001). Traumatic grief as a distinct disorder: A rationale, consensus criteria, and a preliminary empirical test. In M. Stroebe, W. Stroebe, R. O. Hansson, & H. Schut (Eds.), *Handbook of bereavement research: Consequences, coping, and care* (pp. 613-645). Washington, DC: American Psychological Association Press.

Rubin, S. (1992). Adult child loss and the Two-Track Model of Bereavement. *Omega, 24*(3), 183-202.

Rubin, S. (1999). The Two-Track Model of Bereavement: Overview, retrospect and prospect. *Death Studies, 23*(8), 681-714.

Rubin, S., & Malkinson, R. (2001). Parental response to child loss across the life-cycle: Clinical and research perspectives. In M. Stroebe, W. Stroebe, R. Hansson, & H. Schut (Eds.), *Handbook of bereavement research: Consequences, coping, and care* (pp. 219-240). Washington, DC: American Psychological Association Press.

Rubin, S., Malkinson, R., & Witztum, E. (2000). An overview of the field of loss. In R. Malkinson, S. Rubin, and E. Witztum (Eds.), *Traumatic and nontraumatic loss and bereavement: Clinical theory and practice* (pp. 5-40). Madison, CT: Psychosocial Press.

Rubin, S., Malkinson, R., & Witztum, E. (2003). Trauma and bereavement: Conceptual and clinical issues revolving around relationships. *Death Studies, 27*, 1-23.

Schuster, M. A., Stein, B. D., Jaycox, L. H., Collins, R. L., Marshall, G. N., Elliott, M. N. et al. (2002). A national survey of stress reactions after the September 11, 2001, terrorist attacks. *The New England Journal of Medicine, 345*(20), 1507-1512.

Shalev, R. (1999). *Comparison of war bereaved and motor vehicle accident bereaved parents*. Unpublished master's thesis, University of Haifa. (Hebrew).

Shear, M. K., & Smith, K. (2002). Traumatic loss and the syndrome of complicated grief. *PTSD Research Quarterly, 13*(1), 1-6.

Silverman, G. K., Johnson, J. G., & Prigerson, H. G. (2001). Preliminary explorations of the effects of prior trauma and loss on risk for psychiatry disorders in recently widowed people. *Israel Journal of Psychiatry, 38*(3-4), 202-215.

Stroebe, M. S., Schut, H., & Finkenauer, C. (2001). The traumatization of grief? A conceptual framework for understanding the trauma-bereavement interface. *Israel Journal of Psychiatry, 38*(3-4), 185-201.

Witztum, E., & Roman, I. (2000). Psychotherapeutic intervention in complicated grief: Metaphor and leave-taking ritual with the bereaved. In R. Malkinson, S. Rubin, & E. Witztum (Eds.), *Traumatic and nontraumatic loss and bereavement: Clinical theory and practice* (pp. 143-172). Madison, CT: Psychosocial Press.

Voice:
Elizabeth Neuffer:
In Memoriam

Peter S. Canellos

Firefighters can't be firefighters without entering burning buildings. Journalists can calmly ply their trade from behind a desk. It takes a certain kind of journalist to get out from behind the desk and visit the blazing buildings, markets, and roadsides laid to waste by international terrorism. Those outside the journalism profession often assume it's part of the job, the urge to tell the story. But there are other ways to tell a story, and other stories to tell.

The journalists who dedicate their lives, and sometimes lose their lives, bearing witness to the pain of the victims of the world's greatest atrocities choose their work for personal, not professional, reasons. Their commitment springs from a deeper well than journalistic curiosity or ambition. They stand with the victims of terrorism because they believe it is where they should stand.

Elizabeth Neuffer, who reported for *The Boston Globe* from Kuwait, Bosnia, Kosovo, Rwanda, Iran, Afghanistan, and the World Trade Center be-

---

Address correspondence to: Peter S. Canellos, Washington Bureau Chief, *The Boston Globe*, 1130 Connecticut Avenue NW, Washington DC, 20036 USA (E-mail: canellos@globe.com).

The author dedicates this contribution to his beloved partner of 13 years, Elizabeth Neuffer, an award-winning journalist and author whose voice would have been a part of this book, who died May 9, 2003, in a car crash in Iraq.

[Haworth co-indexing entry note]: "Voice: Elizabeth Neuffer: In Memoriam." Canellos, Peter S. Co-published simultaneously in *Journal of Aggression, Maltreatment & Trauma* (The Haworth Maltreatment & Trauma Press, an imprint of The Haworth Press, Inc.) Vol. 10, No. 1/2, 2005; and: *The Trauma of Terrorism: Sharing Knowledge and Shared Care, An International Handbook* (ed: Yael Danieli, Danny Brom, and Joe Sills) The Haworth Maltreatment & Trauma Press, an imprint of The Haworth Press, Inc., 2005.

fore losing her life in a car crash in Samarra, Iraq, wrote, "After watching an elderly woman gunned down in front of me in Sarajevo, in full view of two UN peacekeepers, with orders not to return fire, my grief vanished, replaced by outrage" (Neuffer, 2001, p. xvii).

Elsewhere in her book, *The Key to My Neighbor's House*, she wrote, "Like everyone I met in Bosnia, I wanted something that would assuage my guilt, answer my fears, and punish those who were responsible" (p. xiv).

She, like some others who journey to the world's most dangerous and tormented places, felt a special empathy for victims of random violence. After a happy childhood, her placid existence was shattered by losses beyond her control. It gave her a powerful sense of how average Americans, in the calmness of their own lives, were blinded to deeper truths about life itself: The reality of shocking and unpredictable losses. The awareness that at any moment the floor could fall away, and all that one knows or holds dear could crumble in an instant.

This is how Neuffer would cover terrorism. She'd insist that her readers see the victims as individuals, with the same likes, dislikes, virtues, and flaws as anyone in the world. She'd insist that their loss mattered by itself, divorced from politics or history. But she'd want her readers to know the politics and history so they might be able to do something to prevent such crimes in the future.

At Elizabeth's memorial service, on May 30, 2003 in Wilton Congregational Church in Wilton, Connecticut, Barbara Demick, a friend and fellow war correspondent who saw the evils that she saw, said, "If she would occasionally cry while interviewing somebody with a particularly tragic tale, the empathy would last long after her story was published and the newspaper discarded. She truly believed that powerful writing and reporting could make the world a better place, that evil when exposed to the light of day could be rooted out."

She wasn't alone. Wherever there is an act of terrorism, there are those who bear witness. They tell the world what they saw, and try to make people everywhere confront it. What happens to some of us happens to all of us, to all humankind. Violence is as much a shared experience as a moon landing or the discovery of a cure for a deadly disease.

There's a photograph of Elizabeth Neuffer sitting in a Bosnian field, encircled by women who lost family members in the Srebrenica massacre. The story of the massacre is written on their faces, their desperate sorrow shrouded by their headscarves. Elizabeth is looking into the eyes of a woman as she tells her story. One of Elizabeth's hands holds tight to that of the woman. Her other hand holds a pen. This picture, this tableux, conveys the work of a reporter covering terrorism. It reveals the true spirit of journalism, which is in every sense the true spirit of humanity.

REFERENCE

Neuffer, E. (2001). *The Key to My Neighbor's House: Seeking Justice in Bosnia and Rwanda.* New York: Picador.

Voice:
In Memoriam:
Daniel Pearl

Tamara Pearl

As Daniel Pearl's[1] sister, I have experienced the effects of terrorism in a direct and uncommon way. To simply lose someone you love is profoundly painful. To have to also face the public nature of his ordeal, to watch him on television, to endure the torture of wondering what would happen to him at the hands of his captors, made his death an unbelievable nightmare for our whole family.

After we found out that Danny was dead, the ordeal continued with frustrating and elusive updates about the trial and the ongoing investigation, maddening reports from Pakistan detailing the popular glorification of the murderers, painful phone calls with the military coroners, and seemingly endless tears. Along with this came the questions that gnawed at me. How could anyone lose their humanity enough to want to inflict so much pain on others? How can I still embrace this world after experiencing the worst side of human nature?

I remember when I first saw my best friend after Danny's death, I blurted out to her, "But life is still good." What a strange thing to say. Somehow, I must have known that I would spend many months wrestling with the question of whether life was good or not.

Address correspondence to: Tamara Pearl, The Daniel Pearl Foundation, 16161 Ventura Boulevard # 671, Encino, CA 91436 USA (E-mail: tamara@danielpearl.org).

[Haworth co-indexing entry note]: "Voice: In Memoriam: Daniel Pearl." Pearl, Tamara. Co-published simultaneously in *Journal of Aggression, Maltreatment & Trauma* (The Haworth Maltreatment & Trauma Press, an imprint of The Haworth Press, Inc.) Vol. 10, No. 1/2, 2005; and: *The Trauma of Terrorism: Sharing Knowledge and Shared Care, An International Handbook* (ed: Yael Danieli, Danny Brom, and Joe Sills) The Haworth Maltreatment & Trauma Press, an imprint of The Haworth Press, Inc., 2005.

Danny himself has helped me to answer this question. Throughout his travels around the world as a reporter, he maintained a strong faith in humanity, a deep respect for people, and a healthy sense of humor about himself and human nature. In an e-mail he wrote to my mom not long before he died, "working on the same old terrorism story." Terrorists and their activities were just not as interesting to Danny as the myriad of other ordinary and extraordinary people he wrote about. I think it was because he knew the terrorists did not know how to really live life, something Danny did better than anyone I know.

He was gentle and kind; he valued his friendships tremendously; and he made the most out of every moment. Many people who saw his photo wrote to say that they were inexplicably moved by his smile. Letters and e-mails from people who had been helped or touched by Danny came from all around the world. A woman in India whom Danny had helped with her young son, colleagues who loved working with him and remembered his uplifting "hi!" from his cell phone, college friends who recalled how he never cared if they won or lost a football game, how he only appreciated being with friends outside on a sunny day.

This is why even after what happened to him, I firmly believe that he would still have the same faith in humanity, and the same joy for life that he always had. It was simply his nature. Even in the face of so much hatred he didn't doubt himself and he maintained his dignity; we can see it in his eyes. No band of murderers could change that.

As Jews, we have experienced other hate-driven deaths in our family and culture, particularly in the Holocaust. There are always choices in how to respond to these horrors, and my family has gone through some of these. One is to succumb to despair, and turn our backs on a world that is capable of such cruelty. Another choice is to try to fight hatred and injustice in the spirit of Tikkun Olam (healing the world). One more choice is to sit firmly in our own humanity, facing and embracing life with all its facets. To do this we have had to learn to create an internal process to transform the pain that we feel, transforming the horror into something life-affirming. This choice not only honors the spirit of Danny, but also helps us to fully go on.

To that end, together we have created the Daniel Pearl Foundation,[2] which uses the humane international response to the tragedy to help build cultural bridges. The foundation has brought a Pakistani journalist to the *Wall Street Journal*, conducted an essay contest on tolerance for youth, and connected musicians and music lovers around the world on an annual day of music for humanity on Danny's birthday.

At Danny's memorial service my father recalled, "He was not intimidated even when one teacher stuck a swastika in his face and said, 'You are wearing the Star of David, Danny? Look what I am wearing!'" We were terribly upset, but Danny just narrated the incident in his matter-of-fact way, as if saying: "Upset? Why would I get upset if a teacher makes a fool of himself?"

That was Danny's deepest teaching, part of the palpable knowing and dignity that surrounded him. To honor him, and to prevent the terrorists from prevailing, we have chosen to live our lives fully, love each other deeply, and to feel our own humanity every day. Ultimately, I have found out that what I said to my friend in my initial dazed state of shock is true. The world is still good.

NOTES

1. *Wall Street Journal* reporter Daniel Pearl became the focus of international concern when he was kidnapped and murdered by Islamic terrorists while working on a story in Pakistan in February 2002. A videotape of his murder shows that he was killed because he was Jewish and American. In defiance, his parents Judea and Ruth Pearl published an anthology entitled *I am Jewish–Personal Reflections Inspired by the Last Words of Daniel Pearl* (Jewish Lights, 2004).

2. www.danielpearl.org

SECTION V
SCHOOL- AND COMMUNITY-BASED INTERVENTIONS IN THE FACE OF TERRORIST ATTACKS

Building Resilience:
A School-Based Intervention for Children Exposed to Ongoing Trauma and Stress

Naomi L. Baum

SUMMARY. The context for the National School Intervention Project-Israel has been the ongoing security situation that has exposed the entire civilian population to extremely high levels of trauma. This project places itself within the framework of the resilience literature, focusing on characteristics of resilience that can be brought into the classroom and empower school staff. This article highlights the Building Resilience project, a series of teacher workshops. An initial evaluation of

Address correspondence to: Naomi L. Baum, PhD, The Israel Center for the Treatment of Psychotrauma, P.O.B. 35300, Jerusalem 91351, Israel.

[Haworth co-indexing entry note]: "Building Resilience: A School-Based Intervention for Children Exposed to Ongoing Trauma and Stress." Baum, Naomi L. Co-published simultaneously in *Journal of Aggression, Maltreatment & Trauma* (The Haworth Maltreatment & Trauma Press, an imprint of The Haworth Press, Inc.) Vol. 10, No. 1/2, 2005; and: *The Trauma of Terrorism: Sharing Knowledge and Shared Care, An International Handbook* (ed: Yael Danieli, Danny Brom, and Joe Sills) The Haworth Maltreatment & Trauma Press, an imprint of The Haworth Press, Inc., 2005.

teachers participating in the Building Resilience project found change in knowledge, skills, and willingness to use tools learned with their students in the classroom.

KEYWORDS. School-based intervention, resilience, children, trauma

In the past three years, Israeli society has been subjected to increasing numbers of terrorist attacks, suicide bombers, drive-by shootings, and mortar attacks. In addition to physical wounds and casualties, the resulting trauma and stress to large segments of the population is difficult to estimate. Terrorism seeks to wreak havoc in our day-to-day lives. As Pfefferbaum (2001) notes:

> The intent of terrorism, evident in the word itself, is not the death and injury of direct victims, the sorrow and grief of their loved ones, the wreckage of property, or even the disruption of government, business, and travel. It is rather the emotional consequences that result from the terrorism that accompanies the altered environment in which we will now lead our lives. (p. 940)

In conceptualizing the vulnerability of populations that have been affected by attacks on civilians, it is convenient to picture four concentric circles, sometimes referred to as "circles of vulnerability" (Ayalon & Lahad, 2001). At the epicenter are the people who have been directly injured or killed. The second circle contains those closest to the injured or deceased: family members, close friends, co-workers, and people who fall in the "near miss" category. The third circle consists of community members, neighbors, and classmates. In the outer circles are people who may have had occasional contact with the victims, may have been at the scene ten minutes before or stepped off the bus minutes before it blew up (commonly referred to as "near-miss"), as well as people who have been exposed to media coverage of the event. Pfefferbaum, Pfefferbaum, North, and Neas (2002) have written extensively about the effects of media exposure and its apparent relationship to post traumatic symptomatology. The entire population of Israel is exposed to graphic and detailed accounts broadcast live from the scene of the attack and must be considered when planning for the mental health needs of the country.

The concept of circles of vulnerability implies that even those not directly exposed to the terrorist attacks, and with no contact with the victims, may suffer significant symptoms relating to trauma and stress. As a result of this current state of national trauma, many people avoid public places, shopping malls, theatres, places of entertainment, and downtown areas. Others refuse to ride buses and trains. A review of research documenting the effects of exposure to terrorism and trauma can be found in Pat-Horencyzk (this volume). The effects of terrorism on this large group of victims in the second, third, and fourth circles of vulnerability go largely unreported and unrecognized.

The security situation in Israel and its impact on the population at large formed the impetus for the National School Intervention Project (NSIP). Concern about the long-term impact of stress and exposure to terrorism that go largely unrecognized and untreated spurred the development of this project. It focused on the entire school population, a decidedly non-clinical audience, yet one that has been exposed along with the entire Israeli population. As such, the frame of reference chosen was one of resilience and wellness in contrast to one of pathology, risk, and treatment. Being informed by the "psychology of wellness" and the positive psychology movement (Cowan, 1991; Seligman & Csikszentmihalyi, 2000) helped focus on questions such as: What is optimal functioning during periods of long-term exposure to stress and terrorism? How can we facilitate this functioning?

EFFECTS OF EXPOSURE TO TERRORISM

Summaries of the effects of exposure to terrorism on civilian populations both in Israel and the world can be found extensively in this volume. In attempting to understand the effect of terrorism on the lives of everyday citizens in general and children in particular, the extensive psychological literature on stress can point the way. Terrorism can be perceived as a "stressor" as defined by Grant, Compas, Stuhlmacher, Thurm, McMahon, and Halpert (2003): "environmental events or chronic conditions that objectively threaten the physical and/or psychological health or well-being of individuals of a particular age in a particular society" (p. 452). In a recent review article summarizing over 1500 empirical investigations of the relation between stressors and psychological symptoms among children and youth conducted in the last 15 years, the relationship between stressors and the development of psychopathology has been well documented (Grant et al., 2003). Most significant are the results highlighting the effect of effective parenting on mediating between stressors and healthy child development. Hammen and Rudolph (1996) found that stressors influence the mental health of children and adolescents through the disruption of important interpersonal relationships and interactions including, but not limited to, parent-child relationships. Conger, Conger, Elder, Lorenz,

Simons, and Whitbeck (1993) found that when parents are involved in coping with their own significant stressors, they are unavailable to their children, thereby greatly reducing the mediating effect of the parent-child relationship in buffering reactions to stress. Children thus experience more parental harshness and rejection, reduced nurturing, and less consistent discipline.

Coping and Resilience

Coping and resilience in the face of significant ongoing stressors bring two different frames of reference into the spotlight. Coping mechanisms emphasize what a person does when encountering stress. Resilience, in contrast, focuses on assets and resources that serve a protective purpose in adverse conditions. Norris, Friedman, Watson, and Byrne (2002) note that coping appears when there is distress. While the notion that coping reduces stress is prevalent, most studies have found a relationship between rates of coping and distress that make it difficult to draw this causal relationship and conclude that mobilizing coping resources reduces stress. Norris et al. suggest that coping strategies are mobilized when a person faces stressful situations. Most individuals use many different types of coping simultaneously. What works in one situation may not work in another, what works for one person may not work for another, and what works at one point in time may not work at another point in time for the same individual. Interestingly, a belief in one's ability to cope appears to matter more than what coping mechanisms are actually used.

In a recent review article, Compas, Connor-Smith, Saltzman, Harding Thomsen, and Wadsworth (2001) come to different conclusions. They reported on more than 60 studies suggesting that coping increases psychological adjustment of children and adolescents who have been exposed to stress. They note that the original conceptualization of problem-focused versus emotion-focused coping (Lazarus & Folkman, 1984) is insufficient to capture the complex and diverse reactions of children and adolescents. They conceptualize the coping process as consisting of three major factors: (a) Active coping that helps the person achieve a sense of personal control over the stressful aspects of the environment and one's emotions; (b) Adaptation to the situation, primarily through cognitive methods such as reframing, acceptance, or distraction through positive activities or thoughts; and (c) Avoidance or disengagement from the stressful situation.

Active coping and adaptive coping appear to be associated with better adjustment, while avoidance or disengagement is related to poorer adjustment overall. There are a few studies, however, that show that in uncontrollable situations avoidance or disengagement may be preferable. A recent study

(Ginzburg, Solomon, & Bleich, 2002) suggests that repressive coping may be adaptive in both the short- and long-term aftermath of a single traumatic event.

In contrast to the coping literature, which has focused on the search for specific strategies and behaviors to deal with stress, the resilience literature (Conger & Conger, 2002; Masten, 2001; Masten & Powell, 2003; Mills, 1997) has examined how children develop normally and successfully despite adverse conditions. Resilience is sometimes referred to as "bouncing back" like a spring to our former pre-crisis or pre-trauma behavior. Walsh (2002) has suggested that the term "bouncing forward" may be more appropriate, since people are inevitably and profoundly changed by trauma. The guiding assumption of resilience is that it is "ordinary magic," an underlying, perhaps evolutionary protective process that shields children exposed to adversity in their developing years. This is not to say that all children are resilient and that we need do nothing to help children achieve healthy adulthood, particularly under adverse conditions. As Masten (1997) notes, "in cases of massive trauma due to war or chronic child abuse, resilience refers to good recovery after trauma has ended. Moreover, it is possible for a child to be resilient and still suffer from residual effects of trauma. Resilience does not mean 'invulnerable or unscathed' " (p. 1). In fact, resilience puts the emphasis on protective factors that promote health and normal development. These components may include, but are not limited to, a sense of personal safety, empathy, social (and familial) support, belonging, a sense of control, meaning in life, optimism, hope, faith or religious affiliation, and humor.

An assessment model based on resilience would focus on assets and potential resources, not only on problems, risks, and symptoms. An intervention model based on resilience would stress strategies of enhancement of assets, facilitation of protective processes, and competence promotion rather than reductions of risks and stressors. In the current security situation in Israel, where the risks and stressors are largely uncontrollable, this model seems particularly appropriate.

SCHOOL-BASED INTERVENTIONS AFTER EXPOSURE TO TRAUMA

Chemtob and Taylor (in press) reviewed comprehensively the literature documenting treatment of children with PTSD; this included approximately 80 primarily anecdotal studies, several of them school-based. For the most part, these studies concluded that psychological treatment, both group and individual, is helpful in the reduction of posttraumatic symptoms in children. Chemtob, Nakashima, and Carlson (2002) and Chemtob, Nakashima, and Hamada (2002) noted that most disaster recovery often takes substantially longer than previously thought. Disaster interventions typically take place within the year of the event, while the long-term effects of disaster are ignored or over-looked. Children often keep their own symptoms hidden for fear of overtaxing their already burdened parents. It is for this reason that large-scale school screenings and interventions are particularly appropriate.

The National School Intervention Program

The seeds of the National School Intervention Project (NSIP) began in October 2000 in response to the outbreak of hostilities against the civilian population of Jerusalem. Initial workshops with teachers and school staff underscored the needs of the educational system in dealing with both emergency situations, such as attacks, casualties, hospitalization, and bereavement, as well as ongoing exposure to terrorism and long-term stress experienced by both the student and adult populations in schools. In examining needs and resources of the education system, it became apparent that emergency situations were being addressed on a systemic level with in-service workshops and psycho-education efforts in dealing with immediate crisis situations (Klingman, 1990, 1997; Klingman, Raviv & Stein, 2000). There was little to no response in addressing the long-term effects of terrorism, the media barrage of reports from scenes of terrorism, and the consequent high levels of stress experienced by the entire civilian population of Israel. Our concern was specifically the long-term effects of this exposure on children and adolescents. This concern was based both on professional literature and clinical experience that highlights the fact that children who are exposed to terrorism and trauma are at a particularly high risk for developing posttraumatic symptoms and stress disorders (Chemtob & Taylor, in press; Norris et al., 2002) that, untreated, may accompany them a lifetime.

The NSIP developed a mission to educate and prepare professionals involved in educational settings for crisis, disaster, and trauma with the following underpinnings: (a) a developmental perspective that takes into account the different needs of children at different ages; (b) the active participation of program recipients in designing the program for their schools or professional communities; (c) a focus on the ongoing long-term nature of stress and trauma and the preparation of school professionals to be available long after the "crisis team" has moved on; and (d) the development of multi-level programs for the entire educational system to ensure system-wide change in implementation of programs dealing with the effects of exposure to trauma and stress on children. The work of the NSIP posited that preventive mental health efforts can help large segments of the population deal with ongoing stress resulting from exposure to terrorist acts. In addition, adequate education and preparation can mitigate the traumatic after-effects of terrorism.

The project focused on the full spectrum of the education system, from pre-school through high school. A plan was developed to work with teachers, principals, guidance counselors, and school psychologists within the educational system, as these professionals are at focal points in dealing with large numbers of children. In addition, efforts were made to involve policy makers, specifically professionals in the hierarchy of the Ministry of Education, in both planning and decision making processes. Supervisory staff participated in introductory workshops introducing the program as well.

The NSIP had several facets or "mini projects" under its umbrella. All mini-projects shared the foundations reported upon above. Our approach to the school system was from macro to micro, from the entire school population to the individual student suffering from PTSD. The first facet of the project focused on the entire school population, and was entitled "Building Resilience: A Program for Teachers and Students." Additional facets of the program included a school-wide screening program (see Pat-Horenczyk, this volume) implemented to identify students suffering from moderate to high levels of posttraumatic symptoms as well as PTSD. As an outgrowth of the screening program, school mental health professionals (counselors and psychologists) were trained in identifying symptoms of post trauma, as well as in clinical interviewing, used as follow-ups to the original screening process. Consequently, for children with moderate posttraumatic symptoms, a six-session coping and stress management group was developed; for those with severe symptoms of PTSD, a 12-session treatment group focusing on processing the traumatic events using methods of CBT and exposure was established.

A parent component was also offered to schools, and was an integral part of the project. This component included elements of psycho-education about the effects of trauma exposure and high levels of stress on children, as a workshop on stress management skills for personal use.

An In-Depth Look at the "Building Resilience" Project

This project was conceived as a response to the tremendously high levels of stress experienced by the entire civilian population of Israel beginning in September 2000 and continuing more or less steadily to the time of the current writing of this article (2004). Both teachers and students are members of this civilian population and as such, it was felt that the needs of both groups should be addressed. The resilience model adapted from the work of Masten (2001) and others (see Cowan, 1991; Luthar & Ziegler, 1991; Richardson, 2002) focuses on the paradigm shift from looking at risk factors and psychopathology to the identification of strengths, and the development and deepening of resources to allow for normal development and healthy adaptation. Many factors have been identified as being protective and promoting resilience. While the field of resilience is still in its early childhood, there is a general consensus that these factors include self-esteem, coping strategies, social support, hope and meaning, optimism, and humor. Teachers were chosen as the focus of this program because they are the ones in daily contact with children and can therefore provide the most direct and ongoing support to children experiencing high levels of stress and exposure to trauma. Teachers, in general, are experienced and trained professionals with a working knowledge of child development and well honed interactive group skills. The purpose of the workshop was to provide teachers with skills and knowledge in the areas of resilience, stress, and exposure to trauma, in order for them to develop the self-confidence necessary to interact with children in the classroom around difficult issues such as fear, loss, and dealing with trauma.

The *Building Resilience* project began with an initial visit to the school and a planning meeting with the school principal and leading team consisting of school mental health professionals and additional key staff members. A school trauma history was taken and a needs assessment performed. The program was explained to the staff, and necessary logistical and strategic plans for involving staff were set out. Responsibilities of the various parties were mapped out, and two follow-up sessions with the leading team were set up, one during the course of the workshops and one several weeks after the workshop completion.

The workshop consisted of three sessions of three hours each working with teachers in small groups of approximately 15. Group facilitators were experienced educational or clinical psychologists with training in both group work and trauma treatment. The workshop began with an introductory lecture (20 minutes) introducing the concept of resilience, and pre-intervention evaluation forms were filled out. The remainder of the workshop was spent in the small group sessions. Each teacher participant received a Teachers Manual consisting of twelve classroom activities, an article about the effects of trauma exposure and long-term stress on children, and several information sheets highlighting various aspects of psycho-education (e.g., identification of children with posttraumatic symptoms, how to help people who have experienced a traumatic event). In preparing the Teachers Manual, an attempt was made to include several of the factors deemed important in developing resilience. Because the teacher workshops were limited to three sessions, in order to allow for a wide implementation of this project it was necessary to pare down the number of factors eventually included. The classroom activities that were finally included in the Teachers Manual centered on the following themes: (a) Relaxation; (b) Exploring Fears in particular, and Feelings, in general; (c) Building of Resources; and (d) Finding Hope and Meaning in Difficult Situations. These themes were chosen as being particularly relevant and lending themselves to classroom activities.

Our intervention project developed a three-phase approach to developing resilience: focus on the teacher (Phase 1); simulation of classroom activities (Phase 2); and application of classroom activities and follow-up (Phase 3). At the first phase, the focus was on the teacher and allowed time and space for the teacher to develop self awareness as to the effects of stress and exposure to trauma on his or her own life. The importance of this stemmed from our understanding that before teachers could approach their students and begin to apply the resilience-building classroom activities within their own classrooms, they needed to spend some time identifying their own strengths and weaknesses and building personal resources. Workshop activities geared to these goals were planned and implemented in the first group meeting with the teachers. In addition, relaxation exercises were introduced and practiced.

The second phase focused on simulation of recommended classroom activities geared to building resilience. Two activities were chosen, one from the category of Exploring Fears and the other from the category of Hope and Meaning. The group facilitator explained the activity and then simulated the activity, with the facilitator acting as teacher and the teachers acting as students. The teachers were able to bring to the simulation exercises their personal experiences and continue the processing begun in the first session, all the while gaining confidence in implementing these classroom activities in their own classroom. At the conclusion of the session, a relaxation exercise geared for young children was introduced and practiced.

The third phase of the workshop consisted of application of the classroom activities and follow-up. At the close of the second workshop session, teachers were given the assignment of returning to their classrooms and choosing two activities to implement in their classrooms. They were encouraged to choose activities that they felt comfortable with and that they felt suited their students' needs and abilities. They were given reflective worksheets to report on the classroom activities they chose to implement and were asked to bring them to the third and final session of the workshop.

The third workshop session was scheduled between two and four weeks after the second one to allow teachers enough time to implement activities in the classroom. Teacher responses were very positive and over 90% of teachers reported implementing at least one activity in the classroom. The activity most often implemented was relaxation exercises. These were found to be both easy to implement, and took a minimal amount of classroom time and preparation on the part of the teacher. Student responses to the relaxation exercises, as reported by the teachers at all grade levels, was extremely positive.

In the third and final workshop session, the first half of the session was dedicated to sharing of experiences in implementing activities in the classroom. The final half of the session was spent simulating additional activities, and the session concluded with an additional relaxation exercise. Feedback, both oral and written, as well as post intervention evaluations concluded the workshop session. Evaluation measures focused on knowledge and skills of participants in dealing with the effects of trauma and long-term stress in the classroom, as well as on teachers' in-classroom behavior related to these concepts. Feedback focused on the content of the workshop as well as the manner of presentation and the perceived impact on participants.

Initial analysis of the evaluation data from the first 40 participants in this workshop indicated that teachers showed significant changes in the items measuring knowledge about trauma and stress, and the perceived amount of tools they had available for use in the classroom. Their willingness to talk with students about issues related to trauma and to implement classroom activities also showed significant change in the expected direction. Because of its preliminary nature, this evaluation should be taken with caution.

CONCLUSION

This article briefly reviewed the context within which the National School Intervention Project developed. Building on a clinical understanding of the long-term effects of exposure to trauma and stress on children and adolescents, yet accepting the premise that resiliency in children is not unusual, we set out to bolster the existing resources of the school community and apply our professional expertise in places where it could be utilized to maximum effect. Our early evaluation results are promising, but clearly more thorough examination of the usefulness and impact of these interventions is needed. Empowering teachers through workshops that provide information, skills, confidence-building activities, and support turns teachers into natural partners of mental health professionals working in schools, and creates an environment that can support resiliency and wellness among the student body.

REFERENCES

Ayalon, O., & Lahad, M. (2001). *Life on the edge 2000: Stress and coping in high risk situations.* Haifa: Nord Publications. (Hebrew).

Chemtob, C. M., Nakashima, J., & Carlson, J. G. (2002). Brief treatment for elementary school children with disaster-related posttraumatic stress disorder: A field study. *Journal of Clinical Psychology, 58,* 99-112.

Chemtob, C. M., Nakashima, J., & Hamada, R. (2002). Psychosocial intervention for postdisaster trauma symptoms in elementary school children. *Archives of Pediatric and Adolescent Medicine, 156*, 211-216.

Chemtob, C. M., & Taylor, T. L. (in press). Treatment of traumatized children. In R. Yehuda (Ed.), *Trauma survivors: Bridging the gap between intervention research and practice*. Washington, DC: American Psychiatric Press.

Compas, B. E., Connor-Smith, J. K., Saltzman, H., Harding Thomsen, A., & Wadsworth, M. E. (2001). Coping with stress during childhood and adolescence: Problems, progress, and potential in theory and research. *Psychological Bulletin, 127*, 87-127.

Conger, R. D., & Conger, K. J. (2002). Resilience in midwestern families: Selected findings from the first decade of a prospective, longitudinal study. *Journal of Marriage and Family, 64*, 361-373.

Conger, R. D., Conger, K. J., Elder, G. H. Jr., Lorenz, F., Simons, R. & Whitbeck, L. (1993). A family process model of economic hardship and adjustment of early adolescent girls. *Developmental Psychology, 29*, 206-219.

Cowan, E. L. (1991). In pursuit of wellness. *American Psychologist, 46*, 404-408.

Ginzburg, K., Solomon, Z., & Bleich, A. (2002). Repressive coping style, acute stress disorder, and posttraumatic stress disorder after myocardial infarction. *Psychosomatic Medicine, 64*, 748-757.

Grant, K. E., Compas, B. E., Stuhlmacher, A. F., Thurm, A. E., McMahon, S. D., & Halpert, J. A. (2003). Stressors and child and adolescent psycopathology: Moving from markers to mechanisms of risk. *Psychological Bulletin, 129*, 447-466.

Hammen, C., & Rudolph, K. D. (1996). Childhood depression. In E. J. Mash & R. A. Barkley (Eds.), *Child psychopathology* (pp. 153-195). New York: Guilford Press.

Klingman, A. (1990). *Hitarvut psycho-hinuchit le-ahar ason* [Psycho-educational intervention after disaster]. Jerusalem: Ministry of Education.

Klingman, A. (1997). *Coping with crises in schools: Emergency kit*. Jerusalem: Ministry of Education.

Klingman, A., Raviv, A., & Stein, B. (Eds.) (2000). *Yeladim belahats veherum* [Children in emergencies and stress]. Jerusalem: Ministry of Education.

Lazarus, R. S., & Folkman, S. (1984). *Stress, appraisal and coping*. New York: Springer.

Luthar, S. S., & Ziegler, E. (1991). Vulnerability and competence: A review of research on resilience in childhood. *American Journal of Orthopsychiatry, 61*, 6-22.

Masten, A. S. (1997, Spring). Resilience in children at risk. *Research/Practice: Center for Applied Research and Educational Improvement, 5*. Retrieved July 10, 2003 from, www.education.umn.edu/carei/Reports/Rpractice/Spring97/resilience.htm

Masten, A. S. (2001). Ordinary magic: Resilience processes in development. *American Psychologist, 56*, 227-238.

Masten, A. S., & Powell, J. L. (2003). A resilience framework for research, policy and practice. In S. S. Luthar (Ed.), *Resilience and vulnerability: Adaptation in the context of childhood adversities* (pp. 1-25). New York: Cambridge University Press.

Mills, R. C. (1997, Spring). Tapping innate resilience in today's classrooms. *Center for Applied Research and Educational Improvement, 5*, 12. Retrieved July 15, 2003 from www.education.umn.edu/CAREI/Reports/Rpractice/Spring97/tapping.html

Norris, F. H., Friedman, M. J., Watson, P. J., & Byrne, C. M. (2002). 60,000 disaster victims speak: Part I. An empirical review of the empirical literature, 1981-2001. *Psychiatry, 65*, 207-239.

Pat-Horencyzk, R. (2004). Post-traumatic distress in adolescents exposed to ongoing terror: Findings from a school-based screening project in the Jerusalem area. *Journal of Aggression, Maltreatment & Trauma, 9*(1/2/3/4), 337-348.

Pfefferbaum, B. (2001). Special report: Lessons from the 1995 bombing of the Alfred P Murrah Federal Building in Oklahoma City. *Lancet, 358*, 940.

Pfefferbaum, B., Pfefferbaum, R. L., North, C. S., & Neas, B. R. (2002). Does television viewing satisfy criteria for exposure in posttraumatic stress disorder? *Psychiatry, 65*, 306-310.

Richardson, G. E. (2002). The metatheory of resilience and resiliency. *Journal of Clinical Psychology, 58*, 307-321.

Seligman, M. E. P., & Csikszentmihalyi, M. (2000). Positive psychology: An introduction to a special issue. *American Psychologist, 55*, 5-14.

Walsh, F. (2002). Bouncing forward: Resilience in the aftermath of September 11. *Family Process, 41*, 34-36.

Community-Based Interventions in New York City After 9/11: A Provider's Perspective

Jonas Waizer
Amy Dorin
Ellen Stoller
Roy Laird

SUMMARY. The horrors of 9/11 have created tremendous psychosocial needs in the population of New York. For all major providers in this field, this has meant taking up the challenge of learning within the new situation, creating new frameworks for intervention, and implementing programs that previously had not been a part of the traditional social services environment. In this article, we will describe the process of transforming this challenge into an opportunity for organizational, professional and conceptual growth.

Address correspondence to: Jonas Waizer, PhD, F.E.G.S., 315 Hudson Street, New York, NY 10013 USA (E-mail: jwaizer@fegs.org).

[Haworth co-indexing entry note]: "Community-Based Interventions in New York City After 9/11: A Provider's Perspective." Waizer, Jonas et al. Co-published simultaneously in *Journal of Aggression, Maltreatment & Trauma* (The Haworth Maltreatment & Trauma Press, an imprint of The Haworth Press, Inc.) Vol. 10, No. 1/2, 2005; and: *The Trauma of Terrorism: Sharing Knowledge and Shared Care, An International Handbook* (ed: Yael Danieli, Danny Brom, and Joe Sills) The Haworth Maltreatment & Trauma Press, an imprint of The Haworth Press, Inc., 2005.

KEYWORDS. Traumatic stress, traumatic grief, mental health, crisis counseling, September 11, community-based services, Project Liberty

The monumental impact on New York City (NYC) of the events of September 11, 2001, has been widely written about from many perspectives. Nearly 3,000 individuals were killed and another 4,000 local residents were displaced. In the year that followed, more than 80,000 people contacted the NYC Mental Health Association's crisis hotline, 1-800-LIFENET, and more than 170,000 people called Safe Horizon, a clearinghouse for care management services.

Federation Employment and Guidance Service (F.E.G.S.), currently called F.E.G.S. Health and Human Services System, is one of New York's largest community-based not-for-profit agencies that provides an array of health and human services, employing close to 3,000 people with an annual budget exceeding $160 million. F.E.G.S. is headquartered ten blocks north of where the World Trade Center (WTC) once stood. On that fateful day, hundreds of F.E.G.S. employees and clients looked on in shock with a direct view of the attack. Our response to the terrorist attack began at once.

THE DEMAND FOR SERVICES

A variety of services were requested immediately after the WTC towers fell. Beyond meeting the needs of our own thousands of clients, we received requests for help from the government, local businesses, and residents. Within days, we began on-site work in lower Manhattan, eventually conducting more than 10,000 individual, group and public education sessions throughout greater New York under Project Liberty alone. At its peak, the F.E.G.S. 9/11 disaster programs employed more than 135 counselors, care managers, and employment staff who reached individuals and communities throughout New York. In the year prior to 9/11, F.E.G.S. served more than 70,000 New Yorkers through a network of behavioral health, employment, education, residential, home care and economic development services. In the year following 9/11, F.E.G.S. reached an additional 125,000 people with crisis and counseling services.[1]

The government called upon many New York community agencies and hospitals to supply disaster relief services. In addition to crisis debriefing, community providers were contracted by various sources to provide care management for New Yorkers financially devastated by the attacks, employment services for displaced workers in New York and on Long Island, and community rebuilding for local residents. This article reviews the Project Liberty activities in detail from the perspective of this community provider. Further, it touches on other disaster-related initiatives by government, private foundations, and the private sector. It also discusses the role of the behavioral health agency in dealing with community response to terrorist attacks or other disasters.

PROJECT LIBERTY: "FEEL FREE TO FEEL BETTER"

In October 2001, the Federal Emergency Management Agency (FEMA) and the Community Mental Health Service (CMHS) established Project Liberty, the largest disaster counseling effort ever. With $132 million in funding, Project Liberty contracted with more than 70 providers to offer public education, group crisis counseling and individual counseling services to New Yorkers. Phase one involved the award of licenses by Project Liberty to conduct outreach, public education, and crisis debriefing. F.E.G.S. employed a contingent of part-time, fee-for-service clinicians. Within six months, by the spring of 2002, Project Liberty shifted from licenses to cost-based contracts. Providers shifted from fee-for-service to hiring regular staff. F.E.G.S. organized its responders according to the populations they served.

The rules established by FEMA for funding by Project Liberty were very limiting as funds could only be used for prescribed services that emphasized a health care approach to crisis debriefing and public health education. Soon, other funding sources were required to supplement Project Liberty services.

The experience of the F.E.G.S. teams with Project Liberty and the array of funding sources led to many successes, and many surprises. Their stories generate the lessons learned from this challenging experience from the perspective of a community provider agency.

The Lower Manhattan Healing Project Team. By early 2002 the September 11th Fund of The New York Community Trust and The United Way of New York City agreed to underwrite a special effort to assist people living, working, or attending schools in lower Manhattan. F.E.G.S. staff met with groups of local residents, business leaders and school officials at their sites to determine and meet their needs. Many employees preferred receiving private counseling at their office locations during the workday. Residents wanted information and support groups in their buildings. As a response to several requests by local residents who stated adamantly: "I don't want therapy! I want to talk to my neighbors," the "Time To Share" community support group for lower Manhattan was established. New York residents met for the first time and continued meeting for nearly two years.

The "New Americans" Team. Bilingual/bicultural staff members reached out to various sectors of New York's substantial foreign-born community. A Chinese-American counselor discovered a group of isolated Chinese residents in a housing complex a few blocks from Ground Zero. A South Asian counselor reached out to Hindus and others targeted by anti-Muslim bias. An African-born, Swahili-speaking counselor found that some African families had lost family members they could not claim because they or their family members were undocumented immigrants who were ineligible for many of the available benefits or were fearful of applying for benefits to which they were entitled.

Others who had survived horrifying experiences before their escape from war-torn countries were deeply re-traumatized. Russian-speaking counselors reached out systematically to thousands of Jewish émigrés from the former Soviet Union. A Spanish-speaking former Red Cross employee sought out Hispanic enclaves in Brooklyn and the Bronx that other providers had overlooked. Staff also reached out to New York's gay, lesbian, bisexual and transgender community. One counselor reported that:

> C's[2] partner died on 9/11, but none of his friends, family or co-workers knew he was gay. C therefore could not participate in ceremonies or in his partner's friends' grief. He was also unable to apply for any financial benefit he could have claimed, had they been married.

The Jewish Community Outreach Team. Because of F.E.G.S.' strong ties to many sections of the Jewish community, Project Liberty services were offered with a deep understanding of their unique needs. A Project Liberty team of rabbis, chaplains, social workers, and paraprofessionals was recruited from several traditions, including the Orthodox, Hasidic, Reform, and Sephardic communities, to accord services to their various needs. Two rabbis, trained as chaplains, visited homebound elderly Jews, many of whom were Holocaust survivors, to offer understanding and solace.

Local Colleges Team. Many students at John Jay College of Criminal Justice of the City University of New York are police officers seeking to improve their careers. More than 100 graduates died on 9/11. F.E.G.S. trained John Jay College counseling staff in the FEMA model of crisis counseling and they offered services directly to students. One counselor reported that:

> D, a four-year veteran of the New York Police Department (NYPD), was pursuing a B.S. in Criminal Justice. After a classroom presentation on the effects of traumatic stress, he approached the teacher, an experienced therapist, and they met privately, more than a dozen times, to discuss D's reactions. He had resisted counseling, fearing the consequences for his

career if it became known, but he felt safe meeting with his teacher. "As far as anyone can tell, when I see you, you're advising me on my program for next semester," he said, "It's not like I'm sick or anything; it's just that there aren't a lot of places where you can really talk about this stuff."

Another F.E.G.S. counselor, pursuing a PhD in clinical psychology at City College, set up shop in the cafeteria, displaying materials on a table off by itself to avoid being overheard. This counselor reported that:

E approached the table out of curiosity in the fall of 2002. When she saw materials about 9/11, she shared her sad, empty feelings about that day. Returning in the following week, she told of promiscuity she seemed unable to control since 9/11. Anna suggested arranging to meet at a more private location, but E wasn't interested. "You're not a shrink or anything, right? I don't need that. We're just talking."

Department of Education Unit. By May, 2003, arrangements were completed to fund Project Liberty services in the public schools. F.E.G.S. formed a partnership with the Bronx Division of High Schools to work with local counselors in 16 high schools. One counselor reported that N, a 10th grade Muslim girl, described numerous incidents of harassment by classmates who called her "Mrs. Osama" and similar degrading names.

LESSONS LEARNED

Crisis Counseling Is Different. To a hammer, it is said, everything looks like a nail. Many seasoned clinicians approached Project Liberty as just another opportunity for clinical practice, only to face a rude awakening. Rather, the federal model of crisis counseling is best understood as a "Public Health" model of service. Crisis counselors provide education and counseling to the general public by using standard techniques such as reflective listening and psychoeducation. Participants are helped to recover their pre-disaster level of functioning. The objective is to reach all afflicted individuals in the community.

Traditional mental health practice is inconsistent with the FEMA model. The clinical paradigm starts with the assumption that something is wrong with the patient. The goal of treatment is to relieve symptoms, to intervene and change behavior. In contrast, the Project Liberty crisis counselor and participant share the view that the problem is a normal, expectable reaction to overwhelming stress. There is no need to establish a diagnosis, formal objectives or treatment plans. Counseling that focuses on processing the traumatic material and developing coping strategies can help recover the level of functioning participants enjoyed before the disaster. People with serious disorders should be referred to traditional mental health professionals or clinics. FEMA outlined the differences between the clinical approach and the public health approach (see Table 1).

We knew that many "mental health professionals assume that extreme emotional and psychopathological reactions are typical consequences of disasters" (Quarantelli, 1985, p. 173). We also knew that evidence does not support this belief. Crisis experts note that traditional mental health professionals may not succeed as crisis counselors unless they possess the following attributes: (a) They can assimilate a revised conceptualization of mental health services that is different from their traditional training and function (e.g., lack of diagnosis, interventions in very non-traditional settings, role ambiguity); (b) They are comfortable working with paraprofessionals or trained nonprofessionals; and (c) They are able to incorporate crisis counseling theory and practice into the theoretical construct that usually guides their practice (e.g., psychoanalytical, cognitive/behavioral, insight-oriented approaches) (FEMA, 2000).

THREE CRUCIAL STAFF CHARACTERISTICS: INDIGENOUS, HUMANISTIC, AND INDEPENDENT

Our original trauma response teams included many senior managers and supervisors. We then added seasoned, carefully screened clinicians through a temporary employment agency using a fee-for-service arrangement. Then we hired counselors from communities affected by the crisis who were essential to meeting the needs of hard-to-reach populations: they had immediate credibility and access into their respective communities. Throughout New York City and Long Island, local individuals were employed to work in their own communities.

We followed FEMA's recommendation to use indigenous paraprofessionals. Outreach workers also had to understand basic human services approaches to interacting with the public: active listening, empathy and other fundamental interviewing skills. In addition, they had to be enthusiastic, independent entrepreneurs who could devise and implement successful outreach strategies within their communities. Successful staff also were self-starters who did not define themselves by their schooling or degree. They came from highly diverse backgrounds including a photojournalist, an art therapist, an Ethiopian lawyer, rabbis, yoga instructors, retired people, teachers, social workers, psychologists and

TABLE 1. Differences Between the Clinical and the Public Health Approach

"Traditional" Mental Health Practice	Crisis Counseling
• Usually office based. • Focuses on diagnosis and treatment of a mental illness. • Attempts to impact the baseline of personality and functioning. • Examines content. • Encourages insight into past life experiences and their influence on current problems. • Has a psychotherapeutic focus.	• Primarily home and community based. • Focuses on assessment of strengths, adaptation of existing coping skills and development of new ones. • Seeks to restore people to pre-disaster levels of functioning. • Accepts content at face value. • Validates appropriate reactions to the event and aftermath; normalizes the experience. • Has a psycho-educational focus.

Source: FEMA

students. They were extroverts who could walk into businesses, schools and residences to market themselves with credibility.

APPROACHING THE CLIENT IN THE FIELD

Staff was deployed into the community rather than waiting for the community to appear at a fixed site for services. They spoke to the downtown residential and business communities, held support groups at stores and apartment complexes. In contrast, a storefront drop-in center we established went unused.

When counselors leave the safety of the clinic, they leave behind important supports including their office, desk, and receptionist. In this amorphous setting, counselors must focus carefully on maintaining appropriate professional boundaries. One counselor visited a homebound man who had requested individual counseling. As she was leaving, he asked, "Next time, send one of the pretty young ones, eh?"

DEAL SENSITIVELY WITH PRE-EXISTING CONDITIONS

Inevitably, a public health outreach effort such as Project Liberty, dealing with mental and emotional distress, will encounter individuals with untreated mental, emotional and behavioral problems that predate the critical event. Obviously, crisis counselors who discover such individuals should refer them for appropriate services. One counselor shared that:

A's client asked to meet at a local diner. While sharing her concerns that her husband was having an affair, she became increasingly preoccupied and distant, finally lapsing into a trance-like state, sitting in a slack and unresponsive manner. A reached the husband at work, and together they took her to the hospital.

When Project Liberty came to an end, some chronically unstable participants finally accepted referral to conventional mental health treatment. Others did not, and now remain untreated, just as they, and many others, were on September 10, 2001.

WORK CREATIVELY WITH CRISIS COUNSELING STAFF

The crisis counselor often works alone, reaching out to gatekeepers in key communities and meeting with clients in their homes or communities. We had deliberately selected staff with an affinity for "in-country" work, but they still needed support and guidance. The challenge was how to provide a useful structure without squelching their essentially independent spirit. Clinical supervision always involves balancing staff's personal challenges with professional roles. The line between professional and personal was even more difficult to draw with crisis counselors who were continually re-traumatized, reliving their own experience repeatedly while absorbing the unimaginably harrowing, tragic and grotesque stories their clients needed to tell.

FEMA recommends establishing teams of counselors and outreach workers. We supplemented individual supervision with the teams described above. We combined professionals and para-professionals in a "generalist" model. Team meetings served as informal "grand rounds," where team members presented cases and engaged in guided group supervision. Staff also shared their outreach strategies, collaborated in larger ventures, and brainstormed about new approaches. By expressing enthusiasm for the best of these ideas, we subtly encouraged competition among staff, using positive feedback. One counselor shared that:

> I had worked with many non-uniformed rescue and recovery workers–construction tradesmen who worked side by side with police and firefighters at the site they called "The Foxhole." Many of my clients have disabling respiratory conditions, but were left out of the recognition and other benefits that uniformed workers received. On my last day I said, "I've never had a job like this. You trusted me to do things I didn't know I could do–and I did!"

CARE MANAGERS ARE COUNSELORS TOO

In the wake of a disaster, even the most well organized person can lose the ability to function. After 9/11, a generous but bewildering array of services and entitlements became available to victims and their families, including dozens of sources of cash and support. Care managers provided compassionate, practical and focused advocacy and support to individuals directly affected by 9/11, helping them to find and secure needed services as they coped with their guilt, anger and grief. Care managers became the hub of many people's lives. One counselor reported that:

> Six months after the event, M received a $25,000 grant that enabled her to keep her apartment. She called her care manager. "I should be happy," she said. "How come I feel like crying for the first time?" The quest for survival having finally ended, she could now face her memories of and feelings about the event.

CONFRONT COMPASSION FATIGUE

Human services work is emotionally challenging by nature, but staff members who work with trauma victims on a day-to-day basis are particularly vulnerable. There is the challenging nature of listening empathetically to tragic and upsetting stories. Like all New Yorkers, the Project Liberty and care management staff had directly experienced the destruction of the Twin Towers, and struggled with what Danieli (1988; this volume) has called "event countertransference." Finally, counselors had particularly close connections to the people they counseled in their communities. Ironically, staff members who fit most closely our criteria of being deeply connected to an afflicted community were most at risk.

To deal directly with "compassion fatigue," we incorporated elements of the group crisis-counseling model into group supervision. A trauma expert conducted monthly workshops with staff (Danieli, 1994; this volume). These were designed to make them more aware of themselves in the process of crisis counseling, to see their role as facilitators rather than fixers, and to care for themselves. We also offered a creative writing workshop and sent staff to special retreats for 9-11 caregivers, support groups and healing workshops.

FOCUS ON STAFF TRAINING

One of the themes stressed in public health presentations was, "Knowledge Is Power," the idea that one can mindfully confront the experience of stress and utilize a range of coping strategies. F.E.G.S. brought in experts on traumatic stress to provide our team members with information and skills they could use to work more effectively with clients and the community. Shortly after the attack, staff needed to learn forms of crisis intervention. At a later stage, we invited experts from Israel, where community resilience programs have been developed for many years (Lahad & Cohen, 1998), to provide advanced training. Experts from our for-profit affiliates provided additional expertise and service.

DISPLACED WORKERS RESIST COUNSELING SERVICES

By March 2003, the U.S. Department of Labor estimated that over 180,000 jobs had been lost in New York as a direct result of the 9/11 attack. The crisis brought the unemployment rate in New York to 8.6%, the highest in the nation (Eaton, 2003).

F.E.G.S. mounted a massive effort that helped displaced workers develop more effective job search strategies, package themselves more successfully and, in some cases, retrain for new careers. Those who were unable to succeed increasingly reported feelings of despair and hopelessness, or became irritable or distraught at the least provocation. Yet, attempts to refer such individuals for mental health treatment generally failed. One F.E.G.S. employee reported that:

> To attempt to bridge this gap, one counselor working in the Employment Division of the 9/11 program pursued three objectives: public education, direct individual counseling for self-identified participants, and working with staff to assess cases and make referrals. By offering a series of stress management seminars, she attracted consumers in a non-threatening way, as "stress" was a more palatable concept to them than "mental health."

INFRASTRUCTURE MATTERS

F.E.G.S. believes that community agencies must be better prepared to provide quality services at lower cost, and to assess rapidly an emerging situation, possess the confidence to overcome bureaucratic barriers, demonstrate a willingness to experiment with new approaches and discard what is not working (Miller, 1993). We live in an age of public fiscal restraint and, at the same time, increasing demands for ever-higher standards at ever-lower reimbursement. To prepare for agile response to opportunities, over the past decade F.E.G.S. built an infrastructure based on partnerships with other non-profits as well as private, for-profit affiliates. The use of shared infrastructure is essential to the survival of non-profit agencies. Moreover, it proved a vital factor in the agencies' successful response to the terrorist attack on 9/11 and the development of an array of services.

In the last decade, F.E.G.S. partnered with others to set up a group of independent, for-profit affiliates that handled functions such as personnel management, information technology services, temporary staffing, home care, and staff development and training. Two corporations, HR Dynamics and All Sector Technologies, Inc., developed wide independent customer bases to lower the unit cost of the respective technology for each agency. As these grew, they provided high quality services at lower cost than a freestanding community agency could afford on government financing.

Each of these partnerships helped F.E.G.S. respond to the events of 9/11 and the expansive infrastructure proved indispensable when the need for agility presented itself on 9/11. When program grants became available, we were able quickly to identify and process a large pool of applicants, hire and put them to work and pay them while awaiting final contracts.

As disaster relief programs proliferated, each of the many contracts from government and foundations came with its own complex performance rules and reporting requirements. The billing and accountability for these disaster relief services were new and stringent, requiring quick adaptation by providers. F.E.G.S. immediately turned to its for-profit affiliate, AllSector Technologies, to build computerized accountability systems that met the funding sources' requirements. In contrast, many agencies reported that they found the challenge of meeting the public demands for accountability and reporting too difficult.

Another affiliate, XBRM (Extreme Behavioral Risk Management) Associates, works with corporations, businesses and organizations to develop threat management strategies, and lent considerable expertise to the development of F.E.G.S. crisis services to the business community.

STRENGTHEN COMMUNITY AND INDIVIDUAL RESILIENCE

The FEMA approach emphasizes the power of human resilience and natural recovery following a disaster, whether natural or man-made. Yet most crisis counseling experts agree that it is as important to strengthen community support networks as it is to respond to individual need. In fact, some argue against widespread individual services to "assist" a recovery that in most cases will occur anyway (Quarantelli, 1985). Most would agree, however, that building resilience in a community is very important. As we initiated our outreach to members of communities out of the mainstream, we began by seeking out their gatekeepers. Similarly, as we planned our exit in late 2003, we returned to these individuals, summing up, making sure they knew of available resources.

DON'T BE INDISPENSABLE: AVOIDING DEPENDENCY

Disastrous events arouse a universal, overpowering urge to help. After 9/11, people spent hours standing on line to give blood that eventually had to be thrown away. Human services professionals are strongly motivated to help. At times it was difficult to preserve professional boundaries, but we knew that we were "building a bridge from yesterday to tomorrow, and we want to do it with the community's own materials. We don't want to be the brick that holds that bridge together" (Lahad, personal communication, July 22, 2003).

> J., a Chinese-American Educator, joined the FEGS/Project Liberty team and soon discovered a group of several hundred Chinese-Americans living across the Bowery from Chinatown, in a large housing development. She organized a series of monthly public education meetings in the community room, which turned into monthly socials that continued even after she moved on from Project Liberty in July, 2003, and led to the formation of the Chinese-American Residents Association. She had helped them find their own strength, and they didn't need her any more.

CONCLUSION: TRANSFORMED BY 9/11

Traumatic stress often produces positive as well as negative outcomes (Bloom, 1998). For F.E.G.S., participation in Project Liberty and other disaster services provided an opportunity to refine our approach to behavioral and infrastructure services. First, F.E.G.S. learned that blending a public health model would serve the affected population better. Second, the experience confirmed the capacity to respond more quickly in a time of crisis because the for-profit affiliates were able to adapt rapidly to the demands of new contracts for staffing and technology. Third, our Israeli colleagues, with experience in other terrorist attacks and disasters, taught us new approaches to staff training and a more flexible mix of mental health practice and public health outreach.

Based on the acquired experience, F.E.G.S. now participates in initiatives preparing behavioral responses to future crises. We are collaborating with the New York City Department of Health and Mental Hygiene's newly established Department of Behavioral Preparedness to utilize the lessons learned from this monumental event. We also participate with UJA Federation of New York in a Bi-National Israel/U.S. learning community to become better prepared through research and program exchanges. In addition, we have expanded our commitment to XBRM as a for-profit initiative that prepares the corporate sector for business recovery after a disaster.

Even when the impact is broad, disasters are local events. The central element of our Project Liberty effort was to recruit culturally and ethnically diverse staff that could reach out as "insiders" in their communities. Even in the "sophisticated" community of New York City, with the world's largest concentration of psychiatrists and mental health professionals, we learned that there are many people who are ashamed to seek mental health services when they need them. For most, a crisis is both emotional and economic in its consequences. By working within communities to build future resilience and assisting in rebuilding and strengthening their own networks, we were able to reach and help with both behavioral and employment services many people who would otherwise have gone unattended. We are now also positioned better to spring into action at the local level, and throughout metropolitan New York, in the event of another crisis.

NOTES

1. F.E.G.S. is proud to have been honored with an *Eli Lilly and Comprehensive NeuroScience, Inc. Behavioral Leadership Award* in 2002 for its "Leadership in the Time of Disaster" following 9/11, and the International Association of Jewish Vocational Services 2003 Distinguished Program Award in Recognition of F.E.G.S.' September 11th Initiative.
2. All names have been changed to protect the identities of the people written about in this article.

REFERENCES

Bloom, S., & Reichert, M. (1998). *Bearing witness: Violence and collective responsibility*. Binghamton, NY: The Haworth Press, Inc.

Danieli, Y. (1988). Confronting the unimaginable: Psychotherapists' reaction to victims of the Nazi Holocaust. In J. P. Wilson, Z. Harel & B. Kahana (Eds.), *Human adaptation to extreme stress* (pp. 219-238). New York: Plenum Press.

Danieli, Y. (1994). Countertransference, trauma and training. In J. P. Wilson & J. Lindy (Eds.), *Countertransference in the treatment of post-traumatic stress disorder* (pp. 368-388). New York: Guilford Press.

Danieli, Y. (2004). Some principles of self-healing. *Journal of Aggression, Maltreatment & Trauma, 10*(1/2/3/4), 663-665.

Eaton, L. (2003, March 14). Job losses in New York City since 9/11 continue to grow. *The New York Times*, p. B-3 column 1.

Federal Emergency Management Agency. (2000). *Crisis counseling and mental health treatment similarities and differences* [Brochure]. Rockville, MD: Center for Mental Health Services.

Lahad, M., & Cohen, A. (1998). Eighteen years of community stress prevention. *Community Stress Prevention, 3*, 1-9.

Lahad, M., & Cohen, A. (1998). Critical incident stress debriefing, the Israeli experience. *Community Stress Prevention, 3*, 10-13.

Miller, A. (1993). Continuity and change: A challenge for Jewish communal service. *Journal of Jewish Communal Services, 70*, 5, 4-9.

Quarantelli, E. L. (1985). An assessment of conflicting views on mental health: The consequences of traumatic events. In C. Figley (Ed.), *Trauma and its wake* (Vol. 1, pp. 173-218). New York: Brunner/Mazel.

The September 11th Fund. (2002). *The September 11th fund: One year later.* [Annual report]. New York: Author.

An Ecological Community-Based Approach for Dealing with Traumatic Stress: A Case of Terror Attack on a Kibbutz

Rony Berger

SUMMARY. This article presents our ecological approach toward building community resilience in the aftermath of a traumatic event and its application in the case of a terror attack on a Kibbutz. It delineates the various principles guiding our framework, outlines the phases of our community intervention, describes the intervention processes, and addresses some dilemmas relevant for such interventions.

KEYWORDS. Trauma, terrorism, community-based intervention, crisis-intervention, resilience

---

Address correspondence to: Rony Berger, PsyD, Natal, The Israel Trauma Center for Victims of Terror and War, P.O. Box 4170, Tel Aviv 61041, Israel (E-mail: riberger@netvision.net.il).

The author would like to thank Ms. Varda Oshpeez and Mr. Danny Shandor for their valuable comments and his community staff at Natal for their dedicated work with these Kibbutzim.

[Haworth co-indexing entry note]: "An Ecological Community-Based Approach for Dealing with Traumatic Stress: A Case of Terror Attack on a Kibbutz." Berger, Rony. Co-published simultaneously in *Journal of Aggression, Maltreatment & Trauma* (The Haworth Maltreatment & Trauma Press, an imprint of The Haworth Press, Inc.) Vol. 10, No. 1/2, 2005; and: *The Trauma of Terrorism: Sharing Knowledge and Shared Care, An International Handbook* (ed: Yael Danieli, Danny Brom, and Joe Sills) The Haworth Maltreatment & Trauma Press, an imprint of The Haworth Press, Inc., 2005.

The ecological community-based model for coping with traumatic stress was developed in Natal: Israel Trauma Center for Victims of Terror and War (Berger, 2002a) as a response to the unprecedented number of terror attacks since the beginning of the latest Palestinian Intifada (uprising). The model is based on Bronfenbrenner's (1979) ecological theory and Hobfoll's (1989) Conservation of Resources (COR) theory. It posits that traumatic stress is a bio-psycho-social phenomenon embedded in multi-systemic levels, which impact the individual, the family, the community and the society at large. The changes resulting from the traumatic incident and the resources needed to cope with it determine the various levels of intervention.

Following Belsky (1980), our levels of analysis and intervention are: (a) The Ontogenic Development Level which is the way the survivor copes with the incident depending on his or her biological predisposition, personality structure and history of coping with stress; (b) The Micro-Systemic Level or the way the family copes with the incident depending on its structure, communication and resources; (c) The Exo-Systemic Level which is the way the community copes with the incident depending on its leadership, the inter-relationships between its members and the various subgroups, its cohesion and resources; and (d) The Macro-Systemic Level which is the way in which the country copes with this incident depending on the formal and non-formal leadership, the narratives and myths formulated around the event and the country's resources.

The COR theory postulates that community resilience is a function of the way the community utilizes, preserves and develops its resources. Hence, in planning our intervention we assess the community's existing resources and help its members to both build new ones and expand their previous resources.

PRINCIPLES

The principles guiding our intervention are as follows: (a) Ecological orientation; this program addresses all systemic levels mentioned above; (b) Preventive orientation; the program deals with primary, secondary and tertiary prevention (Caplan, 1964); (c) Holistic orientation; the program incorporates physiological (bodily), mental, and spiritual components; (d) Salutogenic orientation; the program acknowledges the importance of activating health-oriented resources (Antonovsky, 1979); (e) Proactive orientation; the program attempts to reach out actively to the affected community; and (f) Phase Orientation; the program is designed according to 3 phases: immediate phase (hours/few days after the event), early phase (days/few weeks after the event) and rehabilitation phase (weeks and months after the event).

THE PROCESS OF INTERVENTION WITHIN THE COMMUNITY

Our approach comprises several stages (see Figure 1). The first is the engagement stage, where the primary task of the helpers is to join the community in its suffering and to communicate genuine concern and desire to help. One of the major issues at this point is how to establish trust with the community's formal and informal leadership and to create a productive cooperative relationship. The hesitant response and occasional vehement resistance of the community often surprises helpers with good will who fail to engage the community sensitively. It is also important to enlist support from as many stake holders as possible as they tend also to serve as gatekeepers.

Another important issue is how to coordinate the various agencies that often rush to the scene to provide assistance and how to avoid the destructive phenomena of professionals' turf war. The next stage of mapping community needs and resources is often overlooked or rushed through by professionals who are urged to intervene reflexively due to the emergency or by helpless stake holders who need to demonstrate their control over the situation. It is important to be aware of these pressures while, at the same time, slowing down this process and maintaining our professional integrity.

Traumatic situations also tend to mobilize a great deal of energy in helping professionals that is channeled toward instinctive rather than reflective action. Our experience over the past three years has also "forced" us to acknowledge the fact that, at times, our immediate reactions during emergency situations serve our sense of grandiosity while simultaneously assuaging our own helplessness.

Central to this stage are the questions: (a) who assesses? (b) whose needs? and (c) by what means? Unfortunately, too often, the strong populations who are well represented in the community are the ones who are attended to while marginalized groups tend to be neglected.

We believe that a more thorough needs assessment including non-official informers and marginalized groups and utilizing non-conventional assessment methods can give us a better picture of the true needs of the whole community. Additionally, in performing need assessment, it is useful to prioritize community needs according to their importance and urgency (i.e., immediate, short-term and long-term).

The second major task at this stage is to map the existing resources in the community. This aspect of the assessment is essential for many reasons, including providing immediacy and proximity of intervention (Salmon, 1919), establishing continuity of treatment (Omer & Alon, 1994) and, perhaps most importantly, insuring the efficiency of the intervention. We categorize these resources into two types: internal/external and potential resources.

FIGURE 1. The Process of the Ecological Community-Based Model

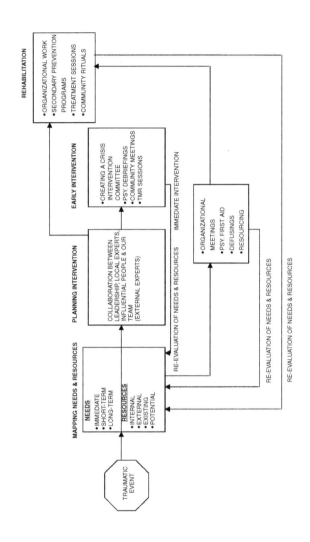

516

Following this assessment, we designed a community-oriented intervention plan. This plan should be formulated through collaboration among formal community leaders (command center), community local experts, informal community leaders and our team (the outside experts). While organizing such a planning committee seems rather complex, it is our experience that this effort is essential to the success of the intervention. In disasters, as in community celebrations, powerful constituencies tend to assert their control. Hence, excluding key figures will lose their cooperation and eventually prove counterproductive.

The next stage involves a tripartite intervention plan, which consists of immediate intervention, early intervention, and long-term intervention (rehabilitation). It should be noted that, while these stages are presented as separate, in reality they overlap. The immediate intervention, which aims at providing emergency organization and psychological first-aid, is often initiated before a comprehensive assessment is completed and the full intervention plan is designed. Hence, we tend to adopt non-intrusive and supportive methods such as defusing and resourcing rather than psychological debriefing (see our case study below). This approach helps us both to engage the community and to map further its needs and resources.

In the early intervention, we establish an operative crisis-intervention team, perform modified psychological debriefings (Berger, 2002b), help assemble community meetings, and provide individuals at risk with Traumatic Memory Restructuring (TMR) sessions (Berger, in press). Our overall goal at this stage is to restore the community's normal functioning and prevent the long-term adverse reactions of individuals and groups. Finally, our model proposes long-term community rehabilitation by providing organizational support to the leadership, secondary preventive programs for affected groups, treatment sessions for symptomatic individuals and families, and community rituals commemorating those who were lost and/or community healing celebrations.

A TERROR ATTACK ON A KIBBUTZ: A CASE STUDY[1]

Our intervention took place in a Kibbutz (a collective agricultural settlement) in northern Israel, established sixty years ago by young, idealistic Zionists from Eastern Europe. They were determined to replace their lives as bourgeois Jews in the Diaspora with lives of enlightened proletarian Jews, galvanizing their tie to their historical Jewish homeland by working the land in a socialistic communal framework. Overcoming tremendous difficulties, ranging from poor health conditions and poverty to hostilities perpetrated by their Arab neighbors, the Kibbutz founders managed to survive and build a stable and self-sufficient community. Since one of the major ideals of the Kibbutz founders was working the land by manual labor, the Kibbutz economy centered on agriculture, crops, and livestock. Between the 1950s and 1970s, the Kibbutz expanded (to approximately 750 residents) and prospered economically. The revolutionary social experiment of the Kibbutz phenomenon succeeded beyond imagination and served as an exemplary model of a strong and healthy Israeli community. However, with the rapid, revolutionary changes in Israeli society and its economy (toward a free-market economy) during the 1980s and 1990s, Kibbutzim in general were forced to adjust by abandoning some of their original principles (e.g., employing workers from outside the Kibbutzim, who were "hired labor" and not communal owners).

This schism within the Kibbutz movement grew even further in recent years, as the notion of privatization (moving from equal division of resources toward a division based on the value of each member's work) was introduced as a solution to the growing economic difficulties of the Kibbutzim. Many Kibbutz members felt that this change represented the elimination of the Kibbutz as a socialist system and the destruction of its basic values. Furthermore, privatization threatened those Kibbutz members (particularly the older members) who were not as economically productive as others.

A major issue with which the Kibbutz grappled in the aftermath of the terror attack was the imminent security threat. Throughout the long-standing Israeli-Palestinian conflict, this Kibbutz had always maintained close relationships with its Arab neighbors and managed to remain somewhat insulated from the conflict. Unlike many Israelis who moved toward a non-reconciliatory political position during the Intifada, members of this Kibbutz maintained their political orientation leaning towards the left. The terrorist attack shattered the Kibbutz members' sense of security as well as challenged their political views. Furthermore, it sent shock waves into the fragile relationships between the Kibbutz and its neighboring Arab villages, who were suspected by some members to be collaborators with the terrorists. In sum, a few days after a horrific terror attack on this Kibbutz, our team found a traumatized community. It was ridden by ideological, social, and economic crises and facing a security threat of existential proportion.

The Incident: Terror Attack on the Kibbutz

This incident began when a ring of three heavily armed Palestinian terrorists invaded the Kibbutz during the early evening when most members were eating supper with their families. The terrorists began a killing spree, which lasted until they were killed by the security forces. The incident lasted approximately six hours and ended with the cold-blooded murder of eight residents of the Kibbutz, including three young children. Among those slaughtered were a grandmother, her daughter and her young son (three generations of one of the Kibbutz's founding families), a father with his two daughters, one of the key leaders of the Kibbutz, and a revered, elderly figure in the Kibbutz.

During these six horrifying hours, Kibbutz members, who heard the shooting but were not aware of precisely what was happening, were instructed to turn off all lights, close doors and windows and wait until the security forces, who arrived late to the scene, cleared the area. From interviews of Kibbutz residents, we learned that many were terrified and extremely confused about what had happened; while many Israelis followed real-time media coverage of the event, they were "in the dark" in more than one way.

When the incident was finally over, many of the Kibbutz members, realizing the severity of the tragedy, were in total shock and grief. Over the next few days, many dignitaries from the government, the army, and the police, came to pay their condolences to the families and to show support for the Kibbutz. Simultaneously, the Kibbutz members were accosted by scores of local and foreign print and television reporters, hounding them for interviews, as often happens in such tragic situations.

The Initial Contact

Hours after the attack, a team from Natal contacted the local social welfare department expressing both our support and concern. We also offered the director our assistance and asked her to perform a preliminary evaluation of the community needs. Since our agency is rather well known throughout Israel (we have trained many social welfare agencies in dealing with traumatic stress), the initial contact was much appreciated.

Following up two days later, we found the director eager to explore with us how to develop an action plan based on the various needs she discovered. During this phone consultation, we decided collaboratively to immediately provide a defusing session to the Kibbutz key leadership (four individuals) who seemed shaken by the event, an organizational session with the helping professionals who were involved in the aftercare, and psychological first-aid to one of the families who was reported to be in serious crisis.

The Immediate Intervention

Two teams of four people each were immediately dispatched to the affected area. The senior team met with the leadership and the helping professionals while the other team went to meet with the family.

The defusing session with the key leaders focused on the personal difficulties experienced by these individuals as well as on identifying the most pressing needs of the community. This was a very painful session in which all participants expressed their devastation, confusion, loss, and deep sense of horror. From our observation, it seemed that this was the first chance for those individuals to attend to their emotional needs and to allow themselves to be out of their leadership role. We normalized their reactions, stressed their wise choices, reframed their self-derogatory comments and generally gave them a great deal of encouragement for the superb job they performed during these difficult days. Conflicts and disagreements were purposefully diffused, and instead, we focused on their common mission as leaders of the community. It should also be emphasized that the participants were discouraged from recounting the specific details of the tragic event (unlike in psychological debriefing).

The second part of this meeting was devoted to identifying their immediate needs. Issues like the lack of security around the Kibbutz, grievances against the government, psychological assistance to various groups and economic problems were brought up. Significant organizational issues within the leadership (like long-term conflicts among groups in the Kibbutz) were also noted by the team but were not dealt with in this session. The session ended with decisions, including: establishing an extended committee to deal with this crisis (comprised of the leadership and key position holders within the Kibbutz), arranging a meeting with the local security forces (army and police), applying for emergency economic assistance from various agencies, arranging immediate support for the bereaved families, and nominating a Kibbutz spokeswoman responsible for handling the media. It was agreed that a team from Natal would perform a more thorough assessment of community needs.

Following this session, the team met with the helping professionals involved in the crisis. Similarly, we began with the workers airing their feelings and then focused on identifying individuals, families, and groups in crisis as well as on coordinating the efforts to provide them with appropriate services. Despite some historical tensions among various helping professionals, they all agreed on designing a mechanism to ensure coordination and exchange of information. The roles of each unit, including the Natal group, were clearly defined and the immediate tasks were identified and divided according to these definitions.

Finally, the other Natal team worked with a family in the Kibbutz. This single-mother family, neighbors of the family who was murdered, experienced a great deal of distress and grief over the loss of their friends. Both the mother and her daughters exhibited significant posttraumatic reactions. After spending three hours with the family, the team managed to stabilize their condition utilizing crisis-intervention techniques. They decided to refer them to a therapist with whom the family had previous contact.

Mapping the Needs and Resources of the Community

Two members from the Natal community team, with both clinical and organizational backgrounds, preformed the assessment. The needs of the community were evaluated in two days of phone surveys with random members of the community, focused individual interviews with position holders, and group meetings with nursery personnel, school staff, factory workers and security forces. Assessment of the community's available resources was derived from our previous meeting with the professionals and from interviews with the Kibbutz medical clinic personnel. Both needs and resources were charted utilizing Ayalon's (in press) diagram of "circles of vulnerability and support" (see Figure 2).

Based on the data from these various sources the team identified and prioritized the community needs according to the following areas:

1. Instrumental needs: improving local and regional security, providing financial assistance for emergency tasks, supplying the concrete needs of bereaved families and maintaining the Kibbutz routines (including replacing the tasks of the murdered members).
2. Organizational needs: clarifying the leadership's primary task, defining leaders' roles, setting boundaries, and improving their cooperative functioning, establishing communication patterns between the Kibbutz position holders and the leaders as well as between the leaders and the members.
3. Emotional needs: trusting the leadership, providing emotional support to each other, expressing feelings related to the incident (pain, sadness, loss, anger, anxiety and guilt) and processing the traumatic experience.
4. Spiritual/ideological: strengthening the value system of the community, commemorating the murdered members and exploring the relationship with the Arab neighbors.

Planning the Intervention

The information gathered by the assessment team was summarized in a report and was presented to a group comprised of the extended crisis-intervention committee (12 key members of the community), several invited community members (with the leadership's agreement), and representatives of the local service provider agencies (welfare department, educational system

FIGURE 2. Circles of Vulnerability and of Support (based on Ayalon, 2003)

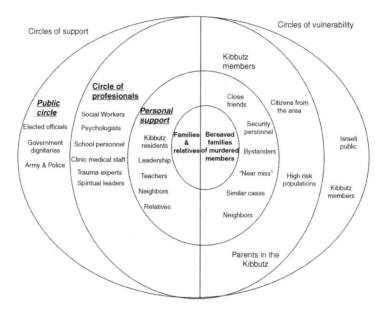

and local medical clinic). After a long brainstorming session with the Natal team all parties agreed upon the following intervention goals:

1. To fortify the Kibbutz's security system.
2. To set-up a modified psychological debriefing for the Kibbutz security personnel who experienced anxiety and guilt.
3. To call for a general Kibbutz meeting in order to acknowledge publicly their tragedy, give an opportunity to raise grievances and concerns and, most importantly, to inform members of the team's course of action in the next days and weeks.
4. To ensure psychological assistance to members at local and outside agencies.
5. To arrange a lecture for parents with young children who seemed to be in distress.
6. To provide consultation for medical personnel who reported a significant increase in clinic visits.

Early Intervention

The next day, the Kibbutz social worker (who was familiar with our de-briefing model) and a member of Natal, led a modified psychological debriefing with the Kibbutz security personnel. Unlike the Critical Incident Stress Debriefing (Mitchell & Everly, 1995) we pre-selected individuals for the session (based on their coping styles) and worked according to the Traumatic Memory Restructuring (TMR) principles. The security personnel expressed sadness and grief over murdered members, guilt over what they considered their faulty functioning, anxiety for their well-being and for the well-being of other Kibbutz residents, and a general sense of overwhelming helplessness. Their reactions were normalized and their narratives were reconstructed (Berger, in press).

A committee composed of the Kibbutz head of human resources, the social worker and the director of the clinic identified the emotional needs of individuals and groups within the community. In consultation with Natal, they built programs to address those needs (e.g., home visits for the elderly, activities for anxious children). Several Kibbutz members were referred for private TMR sessions with Natal staff in order to deal with their acute symptoms. They were seen for 2-6 sessions and were discharged after their symptoms reduced significantly and their functioning restored. Additionally, a Natal member gave a short workshop for the Kibbutz medical personnel addressing how to assess posttraumatic reactions and how to provide psychological first-aid. Most importantly, however, the Natal team met with the Kibbutz crisis-intervention committee to establish a working relationship, define their primary task, prioritize the suggestions offered in the planning session and begin to formulate specific action plans. Since some of the murdered residents were very close friends of the team members, the team decided that we would first help them process their grief experiences. Utilizing our "letter writing technique" (dividing the group into couples, writing "good bye" letters to the lost object, sharing them with the partners and then having the partner write back an answer to the letter), the Kibbutz team shared their pain, guilt and deep loss. This was an extremely painful and touching session, which left many of the participants emotionally vulnerable, yet brought the team closer together (in retrospect, we feel that this session might have been held prematurely).

The next step focused on fostering the strengths of the committee. Utilizing guided imagery, art therapy materials and small group processes (for more details see Berger, 2002a) the Kibbutz team began to identify its individual and collective resources but also discovered some of their deficits and shortcomings. They defined their primary mission as providing security and safety to ALL Kibbutz members and restoring the sense of mutual trust and involvement in the communal living, and set specific objectives for overcoming the current Kibbutz difficulties. However, since unresolved conflicts, disagreement regarding role definitions, lack of clear boundaries, and problematic communication patterns surfaced strongly within the leadership, a collaborative decision was made to work on those issues.

In the next several weeks, the underlying roots for these tensions were explored utilizing organizational counseling techniques. Committee members began to deal honestly with their interpersonal conflicts and their ideological disagreements and to develop some organizational structures to confront them. They were also taught productive communication and problem-resolution skills and practiced them in these sessions. Consequently, the relationship between the committee members improved dramatically and they began to work productively on the tasks at hand. Small sub-committees were formed and began to design what they termed "community-support projects" (such as dealing with the issue of privatization, supporting Kibbutz members with economic problems, encouraging members' productivity, commemorating those who were murdered, and developing the "Kibbutz culture").

Long-Term Intervention

After six weeks of intensive intervention, the situation of the Kibbutz stabilized and most of the members returned to their previous level of functioning. However, ongoing assessment during this period revealed that many residents felt some degree of dissatisfaction and that the general atmosphere in the Kibbutz was gloomy. The members still reported experiencing a significant existential threat (due to security and economic fears), a sense of being isolated (from other members and from the Israeli society at large) and, perhaps most importantly, a sense of hopelessness about their future. In analyzing the situation, our team concluded that part of the problem was related to the fact that the Kibbutz was still under the impact of the tragedy and that not enough time was given for the committee to pursue their proposed projects. However, there was also the sense that many of the Kibbutz difficulties were related to lingering unresolved issues from the past (such as ideological conflicts between socialists and modernists and political disagreement related to the security problem) that were exacerbated by the tragedy.

The team met with the committee and gave them their analysis regarding the Kibbutz problems. The committee urged our team to support the Kibbutz and continue the work with them. We decided to put more pressure on the committees to pursue their community plans and to make more effort to enlist residents' cooperation. We also recommended that the leadership hire immediately external economic experts to help them design a viable rehabilitation plan for the Kibbutz. They were also suggested to inform the members via a Kibbutz meeting and to reassure the residents that all decisions will be taken by a vote of a significant majority only.

These plans were instituted within weeks. The security committee invited army officials to share with residents the security plans and to answer their concerns. The cultural committee put together a plan for yearly cultural events, which was sent to each Kibbutz family. The special needs committee arranged several activities for the elderly and for children. Finally, the economic committee hired a consulting group and began to design several plans for rehabilitation.

Our organizational work with the leadership continued at the same time, focusing on resolving long-standing conflicts, strengthening their relationship and supervising the application of their work within the community. Though our work is still in progress, a survey has already demonstrated significant changes suggesting improved residents' satisfaction and more optimism. This progress was confirmed by objective measures of improved residents' productivity and larger attendance in communal activities.

CONCLUSION

The ecological approach for dealing with traumatic stress was demonstrated in working with this traumatized Kibbutz. As it is often manifested in traumatized individuals and families, the existing systemic difficulties (in our case, the ideological, social, security and economic problems) were amplified by the traumatic experience leading the community to a crisis of existential proportion. Consequently, the trauma further polarized the Kibbutz members threatening the cohesiveness of this already fragile community. Adopting a multi-systemic approach and combining crisis-intervention techniques, trauma-focused treatment and organizational work seem to be effective, not only in dealing with individuals and families, but also in changing the mood and functioning of the community. While experience in working with several traumatized communities led us to believe that this community-based approach bears promise, it clearly needs further empirical evidence.

NOTE

1. This case study is based on a composite of several traumatized Kibbutzim communities with which we have dealt in the past three years.

REFERENCES

Antonovsky, A. (1979). *Health, stress and coping.* San Francisco: Jossey-Bass.
Ayalon, O. (2003, October). The macro and micro of helping the helpers during mass disasters. In R. Berger (Chair), *Helping the helpers. Children responses to terrorist attacks.* Symposium conducted at the Conference for Early Interventions in the Aftermath of Terror Attacks, Haifa, Israel.

Belsky, J. (1980). Child maltreatment: An ecological integration. *American Psychologist, 35*, 320-335.

Berger, R. (2002a). *An ecological model for community-based intervention during traumatic stress: A manual.* Tel Aviv: Natal. (Hebrew).

Berger, R. (2002b, April 15) *Children and parents in the shadow of terrorism.* Retrieved on April 18, 2002 from, www.natal.org.il.

Berger, R. (in press). Early intervention with survivors of terrorism: The Traumatic Memory Restructuring (TMR) model. In D. Knafo (Ed.), *Living with terror, working with trauma: A clinician handbook.* Northvale, NJ: Jason Aronson.

Bronfenbrenner, U. (1979). *The ecology of human development.* Cambridge, MA: Harvard University Press.

Caplan, G. (1964). *Principles of preventative psychiatry.* New York: Basic Books.

Hobfoll, S. E. (1989). Conservation of resources: A new attempt at conceptualizing stress. *American Psychologist, 44*, 513-21.

Mitchell, J. T., & Everly, J. S. (1995). *Critical incident stress debriefing: CISD–An operational manual for prevention of traumatic stress among emergency service and disaster workers.* Elliot City, MD: Chevron Publishing Corp.

Omer, H., & Alon, N. (1994). The continuity principle: A unified approach to disaster and trauma. *Psychologia, 4*, 20-28. (Hebrew).

Salmon. T. W. (1919). War neurosis and their lesson. *New York Medical Journal, 109*, 993-1090.

SECTION VI
A MULTICOMPONENT MODEL
OF PREPARING PROVIDERS
IN COMMUNITIES AFFECTED
BY TERRORISM

Toward a Public Mental Health Approach
for Survivors of Terrorism

Matthew J. Friedman

SUMMARY. Although most people exposed to bioterrorism or mass casualties will be extremely distressed during the immediate aftermath, only a minority (approximately 30%) will develop clinically significant psychiatric disorders. From a public mental health perspective, the challenge is to provide both preventive programs for the entire population and early detection and intervention for those at greatest risk for PTSD or other post-traumatic psychiatric disorders. Both individual and soci-

Address correspondence to: Matthew J. Friedman, MD, PhD, National Center for PTSD (116D), VA Medical & Regional Office Center, 215 North Main Street, White River Junction, VT 05009 USA (E-mail: Matthew.Friedman@Dartmouth.edu).

[Haworth co-indexing entry note]: "Toward a Public Mental Health Approach for Survivors of Terrorism." Friedman, Matthew J. Co-published simultaneously in *Journal of Aggression, Maltreatment & Trauma* (The Haworth Maltreatment & Trauma Press, an imprint of The Haworth Press, Inc.) Vol. 10, No. 1/2, 2005; and: *The Trauma of Terrorism: Sharing Knowledge and Shared Care, An International Handbook* (ed: Yael Danieli, Danny Brom, and Joe Sills) The Haworth Maltreatment & Trauma Press, an imprint of The Haworth Press, Inc., 2005.

etal preventive and early intervention approaches are reviewed. Utilization of the media, especially television, is presented as an example of one of many potential community/societal public mental health approaches.

KEYWORDS. PTSD, public mental health, prevention, intervention, media, disaster response

Progress in any field is a double-edged sword. Each time we wrest a new bit of information from our enigmatic Mother Nature, we achieve a much clearer perspective on other secrets she continues to keep to herself. Indeed, the more we think we know about certain things, the more certain we become about our ignorance in other matters.

Recent events have forced me to acknowledge the limited applicability of traditional clinical approaches for most people exposed to terrorism, mass casualties, and large-scale disasters. Although I remain a firm believer in evidence-based treatments for individuals with post-traumatic psychiatric disorders (Foa, Keane, & Friedman, 2000; Wilson, Friedman, & Lindy, 2001) that meet DSM-IV (American Psychiatric Association, 2000) diagnostic criteria, I now recognize that they represent a small minority of the men, women, and children who survive such disasters.

POST-TRAUMATIC REACTIONS: A POPULATION PERSPECTIVE

From a public health perspective, most people exposed to traumatic events do not develop depression, PTSD, alcoholism, or some other DSM-IV psychiatric disorder. Indeed, a recent review of 160 studies on disaster victims suggests that two-thirds will not develop a clinically significant chronic psychiatric disorder (Norris, Friedman, & Watson, 2002; Norris, Friedman, Watson, Byrne, Diaz, & Kaniasty, 2002). In a recent study of 2,509 Mexican adult trauma survivors, Norris and associates (Norris, Murphy, Baker, & Perilla, 2003) found that whereas 95% of exposed individuals experienced some degree of post-traumatic psychological distress, only 29% experienced acute reactions deemed serious from a clinical perspective and only 30% experienced chronic symptoms lasting more than a year.

When considering the impact of terrorism, the prevalence of psychological distress appears to be considerably higher than for natural disasters. A random-digit dialing national survey of Americans completed within three to five days of the September 11th terrorist attacks indicated that 44% of respondents reported one or more substantial symptoms of severe distress, while 90% reported at least moderate distress (Schuster et al., 2001). Similar findings were reported from a web-based survey of a national probability sample conducted two months after the World Trade Center attacks, which indicated that 17% of the U.S. population outside of New York reported symptoms of September 11-related post-traumatic stress (Silver, Holman, McIntosh, Poulin, & Gil-Rivas, 2002). Finally, it is noteworthy that rates of post-traumatic distress detected among New Yorkers within weeks of the World Trade Center attacks that were reported in both of these studies are considerably higher than the prevalence of PTSD and depression, 7.5% and 9.7%, respectively (Galea et al., 2002).

These examples show that terrorism is not only an effective means of waging psychological warfare but that its impact extends far beyond the immediate vicinity of such attacks. In addition, they indicate that most people with significant traumatic distress do not develop PTSD or some other DSM-IV diagnosis. Elsewhere we have suggested that the major weapon wielded by terrorists is fear (Friedman, Hamblen, Foa & Charney, in press). Fear is highly toxic; it is very contagious and immediately transmissible to large numbers of the population who were never in any physical danger from a specific terrorist attack. Indeed, according to Solomon (1995), there is at least one documented example that fear can be lethal. Eleven Israelis who were never in danger of SCUD missile attacks during the 1991 Gulf War died because of fear after the air raid alerts were sounded: 7 by suffocation from faulty use of gas masks and 4 from heart attacks.

PUBLIC MENTAL HEALTH CHALLENGES

The goals of public mental health are: (a) protection of the general population through preventive measures; (b) early detection of and intervention for populations at risk; and (c) reducing symptom severity and functional impairment among people with chronic psychiatric disabilities. The focus in this article is on the first two objectives, since the third has received attention elsewhere (Foa et al., 2000; see also, Kinzie, this volume; Waizer, Dorin, Stoller, & Laird, this volume). Unfortunately, we know very little about preventive or early intervention measures that might help formulate public mental health policy concerning the threat and impact of terrorism.

Prevention

The best way to protect against post-traumatic distress would be to prevent all future attacks perpetrated by terrorists. It would be the psychological equivalent of draining the swamps to wipe out yellow fever (Friedman, 1981). Given the unlikelihood of successfully implementing such a strategy, the next best approach would be to promote resilience at the societal, community, family, and individual levels. At the societal level, this would mean developing laws, policies, and practices to ensure optimal preparation for and public responses to terrorist attacks.

At the individual level, this might mean promoting psychological and psychobiological resilience through provision of psychological "vaccines," when indicated, to the population at large. Epidemiological data indicate that more than half of adult Americans will be exposed to at least one traumatic event during their lifetimes (Kessler, Sonnega, Bromet, Hughes, & Nelson, 1995). Many more individuals will be thus exposed from nations in conflict, such as Algeria, Palestine, and Bosnia (de Jong et al., 2001). Therefore, the psychological and physical consequences of traumatic exposure constitute a major public health challenge throughout the world (Green et al., 2003; Schnurr & Green, 2003). From this perspective, it is very important to search for effective psychological vaccines and to consider providing them to children and adults as part of an overall public health strategy. Perhaps the most effective vaccine for most children and adults would be a proactive psychoeducational approach provided in school, workplace, and community settings.

Since epidemiologic research has shown that people differ in their vulnerability to (or resilience against) post-traumatic distress (Norris, Friedman, & Watson, 2002; Norris, Friedman, Watson, Byrne et al., 2002), another preventive public mental health strategy might be to identify individuals at greatest risk for such severe, chronic, and debilitating post-traumatic reactions, and provide prophylactic interventions in addition to the vaccines provided to the general populace. For example, a more intensive approach for populations at risk might include stress inoculation training or psychobiological strategies for prevention of post-traumatic distress or for promotion of resilience outlined elsewhere (Friedman, 2002).

Early Detection and Intervention

As discussed previously, most people exposed to a terrorist attack will exhibit psychological distress. For some, this will be a transient reaction that may be briefly incapacitating, at most. For others, this may be the start of a severe, chronic, and potentially incapacitating psychiatric disorder. The public health problem (Friedman, Foa, & Charney, 2003; Friedman et al., in press) is that we cannot distinguish vulnerable from resilient individuals during the immediate aftermath of a terrorist attack, mass casualty, or natural disaster. A number of prognostic categories have been proposed as early indicators of future chronicity, such as functional impairment (Norris et al., 2003), elevated heart rate (Shalev, Peri, Canetti, & Schreiber, 1996), and negative cognitions (Ehlers & Clark, 2003). Unfortunately, none of these have been tested sufficiently. In addition, the new DSM-IV diagnosis, Acute Stress Disorder, has had only limited usefulness as a screening criterion for the general population since the majority of people who develop PTSD will not have met ASD criteria beforehand (Bryant, 2003). This is obviously a major concern for public mental health planners who, understandably, do not want to pathologize normal and transient post-traumatic distress and who do not want to use scarce and expensive clinical resources for individuals who will recover spontaneously or with minimal assistance.

Early detection is also important because different interventions may be indicated for people who are situated at different points along the vulnerability to resilience continuum. For example, very vulnerable survivors might be most susceptible to the potentially deleterious effects of psychological debriefing offered shortly after a terrorist attack (Rose & Bisson, 1998). They might do better if treatment is delayed for a minimum of several weeks, after which they should be offered a brief course of cognitive behavioral treatment (Bryant, 2003; Ehlers & Clark, 2003). In contrast, the most resilient survivors might benefit most from family/peer group support or from psychoeducational information provided through the media rather than from any formal intervention during the acute post-traumatic aftermath.

To summarize, there appear to be many differences among individuals with regard to post-traumatic vulnerability vs. resilience, to the likelihood of transient vs. chronic post-traumatic reactions, and to the best choice of pre-traumatic preparation and post-traumatic interventions.

Conceptual Approach: Inverted Psychosocial Pyramid

As indicated by the previous examples, terrorism is psychological warfare against society as a whole. Therefore, it must be approached from a societal rather than a traditional clinical perspective. A useful conceptual mode within which to frame a public mental health perspective is the inverted psychosocial pyramid (de Jong, 2002; Fairbank, Friedman, de Jong, Green, & Solomon, 2003; Marsella, 1998), which defines four levels of intervention (see Figure 1). At the top, *societal* interventions are preventive cost-effective interventions designed for the whole population. With respect to terrorism, these include international and national laws, public policy, and public institutions supporting basic human needs, safety, security, and education. Reestablishing safety and security after a mass casualty can be considered a societal mental health intervention. An effective national health and mental health care system is also a societal intervention, as is a national emergency medical disaster system equipped to provide needed services. As discussed subsequently, societal interventions might also include policy and practice concerning the media and risk communication.

Community interventions also target the general population rather than individuals at risk. They foster individual resilience and rejuvenate communities following catastrophic events by restoring support networks, re-establishing communication, providing public education, empowering communities so that individuals can help themselves, and providing training to indigenous survivors so that they can participate more effectively in the post-traumatic recovery (Fairbank et al., 2003). Obvious community sites for such interventions include schools, religious settings, labor unions, employee assistance programs, and ethnic communities.

Family interventions rely on natural helping networks and focus primarily on informal support systems of family, friends, peers, neighbors, and local community organizations. Since the whole family is affected even if only one of its members has been severely traumatized, and the legacy of traumatic exposure is often transgenerational in nature, family interventions are extremely important (Danieli, 1998).

Individual interventions are most familiar to clinically trained professionals. They should be reserved for the most seriously impaired whose post-traumatic stress is clinically significant and functionally incapacitating (Foa et al., 2000; Wilson et al., 2001).

The inverted pyramid depicted in Figure 1 (Green et al., 2003) is essentially a public mental health model to promote wellness rather than a clinical model to treat illness. It is predicated on the following set of assumptions:

a. Most people exposed to terrorism will exhibit fear and a predictable array of post-traumatic symptoms. The geographic distribution of such psychological distress will far exceed the physical danger of such a terrorist attack, potentially affecting a community, city, or entire nation (as shown by the aforementioned post-9/11 epidemiological research findings).
b. Most people exposed to such attacks will recover from their initial post-impact distress, although such recovery may take weeks or months (for a thorough discussion of recovery from traumatic grief, see Pivar & Prigerson, and Malkinson, Rubin, & Witztum, this volume).
c. In the immediate aftermath of a terrorist attack, almost everyone will be very upset, and it will be difficult to distinguish those who will have transient post-traumatic reactions from those who will develop chronic, incapacitating psychiatric disorders.
d. A reasonable public health approach will be to prepare the population-at-large as much as possible before such attacks occur, to provide

effective risk communication (see U.S. Department of Health and Human Services, 2002) and education immediately afterward, and to conduct early detection and intervention for those most in need.

e. It is expected that societal and community interventions before and immediately after terrorist attacks will accelerate the recovery of resilient individuals but this assumption must be tested empirically.

f. Effective implementation of a wellness-promoting public mental health approach at the societal, community, and family levels should reduce the number of people seeking traditional clinical interventions for post-traumatic psychiatric disorders. Such an approach makes sense clinically and economically: clinically, to avoid needless treatment for people who will recover without formal assistance; and economically, to avoid the high costs of utilizing scarce professional resources.

FIGURE 1. Inverted Psychosocial Pyramid (*modified from Fairbank et al., 2003) illustrates a conceptual model within which to frame a public mental health strategy following mass casualties or disasters. Societal level strategy of interventions might involve public policy or education whereas individual level interventions include clinical treatment. *Trauma Interventions in War and Peace: Prevention, Practice, and Policy.* Green et al., 2003. Kluwer Academic/Plenum Publishers. Printed with permission.

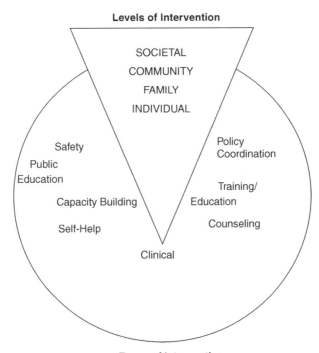

Levels of Intervention

SOCIETAL
COMMUNITY
FAMILY
INDIVIDUAL

Safety
Public
Education

Policy
Coordination

Capacity Building

Training/
Education

Self-Help

Counseling

Clinical

Types of Intervention

An Example: Utilizing the Media for Societal/Community Interventions. A concrete example of a large-scale societal level intervention to help achieve the public health goals described above might enhance our understanding of the issues. Such an intervention must be available to the population at large, be relatively inexpensive, have the capacity to facilitate preparation for the impact of terrorism, have the potential to ameliorate widespread distress during the immediate aftermath of a terrorist attack, and be an effective tool for reaching vulnerable individuals with clinically significant post-traumatic reactions. Although there are many examples from which to choose (Green et al., 2003), I will focus on the media because they are very well situated to play a key role in this regard.

Experience in New York City following the September 11th attacks has shown the power of media exposure either to exacerbate or attenuate post-traumatic distress on a massive scale. Regarding adverse effects, two reports have documented a close response relationship between post-traumatic distress and exposure to televised material on the World Trade Center and Pentagon attacks (e.g., airplanes hitting the Twin Towers, human casualties, flames, smoke, falling debris, interviews with acutely bereaved individuals). In a survey conducted three to five days after September 11th, Schuster and associates (2001) observed that substantial post-traumatic distress was more likely among those who spent the most time watching televised coverage of these events. Similar findings were reported in a web-based nationally representative sample, which also found that the magnitude of PTSD symptom levels was associated with the number of hours of watching coverage of the September 11th events (Schlenger et al., 2002).

Research has produced similar findings with regard to television viewing of traumatic material by American children after the Oklahoma City bombing (Pfefferbaum et al., 2001; Pfefferbaum, Pfefferbaum, North, & Neas, 2002) and by Kuwaiti children exposed to military occupation during the Gulf War (Nader, Pynoos, Fairbanks, Al-Ajeel, & Al-Asfour, 1993). Interpretation of these findings is by no means obvious. On the one hand, they suggest that television viewing, itself, may be toxic due to its capacity to instigate or exacerbate post-traumatic distress. Indeed, there is evidence to suggest that repeated exposure to televised traumatic images might interfere with the normal recovery process during the immediate aftermath of a traumatic event (Ehlers & Clark, 2003). On the other hand, it may be that people who are already most distressed are those who watch the most television, possibly as a coping mechanism to understand the event better (Newman, Davis, & Kennedy, in press; Schlenger et al., 2002).

Whatever the reasons, the data clearly indicate that the most distressed people watch the most television. This is a golden opportunity for a societal/community level mental health intervention since we can be reasonably confident that we can gain access to the most vulnerable individuals through television. This is an opportunity to provide televised information about the nature of a post-traumatic event, and for public officials, celebrities, experts, parents, and others to appear on television to provide such information to the population at large. An additional possibility is for the media to help people regulate post-traumatic anxiety and arousal (see G. Ross's Guide, this volume). As days go by, information about abnormal reactions and where to get help might also be aired so that viewers can make accurate assessments of their own (or a loved one's) psychological state. In this way, vulnerable individuals might be self-identified as soon as possible and directed to appropriate professional assistance.

Another key role in which television (and other media) can participate is in risk communication. How information is communicated before, during, and after a catastrophe can have a major impact on the level of distress experienced by the general population. Although it is the responsibility of public officials to ease public concern and to provide guidance on how best to respond to a crisis, the media are in the best position to educate the public, provide accurate and timely information about the extent and likely danger from a terrorist attack, provide a forum for experts who can knowledgeably address public concerns, and check sources carefully before airing information that may heighten public anxiety.

There are many complex issues that need to be addressed before television (and other media) can be enlisted as a hard-wired component of a public mental health response. Journalists have a primary responsibility to report the news objectively and many would object strongly to modifying their coverage to meet a non-journalistic objective such as public mental health (Newman et al., in press). However, journalistic policy is not fixed and immutable. Differences in editorial policy on television coverage of the recent war in Iraq illustrate this point since there was a great divergence in the graphic death and destruction imagery shown on different stations. Therefore, an acceptable middle ground can be achieved between journalistic prerogatives to report the news objectively and media participation in a coordinated public mental health outreach initiative. Although these two roles are not mutually exclusive, a thoughtful dialogue must take place between media and public health officials before the parameters of these two roles can be defined better.

The recent experience of New York City's post-9/11 disaster mental health program, Project Liberty, shows how effective media-public health partnerships can benefit the general public after a major catastrophe. In her description of a broad scale public media campaign as a post-9/11 mental health outreach strategy, Naturale (in press) lists four objectives of such an initiative:

(a) branding a disaster response program to provide recognition of available services; (b) broadcasting the overall message that post-traumatic distress is a normal reaction; (c) promoting a sense of security for the community at large by announcing that mental health services are available to those in need; and (d) identifying and legitimizing outreach staff conducting face-to-face and door-to-door outreach services. Two additional objectives can be added to this list: (e) alleviating unnecessary public anxiety through thoughtful programming; and (f) helping guide public empowerment by identifying constructive courses of action.

Project Liberty developed a 30-second television commercial that aired within two weeks of the terrorist attacks and which directed the public to available mental health services. Equally impressive information about societal/community interventions implemented by Project Liberty concern radio announcements, printed brochures, utilization of a cost-free "800" phone number, and information provided through the internet. In addition, Project Liberty's community-directed interventions were tailored specifically for school children, the elderly, the workplace, and for many distinct ethnic communities. For purposes of this article, any one of these interventions could have been selected as examples of cost-effective, broad-based, societal/community public mental health interventions. The present focus on television should be understood as one of many possible concrete examples of a public mental health strategy designed to foster wellness, ameliorate psychological distress, accelerate normal recovery, facilitate identification of people who require clinical attention, and to help people find appropriate professional help when needed.

CONCLUSION

Focusing on a public mental health approach to terrorism, this article has discussed effective and efficient strategies of prevention, promoting resilience, and a post-traumatic intervention strategy that will reach the general public. Television has been explored as one of many potential vehicles through which such societal interventions might be implemented. This is new territory for traditional clinicians, but one that addresses the needs of the population-at-large rather than self-selected individuals in distress who seek conventional, office-based treatment. This approach emphasizes wellness rather than illness and is completely consistent with the general objectives of any public health program.

It is important to emphasize that I have only presented a conceptual framework, with no data. Clearly, that is the next challenge. We must test the hypotheses spawned by a public mental health approach with the same scientific rigor we have utilized to evaluate psychosocial and pharmacological treatments developed for people with DSM-IV psychiatric disorders. With respect to television, we must begin to carry out careful dismantling studies in order to understand which components of televised messages are toxic and which are salutary. We need to test systematically a wide variety of qualitative and quantitative aspects of televised presentations to determine which are most effective and what outcomes they may be expected to produce. We must also seek to discover how to translate the successful lessons of clinical practice into useful interventions for society as a whole.

REFERENCES

American Psychiatric Association. (2000). *Diagnostic and statistical manual of mental disorders* (4th ed., text revision). Washington, DC: Author.

Bryant, R. A. (2003). Early predictors of posttraumatic stress disorder. *Biological Psychiatry, 53,* 789-795.

Danieli, Y. (Ed.). (1998). *International handbook of multigenerational legacies of trauma.* New York: Plenum.

de Jong, J. T. V. M. (2002). Public mental health, traumatic stress and human rights violations in low-income countries: A culturally appropriate model in times of conflict, disaster and peace. In J. T. V. M. de Jong (Ed.), *Trauma, war and violence: Public mental health in sociocultural context* (pp. 1-91). New York: Kluwer/Plenum.

de Jong, J. T. V. M., Komproe, I. H., Van Ommeren, M., El Masri, M., Mesfin, A., Khaled, N. et al. (2001). Lifetime events and posttraumatic stress disorder in 4 postconflict settings. *Journal of the American Medical Association, 286,* 555-562.

Ehlers, A., & Clark, D. M. (2003). Early psychological interventions for adult survivors of trauma: A review. *Biological Psychiatry,* 53, 817-826.

Fairbank, J. A., Friedman, M. J., de Jong, J., Green, B. L., & Solomon, S. D. (2003). Intervention options for society, communities, families, and individuals. In B. L. Green, M. J. Friedman, J. de Jong, S. Solomon, T. Keane, J.A. Fairbank et al. (Eds.), *Trauma interventions in war and peace: Prevention, practice and policy* (pp. 57-72). Amsterdam: Kluwer Academic/Plenum.

Foa, E. B., Keane, T. M., & Friedman, M. J. (Eds.). (2000). *Effective treatments for post-traumatic stress disorder: Practice guidelines from the international society for traumatic stress studies.* New York: Guilford Press.

Friedman, M. J. (1981). Post-Vietnam syndrome: A delayed stress reaction. *Psychosomatics, 22,* 931-943.

Friedman, M. J. (2002). Future pharmacotherapy for post-traumatic stress disorder: Prevention and treatment. *Psychiatric Clinics of North America, 25,* 427-441.

Friedman, M. J., Foa, E. B., & Charney, D. S. (2003). Toward evidence-based early interventions for acutely traumatized adults and children. *Biological Psychiatry, 53,* 765-768.

Friedman, M. J., Hamblen, J. L., Foa, E. B., & Charney, D. S. (in press). Commentary: Fighting the psychological war against terrorism. *Psychiatry.*

Galea, S., Ahern, J., Resnick, H. S., Kilpatrick, D. G., Bucuvalas, M. J., Gold, J. et al. (2002). Psychological sequelae of the September 11 terrorist attacks in New York City. *New England Journal of Medicine, 346,* 982-987.

Green, B. L., Friedman, M. J., de Jong, J., Solomon, S., Keane, T., Fairbank, J. A. et al. (2003). *Trauma interventions in war and peace: Prevention, practice, and policy.* Amsterdam: Kluwer Academic/Plenum.

Kessler, R. C., Sonnega, A., Bromet, E., Hughes, M., & Nelson, C. B. (1995). Posttraumatic stress disorder in the national comorbidity survey. *Archives of General Psychiatry, 52,* 1048-1060.

Kinzie, J. D. (2004). Some of the effects of terrorism on refugees. *Journal of Aggression, Maltreatment & Trauma, 9*(1/2/3/4), 411-420.

Malkinson, R., Rubin, S., & Witztum, E. (2004). Terror, trauma, and bereavement: Implications for theory and therapy. *Journal of Aggression, Maltreatment & Trauma, 9*(1/2/3/4), 467-477.

Marsella, A. J. (1998). Toward a "global-community psychology": Meeting the needs of a changing world. *American Psychologist, 53,* 1282-1291.

Nader, K., Pynoos, R., Fairbanks, L., Al-Ajeel, M., & Al-Asfour, A. (1993). A preliminary study of PTSD and grief among the children of Kuwait following the Gulf crisis. *British Journal of Clinical Psychology, 32,* 407-416.

Naturale, A. J. (in press). Mental health outreach strategies: An experiential description of the outreach methodologies utilized in the New York 9/11 disaster response. In E. C. Ritchie, M. J. Friedman, & P. J. Watson (Eds.), *Mental health intervention following disasters and mass violence.* New York: Guilford Press.

Newman, E., Davis, J., & Kennedy, S. (in press). Journalism and the public during catastrophes. In Y. Neria, R. Gross, R. Marshall, & E. Susser (Eds.), *Public mental health in the wake of a terrorist attack.* Cambridge, UK: Cambridge University Press.

Norris, F., Friedman, M., & Watson, P. (2002). 60,000 disaster victims speak, Part II: Summary and implications of the disaster mental health research. *Psychiatry, 65* 240-260.

Norris, F., Friedman, M., Watson, P., Byrne, C., Diaz, E., & Kaniasty, K. (2002). 60,000 disaster victims speak, Part I: An empirical review of the empirical literature, 1981-2001. *Psychiatry, 65,* 207-239.

Norris, F. H., Murphy, A. D., Baker, C. K., & Perilla, J. L. (2003). Severity, timing and duration of reactions to trauma in the population: An example from Mexico. *Biological Psychiatry, 53,* 769-778.

Pfefferbaum, B., Nixon, S., Tivis, R., Doughty, D., Pynoos, R., Gurwitch, R. et al. (2001). Television exposure in children after a terrorist incident. *Psychiatry, 64,* 202-211.

Pfefferbaum, B., Pfefferbaum, R. L., North, C. S., & Neas, B. R. (2002). Commentary: Does television viewing satisfy criteria for exposure in posttraumatic stress disorder? *Psychiatry, 64,* 306-309.

Pivar, I., & Prigerson, H. (2004). Traumatic loss, complicated grief, and terrorism. *Journal of Aggression, Maltreatment & Trauma, 9*(1/2/3/4), 277-288.

Rose, S., & Bisson, J. I. (1998). Brief early psychological interventions following trauma: A systematic review of the literature. *Journal of Traumatic Stress, 11,* 697-710.

Ross, G. (2004). Guide. Media guidelines: From the "trauma vortex" to the "healing vortex." *Journal of Aggression, Maltreatmemt, & Trauma, 9*(1/2/3/4), 391-394.

Schlenger, W. E., Caddell, J. M., Ebert, L., Jordan, B. K., Rouke, K. M., Wilson, D. et al. (2002). Psychological reactions to terrorist attacks: Findings from the national study of American's reactions to September 11. *Journal of the American Medical Association, 288*, 581-588.

Schnurr, P. P., & Green, B. L. (Eds.). (in press). *Trauma and health: Physical health consequences of exposure to extreme stress.* Washington, DC: American Psychological Association.

Schuster, M., Bradley, D., Stein, M., Jaycox, L. H., Collins, R. L., Marshall, G. N. et al. (2001). A national survey of stress reactions after the September 11, 2001, terrorist attacks. *New England Journal of Medicine, 345*, 1507-1512.

Shalev, A. Y., Peri, T., Canetti, L., & Schreiber, S. (1996). Predictors of PTSD in injured trauma survivors. *American Journal of Psychiatry, 153*, 219-225.

Silver, R. C., Holman, E. A., McIntosh, D. N., Poulin, M., & Gil-Rivas, V. (2002). Nationwide longitudinal study of psychological responses to September 11. *Journal of the American Medical Association, 288*, 1235-1244.

Solomon, Z. (1995). The pathogenic effects of war stress: The Israeli experience. In S.E. Hobfall & M.W. de Vries (Eds.), *Extreme stress and communities: Impact and intervention* (pp. 229-246). Amsterdam: Kluwer Academic.

U.S. Department of Health and Human Services. (2002). *Communicating in a crisis: Risk communication guidelines for public officials.* Rockville, MD: Author.

Waizer, J., Dorin, A., Stoller, E., & Laird, R. (2004). Community-based interventions in New York City after 9/11: A provider's perspective. *Journal of Aggression, Maltreatment, & Trauma, 9*(1/2/3/4), 499-511.

Wilson, J. P., Friedman, M. J., & Lindy, J. D. (Eds.). (2001). *Treating psychological trauma and PTSD.* New York: Guilford Press.

The Primary Care Health System as a Core Resource in Response to Terrorism

Margaret Heldring
Harold Kudler

SUMMARY. Living through a terrorist event or under threat of attack affects both mental and physical health. A nation's primary care system plays a critical role under such circumstances. This article reviews the American experience after September 11, 2001 and advocates for integration of mental and physical health services in primary care settings as a key counter-terrorism strategy. Americans put their trust in primary care providers. The nation's healthcare system must develop and implement a strategy that informs and supports primary care providers in meeting the mental health needs of a nation confronted by terrorism.

KEYWORDS. Terrorism, mental health, primary care, collaborative care, mind-body interactions

---

Address correspondence to: Margaret Heldring, America's HealthTogether, 505 C Street NE, Washington, DC, 20002 USA (E-mail: Mheldring@aol.com).

The authors acknowledge the contributions of F. Thurston Drake, of America's HealthTogether and Princeton University Project 55, to this article.

[Haworth co-indexing entry note]: "The Primary Care Health System as a Core Resource in Response to Terrorism." Heldring, Margaret, and Harold Kudler. Co-published simultaneously in *Journal of Aggression, Maltreatment & Trauma* (The Haworth Maltreatment & Trauma Press, an imprint of The Haworth Press, Inc.) Vol. 10, No. 1/2, 2005; and: *The Trauma of Terrorism: Sharing Knowledge and Shared Care, An International Handbook* (ed: Yael Danieli, Danny Brom, and Joe Sills) The Haworth Maltreatment & Trauma Press, an imprint of The Haworth Press, Inc., 2005.

Americans tend to conceptualize homeland security in terms of maintaining surveillance, guarding against weapons of mass destruction, and countering specific infections or injuries. It is, however, inadequate to frame terrorism in terms of physical assaults because terrorism is primarily a psychological weapon, aimed at inflicting psychological trauma on a community or nation in order to gain control over it. This definition accounts for terrorism's terrible economy and reach. The killing of a single soldier in Iraq can affect millions of people on the other side of the planet. None of these people are within range of bullets or bombs but all are well within the range of terrorism because they can be made to feel vulnerable and overwhelmed. Mere threats can assure success. Because terrorists wield psychological trauma as a weapon, terrorism is very much a mental health issue.

On the other hand, the American mental health system, while relatively robust, is not capable of meeting the medical challenge of terrorism on its own. It cannot deal with the direct medical and surgical consequences of terrorism nor with the indirect but very real effects on physical health that can be produced by exposure to terrorism (Hassett & Sigal, 2002; Holman, Silver, & Waitzkin, 2000; Silver, Holman, McIntosh, Povlin, & Gil-Rivas, 2002). Neither are mental health resources available everywhere terrorism might strike. Community resilience demands *integrated* care for mind and body.

This chapter considers the new demands on the American healthcare system following the events of September 11, 2001. While we have largely confined ourselves to the effects on one nation, our remarks are relevant for healthcare providers and leaders in other nations as well.

MENTAL HEALTH AND THE RESPONSE
TO THE SEPTEMBER 11 ATTACKS

David Satcher, MD, former U.S. Surgeon General and a family physician, provided the following principles and core recommendations in his landmark *Report on Mental Health* (U.S. Department of Health and Human Services, 1999): (a) Mental health is fundamental to good health, (b) Mental health should flow in the mainstream of healthcare, and (c) The destructive split between mental and physical health should be mended. Based on the recent American experience with homeland terrorism, we can add the following: (d) The aftermath of September 11, 2001 revealed a need for comprehensive mental health planning and services in response to the impact of terrorism on individuals, families, and the larger community, (e) Local mental health plans must be carefully integrated into national systems of response and coordinated with activities of governmental and non-governmental agencies, and (f) Mental health issues continue to be obscured by widespread ignorance, misunderstanding, and stigma which limit effective response to terrorism.

Living with the possibility of homeland terrorism on a national scale is a new American experience. In truth, we have no blueprint for the unfolding mental health story following September 11th. We cannot extrapolate from the literature on responses to natural disasters such as floods or hurricanes. We are used to consuming such events in the process of reading our morning papers; they no longer have the power to terrify us. We can draw important lessons from certain seminal events such as the bombing of the Murrah Federal Building in Oklahoma City and the mass shooting of high school students by their own classmates in Columbine, Colorado. Still, these were tragedies of a different scale and each occurred within a discrete time frame and a particular geography. And, while we can benefit by reviewing critical lessons from nations with longer histories of terrorism, we cannot entirely import their experiences. America has its own culture (or set of diverse cultures). We need to plumb our own national experience in order to develop an appropriate plan of action.

What was the impact of September 11 on mental health? Galea et al. (2002) found that in the 5-8 weeks after September 11th, 13% of people in Manhattan met criteria for Post Traumatic Stress Disorder (PTSD) and/or depression. This rate jumped to 20% in the immediate vicinity of the World Trade Center. The same study showed that 29% of New Yorkers acknowledged increased use of substances during those first weeks. Hoven (2002) found that 10.5% of New York City school children experienced posttraumatic stress. Local responses were mirrored across America. Silver et al. (2002) conducted a nationwide longitudinal study and found that global distress remained high across the country at two and six months after the attacks. In 2003, a national survey of primary care providers found that nearly 80% noted new or increased physiological or physical symptoms of terrorism-related stress in their patients (America's HealthTogether & The Robert Wood Johnson Foundation, 2003).

In a national survey in October 2001, The Harvard School of Public Health found that Americans had quickly adapted to terrorism by taking new precautions (Blendon et al., 2001). For example, Americans believed that they were more likely to get the flu (73%) than be exposed to anthrax (14%) or smallpox (9%) within the next twelve months, yet 57% had begun opening mail more carefully and maintaining emergency supplies at home. This study also showed that the majority of Americans could not identify a national figure or agency they could trust for reliable information in the event of a bioterrorist attack. When asked who they would trust for information within their own community, 61% of respondents indicated significant confidence in their fire department, 53% in the police, and, most importantly in this context, 77% of people indicated a great deal or quite a lot of trust in their own doctor.

Since September 11, the U.S. government's medical responses have primarily focused on anticipating nuclear, biological and/or chemical acts of terrorism. Countless reports, public lectures, consumer bulletins, and website postings describe the presentation, course, and treatment of specific physical vectors (including radioactive iodine, weapons-grade anthrax, and a host of organophosphates). Much less attention has been devoted to understanding and dealing with psychological responses to terrorism. This flies in the face of evidence that psychological causalities from terrorism tend to outnumber physical casualties. For example, in the Aum Shinrikyo poison gas attack on Tokyo subway commuters, twelve people were killed but more than 5,000 sought care for presumed exposure (Ursano, 2002; see Lifton, this volume). While some of those 5,000 may have been exposed to sub-lethal levels of nerve gas or otherwise physically injured during the attack, it is reasonable to assume that a much larger proportion were seeking medical attention for what was primarily a psychological injury. Health planners sometimes worry how they will distinguish "real casualties" (those who have been physically affected) from those who "have nothing really the matter with them" (psychological casualties) after a terrorist attack. They are less likely to develop a plan to respond to the very real and legitimate needs of psychological casualties. Further, in the rush to provide immediate, effective medical and surgical treatment for survivors, healthcare providers often overlook the fact that those who are physically injured may also require psychological help, as may their families and their community.

In order to meet the challenge of terrorism, the nation's healthcare system must be based on a biopsychosocial model. Different disciplines must work together to promote physical, mental and community health (Blount, 1998; Engel, 1997; Katon et al., 2002). In responding to terrorism, it is neither possible nor desirable to decide if pathology resides in the mind or in the body: the problem resides in the person and, ultimately, in the community.

THE ROLE OF THE PRIMARY HEALTHCARE SYSTEM IN PROVIDING MENTAL HEALTHCARE

In point of fact, more than 50% of all mental healthcare visits in the United States are made to primary healthcare providers (deGruy, 1996). When stressed or anxious, demoralized or bereaved, more people turn to their primary care provider for help than to specialized mental health providers (Pincus, 2003; Regier, 1978). The nation's primary healthcare system is increasingly recognized as its de facto mental health system (Frank, McDaniel, Bray, & Heldring, 2003; Perrin, 1999).

How Widespread Are Mental Health Issues in Primary Care? In a representative sample of 2,160 outpatients followed in Boston area outpatient programs of the US Department of Veterans Affairs (VA), 40% screened positive for at least one current mental health disorder. Twenty percent of the entire sample screened positive for PTSD (Hankin, Spire, Miller & Kazis, 1999). Taubman-Ben-Ari, Rabinowitz, Feldman, and Vaturi (2001) reported that 23% of primary care patients have been exposed to traumatic events and that 39% of those met full criteria for a diagnosis of posttraumatic stress disorder. Twenty-four percent of patients presenting to primary care providers suffer from a well-defined ICD-10 mental disorder. The majority of these patients (69%) present to providers with physical complaints (World Health Organization, 2000).

A 2003 national survey conducted by America's HealthTogether (a non-profit organization promoting health policy) and The Robert Wood Johnson Foundation showed that primary care providers identified an increased need for mental health services and advocated a collaborative model that integrates mental healthcare into primary care practice. Their patients included families of September 11th victims, rescue workers, displaced employees and their families, military personnel and their families, and a wide range of Americans affected by those events.

Not every person who survives a traumatic event will require specialty mental health treatment but most will benefit from skilled and sensitive assistance. According to the Harvard Program in Refugee Trauma (2002), 85% of trauma survivors return to baseline psychological function with time and the support of family and friends, while only 15% require professional assistance. Even among Vietnam War combat veterans, there was only a 30% lifetime prevalence of PTSD (Kulka et al., 1990). Half of these veterans no longer met full PTSD criteria by the late 1980s.

PTSD is only one of many possible medical sequelae of psychological trauma. When survivors present for medical help, their responses tend to be complex (Kroll, 2003). They may report anxiety, depression, loss of interest in work or recreation, memory loss, intrusive memories or fear for the safety of family members and friends. Psychological trauma may also surface indirectly as an exacerbation of chronic physical ailments (shortness of breath in an asthmatic, increased pain in a person with arthritis). It may be expressed in new somatic and/or behavioral symptoms (i.e., headaches, abdominal pain) or as new or exacerbated substance abuse. It may remain masked behind vague complaints of malaise or loss of energy or an upswing in family friction or workplace stress. Individuals with prior history of trauma may re-experience symptoms and signs referent to that earlier stressor. Individuals with pre-exist-ing mental illness may experience exacerbation/relapse.

Even though primary care providers are first-line mental health providers, their circumstances frequently preclude their making effective mental health interventions (Escobar et al., 1998; Katon et al., 1991; North, 2002). Most have only scant training in mental health and many face considerable disin-centives to open such issues with patients and families. Providers may not have adequate time in their hectic clinic schedules. There may be no screening process to trigger in-depth review of traumatic experiences and responses. There may be a dearth of mental health consultation services in the clinic or even in the community. Primary care clinicians may also find the communica-tions of the mentally ill confusing and frustrating because they are often framed in vague terms and patients may be hesitant to discuss them openly. Consequently, mental health issues frequently go undetected and untreated in primary care settings. Acute reactions are thus more likely to become chronic conditions. The result is increased human suffering and inefficient healthcare utilization (Katon et al., 2003).

Integrating Mental Health and Primary Care

American medicine can learn from recent experience in post-war Kosovo. Stemming, in part, from their need to respond to widespread trauma, the Kosovar Family Professional Education Collaborative launched a strategic plan in 2000 to address mental health and psychosocial needs by stressing col-laboration between family medicine and mental health practitioners (Cardozo, Vergara, Agani, & Gotway, 2000). The Rand Corporation and the Interna-tional Society for Traumatic Stress Studies (ISTSS) are building on that expe-rience, in collaboration with the Kosovo Federal Ministry of Health and other national and international governmental and non-governmental agencies, to produce a *Guideline for International Trauma Training of Primary Care Pro-viders* (Eisenman, Agani, & Rolland, 2003). The guideline will lay out a cur-riculum for basic mental health training for primary care providers (i.e., physicians, nurses), which supports their efforts in response to traumatic situa-tions. It will provide a rich information infrastructure and a crucial set of link-age and referral options. The Kosovars have demonstrated that a nation's primary healthcare system can serve as an effective biopsychosocial resource during times of national trauma.

America is still in the process of developing a national model of integrated care that promotes resilience to terrorism. In order to provide integrated care, several health disciplines must combine perspectives and expertise to better serve individuals, families, and communities (Katon et al., 2002). This is a logical application of the biopsychosocial medical model. It is a patient-centered approach in which systems of care are designed to suit the needs of patients rather than making them migrate from clinic to clinic and discipline to discipline. Such integration can be expected to lead to better care and greater efficiency. One example would be inclusion of a mental health provider within a primary care team. This makes good sense because mental health providers are most helpful to primary care providers and their patients when they are fully acquainted with primary care settings and have had time to develop rapport and trust with providers in those settings (McDaniel, Campbell, & Seaburn, 1995).

The Clinical Practice Guideline (CPG) for the Management of Post-Traumatic Stress, developed jointly by the U.S. Departments of Veterans Affairs (VA) and Defense (DoD) (2003) offers a template that integrates health system responses for military men and women and veterans who have been exposed to combat, hazardous peacekeeping missions, and sexual trauma and other stressful events. CPG's are recommendations for the performance or exclusion of specific procedures or services for specific disease entities. They integrate evidence-based care into clinical algorithms, a set of rules, in flowchart format, for solving a problem in a finite number of steps. CPG's function like textbooks or journals but are more user-friendly in clinical settings. They are meant to inform care without constraining it: they must always be applied within the context of the individual provider's clinical judgment for the care of a particular patient.

The VA/DoD CPG for Post-Traumatic Stress addresses screening, diagnosis, and treatment in mental health and primary care settings. It was designed by a multidisciplinary group including mental health and primary care practitioners, pharmacists, occupational therapists and chaplains in order to be maximally accessible across care settings. Its decision tree for clinical management addresses a wide range of posttraumatic responses. Particular emphasis was placed on educating and supporting families, military units, and communities as a critical element of care for the individual. Whenever possible, CPG recommendations were tied to research findings but, where no good evidence base exists, recommendations reflect expert consensus. Evidence tables identify the authority for each recommendation, the quality of the evidence, and the strength of the recommendation. Separate modules address care in primary care and mental health settings and provide a cross-walk between these settings based on patient needs and provider skills and preferences. Other modules address post-traumatic reactions in acute situations and in ongoing combat situations.

A core element of the Joint VA/DoD CPG is a brief, problem-focused PTSD screening tool validated in primary care settings (Prins et al., 2004). It consists of the following questions: In your life, have you ever had any experience that was so frightening, horrible, or upsetting that, in the past month, you: (a) Have had nightmares about it or thought about it when you did not want to? (b) Tried hard not to think about it or went out of your way to avoid situations that reminded you of it? (c) Were constantly on guard, watchful, or easily startled? or (d) Felt numb or detached from others, activities, or your surroundings?

The PC-PTSD screen is scored "positive" if a patient answers "yes" to any two items. If the screen is positive, the CPG guides the clinician through the process of making a diagnosis and instituting an integrated biopsychosocial treatment plan. By mandating routine screening in primary care and mental health settings and additional screening following stressful events, the CPG aims to increase provider awareness of posttraumatic problems and galvanize clinical response to them.

There is, to date, insufficient evidence that early intervention can prevent the development or progression of PTSD. There is, however, strong evidence that those who develop Acute Stress Disorder are more likely to go on to develop PTSD (Bryant, 2003). In addition, numerous studies (reviewed by Schnurr & Jankowski, 1999) indicate a substantial increase in healthcare utilization among people who have survived traumatic events. It therefore makes good clinical sense to ensure that people exposed to traumatic events are screened in order to identify those at greatest risk for severe and/or chronic reactions including PTSD, if only to do a better job of identifying patients who will need additional follow-up. Appropriate interventions may include psychopharmacological intervention, education about normal responses to traumatic events (which may help survivors normalize their responses), individual, group, and/or family support programs, and identification of resources for follow-up. With such systems in place, it may be possible to prevent or mitigate some of the biopsychosocial morbidity of psychological trauma.

Promoting Integration of Mental Health and Primary Care

The VA/DoD CPG serves the needs of a special subpopulation of traumatized Americans seeking comprehensive healthcare but a national strategy is needed as well. In 2002, The Robert Wood Johnson Foundation responded to this challenge by funding *Facing Fear Together (FFT)*, an initiative that researches health needs of Americans post-September 11th and works to strengthen the capacity of the nation's primary healthcare system.

FFT has interviewed more than 500 primary care providers about their professional and personal experiences in the wake of September 11th and in the context of ongoing threats. They concluded that: (a) September 11th changed the nation's emotional and psychological landscape. September 11th and subsequent national stressors have created ongoing psychological distress and cascading trauma. Individuals with greater physical proximity to these events, pre-existing physical or mental illnesses, refugees, recent immigrants, children, and those with prior trauma exposure were particularly vulnerable; (b) Primary care providers feel ill equipped to handle the changing health and mental health needs of patients. As people seek physical and mental healthcare from their primary care providers, practitioners reported limited mental health support and apprehension about their capacity to handle increased workload associated with future terrorist acts. The frayed mental healthcare system in the U.S. results in overburdened primary care providers and poorly served patients. The new context of terrorism has made primary care providers' needs for more time, information, and resources even more urgent; and (c) Primary care providers are calling for more support and education in addressing mental health issues. While the Centers for Disease Control and Prevention (CDC) is readily identified as a valuable source of expert information on biomedical aspects of terrorist threats, many primary care providers cannot identify a trusted resource that addresses the mental health dimension of terrorism.

This expertise does, however, exist in the VA's National Center for PTSD. Its website (www.NCPTSD.org) is a source of information on trauma survivors and is available to all providers and the public. The VA has also produced a Veterans Health Initiative manual on PTSD in Primary Care (available to providers as a web-based independent study program at http://www.appc1.va.gov/vhi_ind_ study/ptsd/index. cfm) that offers comprehensive clinical guidance in a format crafted for use by primary care clinicians.

The *Facing Fear Together* initiative (www.facingfeartogether.org) continues to foster collaboration between primary care providers and mental health providers through the development of public and professional educational and training materials that increase the capacity of primary care providers to meet the mental health needs of patients and bolster the psychological resilience of individuals, families, and communities.

CONCLUSION

As the nation copes with the biopsychosocial challenge of terrorism, it makes good sense to meet patients where they are and to remember the maxim, "the public will not take the pill if it does not trust the doctor." Americans put their trust in their primary care providers. To honor that trust, the nation's healthcare system must develop and implement a strategy that informs and supports primary care providers in meeting the mental health needs of a nation confronted by terrorism.

REFERENCES

America's HealthTogether and the Robert Wood Johnson Foundation (2003). *The Blueprint Report: Mental health and primary care in a time of terrorism.* Available from, http://www.facingfeartogether.org

Blendon, R. J., Benson, J. M., DesRoches, C. M., & Hermann, M. J. (2001). *Harvard School of Public Health/Robert Wood Johnson Foundation Survey Project on Americans' Response to Biological Terrorism, Oct 24-Oct 28, 2001.* Results available from, http://www.hsph.harvard.edu/press/releases/blendon/report.pdf

Blount, A. (1998). *Integrated primary care: The future of medical and mental health collaboration.* New York: Norton.

Bryant, R.A. (2003). Early predictors of post traumatic stress disorder. *Biological Psychiatry, 53,* 789-795.

Cardozo, B. L., Vergara, A., Agani, F., & Gotway, C. A. (2000). Mental health, social functioning, and attitudes of Kosovar Albanians following the war in Kosovo. *Journal of the American Medical Association, 284,* 569-577.

DeGuy, F. (1996). Mental health in the primary care setting. In M. S. Donaldson, K. D. Yordy, K. N. Lohr, & N. A. Vanselow (Eds.), *Primary care: America's health in a new era* (pp. 285-311). Washington, DC: Institute of Medicine, National Academy Press.

Eisenman, D., Agani, F. & Rolland, J. (2003, October). *International trauma training of primary care providers.* Presented at the 19th Annual Meeting of the International Society for Traumatic Stress Studies, Chicago, IL.

Engel, G. (1997). From biomedical to biopsychosocial: Being scientific in the human domain. *Psychosomatics, 38,* 521-528.

Escobar, J. I., Gara, M., Cohen-Silver, R., Waitzkin, H., Holman, A., & Compton, W. (1998). Somatization disorder in primary care. *British Journal of Psychiatry, 173,* 262-266.

Frank, R. G., McDaniel, S. H., Bray, J. M., & Heldring, M. (2003). *Primary care psychology.* Washington, DC: American Psychological Association.

Galea, S., Ahern, J., Resnick, H., Kilpatrick, D., Bucuvalas, M., Gold, J. et al. (2002). Psychological sequelae of the September 11 terrorist attacks in New York City. *New England Journal of Medicine, 346,* 982-987.

Hankin, C. S., Spire, A., Miller, D. R., & Kazis, L. (1999). Mental disorders and mental health treatment among U.S. Department of Veterans Affairs outpatients: The veterans health study. *American Journal of Psychiatry, 156,* 1924-1930.

Hassett, A., & Sigal, L. H. (2002). Unforeseen consequences of terrorism: Medically unexplained symptoms in a time of fear. *Archives of Internal Medicine, 162,* 1809-1813.

Holman, E. A., Silver, R. C., & Waitzkin, H. (2000). Traumatic life events in primary care patients: A study in an ethnically diverse sample. *Archives of Family Medicine, 9,* 802-810.

Hoven, C. W., Duarte, C. S., Lucas, C. P., Mandell, D. J., Cohen, M., Rosen, C. et al. (2002). *Effects of the World Trade Center attack on NYC public school students–Initial report to the New York City Board of Education.* New York: Columbia

University Mailman School of Public Health-New York State Psychiatric Institute and Applied Research and Consulting, LLC.

Katon, W., Lin, E., Russo, J., & Unutzer, J. (2003). Increased medical costs of a population-based sample of depressed elderly patients. *Archives of General Psychiatry, 60*, 897-903.

Katon, W., Russo, J., Von Korff, M., Lin, E., Simon, G., Bush, T., Ludman, E., & Walker, E. (2002). Long-term effects of a collaborative care intervention in persistently depressed primary care patients. *Journal of General Internal Medicine, 17*, 741-748.

Katon, W., Lin, E., Von Korff, M., Russo, J., Lipscomb, P., & Bush, T. (1991). Somatization: A spectrum of severity. *American Journal of Psychiatry, 173*, 198-202.

Kroll, J. (2003). Posttraumatic symptoms and the complexity of responses to trauma. *Journal of the American Medical Association, 290*, 667-670.

Kulka, R. A. Schlenger, W. E., Fairbank, J. A., Hough, R. L., Jordan, B. K., Marmar, C. R. et al. (1990). *Trauma and the Vietnam War generation: Report of findings from the National Vietnam Veterans Readjustment Study*. New York: Brunner/Mazel.

Lifton, R. J. (2004). Aum Shinrikyo: The threshold crossed. *Journal of Aggression, Maltreatment, & Trauma, 9*(1/2/3/4), 57-66.

McDaniel, S. H., Campbell, T. L., & Seaburn, D. B. (1995). Principles for collaboration between health and mental health providers in primary care. *Family Systems Medicine, 13*, 283-298.

North, C. S. (2002). Somatization in survivors of catastrophic trauma: A methodological review. *Environmental Health Perspectives, 110*, 637-640.

Perrin, E. C. (1999). Collaboration in pediatric primary care: A pediatrician's point of view. *Journal of Pediatric Psychology, 24*, 453-458.

Pincus, H. A. (2003). The future of behavioral health and primary care: Drowning in the mainstream or left on the bank? *Psychosomatics, 44*, 1-11.

Prins, A., Ouimette, P., Kimerling, R., Cameron, R. P., Hugelshofer, D. S., Shaw-Hegwer, J. et al. (in press). The primary care PTSD screen (PC-PTSD): Development and operating characteristics. *Primary Care Psychiatry*.

Regier, D. A., Goldberg, I. D., & Taube, C. A. (1978). The de facto U.S. mental health services system: A public health perspective. *Archives of General Psychiatry, 35*, 685-693.

Schnurr, P. P., & Jankowski, M. K. (1999). Physical health and post traumatic stress disorder: Review and synthesis. *Seminars in Clinical Neuropsychiatry, 4*, 295-304.

Silver, R., Holman, E., McIntosh, D., Povlin, M., & Gil-Rivas, V. (2002). Nationwide longitudinal study of psychological responses to September 11. *Journal of the American Medical Association, 288*, 1235-1244.

Taubman-Ben-Ari, O., Rabinowitz, J., Feldman, D., & Vaturi, R. (2001). Post-traumatic stress disorder in primary-care settings: Prevalence and physicians' detection. *Psychological Medicine, 31*, 555-560.

Ursano, R. J. (2002). Post-traumatic stress disorder. *New England Journal of Medicine, 346*, 130-132.

U.S. Department of Health and Human Services, Substance Abuse and Mental Health Services Administration, Center for Mental Health Services, National Institutes of Health, National Institute of Mental Health. (1999). *Mental health: A report of the Surgeon General.* Rockville, MD: Author.

U.S. Department of Veterans Affairs. (2002). *Veterans health initiative: Post traumatic stress disorder: Implications for primary care.* Washington, DC: Author.

U.S. Department of Veterans Affairs/Department of Defense Clinical Practice Guideline Working Group. (2003). *Management of posttraumatic stress.* Washington, DC: Veterans Administration, Department of Veterans Affairs, Department of Defense, Office of Quality and Performance Publication 10Q CPG/PTS-03.

World Health Organization. (2000). *WHO guide to mental health in primary care.* London: WHO Collaborating Centre for Mental Health Research and Training, Institute of Psychiatry.

Identification and Follow-Up by Primary Care Doctors of Children with PTSD After Terrorist Attacks

Moshe Vardi

SUMMARY. Many children and adolescents were among the victims of the suicide bomb attacks in Israel since March, 2000. While the number with emotional and behavioral symptoms was expected to be high, very few children who developed terrorism-related posttraumatic stress disorder (PTSD) were actually referred to mental health professionals for assessment or treatment. Prolonged exposure to terrorism lowers even further the number of children who remain in treatment. This article discusses reasons and presents a training program for primary care providers (pediatricians, family doctors) in identifying PTSD in child victims, and for mobilizing them to carry out long-term follow-up of these children.

Address correspondence to: Moshe Vardi, MD, Lowenstein Hospital Rehabilitation Center, 278 Achuza Street, Raanana 43100, Israel (E-mail: moshev@clalit.org.il).

[Haworth co-indexing entry note]: "Identification and Follow-Up by Primary Care Doctors of Children with PTSD After Terrorist Attacks." Vardi, Moshe. Co-published simultaneously in *Journal of Aggression, Maltreatment & Trauma* (The Haworth Maltreatment & Trauma Press, an imprint of The Haworth Press, Inc.) Vol. 10, No. 1/2, 2005; and: *The Trauma of Terrorism: Sharing Knowledge and Shared Care, An International Handbook* (ed: Yael Danieli, Danny Brom, and Joe Sills) The Haworth Maltreatment & Trauma Press, an imprint of The Haworth Press, Inc., 2005.

KEYWORDS. Children, terrorism, PTSD, service utilization, primary care

Trauma and post-trauma have become over recent years one of the main topics in research and treatment due to increasing violence and terrorism against civilian populations around the world. Studies conducted after terrorist attacks in Oklahoma City (Pfefferbaum, Nixon, & Krug, 1999), New York City (Hoven et al., 2002; Schuster et al., 2001), Israel (Bleich, Gelkopf, & Solomon, 2003), and elsewhere showed that 10-16% of adults and children suffered from chronic PTSD that caused significant difficulties in functioning. The vast media exposure after the 9/11 attack in New York also increased the number of people with PTSD (Cantor, 2000; Stuber et al., 2002). On the other hand, a very small number of people, especially children, received psychological treatment in the sub-acute and chronic stages of PTSD.

The worldwide wave of terrorism is likely to last for many more years, and might become more severe. The number of adults and children suffering from chronic PTSD will thus increase and with it the gap between the need for psychological treatment, service need, and the utilization of psychological services, service utilization, in the field of trauma. This gap is more striking in children and adolescents who suffer from PTSD (Hoven et al., 2002).

Koenen, Goodwin, Struening, Hellman, and Guardino (2003) examined factors related to PTSD and help-seeking in a large national sample ($n = 15,606$) in the United States. This study used a behavioral model of health service, which posits that there are three types of factors involved in whether or not individuals seek services: (a) Predisposing factors (i.e., demographics, social structure variables and beliefs about treatment); (b) Enabling factors (means by which one accesses treatment, including insurance, finances and knowledge about where treatment is available); and (c) Need factors (the level of an individual's illness manifested by the degree to which symptoms interfere with daily life and other diagnoses. More interference by symptoms in their daily life and having an additional diagnosis, specifically Panic Disorder, were associated with seeking mental health services).

The authors note that a high degree of impairment and other diagnoses was also found among individuals who had never sought treatment. Additionally, they found it striking that minority individuals with PTSD were less likely to have received mental health treatment. Participants with PTSD were more likely to provide the following reasons for not seeking treatment than those with other anxiety disorders: (a) being "afraid of what others might think," or (b) they were "not sure where to get help," and (c) they just "couldn't afford treatment."

Studies of service use provide information on the success or failure of the health care system in addressing the needs of its target population. Some have focused on the high levels of service use among people with PTSD (Switzer et al., 1999). Other studies demonstrated considerable under-utilization of services (Amaya-Jackson et al., 1999; Hoven et al., 2002). The study conducted by Kulka et al. (1990) is best known for documenting the high prevalence of PTSD in Vietnam Veterans. This study also documented dramatically low rates of service utilization among veterans and helped stimulate the development of a national network of specialized VA services for PTSD.

Effectiveness studies help us understand the performance of services as they are actually delivered by healthcare providers in real-world healthcare systems. Consequences of exposure to trauma are enormously costly, not only to the victims, but also to our health care system and to society. It is not a question of dollars versus healthcare, but of using dollars in the best service of healthcare. Rosenheck and Fontana (1996) compared outcomes among patients who received high-intensity outpatient treatment and patients who received lower-intensity treatment. Here, too, evidence that lower-intensity services offered greater value (i.e., more clinical benefit per dollar) suggests an approach to treatment that can provide benefits to larger numbers of patients. Only systematic research and evaluation of operating service systems can determine when programs provide either too few or too many services, or inefficient services, thus wasting limited resources.

THE PRIMARY CARE DOCTOR AND THE RELATIONSHIP BETWEEN PTSD AND PHYSICAL HEALTH

Several studies (Drozdek, 2003; Holman, Silver, & Waitzkin, 2000; Schnurr & Jankowski, 1999) showed that in states of stress, crisis, and terror, the morbidity and the number of calls to primary care doctors increased significantly. A sizable number of patients with health problems also suffer from PTSD, which often remains undiagnosed and untreated in medical settings. This may have negative impact on compliance with medical treatment, response to treatment, patient satisfaction, level of health care utilization and cost (Arnow et al., 1999; Walker et al., 1999).

Gebhart and Neeley (1996) encouraged the development of a dialogue between mental health providers with expertise in PTSD and primary care providers. They proposed to assist primary care providers with brief, self-administered screening tools, educational brochures, and effective communication techniques which would decrease their time pressure and daily workload, since these patients often consume the providers' time with frequent visits, multiple complaints, and poor compliance with advice and treatment.

The proposed educational programs would provide helpful changes in primary care practices that could increase detection, enhance appropriate referrals to mental health specialists, and improve clinical management of patients with psychiatric symptoms. Fifer et al. (1999) showed that the dialogue between the mental health and primary health care providers had a positive effect. Taubman-Ben-Ari, Rabinowitz, Feldman and Vaturi (2001) examined the prevalence of PTSD in a national sample in Israel of primary care attendants and primary care physicians' detection of PTSD and general psychological distress in PTSD patients. They concluded that primary care providers may be the first to recognize that a patient with PTSD is entering a related psychosocial crisis. Depending on the severity and disability associated with the crisis, the primary care provider may be obliged to obtain specialty mental health services, even if the patient is reluctant to seek treatment. They suggested that relatively brief but specialized interventions may prevent PTSD effectively in some subgroups of trauma patients and recommended that all patients with PTSD should have a specific primary care provider assigned to coordinate their overall healthcare. Pharmacological management of PTSD or related symptoms may be initiated based on a presumptive diagnosis of PTSD.

Primary care providers should perform a brief PTSD symptom assessment at each visit. The use of a validated PTSD symptom measure, such as the PTSD Checklist, should be considered. Primary care-based supportive counseling for PTSD has received little study to date and cannot be endorsed as an evidence-based psychotherapeutic strategy. However, it may be the sole psychotherapeutic option available for the patient with PTSD who is reluctant to seek specialty mental health care. Elements for primary care-based supportive counseling for PTSD include helping patients solve problems presented by PTSD symptoms and sequelae (e.g., agoraphobia or other phobic avoidance), provision of PTSD-related psycho education, assisting patients in recognizing early signs and symptoms of PTSD relapse, and encouraging initiation of active coping strategies such as physical activity, relaxation strategies, and social and recreational activities.

Taubman-Ben-Ari et al. (2001) called for regular follow-up with monitoring and documentation of symptoms as part of primary care treatment of any chronic disease. Primary care providers should consult with a mental health provider and/or a PTSD Specialty Team regarding all patients with acute or chronic stress disorders. They should continue to be involved in treating these patients. Case management should be provided, as indicated, to address high utilization of medical resources. They should consider referral to mental health agencies if indicated by patient symptoms. The primary care provider and the primary care team (including the Health Care Integrator) have to stay actively involved, in coordination with the mental health specialist, in the care of patients with PTSD.

It is necessary to develop active approaches to screen and reach out to vulnerable subjects who find it hard to ask for help when needed. Among these high-risk populations for PTSD are those who have been directly injured and their families, children and adolescents exposed to horror and terrorism by the media, the elderly, and people who have experienced previous trauma or lived under difficult socio-economic conditions. A short and single diagnosis is not sufficient. It is necessary to follow up and observe the high-risk population for a long time, to check for spontaneous functional recovery, and to see whether the problems and the complaints continue and require professional intervention.

When dealing with children, we know that the younger the age, the bigger the risk of developing PTSD (see Pfefferbaum et al., this volume). It is harder to diagnose and distinguish between the normal anxiety reactions in children and the reactions that require professional treatment. Children are also more reluctant to ask for psychological help. Wells, Kataoka, and Asarnow (2001) found in their studies that primary care appointments were the most effective place to screen children, since most children have some contact with primary care medical services.

The screening and follow-up period should be long and last at least a few years. Schuster et al. (2001) argued that the psychological effects of recent terrorism are unlikely to disappear soon. Many of the respondents in their survey said that they anticipated further attacks and that they thought the attacks could be local. Concern about future attacks could heighten anxiety. Ongoing media coverage may serve as a traumatic reminder, resulting in persistent symptoms. When people are anticipating disaster, their fears can worsen existing symptoms and cause new ones (Kiser et al., 1993; Turner, Nigg, & Paz, 1986).

THE PROJECT

For years, Israelis have lived in a state of terror, which has changed their view of the world drastically. In this case, expecting the unexpected in their life has become a routine phenomenon. People in general, especially parents, are bound to behave according to a "survival mode," where preserving and maintaining their existence, and avoiding threatening situations, such as going out, taking a bus, going to a restaurant, become normative, not pathological, behaviors.

In this situation, it is difficult to distinguish between normative reactions of anxiety and PTSD. Many services and clinics specializing in trauma were opened due to the continued terrorism and national security conditions. However, although the National Insurance Institution and the Health Funds finance the treatment of injuries from terrorist attacks, and although the media encourage the population to seek assistance if needed and provide information on the importance of early diagnosis and treatment, the number of people requesting help is relatively low.

Studies conducted in New York six months after September 11th estimated that 10.5 percent of New York City grade and high school students suffered from PTSD and that 26 percent of these children suffered from other types of disorder related to the terrorist attacks (Hoven et al., 2002). Only one third of the children in this extensive study spoke with a teacher, a counselor or a mental health professional. Considering the frequency and duration of terrorist attacks in Israel, we can assume that the percentage of children suffering from symptoms of PTSD is at least the same which equates to approximately 160,000 school-age children. An unofficial survey of mental health services found that, even after three years of continued exposure to terrorist attacks, only a few dozen children and adolescents were treated in mental health professional units for children for chronic PTSD.

There are several reasons for this phenomenon; some are also seen with other psychiatric disorders and others are specific to PTSD.

- Negative stigma that is associated with psychological treatment.
- The lack of faith in the effectiveness of treatment and the widespread belief that one has to overcome mental problems on his or her own, or that 'only time will cure' (Rosenheck & Fontana, 1995).
- Difficulties finding a suitable professional agency.
- Reluctance to go for treatment as an avoidance reaction. Schwarz and Kowalski (1991) conclude that some individuals may avoid formal mental health services because they might trigger malignant memory retrieval.
- Therapists and primary care providers in times of disaster and terrorism also suffer from posttraumatic symptoms after being exposed to the terrorism and its effects (Figley, 1995; Luce, Firth-Cozens, Midgley, & Burges, 2002). They have difficulties in identifying patients with similar symptoms and referring them to treatment because they are inclined to consider these symptoms as normal reactions that do not need treatment.

Therefore, we decided to utilize the primary care doctors in the community as agents to identify and follow up children that suffer from PTSD in Israel. At the beginning of 2002, we began training primary care doctors (family doctors and pediatricians) to identify PTSD in all children and adolescents that arrive at their clinics requesting routine treatment or check-ups. We held workshops and pilot groups with 500 primary care doctors. Our main goal was to form an efficient approach to recruit and convince doctors to participate in the project, and to identify PTSD reactions actively and over the long-term.

The feedback received from the participating primary care providers in the pilot groups and workshops that lasted for about a year helped us to design, develop, and formulate step by step a program to identify PTSD in children and adolescents due to terrorism. The feedback included:

- The majority of the participating doctors agreed that in times of crisis and terrorism it is important to identify children who suffer from anxiety and PTSD.
- They and their own families are anxious because of the security situation, and many suffer from partial or full PTSD. They also need support and encouragement.
- They complained of the large workload they have in their clinics, the short time they can give to each patient (between 5 to 12 minutes), and the difficulty of taking on even more tasks, assignments and diagnoses, such as administering questionnaires to parents and adolescents.
- They usually avoid talking with their patients about emotion-laden subjects, although they realize that prolonged stress and anxiety increase the medical morbidity and the number of patients requesting help.
- They asked for an easy, practical and short method to diagnose patients that suffer from PTSD.
- They complained that it is hard to find psychiatric units for children and that waiting lists are very long.
- They need clear and exact instructions on how to cope with the patients that are diagnosed with PTSD and refuse psychological referral.
- They need continuous and open lines of communication with coordinators or facilitators from the mental health professions to encourage them to continue the project for several years.

During these workshops, great emphasis was given to the fact that primary caregivers were themselves under stress and tension and, finding it difficult to identify their own anxiety and avoidance emotions, they tend to ignore their patients' anxiety and functional difficulties as symptoms of PTSD. The participating doctors received brief training on psychiatric disturbances during and after crisis and disaster, and were instructed on the relations between these disturbances and the medical disorders they see in their clinics every day (Friedman & Schnurr, 1995). Furthermore, they were instructed how to diagnose PTSD in adults and children of various ages, according to the DSM IV (American Psychiatric Association, 1994).

Clearly, the duty of the primary care doctor is not to replace the psychiatrist, but to screen for patients who are suspected of suffering from PTSD, to follow these patients' condition during their routine visits to the clinic, and refer them to a mental health professional. The primary care doctor who participates in the project (the aim is to recruit all doctors in the country) should check all children arriving at his or her clinic to determine what influence the terrorist attacks had on them. This can be done by asking an essential question: "How does the security situation (or the terrorist attacks) influence your behavior and functioning (or your child's behavior)?" If there is a positive answer (i.e., client expresses significant damage to one of the important functions such as studies, social life, leisure activities, sleep and somatic complaints), the doctor should continue to check and register the symptoms using the brief PTSD questionnaire based on The Primary Care PTSD Screen (PC-PTSD; Prins et al., 1999) with minor changes for children. The PC-PTSD has only four questions and is problem-focused. The physician can ask patients if they have ever had an experience so frightening, horrible, or upsetting that in the past month they have had nightmares or thought about the incident when they didn't want to; tried to avoid situations that reminded them of it; were constantly on guard; or felt numb and detached from others and their surroundings.

A positive response does not necessarily indicate that a patient has PTSD, but it does indicate that a patient may have PTSD- or trauma-related problems and that further investigation of trauma symptoms by a mental health professional may be warranted. A referral or more comprehensive testing should be considered if a patient answers yes to at least two questions, or to the single hyper arousal question.

The doctor can, if the situation allows, continue his check-up thoroughly, according to the PTSD criteria. He or she can also continue the check-up during the next visits of the child, registering the continuation or disappearance of the symptoms. The first registration in the patient's file is very important, when the doctor decides that there is suspicion of an emotional problem due to the security situation. This information will help with the follow-up, until the doctor determines that the complaints are no longer present and that the child functions well in all areas.

We prepared a relatively short manual for doctors, based on the feedback received from them, including information on: (a) Behavioral and functional reactions, adaptive and pathological, in children of different ages and in their parents during periods of emergency and crisis; (b) The symptoms and criteria to identify PTSD in children of different ages, and in adults; (c) Short instructions on how the primary care doctor should perform in his or her clinic when caring for people subjected to continuous terrorist attacks; and (d) Instructions for parents on what to do and how to react or talk with their children of various ages during periods of emergency and terrorism. The manual is also written in a language suitable to the community not expert in psychopathology. It is offered as a handout to parents as well.

THE REGIONAL COORDINATORS

Many doctors expressed their concern that during periods of calm, when priorities change, they would not be able to attend the program continuously and consistently. They proposed that a regional coordinator/facilitator work with them. This person should be a psychologist or a social worker, whose task would be to collect all the accumulated data from the primary care doctors. The coordinators should always be available to instruct, train, and provide consultation if needed. They should maintain a close relationship with mental health care givers in the community and assist the doctors in referring patients who need help. The coordinators should give the doctors feedback on their activities and support them in continuing the project for as long a period of time as needed.

CONCLUSION

Mental disorders, PTSD and access to services among children are a significant public health problem. Many studies link PTSD to increased use of non-mental health care services and low use of mental health care services. This implies a need for screening children for PTSD in primary care clinics. There is a growing body of knowledge on the efficacy of services in research settings (Sansone, Sansone, & Wiederman, 1997), but limited research on the effectiveness of services in community settings. The questions are: (a) Should all children be screened? (b) Is it cost effective? (c) Should we screen only high-risk populations? and (d) Isn't the screening procedure described here too simple and concrete?

Since terrorism, in the form of random and massive killing of innocent civilians, is relatively new in the world, the necessary infrastructure for an effective mental health response to terrorism has to be built largely from scratch. The enormous gap between the service needs rates and the service utilization rates, revealed in various surveys done on PTSD, raises doubt of the clinical validity of the current screening procedures and questionnaires usually used for PTSD. The risk lies perhaps in the tendency to develop complicated and expensive programs to screen and treat PTSD.

We recommend shifting the main clinical focus of professionals who deal with chronic PTSD to reaching out toward those who are today reluctant to go to treatment, and developing simple, innovative and inexpensive methods to bring them to professional caregivers. The screening of children for PTSD due to terrorist attacks, and some forms of treatment intervention and prevention, should occur at the primary care level. Untreated PTSD tends, for the most part, to get worse rather than better, and the effects can be substantial, affecting learning, employment and relationships.

REFERENCES

Amaya-Jackson, L., Davidson, J. R., Hughes, D. C., Swartz, M., Reynolds, V., George, L. K. et al. (1999). Functional impairment and utilization of services associated with posttraumatic stress in the community. *Journal of Trauma Stress*, *12*(4), 709-724.

American Psychiatric Association. (1994). *Diagnostic and statistical manual of mental disorders* (4th ed.). Washington, DC: Author.

Arnow, B. A., Hart, S., Scott, C., Dea, R., O'Connell, L., & Taylor, C. B. (1999). Childhood sexual abuse, psychological distress and medical use among women. *Psychosomatic Medicine*, *61*, 762-770.

Bleich, A., Gelkopf, M., & Solomon, Z. (2003). Exposure to terrorism, stress-related mental health symptoms, and coping behavior among a nationally representative sample in Israel. *Journal of the American Medical Association*, *290*, 612-620.

Cantor, J. (2000). Media violence. *Journal of Adolescent Health*, *27*(Suppl. 2), 30-34.

Drozdek, B., Noor, A. K., Lutt, M., & Foy, D. W. (2003). Chronic PTSD and medical services utilization by asylum seekers. *Journal of Refugee Studies*, *16*(2), 202-211.

Felitti, V. J., Anda, R. F., Nordenberg, D., Williamson, D. F., Spitz, A. M., Edwards, V. et al. (1998). Relationship of childhood abuse and household dysfunction to many of the leading causes of death in adults: The Adverse Childhood Experiences (ACE) Study. *American Journal of Preventive Medicine*, *14*, 245-258.

Fifer, S. K., Mathias, S. D., Patrick, D. L., Mazonson, P. D., Lubeck, D. P., & Buesching, D. P. (1999). Untreated anxiety among adult primary care patients in a health maintenance organization. *Archives of General Psychiatry*, *51*, 740-750.

Figley, C. R. (1995). Compassion fatigue: Toward a new understanding of the costs of caring. In B.H. Stamm (Ed.), *Secondary traumatic stress: Self-care issues for clinicians, researchers, and educators* (pp. 3-28). Lutherville, MD: Sidran Press.

Gebhart, R. J., & Neeley, F. L. (1996). Primary care and PTSD. *National Center for PTSD Clinical Quarterly*, *6*(4), 72-74.

Holman, A. E., Silver, R. C., & Waitzkin, H. (2000). Traumatic life events in primary care patients: A study in an ethnically diverse sample. *Archives of Family Medicine*, *9*, 802-810.

Hoven, C. W., Duarte, C. S., Lucas, C. P., Mandell, D. J., Wu, P. & Rosen, C. (2002). *Effects of the World Trade Center attack on NYC public school students: Initial report of the New York Board of Education.* New York: Applied Research and Consulting, LLC & Columbia University Mailman School of Public Health & New York State Psychiatric Institute.

Kiser, L., Heston, J., Hickerson, S., Millsap, P., Nunn, W., & Pruitt, D. (1993). Anticipatory stress in children and adolescents. *American Journal of Psychiatry, 150,* 87-92.

Koenen, K. C., Goodwin, R., Struening, E., Hellman, F., & Guardino, M. (2003). Posttraumatic stress disorder and treatment seeking in a national screening sample. *Journal of Traumatic Stress, 16*(1), 5-16.

Kulka, R. A., Schlenger, W. E., Fairbank, J. A., Hough, R. L., Jordan, B. K., Marmar, C. R. et al. (1990). *Trauma and the Vietnam War generation: Report of findings from the National Vietnam Veterans Readjustment Study.* New York: Brunner/Mazel.

Luce, A., Firth-Cozens, J., Midgley, S., & Burges, C. (2002). After the Omagh bomb: Posttraumatic stress disorder in health service staff. *Journal of Traumatic Stress, 15*(1), 27-30.

Pfefferbaum, B., DeVoe, E. R., Stuber, J. Schiff, M., Klein, T. & Fairbrother, G. (2004). Psychological impact of terrorism on children and families in the United States. *Journal of Aggression, Maltreatment & Trauma, 9*(1/2/3/4), 307-319.

Pfefferbaum, B., Nixon, S., & Krug, R. (1999). Clinical needs assessment of middle and high school students following the 1995 Oklahoma City bombing. *American Journal of Psychiatry, 156,* 1069-1074.

Prins, A., Kimerling, R., Cameron, R., Oumiette, P.C., Shaw, J., Thrailkill, A. et al. (1999, November). The Primary Care PTSD Screen (PC-PTSD). In A. Prins (Chair), *The primary care PTSD screen: Psychometric properties, operating characteristics, and clinical implications.* Symposium conducted at the annual meeting of the International Society for Traumatic Stress Studies, Miami, FL.

Rosenheck, R. A., & Fontana, A.F. (1995). Do Vietnam era veterans who suffer from posttraumatic stress disorder avoid VA mental health services? *Military Medicine, 160,* 136-142.

Rosenheck, R. A., & Fontana, A. F. (1996). Treatment of veterans severely impaired by PTSD. In R. J. Ursano & A. E. Norwood (Eds.), *Emotional aftermath of the Persian Gulf War* (pp. 501-532). Washington, DC: American Psychiatric Press.

Sansone, R. A., Sansone, L. A., & Wiederman, M. W. (1997). Increased health care utilization as a function of participation in trauma research. *American Journal of Psychiatry, 154,* 1025-1027.

Schnurr, P. P., & Jankowski, M. K. (1999). Physical health and post-traumatic stress disorder: Review and synthesis. *Seminars in Clinical Neuropsychiatry, 4,* 295-304.

Schuster, M. A., Stein, B. D., Jaycox, L. H., Collins, R. L., Marshall, G. N., Elliott, M. N. et al. (2001). A National Survey of Stress Reactions after the September 11, 2001, Terrorist Attacks. *The New England Journal of Medicine 345,* 1507-1512.

Schwarz, E. D. & Kowalski, J. M. (1991). Malignant memories: PTSD in children and adults after a school shooting. *Journal of the American Academy of Child and Adolescent Psychiatry, 30,* 936-944.

Stuber, J., Fairbrother, G., Galea, S., Pfefferbaum, B., Wilson-Genderson, M., & Vlahov, D. (2002). Determinants of counseling for children in Manhattan after the September 11 attacks. *Psychiatric Services, 53*, 815-b822.

Switzer, G. E., Dew, M. A., Thompson, K., Goycoolea, J. M., Derricott, T. & Mullins, S. D. (1999). Posttraumatic stress disorder and service utilization among urban mental health center clients. *Journal of Traumatic Stress, 12*, 25-39.

Taubman-Ben-Ari, O., Rabinowitz, J., Feldman, D., & Vaturi, R. (2001). Post-traumatic stress disorder in primary care settings: Prevalence and physicians' detection. *Psychological Medicine, 31*(3), 555-560.

Turner, R. H., Nigg, J. M., & Paz, D. H. (1986). *Waiting for disaster: Earthquake watch in California.* Berkeley: University of California Press.

Walker, E. A., Unutzer, J., Rutter, C., Gelfand, A. N., Saunders, K., Von Korff, M. et al. (1999). Costs of health care use by women HMO members with a history of childhood abuse and neglect. *Archives of General Psychiatry, 56*, 609-613.

Wells, K. B., Kataoka, S. H., & Asarnow, J. R. (2001). Affective disorders in children and adolescents: Addressing unmet need in primary care settings. *Biological Psychiatry, 49*(12), 1111-1120.

Religious Care in Coping with Terrorism

Zahara Davidowitz-Farkas
John Hutchison-Hall

SUMMARY. Spiritual care has taken an important role in the aftermath of 9/11. The shattering of numerous basic assumptions by this attack has created many spiritual and existential questions. In this article, we explore different aspects of spiritual care after major disasters and the different roles that clergy can fulfill. As the field of spiritual trauma care is in a rudimentary stage, best practices for spiritual care need to be developed. In the second part of the article, different elements of the training for spiritual caregivers are described. In order to assure appropriate caregiving, guidelines for training of clergy need to be developed.

KEYWORDS. Spiritual care, disaster relief, training, trauma

Address correspondence to: Rabbi Zahara Davidowitz-Farkas, 120A East Rocks Road, Norwalk, CT 06851 USA (E-mail: zdavidowitz@mindspring.com). Reverend Hierodeacon John Hutchison-Hall may also be contacted: (E-mail: frjohn@stbasilmonastery.org).

[Haworth co-indexing entry note]: "Religious Care in Coping with Terrorism." Davidowitz-Farkas, Zahara, and John Hutchison-Hall. Co-published simultaneously in *Journal of Aggression, Maltreatment & Trauma* (The Haworth Maltreatment & Trauma Press, an imprint of The Haworth Press, Inc.) Vol. 10, No. 1/2, 2005; and: *The Trauma of Terrorism: Sharing Knowledge and Shared Care, An International Handbook* (ed: Yael Danieli, Danny Brom, and Joe Sills) The Haworth Maltreatment & Trauma Press, an imprint of The Haworth Press, Inc., 2005.

Human beings must posit some prime assumptions about the world in order to survive and keep at bay "the real dilemma of existence, the one of the mortal animal who at the same time is conscious of his mortality" (Becker, 1973, p. 268). Janoff-Bulman (1992) suggests that people need to believe that the world and those who live in it are essentially benevolent, that there is a meaningful causal relationship between events and the individuals they impact, and that we are good and moral individuals and thereby deserving of positive outcomes. These assumptions are emotionally laden and infuse us with positive feelings.

The events of September 11, 2001 shook Americans to the core. The United States was no longer safe. The vulnerability was new and frightening. Our invincibility was revealed to be a myth. When the Towers fell, the positive feelings turned dark. Americans found themselves helplessly facing an unpredictable world over which they had no control. Almost instantaneously, they were bereft of meaning and saw evil in a way that was new and personal. Their pain was not only physical and emotional, but also spiritual and existential (Danieli, Engdahl, & Schlenger, 2003).

At its core, America is a country of faith. Richard Cox, in his book *The Sacrament of Psychology* (2002), quotes Gomes when he says, "To fail to understand the religious dimension of the American culture is to be unable to read that culture or its nuances in any effective way" (p. 217). This is substantiated by a Gallup review of more than a half-century of polling data which concluded that, "the depth of religious commitment often has more to do with how Americans think and act than do other key background characteristics, such as level of education, age, and political affiliation" (Gallup, 1995, as cited in Shafranske, 2000, p. 525).

In this article, we explore different aspects of spiritual care after a major disaster. The experience of 9/11 has taught us many lessons and some of those are reflected here. Disaster spiritual care services is a new and growing field. No systematic studies are known to us about the effectiveness of spiritual care. The religious community is now aware that the appropriate provision of spiritual care in the context of disaster is a learned skill and not one you can assume to be present in all clergy. The issues raised here form the beginning of a conceptual framework for spiritual care, among other forms of care, after major terrorist attacks.

SPIRITUALITY AND HEALTH

Scientific research is currently validating the proposition that a religious and/or spiritual worldview influences physical and psychological well-being.

Focusing on the trauma of illness, this research points to the efficacy of spiritual care in healing and highlights the importance of responding to religious and spiritual concerns when treating holistically a suffering individual.

Studies indicate that as many as 70% of cancer patients are aware of one or more spiritual needs related to their illness (Fitchett, Burton, & Sivan, 1997; Moadel et al., 1999). They are often distressed and fearful and frequently isolated. Many of them can articulate that they are not only suffering in body, but in spirit as well, and that these two elements are not independent of each other.

In a research project involving nearly 600 older, severely ill medical patients, those who sought a connection with God, as well as support from clergy and faith group members, were less depressed and rated their quality of life as higher, even after taking into account the severity of their illness (Koenig, Pargament, & Nielsen, 1998). Further, it has been shown that spiritual well-being helps people moderate feelings of anxiety (Kaczorowski, 1989), hopelessness (Fehring, Miller, & Shaw, 1997; Mickley, Soeken, & Belcher, 1992), and isolation (Feher & Maly, 1999) that accompany illness. As a consequence of the evidence, attention is increasingly being placed on religious affiliation, beliefs, and practices as clinically relevant variables in physical and mental health (Levin, Larson, & Puchalski, 1997; Sloan, Bagiella, & Powell, 1999).

Although the above studies focussed on illness, they do point to the efficacy of spiritual care in the healing of persons suffering distress and illness. It is thus reasonable to suggest that individuals who found themselves feeling hopeless, traumatized, isolated and confronted by something repulsive, out of control, and vastly larger than themselves as a result of experiencing the attacks on 9/11 were also aware of spiritual needs related to their situation. Able to recognize these needs, they sought a spiritual caregiver for support and comfort.

Looking at help-seeking behavior, Jacobs and Quevillon (2001) and Milstein (2003) both reference a national poll commissioned by the American Red Cross less than one month after September 11. The results show that approximately 60% of all the respondents said they would likely seek help from a spiritual counselor, compared to 45% of all the respondents who would likely seek help from their physician and 40% who would seek help from a mental health care professional.

TRAUMA AND THE SEARCH FOR SPIRITUALITY

Although many people are not affiliated with an "official" organized religious structure, they nevertheless experience themselves as spiritual beings in relationship to something greater than themselves. It was no surprise, therefore, that people turned to God, in whatever form, in the aftermath of the World Trade Center tragedy. Some turned for compassion and solace, some turned with anger and outrage, many turned with soul-wrenching confusion.

Following the attacks, people filled public spaces, setting up memorials in parks and in front of fire stations for community and comfort. Desperate to understand and find meaning in the overwhelming terror, people also filled houses of worship beyond capacity. The trauma had exceeded their ability either to comprehend or absorb it. In the deepest part of themselves, perhaps they understood the transcendent nature of their experience.

The nature of terror, its suddenness and unpredictability and its wrathful betrayal of personhood is a complex experience unique unto itself. In the instance of the 9/11 attacks, the situation was further complicated because the acts were perpetrated "in the name of God." Wilson and Moran (1998) describe the spiritual challenge after severe trauma as follows:

> Traumatic life events impact the body, self-structure, and soul of the survivor. Accordingly . . . overwhelmingly traumatic events adversely affect not only the psychological dimension of the self but also the faith systems and spirituality which give meaning to one's life . . . extreme trauma can devastate the psyche and leave the human personality in ruin. Religious faith and spirituality are integral aspects of personality and essential components of one's identity. Accordingly, the psychological trauma caused by natural disasters, accidental disasters, and those of human origin can leave the spiritual domain in complete disarray. (p. 174)

The literature argues that a loss of faith in the order and continuity of life is central to psychological trauma, and that, at least in part, this crisis of faith results from traumatic events shattering a sense of connection between the individual and the community. The capacity for evil in human nature is made manifest and a necessary sense of meaning, safety and control over one's life is shattered. In her 1992 book, *Trauma and Recovery*, Herman states that traumatic events breach attachments, shatter the self, undermine belief systems, and violate faith in a natural or divine order, which can have an impact on one's spiritual life. Grame, Tortorici, Healey, Dillingham, and Winklebaur (1999) echo this when they quote McBride, who states, "It certainly appears to be characteristic of chronic PTSD patients that a wounded self or soul lies at the very core of their being. As a result, they often have a profound sense of spiritual alienation and emptiness" (p. 226).

On the other hand, as has been found with illness, "Trauma acts to increase spiritual development if that development is defined as an increase in the search for purpose and meaning" (Decker, 1993, p. 35). Having reviewed the trauma literature, Decker concludes that:

> [The literature] has included the citing of spiritual/religious issues as an important aspect of understanding psychological responses in trauma. These issues have often been indicated as major determinants in both the development of, and recovery from, post traumatic stress disorder (PTSD) . . . regardless of the presence or absence of trauma-produced personality deterioration there will be an increase in the search for an expanded and more meaningful perspective of existence (i.e., spiritual development) as a result of a traumatic experience. (p. 37)

CATEGORIES OF SPIRITUAL CARE

In the broadest of terms, it is possible to identify four categories through which spiritual care is manifested. *Religion* is the recognised formal structure, institutionally based, through which people identify themselves and their system of belief. *Religious Care* is the provision of specific ritual and prayer within the context of a unique faith tradition. *Spirituality* is the expression of a person's relationship to that which is greater than him/herself and which gives meaning and purpose to his/her life. It is the core through which people relate to themselves, to the world, and to God. Often, spiritual questions are neither formalized nor faith specific. *Spiritual Care* is the support offered to people in a time of crisis. It assists them in drawing upon their spiritual resources in the midst of their pain. Depending upon the context, it may include religious care. In general, such care respects the broad nature of spiritual response by responding to the human search for meaning in non-faith specific language.

The needs of the individual, and the caregiver's assessment of those needs, will determine the nature of the relationship established by the spiritual caregiver. A woman who believes she killed her father because she had left the church has different needs than a young man grieving his brother's violent death. A fire fighter who is trying to maintain his faith (which he says is the only thing that keeps him going) while he extracts body part after body part from the rubble has different needs than the 19-year-old Americorps volunteer who, after many days of hearing stories from the survivors who dodged bodies falling from the sky as they fled the disaster site, no longer feels anything and is worried that she is losing her soul.

CLERGY IN DISASTER RESPONSE

In the United States, the provision of spiritual care in the context of disaster formally began as a result of the Aviation Disaster Family Assistance Act of 1996. The Act created a national spiritual care disaster response team deployable in the event of aviation disasters. Team members were professional chaplains, responsible for organizing and administering the protocol by which community clergy could deliver direct care most effectively. Importantly, the dialogues resulting from the development of the team and its mission led to the creation of standards establishing the guidelines for best practices. Training materials, a code of ethical conduct, a providers' agreement assuring accountability, and a certification process grew out of the process.

Well over 900 community clergy presented themselves to the Spiritual Care Aviation Incident Response Team of the American Red Cross in the weeks immediately following 9/11. They were spontaneous volunteers seeking official endorsement to serve at such designated sites as Ground Zero, the respite centers established for rescue and recovery workers, the shelters, the family assistance centers, and the morgues. Professional chaplains associated with hospitals served heavily in the early days of the disaster and then were recalled to their institutions.

Approximately one quarter of these individuals came from areas outside of the New York City tri-state region and went home soon after. Since they had no local congregational or institutional responsibilities, they could work intensely at the sites but were able to "leave it behind" when they finished for the day. The majority of clergy, however, lived and worked in the areas directly affected by the terrorist attacks and were both personally and professionally immersed in the aftermath of the events.

Clergy found themselves in many roles. They ministered within their congregations and, as identified members of the local community leadership, were looked to for support and comfort by their larger community. Some found themselves performing funeral after funeral. Many also volunteered at disaster sites. They worked amidst the sights and smells of the attacks and then returned home to minister to their faithful. They suffered trauma many times over.

Clergy also served as fire and police chaplains. Given the extraordinary losses suffered by these groups, the toll on their spiritual leadership was enormous. Other clergy, who serve primarily in religious institutions or agencies, frequently acted as spokespersons to the broader community as society looked to them for guidance, comfort, support and meaning. Many of them also volunteered at the sites.

During the course of the disaster response, certain things became clear. It was assumed, for example, that individuals who already had clinical pastoral education training and experience could do the work more effectively than those who did not have this training. Reality showed, however, that previous chaplaincy and/or mental health training did not necessarily make one an appropriate disaster chaplain. Although there are similarities, spiritual care in the context of disaster is different than spiritual care in a hospital or institutional setting. Consequently, a different skill set is required. All spiritual leaders functioning during a disaster, in whatever capacity, need fundamental knowledge to help them in their work with affected individuals and communities.

THE TRAINING OF CLERGY

Many clergy feel inadequate when responding to trauma and grief. They have not been trained to recognize the physical, cognitive, psychological, behavioral, and spiritual responses to each or to understand their nuances and implications. Further, they are often not aware of the impact of trauma and grief on special populations such as children, adolescents, the frail elderly and the disabled. Educators must begin with the basics. There is a need for continuing education in such basic areas as listening skills, the difference between care and counseling, supportive care, helping and coping strategies, spiritual care interventions, and appropriate referral.

In addition, the clergy will have to deal with questions, such as: What is disaster and what is terrorism? How do they manifest? How are they similar and dissimilar? In broad strokes, how might each impact an individual, a family, a community, and a country? For many, the idea of "public trauma" is a new one.

Defining a traumatic event is only the first step. Although the exercise of definition creates a common language, it must also articulate the lifecycle of various traumatic events so that clergy responders can identify what they are witnessing and place it into a context that will help them determine appropriate interventions. Clergy must learn to recognize what can be expected of an individual and a community in the short-term, mid-term and long-term rescue, recovery, relief and healing processes. What are the goals of care immediately following a disaster and what are the post-disaster goals?

Once clergy can anticipate and identify normal reactions to an abnormal situation and can normalize these reactions for others, they will need to develop the skill to demarcate these reactions from those defining extreme, complicated and unresolved grief and mourning. How can one know if a stress/grief/trauma reaction is becoming a mental illness? For example, what is post traumatic stress disorder and its warning signs?

Additional topics to be covered in the training of clergy:

- The experience of working in a chaotic trauma environment
- Disaster response mapping: What are the *local* disaster response agencies and their roles?
- How do the roles of the local response agencies change in the event of a national disaster?
- The culture of national disaster response teams and agencies
- Ritual, prayer, funerals, memorials, sacred space and faith as community support
- Referral as an art, not a failure
- Knowledge of various agents and materials that may be used by terrorists and their implications for clergy response
- Finding, using and sharing religious resources
- Compassion fatigue, secondary traumatization and burnout: How to avoid them
- And last, but not least: Flexibility, flexibility, flexibility

The following are also recommended as part of the overall training:

- Disaster simulations
- Ambulance "ride-alongs"
- Acquaintance with rescue and recovery workers
- Functioning in a designated "crime scene"
- Death notifications and body identification
- Functioning as part of an interdisciplinary team

CARE FOR THE CLERGY AFTER DISASTER

Clergy tend to be "lone rangers," working independently within their own community of faith. The events of 9/11 demonstrated the need for disciplined networking. What should this networking include? Community spiritual leaders need to have a better sense of who their colleagues are and need to build trusting relationships with them.

- Learn who your colleagues are in all faith traditions and establish relationships
- Create a support system for yourself
- Create a comprehensive referral network

- Create relationships with the fire and police departments and other emergency responders that serve your local community
- With your colleagues, plan for immediate, short-term, mid-term and long-term responses
- Be aware of the demographics of your community
- Pool resources

Clergy, themselves victims of 9/11, were faced with a multitude of difficult questions and concerns reflecting both faith and praxis. Some seemed to be direct questions concerning appropriate ritual and practice, such as burial of a body part versus a whole body, or how to determine when the mourning period starts. Other questions appeared to reflect primarily existential and spiritual despair–a tear in the person's very fabric of meaning. These questions don't ask, "How can I cope?" They ask, "How could God have allowed this?" "How can I believe and in what?" "Who am I?" "Why am I here and alive?" Words are limiting. Symbol, ritual, prayer and presence are frequently the only ways to respond to transcendent questions such as these. Even when nothing else is stable, ritual, religious nuance and spiritual longing are. Rituals are also familiar and can remind an individual of other difficult times in which they were helped to cope and survive. They can foster a sense of continuity between the past, distant or recent, and the present and in this way facilitate a more hopeful outlook on the future. Since the language clergy use is one of symbol, they can point to a place beyond the ugliness they confront.

CHALLENGES OF DISASTER SPIRITUAL CARE

Disaster ministry differs from congregational ministry in very specific ways, and "formal" clergy disaster responders are required to learn the differences. A clergy person working in a faith-specific environment is expected to preach, to answer questions and to articulate their own faith perspective and response. As a disaster responder, the clergy person functions as a spiritual support and comforter for a broad number of individuals representing many faith traditions and cultures. The clergy person becomes a chaplain and should not expect to give answers or to preach. They are also not to bear witness to their own specific faith tradition or to proselytize for it. Rather, they are to function on the level of global spiritual concerns rather than specific religious concerns. If faith-specific questions are raised, then the chaplain is expected to seek out an appropriate spiritual care responder. Cross-cultural knowledge is also important. To be most effective, a chaplain should have a working knowledge of the cultural, ethnic and religious diversity of the impacted community.

An ability to be supervised and to function appropriately in a multifaith environment is an essential requirement for anyone wishing to function as a disaster chaplain. Accountability is key.

Complications about jurisdiction and access to disaster sites after 9/11 occasionally arose because the terms "clergy" and "chaplain" were often confused and used interchangeably by rescue, recovery, and relief officials and workers. In brief, a chaplain is a clergy (or lay) person who is officially attached to an institution such as a branch of the military, fire or police departments, a hospital, a prison, or a governmental agency such as a court. Most clergy are not chaplains, and most individuals generally identified as chaplains are not clinically trained or professionally certified. For our purposes, any individual who was given a badge by an agency such as the American Red Cross or the Office of Emergency Management was automatically given the title "chaplain" while they worked at a disaster related site. This was the only time that they carried this designation. To become a certified, professional chaplain, an individual must have had at least 1600 hours of supervised clinical work. Certified chaplains are specifically trained in the provision of non-sectarian, multifaith, spiritual care.

CONCLUSION

The world community was impacted by the traumatic events of September 11, 2001. An affected person can experience pain and obtain relief in many ways. Physical reactions necessitate medical intervention, and psychological responses require the assistance of a mental health professional. However, either in isolation or in conjunction with the above, there is almost always a spiritual response that requires the help of a trained spiritual care provider.

America is a country of faith, and it responded as such. For many, spiritual suffering defined, at least in part, their experience of the trauma resulting from the horrific events of 9/11. They turned to spiritual care providers in rage and frustration as well as for help. Houses of worship filled, and massive numbers of fundamental and profound questions of meaning came to the forefront. Clergy, themselves victims, were faced with the need to respond. The vast majority ministered with wisdom and compassion; they consoled and they comforted. Some were inappropriate and exacerbated the suffering of the bereaved and the traumatized.

Spiritual caregivers ministered within their own communities and congregations, and/or worked at actual disaster sites. Whether they served their own faith tradition or provided non-sectarian spiritual care to those who required it, even if the person in need was from a different faith tradition or no faith tradition, fundamental training to become effective caregivers in the context of disaster was necessary. This was also true for those who were already certified chaplains or had other mental health training.

Leaders in the field of disaster spiritual care are currently determining "best practices" and have developed standards for certification and training modules to assure appropriate care giving. Acknowledging the existence of a deeply rooted spiritual component in the life of persons, and its importance in the healing of traumatized individuals, clinicians in the field of mental health are asking questions about trauma and its impact on this fundamental aspect of personality. As a result, collaboration between the two disciplines of disaster mental health and disaster spiritual care is moving toward the provision of holistic care for the suffering individual. Such collaboration is reflected in the networking that many communities are undertaking in order to assure preparedness in the event of other catastrophic occurrences.

Ideally, clergy can become integrated into local, state, and federal disaster response protocols. A clear working relationship between the clergy and members of these organizations can be developed so that the first time they meet is not in the middle of a major disaster. Such proactive organizing is valuable for the community on many levels, not the least of which is the confidence born out of a shared sense of preparedness.

REFERENCES

Becker, E. (1973). *The denial of death*. New York: The Free Press.

Cox, R. (2002). *The sacrament of psychology*. Springfield, MO: INSYNC Press.

Danieli, Y., Engdahl, B., & Schlenger, W. E. (2003). The psychosocial aftermath of terrorism. In F. Moghaddam, A. J. Marsella, & A. J. Bandura (Eds.), *Terrorism: Psychosocial perspectives* (pp. 223-246). Washington, DC: American Psychological Association.

Decker, L. (1993). The role of trauma in spiritual development. *Journal of Humanistic Psychology, 33*(4), 33-46.

Feher, S., & Maly, C. (1999). Coping with breast cancer in later life: The role of religious faith. *Psycho-Oncology, 8*(5), 408-416.

Fehring, R., Miller, J., & Shaw, C. (1997). Spiritual well-being, religiosity, hope, depression, and other mood states in elderly people coping with cancer. *Oncology Nursing Forum, 24*(4), 663-671.

Fitchett, G., Burton, L., & Sivan, A. B. (1997). The religious needs and resources of psychiatric in-patients. *Journal of Nervous and Mental Disease, 185*(5), 320-326.

Grame, C., Tortorici, J., Healey, B., Dillingham, J., & Winklebaur, P. (1999). Addressing spiritual and religious issues of clients with a history of psychological trauma. *Bulletin of the Menninger Clinic, 6*(2), 223-239.

Herman, J. (1992). *Trauma and recovery: The aftermath of violence–From domestic abuse to political terror.* New York: Basic Books.

Jacobs, G., & Quevillon, R. (2001, November). *Spiritual care and disaster mental health.* Paper presented at an American Red Cross Disaster Mental Health conference entitled, The Ripple Effect from Ground Zero: Coping with Mental Health Needs in Time of Tragedy and Terror, New York, NY.

Janoff-Bulman, R. (1992). *Shattered assumptions: Towards a new psychology of trauma.* New York: The Free Press.

Kaczorowski, J. (1989). Spiritual well-being and anxiety in adults diagnosed with cancer. *The Hospice Journal, 5*(3-4), 105-116.

Koenig, H., Pargament, K., & Nielsen, J. (1998). Religious coping and health status in medically ill hospitalized older adults. *Journal of Nervous and Mental Disease, 186*(9), 513-521.

Levin, J., Larson, D., & Puchalski, C. (1997). Religion and spirituality in medicine: Research and education. *Journal of the American Medical Association, 278*, 792-793.

Mickley, J., Soeken, K., & Belcher, A. (1992). Spiritual well-being, religiousness and hope among women with breast cancer. *Journal of Nursing Scholarship, 24*(4), 267-272.

Milstein, G. (2003). Clergy and psychiatrists: Opportunities for expert dialogue. *Psychiatric Times, 20*(3), 36-39.

Moadel, A., Morgan, C., Fatone, A., Grennan, J., Carter, J., Laruffa, G. et al. (1999). Seeking meaning and hope: Self-reported spiritual and existential needs among an ethnically diverse cancer patient population. *Psycho-Oncology, 8*(5), 378-385.

Shafranske, E. (2000). Religious involvement and professional practices of psychiatrists and other mental health professionals. *Psychiatric Annals, 30*(8), 525-532.

Sloan, R., Bagiella, E., & Powell, T. (1999). Religion, spirituality, and medicine. *Lancet, 353*, 664-667.

Wilson, J., & Moran, T. (1998). Psychological trauma: Posttraumatic stress disorder and spirituality. *Journal of Psychology and Theology, 26*(2), 168-178.

Responding to Terrorism in the USA: Firefighters Share Experiences in Their Own Words

John K. Schorr
Angela S. Boudreaux

SUMMARY. In this article, career firefighters from Oklahoma City, New York City, and Arlington County, VA, and volunteer firefighters from Pennsylvania, share their on-site experiences and the emotional aftermath of responding to terrorism. The authors acted as facilitators, compilers, and organizers so that major themes firefighters have raised are presented to inform the work of first responders and others seeking to understand the experiences of firefighters during and after terrorist incidents. The authors conclude by presenting survey data indicating high levels of firefighter job satisfaction and the major sources of emotional support they use following exposure to terrorism.

Address correspondence to: John K. Schorr, PhD, Department of Sociology, Stetson University, 421 North Woodland Boulevard, Unit 8263, DeLand, FL 32723 USA (E-mail: jschorr@stetson.edu).

This research is supported under award number MIPT 106-113-2000-020 from the Oklahoma City National Memorial Institute for the Prevention of Terrorism and the Office for Domestic Preparedness, U.S. Department of Homeland Security. Points of view are those of the authors and do not necessarily represent the official position of MIPT or the U.S. Department of Homeland Security.

[Haworth co-indexing entry note]: "Responding to Terrorism in the USA: Firefighters Share Experiences in Their Own Words." Schorr, John K., and Angela S. Boudreaux. Co-published simultaneously in *Journal of Aggression, Maltreatment & Trauma* (The Haworth Maltreatment & Trauma Press, an imprint of The Haworth Press, Inc.) Vol. 10, No. 1/2, 2005; and: *The Trauma of Terrorism: Sharing Knowledge and Shared Care, An International Handbook* (ed: Yael Danieli, Danny Brom, and Joe Sills) The Haworth Maltreatment & Trauma Press, an imprint of The Haworth Press, Inc., 2005.

KEYWORDS. Firefighters, first responders, emergency services, disasters, terrorism, trauma

This article does not present a standard academic treatment of the reactions of first responders to terrorism. Instead, career firefighters from Oklahoma City, New York City, and Arlington County, VA, and volunteer firefighters from Shanksville and Somerset County, PA, share in their own words their on-site experiences and the emotional aftermath of responding to terrorism. The authors have acted as facilitators, compilers, and organizers so that major themes raised by the firefighters can be presented to inform the work of first responders everywhere, as well as scientists and others seeking to understand the experiences of firefighters during and after terrorist incidents.

OVERVIEW OF RESEARCH AND POPULATIONS STUDIED

Our work with first responders began in 1996, one year after the Alfred P. Murrah Federal Building bombing in Oklahoma City. We surveyed, via a questionnaire delivered to fire houses, Oklahoma City Fire Department (OCFD) uniformed personnel who participated in the search, rescue, and recovery (Boudreaux & Schorr, 1996). We received responses from approximately 40% ($N = 325$). We followed the OCFD until 2000, surveying personnel in 1998 and again in 2000 (Schorr & Boudreaux, 2000), with a 38% response rate ($N = 309$) in 2000. In 2000, we revised the open-ended response questions to query firefighters about the insights and advice they would share with other firefighters. This article includes OCFD responses from 1996 and 2000.

Following the September 11, 2001 terrorist attacks, we surveyed fire service personnel who responded at the three sites. Arlington County Fire Department (ACFD) members, who responded to the Pentagon attack in Arlington County, VA, were surveyed in summer 2002 (Schorr & Boudreaux, 2002a), with an 82% response rate ($N = 232$). Shanksville, PA, Volunteer Fire Company (SVFC) and Somerset County, PA, Volunteer Fire Department (SVFD) members, who responded to the United Airlines Flight 93 crash in Shanksville, PA, were surveyed in Fall/Winter 2002 (Schorr & Boudreaux, 2002b), resulting in a combined 68% response rate ($N = 37$). Finally, mail surveys of Fire Department of New York (FDNY) retired firefighters and active fire officers began in summer 2003. The study is ongoing, with approximately 300 responses received by January 2004.

DATA COLLECTION AND MANAGEMENT

The questionnaires used with all fire service groups consisted of many closed-ended and a few open-ended questions. This article is based primarily on responses to the open-ended questions that were first transcribed and then organized by group and theme. The open-ended responses reported here are not representative of all members of the fire departments studied, since not all firefighter respondents completed the open-ended questions. However, having a representative sample of open-ended comments from which we could generalize to populations of firefighters was not our intention. We learned early in our 1996 study that many firefighters had important information to share with other firefighters who might someday respond to terrorism. We recognized that, not being firefighters ourselves, there was little chance that we could design closed-ended questions that would encompass the range of responses firefighters would want to give. Therefore, we simply facilitated the process by asking broad questions that encouraged firefighters to express the insights they thought were most important.

FINDINGS

This article introduces three overarching themes, and then turns to firefighters' comments that illustrate descriptions of the event, its emotional aftermath, and the job (i.e., what it means and why they do it). The article concludes with a presentation of survey results on the subject of job satisfaction and sources of emotional support among firefighters (see Table 1). When necessary, identifying information was omitted to protect the confidentiality of respondents. It is important to note that, outside of the line-of-duty deaths experienced by the FDNY, the themes and sub-themes that emerged from the groups were similar. Given the large differences in the environment and actual work at each of the terrorist attack sites, this may be surprising. As we reflected on this similarity in spite of the diversity of on-site exposure, we realized the importance of the message these firefighters have for others who will face terrorist attacks in the future. A shared philosophy and approach to these types of events is evident. The results show similar levels of job satisfaction and similar sources for emotional support for all groups. Researchers and mental health professionals may find these accounts useful as they try to understand how other emergency services populations may respond to future terrorist events and how best to serve their needs.

We now present each of the overarching themes mentioned above, followed by firefighters' responses illustrative of each.

THE EVENT

OCFD

As a firefighter I knew I would see the worst of certain situations, but this was the absolute worst. I cut people apart to extricate them. I gathered body parts when there was no body around it. The smell was terrible, but we got used to it. You could smell it 2 blocks away! I personally found 2 bodies, 1 male and 1 female. The male victim had to be dismembered to get him out. The female wasn't so bad. It has affected me to a point, but I don't really know how. It just kind of comes up in my mind at least once a day. If you want to talk further please call. . . .

I had a high feeling, and a low feeling. *Low feeling*, after I had worked (at bombing) all day the first day, and they said we were going to look and dig where the children were supposed to be. *High feeling* as we walked past the people standing outside the fence and [were] going to try and walk through the crowd, they just parted the crowd and made us a path to exit and as we walked through they cheered and applauded. I still feel very strange going into the buildings downtown.

First, I was in unbelief when we arrived on scene. Later that day . . . I was chomping at the bit to go back in. The next day when I was home and saw TV, reality set in and I was sad and blue. The 3rd day I was eager to work. The 4th day I was tired. The 5th day I was cold and it was raining and windy. I was mad that I had to work logistics and didn't get to work on the rock pile. The 6, 7, 8, and 9th day I was supposed to be off but I went back and volunteered the 7th day and finally got to dig on the rock pile. I felt great. I took off the 8th and 9th days and was grateful for family and friends. The 10, 12, and 14th days, I was awestruck by the outpouring of love and support from the kids all over the world and from the volunteers from our community, state, and nation. It was overwhelming . . . command, logistics, and rescue . . . were all important and satisfying. I was fortunate to . . . help rescue and care for a lady who lived, and later to visit her.

TABLE 1. Job Satisfaction by Fire Department

	Percentage			
	OCFD 1996 (1 year post incident)	OCFD 2000 (5 years post incident)	ACFD 2003 (1 year post incident)	SVFC/ SVFD 2003 (1 year post incident)
Current overall job satisfaction				
Very high	31	38	21	27
High	44	37	29	41
Moderate	20	21	32	32
Low	5	4	12	0
Very low	1	0	7	0
Change in job satisfaction since incident				
Very positive	5	5	5	19
Positive	22	20	17	41
No change	59	52	45	32
Negative	12	20	23	8
Very negative	2	4	10	0

FDNY

On the morning of 9/11, it started out like any other day. I went to work early that day, most of our guys were in the firehouse. They were going to Pennsylvania to play golf. As they were getting ready to leave, I was taking the new probie [probationary firefighter assigned to a firehouse] around the rig, explaining to him his duties. Then someone yelled a plane hit the WTC. We changed the channel on the T.V. in the kitchen and we all watched. Minutes later the phone rang. It was my daughter, she worked a block away from the WTC when the plane hit. She said, "Daddy what should I do?" I remember telling her that this is no accident, and she should leave her office and start uptown to my son-in-law's office, which she did with the other girls in her office.

Meanwhile everyone in the firehouse was glued to the T.V. . . . That's when the second plane hit. Most of the off duty guys went upstairs and changed knowing it was going to be a long day. At about 9:15 the engine was sent to Manhattan. We didn't see them until the next day. In the next hour, we prepared for the worst. As being the senior man, I had to think like a Lt., I was the chauffeur, with over 20 years in the FD. I had a covering Johnnie Lt., a probie, his first day, a detail from the engine, and two somewhat senior men. And one of them was worried about his brother-in-law who worked at WTC (later found out his brother-in-law was lost.) By 10:30, we were ready to go, we watched the first tower fall, knowing how we operate, we all knew that we just lost a lot of guys. The troops were going to Shea [stadium], as soon as they came in, but we just sat watching.

Then the second tower fell, and we were still waiting to go somewhere. But as all the other companies around us were leaving, we kind of knew we had to stay and protect the rest of the city. Around 5 p.m., the vollies [firefighters from volunteer fire companies] were coming to firehouses, that proved to be another problem. No communications, they could hook up to a hydrant but not the tower ladder. We told them if we get anything that they would fight it from the outside. We were the only ones to go inside. As it was getting near midnight, everyone was still on pins and needles listening to reports and getting secondhand information. I think not knowing has to be the worst.

Around 1 a.m., we got assigned to cover Ladder ##, luckily I had worked downtown because when we got to Canal St., there were no streetlights. It was all dark. We got to Ladder ##, # engine, that's when we found out about their loss. We weren't long before we started taking in calls. We ran all night long all over lower Manhattan. The sun came up and we returned to ladder ##, as we pulled up in front of quarters that's when we saw the wives with their children looking for their husbands. And nobody there to help them. We're just firefighters, what training did we have to handle this situation? None. . . . Around noon we were put back in the system and started to do runs in lower Manhattan. On one run down Broadway we found the wheel of one of the planes.

By mid-afternoon, more wives were outside and still no help for them or the house. . . . We returned home, only to come back the next day. This is my story of what happened to me on that day. One, help should be sent immediately. Trained personnel. Two, supervisors should use their senior personnel no matter what rank. That day, I was a father, counselor, priest, a big brother.

THE EMOTIONAL AFTERMATH

OCFD

Felt horrible about the loss of a friend and of being part of the recovery team who dug her out 10 days into incident, not being able to tell her family we had found her for three days till they were notified. Felt bad that I felt good. Had a sense of direction and purpose after being in clinical depression after a very painful divorce.

I still have dreams about once a week of that morning. Of the first body I saw which was burning and decapitated. Not knowing if I knew anyone who worked there finding out later that my high school coach [and two friends were] . . . now working there and [were] killed.

I wasn't sure how it affected me at first. We were one of the initial response crews. It didn't bother me at all during the first response. I've seen just about all of that before. It's just that when I tried to tell people that are close to me about it, I would break down. I thought that had all gone until this anniversary came along. It has brought up some feelings again but I'm sure they will pass. I do have a restlessness about me now that I don't know is good or bad.

It becomes more difficult to remember what "normal" is or was. The stress and exposure that the bombing subjected us to was of a nature that transforms the sense of normal. After I understood this. . . . Clearly, then I can start to reconstitute my life around a new sense of what is "normal." Our department . . . [has] undergo[ne] a profound change. The old means of daily operation is tainted by comparing it with what occurred during the incident. An intensity of emotion is quietly lurking beneath a lot of routine. We who must administrate are challenged with condensing fact from the vapor of nuance in our charges. . . . I implore you to study us, analyze us, and evaluate us. However, it is a moral imperative for you to HELP US!

. . . How Murrah incident affected me: I was one of the first OCFD units on the scene and entered the structure with another co-worker. I spent the next 16 days and over 250 hours at the site. I have spent the last year working with written reports of this incident. I have felt attached to the incident, as if I had some form of 'ownership' in it. I still have dreams about the incident or related events. I have been unable to physically, mentally or emotionally close it [but] I am ready to do so. . . . Now alone, I have more time to think about things. Tears come easier . . . now than ever before. Feelings of sadness and grief constantly pervade my thoughts. I am angry at the criminal justice system and the criminals who carried out this act of terrorism. But I am proud of our City, State and Nation, and the way we pulled together to meet the challenge of this incident. The Murrah incident has basically been my life for the past year. I have lost those most dear to me, at least it appears so at this point. I feel lost and don't believe I really have any reason to hang around much longer, but know I must. This probably doesn't help your survey, but it helps me a bit. Good luck. I look forward to seeing your results.

SVFC and SVFD

Be prepared for anything. Big things can happen in small places. Take what's thrown at you and do your best. Share your feelings with others. Do not keep things in. Use your fellow firefighters and any counselors necessary if any problems arise. Firefighters are a true brotherhood, use it.

To never say it can't happen here! Never underestimate yourself or other volunteers or even your friends and neighbors, as to what you or they can and will do, when needed. God bless the heroes of Flight 93 and God Bless America. . . .

ACFD

I learned if you have trouble don't be afraid to talk about it because talking to co-workers, friends, and families will make things a lot better.

EAP [Employee Assistance Program] services need to be provided for those seeking help [in all fire departments]. . . . Use case studies to show how they helped the members of the departments.

I appreciate the availability of EAP/counselors to assist me/co-workers with any problems. I don't think my perspective toward life, the universe, and everything has changed. I understand that there are things I cannot change or prevent, no matter what I do.

There is a high level of stress and exhilaration during and right after the incident if it went well. There is a feeling of fatigue and despair if it didn't go well. We need to be prepared to care for our employees right away and for the long term. Spouse/significant others and children need info about what to expect and how to get help early.

I have learned some of the effects that a traumatic incident can have on a person's mental health and well-being. I have seen the effects on personal friends and co-workers who worked at the Pentagon. For the longest time, I always felt that all my co-workers were tough and invincible. I soon learned that we are all just human. We have feelings and emotions. We all have individual reactions to life in stressful situations.

FDNY

I have had a hard time dealing with the grief and guilt when of the 16 personnel and 42 all told, that I forget to remember all of them in my thoughts. Missing them so much that when thoughts of one brother led to thoughts of another and another, you stop and force yourself to think of anything else. . . . Later I feel guilty that I on purpose denied my grief for all of them. I will never forget them and how lucky I was to work with such fine men. I try each day to recall those other than those in my mind the day before. It hurts to think that they might feel forgotten. This sorrow will be a daily part of life until I die. For me a couple a day is easier to grieve than for all each day. It just became too much.

The Dept. was woefully lacking in ability to handle a tragedy of the magnitude of the WTC. I don't blame the Dept. because no one could foresee the enormity that was/is the WTC. I recommend that each and every member treat mental health as they should physical health–that is something to be worked on a regular basis–diet/exercise, etc., relationships, hobbies, interests, etc.

We think of ourselves as "macho men" and we are, but during difficult times all members of the FD should have counseling. As a retired Batt. Chief with 35 years of service, I should have taken advantage of counseling to help me cope with my feelings. I'm sure many recent retired members feel the same way.

I think it would be helpful if counseling service personnel would contact members and families at home during their off duty time and offered services on a regular basis. There are times when you feel you do not need it, but the week or months later you feel like you do.

We should encourage each other to take advantage of counseling services sooner, rather than later.

I also believe that we can depend on each other for assistance, but not the FDNY administration, which still has not realized that they have virtually ignored us for six years.

When we were attacked, I had 28 years on the job. In those years I saw a great deal but I was greatly affected by what happened. However, most or many of the others there were young and could not cope as well. What is needed is immediate counseling, whether it is professionally done or having a senior man or staff officer talk to the men.

I worked too hard at the site and at the landfill and gave myself two minor heart attacks. At the time I thought working hard as I can would make me feel better. Instead it nearly killed me.

Guilt feelings of survival (fate of being on/off duty) will accompany the aftermath of any similar catastrophe for some time to come. It will recede with time, but will linger for some time thereafter. Also have developed more acute sensitivity to behavioral changes of FD coworkers in the aftermath of such an extraordinary event.

The mourning process takes time. 9/11 seems like it happened a long time ago. I think we will survive.

To compartmentalize my 9/11 experience (because most people wouldn't understand) and try to limit its effect on the future.

Since 9/11, I am not the same person mentally and never will be! The experience has ruined my family life and shattered my reason for living!

Do not hesitate to reach out for help. Some of the problems you had before an experience like WTC will escalate and become worse. Try and take advantage of all the help that is offered to you. Giving things time to work themselves out is not the answer. Get help ASAP. Not only has WTC had an impact on my life it had a severe impact on my family's life. Have barely spent quality time with my family in one year between the funerals, memorials, fund raising, and having to steadily work on the side just to make ends meet because of our horrible wages. There should be more family weekend packages offered. . . .

Since I was trapped/caught inside the Marriott on 9/11, I've had "PTSD." I thought the FDNY did what should have been done. They got me a personal psychologist and psychiatrist. But this is because I came forward. What about the others? Are they hiding their emotions and going to blow up soon? Just keep giving counseling to members and try and look for any kind of alcohol or drug abuse. I've been seeing my doctors since 11/01 and am just starting to see an improvement. Keep asking people if they have any kind of problems because of 9/11.

THE JOB:
REFLECTIONS FROM OKLAHOMA CITY FIREFIGHTERS
FIVE YEARS POST-EVENT

Terrorism and natural disasters are going to be part of our world. We didn't cause the destruction but quite possibly, we can mitigate some of the harm by helping those who survive the initial incident.

Firefighting is not for everyone. This is a tough job emotionally and physically. Testing should be geared toward those issues. Leave problems at work, before you enter your home leave anger outside. Take time to talk to your wife and give support to your children. Control anger by remembering who you are mad at.

Although it was a tragic incident, I do not feel that my life or career should be defined by this incident. I have good memories of our response, teamwork, dedication, etc., that seem to overcome any negative images of this tragedy. My only regret concerning either incident is that I wasn't more involved or able to give more of myself to assist in the operation.

We are professionals with a specific job to do. When we are called to a scene, we are called to react to a situation that has already occurred and nothing we can do can change what has already happened. Just pick up the pieces and be sure you do the best job you possibly can for the people you serve.

As shown in Table 1, in spite of the horror of the events described above and the sometimes difficult emotional aftermath, over 80% of each group reported at least moderate levels of job satisfaction, with 75% of Oklahoma City firefighters (one year and five years after the bombing), 68% of the Shanksville/Somerset volunteers, and 50% of the Arlington County firefighters reporting "high" or "very high" levels of job satisfaction. Changes in job satisfaction since each of the incidents was reported to be predominantly positive among Oklahoma City firefighters (both one year and five years after the bombing) and by the Shanksville/Somerset volunteers. Arlington firefighters reported more negative than positive change (33% and 22%, respectively). Our open-ended and closed-ended survey items have suggested to us that firefighters responding to terrorism will be quite resilient. Their philosophy toward their work and their desire to help others probably play an important role in this resilience, but so too might the sources they turn to for emotional support. When asked to indicate the degree to which they received emotional support from a list of possible sources, including co-workers, friends, spouse or significant other, parents and other family, administrators/management, immediate supervisor, community, mental health counselors (EAP for Arlington), religious faith, and the CISD/CISM (Critical Incident Stress Debriefing or Management) team, very similar results were reported. Over 50% of the respondents in all of the groups reported that their spouses/significant others, other family members, and religious faith gave them a "high" or "very high" degree of emotional support. Over 50% of the firefighters in Oklahoma City one year after the bombing reported that their community provided them a "high" or "very high" degree of emotional support. Nearly 60% of

Arlington firefighters found their Employee Assistance Program (EAP) to be a source of a "high" or "very high" degree of emotional support.

CONCLUSIONS

This article allowed the voices of firefighters to be heard in their own words as they describe the work they do and their reactions to responding to terrorism in order to give the reader some insight into the way fire service personnel see their work. The events the firefighters responded to were horrible and their communities suffered great losses. It is thus very encouraging that firefighter job satisfaction remains high one year and, in the case of Oklahoma City, five years after the terrorist incident. The resilient philosophy and orientation of firefighters toward their work is clearly exemplified in their comments. That many also welcome the support of their spouses, family, and faith is illustrated by the comments and the quantitative results of our research. Other important sources of emotional support in at least one of the communities were the sense of community support for firefighters in Oklahoma City and a responsive, prepared team of mental health professionals (the EAP) in Arlington.

The reader should come away with heightened respect for first responders everywhere and their service to their communities. Those charged with administering first responder programs should recognize the resilience of their firefighters, yet at the same time, acknowledge the importance of emotional support sources for building and maintaining that resilience. Emergency services policy makers should make efforts to reinforce and strengthen these sources before a terrorist incident occurs in their community. More effective family programs in fire departments would be a start, as well as more recognition for the role that religion and/or faith plays, perhaps through a volunteer or official chaplain's office. The very high rating of perceived emotional support given by Arlington County firefighters to the county EAP indicates that mental health professionals may also be very useful in helping firefighters after their exposure to terrorism. Effective models for gaining the trust of first responders before an incident and providing behavioral health support during and after an incident should be researched and, where appropriate, emulated.

REFERENCES

Boudreaux, A. S., & Schorr, J. K. (1996). [Oklahoma City firefighter survey]. Unpublished raw data.

Schorr, J. K., & Boudreaux, A. S. (2000). [Oklahoma City firefighter survey follow-up]. Unpublished raw data.

Schorr, J. K., & Boudreaux, A. S. (2002a). [Arlington County firefighter survey]. Unpublished raw data.

Schorr, J. K., & Boudreaux, A. S. (2002b). [Shanksville and Somerset, PA. Volunteer firefighter survey]. Unpublished raw data.

Guide:
Caring for Public Servants

Dodie Gill

When a community develops an infrastructure, it is critical that it includes measures to care for its public servants separately and distinctly from its responses to citizen needs. Public servants are those who are expected to respond to a community's needs during a critical incident. For example, a community's first line of defense during a terrorist attack is its public safety employees. While most people are fleeing danger, public safety employees are rushing in to secure a scene, providing medical assistance, fighting fire, and/or rescuing victims. It is most often a closed culture where people "take care of their own." Outsiders are generally not welcome or they must work hard to earn the trust of these dedicated employees.

To provide services to public safety employees following a critical incident, the work must begin long before the incident occurs. Internal Employee Assistance Programs (EAPs) are uniquely positioned inside work organizations to learn the culture of these employees and earn their trust. When the terrorists attacked the Pentagon on September 11, 2001, the Arlington EAP was in place, was known throughout the County workforce and was able to respond immediately to the needs of the public employees.

Prior to 9/11, the Arlington EAP had been in existence for a number of years. The EAP had set, and was achieving, goals to increase the visibility of

Address correspondence to: Dodie Gill, LPC, LSATP, CEAP (E-mail: dgill@ arlington.k12.va.us).

[Haworth co-indexing entry note]: "Guide: Caring for Public Servants." Gill, Dodie. Co-published simultaneously in *Journal of Aggression, Maltreatment & Trauma* (The Haworth Maltreatment & Trauma Press, an imprint of The Haworth Press, Inc.) Vol. 10, No. 1/2, 2005; and: *The Trauma of Terrorism: Sharing Knowledge and Shared Care, An International Handbook* (ed: Yael Danieli, Danny Brom, and Joe Sills) The Haworth Maltreatment & Trauma Press, an imprint of The Haworth Press, Inc., 2005.

the program and offer services to all public employees. Regarding the public safety employees, the EAP staff participated regularly in relationship building activities, such as station visits, ride-alongs, and live burns (i.e., drills for firefighters under controlled circumstances). Additionally, the staff attended medic classes to understand how their training was structured and to learn about the stress of being a medic. Within one year prior to 9/11, four hours of mandatory training was given to all firefighters and medics regarding stress, PTSD, substance abuse and the EAP. This effort was a way to "immunize" these employees against potential critical incidents. Not only did these activities assist the EAP staff in learning about the culture, but they also enabled public safety employees to build relationships with EAP staff and learn about the services the EAP offered. All of these efforts greatly enhanced the EAP's ability to provide services during and after the attack on 9/11.

Within an hour of the plane hitting the Pentagon, since traffic had come to a standstill, the EAP staff walked to the nearest fire station to be deployed to the Pentagon. During the entire eleven days that Arlington held Incident Command, the EAP staff was inside the perimeter at the Pentagon providing support and comfort to public safety employees. The EAP staff was clear about its role in providing services only to those under their charge. It is important to be clear about boundaries in providing services as a way to mitigate the inevitable chaos in critical incidents and to ensure effective follow-up.

Subsequent to the attack on the Pentagon, it has become clear that, depending on the nature of the event, public safety employees are not the only "first responders." The Arlington EAP has extended its comprehensive approach to all public trades workers, mental health workers and public health officials. Included in this approach is the necessity to coach managers and supervisors throughout the process to assist them in shift development, time of exposure, and communication of expectations. Employees are encouraged to develop their own family emergency response plans so they may be more available to serve. These activities lessen anxiety and are imperative for effective planning, staffing and accountability over the long haul. They also create a foundation upon which to build a resilient community, namely, by instilling the idea that public employees must first take care of their own, before they can take care of the community.

Coping with the Aftermath of Terror–Resilience of ZAKA Body Handlers

Zahava Solomon
Rony Berger

SUMMARY. This study assessed the psychological consequences of body handling in the aftermath of terror attacks on 87 ZAKA volunteers and the implications of coping in attenuating the detrimental effects of prolonged exposure to terror. Subjects reported a low sense of danger and considerable self-efficacy. Only two participants (2.3 percent) met symptom criteria for PTSD, and 16 (18.4 percent) met criteria for sub-clinical posttraumatic disorder. Several possible explanations for the resilience of subjects are altruistic and religious rewards, respect and admiration from society and a tendency for sensation seeking.

KEYWORDS. Body handling, psychological terror, coping

Address correspondence to: Zahava Solomon, PhD, Adler Research Center, Tel-Aviv University, Tel Aviv 69978, Israel (E-mail: Solomon@post.tau.ac.il).

The authors wish to acknowledge the help of Liat Lev Shalem and Danny Horesh in the preparation of the manuscript and Anat Damon for her assistance with data analysis.

[Haworth co-indexing entry note]: "Coping with the Aftermath of Terror–Resilience of ZAKA Body Handlers." Solomon, Zahava, and Rony Berger. Co-published simultaneously in *Journal of Aggression, Maltreatment & Trauma* (The Haworth Maltreatment & Trauma Press, an imprint of The Haworth Press, Inc.) Vol. 10, No. 1/2, 2005; and: *The Trauma of Terrorism: Sharing Knowledge and Shared Care, An International Handbook* (ed: Yael Danieli, Danny Brom, and Joe Sills) The Haworth Maltreatment & Trauma Press, an imprint of The Haworth Press, Inc., 2005.

INTRODUCTION

Intifada Al Aqsa–the Palestinian uprising–is the latest peak in the long term Israeli-Palestinian conflict. The current Intifada commenced in September 2000 and is continuing at the time of this writing. During the 3 years of the Intifada, Palestinian militants set off bombs, many times by suicide bombers, in Israeli shopping malls, buses, restaurants, and other crowded places, killing and maiming many Israeli citizens.

Terrorist attacks have become very common in Israel during the Intifada, blindly striking victims from all facets of society. However, some sectors of society are more prone than others to experience terror-related events. One group whose members are constantly exposed to terror and its consequences is ZAKA (Hebrew initials for "Identification of disaster victims"), a voluntary religious organization that has been part of the Israeli rescue forces since the mid 1990s. During the current Intifada, ZAKA has played a prominent role in carrying out tasks of body removal and providing first aid in the aftermath of terrorist attacks. As a result, ZAKA volunteers have been repeatedly exposed to the most horrific sights of carnage, mutilated bodies, body parts and critically wounded casualties.

Evidence from a large body of literature consistently indicates that such exposure in rescue workers might cause psychological distress. This was found in various contexts, such as wars (McCarroll, Ursano, & Fullerton, 1993) and accidents (Miles, Demi, & Mostyn-Aker, 1984), and among various professions, such as police officers (Greene, 2001), peacekeepers, humanitarian aid and human rights workers, and the media (Danieli, 2002) and forensic pathologists (Tucker, Pfefferbaum, Nixon, & Foy, 1999). A study by Ursano, Fullerton, Kao, and Bhartiya (1995), for example, found that body handlers were suffering from elevated levels of intrusion, avoidance and somatization, as well as from increased hostility levels. Exposure to bodies was also identified as a risk factor for Posttraumatic Stress Disorder (PTSD). A host of other studies (e.g., Sutker, Uddo, Braisley, Vasterling, & Errera, 1994) reported relatively high levels of posttraumatic symptomatology among those carrying out tasks involving exposure to bodies.

Encountering the bodies of the dead and the injured involves several psychological risk factors. Above all, this encounter often forces people to let go of their most basic denial defense and recognize their own biological vulnerability. A common reaction, in this respect, is "it could have happened to me" (Ursano & McCarroll, 1990). Another risk factor has to do with the sensory overload experienced by body handlers (McCarroll, Ursano, Wright, & Fullerton, 1993). The grotesque sights, sounds and smells often encountered by these workers can be extremely stressful and might leave long-lasting psychological scars.

However, while it seems that body handling in general carries the risk of adverse psychological implications, there still seems to be considerable variability among the exposed in terms of their distress. These individual differences may stem from several sources, among which are levels of exposure (Wagner, Heinrichs, & Ehlert, 1998), prior working experience (Dyregrov, Kristoffersen, & Gjestand, 1996) and reasons or motivation for being involved with body handling.

An important factor that may account for the variability in body handlers' emotional responses is their coping mode. The concept of coping has been defined in various ways and according to different theories. A classic conceptualization of coping was offered by Lazarus and Folkman (1984), who defined the term as "constantly changing cognitive and behavioral efforts to manage the specific external and/or internal demands that are appraised as taxing or exceeding the resources of the person" (p. 141). Numerous mechanisms that aim to remove the stressor or to ameliorate its effects are viewed as coping. A comprehensive categorization coupled with a measure of coping was suggested by Carver, Scheier and Weintraub (1989). They posit that coping is a complex, multifaceted concept and devised a measure, COPE, that taps the following dimensions: active coping, planning, suppression of competing activities, restraint coping, seeking instrumental social support, seeking emotional social support, positive reinterpretation, acceptance, turning to religion, venting of emotions, denial, behavioral disengagement, mental disengagement and alcohol/drug disengagement.

The present study aims to assess the psychological consequences of body handling in the aftermath of terror attacks and the implication of coping in attenuating or buffering the detrimental effects of prolonged exposure to terror.

METHOD

Sample

The sample comprised 87 male ZAKA volunteers from three counties who participated in psychological resourcing seminars held by NATAL (Israel Trauma Center for Victims of Terror and War). All but six consented to participate in the study. They were asked to fill out anonymous self-report questionnaires. Their age range was 28-72 years, $M = 43.3$, $SD = 9.89$; most of them are married (96.5 percent) and gainfully employed (82.5 percent); 35.6 percent have income below average, 23 percent average income and 41.4 percent reported above average income. Time in ZAKA ranged from 2 months to 12 years, $M = 5.77$, $SD = 3.78$. Of them, 80.3 percent are body handlers and the rest handle bodies and also provide first aid.

Measures

Sociodemographic Background: Subjects were asked about their age, place of birth, marital status, education, occupation and service in the army and police.

Professional Exposure: Participants were asked about their activities in ZAKA in terms of time, role and number of terrorist attacks in which they were involved.

Personal Exposure: They were asked whether since the beginning of the El Aqsa Intifada they had been exposed to a terrorist attack and whether they had a friend or family member who had been exposed to an attack during this time.

History of Stressful Events: The participants were presented with a list of 11 stressful events (e.g., serious illness, accident; Solomon & Prager, 1992) and were asked to indicate whether they had experienced these events.

Perception of threat, sense of safety and self-efficacy were assessed by a scale devised by Solomon and Prager (1992). The scale comprises 4 measures: perception of threat to personal safety, $\alpha = 0.68$; sense of security stemming from faith in the defense forces, $\alpha = 0.94$; self-efficacy, that is, faith in one's ability to function if caught in a terrorist attack, $\alpha = .82$; and changes in behavior resulting from the Intifada, $\alpha = .41$.

Trauma-related psychiatric symptoms were measured using the PTSD Inventory (Solomon et al., 1993). This scale assesses DSM symptom criteria for PTSD (American Psychiatric Association, 1994). It has acceptable psychometric properties and has been used in trauma-related surveys. The score therefore is not a clinical diagnosis of PTSD but an aggregation of symptom criteria for PTSD.

Psychological Distress: The Brief Symptom Inventory (BSI; Derogatis & Spencer, 1982) was used to assess psychological distress. BSI analysis entails both global indices of distress and a profile of the nine subscales: anxiety, somatization, paranoid ideation, obsessive compulsive, hostility, phobic anxiety, depression, interpersonal sensitivity, social alienation and additional items. This is a widely accepted and used measure with proven psychometric properties (Derogatis & Spencer, 1982).

COPE (Carver, Scheier, & Weintraub, 1989) is a self-report scale to assess coping. The scale reportedly has good psychometric properties and has been used in trauma-related studies (e.g., Carver, Scheier & Weintraub, 1989). In the current study we modified the COPE. Several items were omitted, and factor analysis with Varimax rotation yielded nine coping strategies, as follows: seeking social support ($\alpha = 0.89$), humor ($\alpha = 0.88$), denial ($\alpha = 0.64$), acceptance ($\alpha = 0.58$), taking action ($\alpha = 0.71$), faith ($\alpha = 0.72$), escapism ($\alpha = 0.55$), positive thinking ($\alpha = 0.65$), and monitoring ($\alpha = 0.71$).

RESULTS

Exposure. In the aftermath of terrorist attacks, most participants (61, 80.3 percent) were involved in handling and removal of bodies, while the rest (15, 19.7 percent) took part in both evacuating bodies and providing first aid. Three participants (3.5 percent) have not yet been involved in any body handling, 8 (9.3 percent) assisted in one or two terror attacks, 15 (19.7 percent) in 3-5 attacks, 16 (18.6 percent) in 6-9 attacks, and more than half of the participants (44, 51.2 percent) assisted in 10 attacks or more.

As for exposure to terror attacks, 11 participants (12.6 percent) were personally exposed to such an event. A similar percentage (10, 11.5 percent) had a family member who was exposed to a terror attack, and over half the participants (50, 57.5 percent) reported that someone they knew was exposed to at least one terror-induced event. Finally, 21 participants (24.1 percent) reported having had a past experience that reminded them of the current terrorist attacks.

Perception of Danger. Two aspects of perceived threat were assessed: sense of danger and sense of security. Only 11.5 percent reported sensing some personal danger and only two (2.3 percent) reported feeling considerable danger. With regard to safety, 65.5 percent reported a considerable sense of security related to their faith in Israel's security forces, and 90.8 percent reported some sense of security.

Perception of Self-Efficacy. Two aspects of perceived self-efficacy and changes in behavior were assessed. Of the participants, 67.8 percent reported considerable self-efficacy and 97.7 percent reported some self-efficacy. In other words, the majority of respondents felt confident that they would function adequately if caught in a terror attack. With regard to behavioral changes stemming from the threat of terror, 11.5 percent reported that they have made considerable changes in their lifestyle and behavior as a result of the threat of terror, and 47.1 percent reported that they have made some changes in their lifestyle as a result of such threat.

Psychological Briefing. With regard to stress inoculation training and psychological briefing, most participants (55, 65.5 percent) reported not having received any formal guidance for emotional coping before deployment.

Posttraumatic Symptomatology. Only 2 participants (2.3 percent) met symptom criteria for PTSD. Sixteen (18.4 percent) met criteria for sub-clinical posttraumatic disorder when the latter was defined according to the existence of any one of the following: intrusion *or* avoidance *or* hyper-arousal. When it was defined as endorsement of intrusion *and* avoidance, 11 participants (12.6 percent) met criteria. And, finally, when it was defined as endorsement of intrusion *and* hyper-arousal, 14 participants (16.1 percent) met criteria. Intrusion was found in 53 participants (39.1 percent), hyper-arousal in 35 participants (40.2 percent) and avoidance in only 7 participants (8 percent).

Psychiatric Symptomatology. The scores of the BSI were relatively low. In the absence of a control or comparison group, the participants' BSI scores were compared with norms obtained for the Israeli population (Gilbar & Ben-Zur, 2002). The following are the percentages of participants whose scores exceed the norms for each subscale of the questionnaire: GSI–16 (18.4 percent); obsession-compulsion–28 (32.2 percent); inter-personal sensitivity–18 (20.7 percent); depression–13 (14.9 percent); anxiety–20 (23 percent); hostility–19 (21.8 percent); phobia–12 (13.8 percent); paranoia–16 (18.4 percent); psychoses–24 (27.6 percent); and somatization–9 (10.3 percent). In other words, relatively low percentages of ZAKA subjects reported levels of distress that are indicative of psychopathology. These low rates reveal again the resilience of the participants in this study.

Physical Health. Participants were also asked to rate their physical health. The majority (79, 91.9 percent) reported being in good health, 7 (8.1 percent) defined their physical health as average, and none reported poor health.

Modes of Coping with Terrorist Attacks. The most frequently used modes of coping were trusting in God (98.9 percent of the subjects reported that they used this coping strategy to some extent), 'Asking for God's help' (94.2 percent) and looking for the best in every situation (93 percent). Modes of coping that were used least frequently as a specific coping mechanism were use of tranquilizers (1.2 percent) and consumption of alcohol or drugs (9.6 percent).

Multivariate Analyses. Three hierarchical regression analyses were performed to assess the relative contribution of demographic items, exposure to terrorist attack, and means of coping, which were associated with the outcome measures. The three dependent variables were PTSD, BSI general distress score and sense of safety. The final regression models are presented in Table 1. In the first step, sociodemographic variables (age, number of children, income and level of religious commitment) were entered. The second step comprised the exposure variables: number of past stressful events, years in ZAKA, number of terrorist attacks experienced as a volunteer in ZAKA, role in ZAKA and exposure of family and friends to terrorist attacks. In the third step coping strategies were entered.

Inspection of Table 1 reveals that sociodemographics explain 21.8 percent of the variance of PTSD. Age and income are inversely associated with PTSD. Copings in the form of denial explain an additional 13.3 percent. The model explains 30.3 percent of the variance of PTSD.

With regard to BSI general score, sociodemographic variables explain 25.2 percent of the variance. Age and income are inversely related to BSI. Introduction of exposure variables adds 10.2 percent as past stressful events and exposure of acquaintances to terrorist attacks each make a significant contribution. Finally, coping, entered in the third step, did not make any significant contribution. The model explains 36.7 percent of the variance of BSI.

With regard to sense of safety, sociodemographics explain 11.3 percent. Religious life style is associated with sense of safety. Exposure had no contribution to the explained variance. Introduction of active coping and religious coping in the third step each made a unique and significant contribution to the explained variance. The model explains 27.4 percent of the variance of sense of safety.

DISCUSSION

An interesting and surprising finding reveals a very low level of psychological distress among ZAKA volunteers. Contrary to expectation that these men are at high risk for psychological distress due to their horrific recurrent exposure, only 2 percent reported posttraumatic symptoms. This finding is inconsistent with previous studies, which had reported elevated rates of PTSD among rescue workers (e.g., Ursano et al., 1995). Furthermore, this low rate is even lower than the rate of posttraumatic symptoms found in a representative national sample of the Israeli adult population conducted at the same time (Bleich, Gelkopf, & Solomon, 2003). In other words, our findings negate the notion that ZAKA rescue workers are at increased risk for psychopathology. Furthermore, findings suggest that despite their intense and repeated exposure, these men are particularly resilient.

Several factors may account for these findings. ZAKA work entails repeated exposure to horrific sights, but it also gives rise to positive feelings that stem from altruistic and religious extrinsic rewards. An American study of body handlers revealed that volunteers fared better than other body handlers (McCarroll, Ursano, Fullerton, Liu, & Lundy, 2001). It has been claimed that volunteer work and altruisms are associated with enhanced sense of control and welfare (Thoits & Newitt, 2001) and moderate the noxious effects of stress (e.g., Kishon-Barash, Midlarsky & Johnson, 1999). Furthermore, ZAKA volunteers see their contribution as an ultimate act of religious mission

TABLE 1. Final regression models for PTSD, BSI general distress score and sense of safety

PTSD				BSI				Sense of Security			
step	Variables	β	t	R^2	Variables	β	t	R^2	Variables	β	t	R^2
1	Income	35.-	−3.25**	15.5	Income	−.34	−3.5***	16.5	Religious Life Style	.33	3.26**	11.3
	Age	25.-	−2.34*	6.3	Age	−.26	−2.68***	6.7				
2	---	--	--	--	Income	−.34	−3.5**	17.4	---	--	--	--
					Age	−.35	−3.5**	9.1				
					Past Life Events	.27	2.8**	6.1				
					Exposure of Acquaintances	−.20	−2.1*	4.1				
3	Income	−.40	−4.05***	16.7	--	--	--	--	Religious Life Style	.29	2.75**	14.1
	Denial	.36	3.67***	13.3					Acting Religious	.32	2.95**	4.9
									Religious coping	−.31	−2.84**	8.4

*p < .05, **p < .01, *** p < .001

Total explained variance for PTSD–30.0 percent; for BSI–36.7 percent; and for Sense of Security–27.4 percent

(MIZVA) that entails for ultra-Orthodox Jews considerable spiritual rewards, which, in turn, may promote resilience.

There are also secondary gains to be had. ZAKA volunteers, like other ultra-Orthodox Jews, belong to a small and secluded sector that has a loose and complex relationship with Israeli society. ZAKA's unique contribution, however, is received with great respect and gratitude. The respect and admiration that are bestowed on ZAKA volunteers reinforce their self-esteem and may promote resilience.

Another explanation is related to self-selection into ZAKA. As their work is strictly voluntary, it is likely that only the most resilient volunteer for this tough mission. Studies that had assessed volunteers documented a process of self-selection in which individuals with high sense of welfare tend to volunteer (e.g., Thoits & Newitt, 2001). Other factors may also be related to self-selection of this particular group. In the close-knit ultra-Orthodox society that values learning and prayers, opportunities for actions are limited. It is possible that the volunteers are sensation and action seekers and have very limited outlets other than their activities in ZAKA. The psychologists who led the workshop also felt that these men are active and restless and can be characterized as sensation seekers. Previous studies demonstrated that sensation-seeking serves as a stress buffer (Solomon, Ginzburg, Neria, & Ohry, 1995).

We also assessed the use and contribution of a wide variety of coping modes. Findings show that ZAKA volunteers reported extensive use of what is often described as religious coping (Tix & Frazier, 1998). The role of religion as a stress buffer has consistently been documented. Bettelheim (1961), for example, observed that among concentration camp Holocaust survivors, religious Jews suffered less from adverse psychological effects than non-religious Jews. More recently, a growing number of studies have generally revealed positive consequences for using religious coping during times of stress (Pargament, 1997). Religious coping has been associated with less occupational stress in police officers (Beehr, Johnson, & Nieva, 1995) and with stress-related growth in survivors of the Oklahoma City bombing (Pargament, Smith & Koenig, 1996).

Why is religious coping effective? Religion often provides a sense of control (Tix & Frazier, 1998), an ability to find meaning for a traumatic event (McIntosh, Silver, & Wortman, 1993), and a sense of belonging with others (Frazier, Krasnoff, & Port, 1995). Across different studies, it appears that the use of religious coping may exert its beneficial effects through three general pathways: beliefs that may facilitate cognitive restructuring of the meaning of the traumatic events, the social support of the close-knit religious community, and a sense of divine control over the stressful experiences (see also Davidowitz, this volume).

Another coping mode that was found to be helpful for ZAKA volunteers in mitigating the noxious effects of terror is denial, which is defined as an unconscious attempt to reject unacceptable feelings, needs, thoughts, wishes, or external reality factors. At times, denial is seen as an inappropriate mode of coping. In some studies, denial was found to be associated with psychological distress and elevated levels of posttraumatic symptomatology (e.g., Green, Lindy, & Grace, 1988). The current study, however, which is consistent with a previous study of emergency workers (Grevin, 1996), found that denial helped contain anxiety and served as a useful psychological protective measure. It seems that rescue workers who distort incoming affect and information avoid developing stress syndromes. Denial in these cases helps to block out information that is too affectively stimulating or anxiety provoking. In this ultra-Orthodox group, belief in divine providence may further reinforce denial. The surprisingly low rates of PTSD among ZAKA workers may therefore be attributed, at least in part, to their adaptive use of denial in coping with potentially distressing aspects of their work.

Other coping modes, except active coping, made only marginal contributions to both measures of distress and sense of safety. The beneficial effect of active coping, even in the face of events that cannot be manipulated and altered, has been previously documented. For example, in the 1992 Gulf War, when Israeli cities were repeatedly bombarded and Israeli citizens were confined to their sealed rooms, those who employed active coping fared better than those who did not (Solomon, 1995).

Interpretation of results from this study should be made with some caution. The study sample is drawn from a unique population and suffers from some limitations. These include the relatively small sample size and the sampling procedure. Participants in the workshop are not necessarily representative of ZAKA volunteers. Thus, one cannot negate the possibility that the more vulnerable volunteers did not participate in the workshop and in our study. Despite these limitations, the present study provides valuable information on resilience and the use of religious coping with ongoing terror. Since, unfortunately, human proclivity to aggression continues to give rise to terror, future research should systematically assess the role of these and other coping modes in mitigating the noxious effects of trauma. Finally, the direction taken in the present study should be further developed. More specifically, further research should assess the role of sensation-seeking and religious coping in promoting resilience.

REFERENCES

American Psychiatric Association. (1994). *Diagnostic and statistical manual of mental disorders.* Washington, DC: Author.

Beehr, T. A., Johnson, L.B. & Nieva, R. (1995). Occupational stress: Coping of police and theirs spouses. *Journal of Organizational Behavior, 16,* 3-25.

Bettelheim, B. (1961). *Informed heart.* New York: Free Press.

Bleich, A., Gelkopf, M., & Solomon, Z. (2003). Exposure to terrorism, stress-related mental health symptoms, and coping behaviors among a nationally representative sample in Israel. *Journal of the American Medical Association, 290*(5), 612-690.

Carver, C. S., Scheier, M. F., & Weintraub, I. K. (1989). Assessing coping strategies: A theoretically based approach. *Journal of Personality and Social Psychology, 52,* 267-283.

Danieli, Y. (Ed.) (2002). Sharing the front line and the back hills: International protectors and providers, peacekeepers, humanitarian aid workers and the media in the midst of crisis. Amityville, NY: Baywood Publishing Company, Inc.

Derogatis, L. R., & Spencer, P. M. (1982). *The Brief Symptom Inventory: Administration, scoring and procedures manual.* Baltimore, MD: Clinical Psychometrics Research.

Dyregrov, A., Kristoffersen, J. I., & Gjestand, R. (1996). Voluntary and professional disaster-workers: Similarities and differences in reactions. *Journal of Traumatic Stress, 9*(3), 541-555.

Frazier, P. A., Krasnoff, A. S., & Port, C. L. (1995, August). The role of religion in coping with chronic medical conditions. Paper presented at the 103rd Annual Convention of the American Psychological Association, New York, NY.

Gilbar, O., & Ben-Zur, H. (2002). Adult Israeli community norms for the Brief Symptom Inventory (BSI). *International Journal of Stress Management, 9*(1), 1-10.

Green, B. L., Lindy, J. D., & Grace, M. C. (1988). Long-term coping with combat stress. *Journal of Traumatic Stress, 1*(4), 399-412.

Greene, C. L. (2001). Human remains and psychological impact on police officers: Excerpts from psychiatric observations. *Australasian Journal of Disaster and Trauma Studies, 5*(2), n.p.

Grevin, F. (1996). Posttraumatic stress disorder, ego defense mechanisms, and empathy among urban paramedics. *Psychological Reports, 79*(2), 483-495.

Kishon-Barash, R., Midlarsky, E., & Johnson, D. R. (1999). Altruism and the Vietnam War veteran: The relationship of helping to symptomatology. *Journal of Traumatic Stress, 12*(4), 655-662.

Lazarus, R. S., & Folkman, S. (1984). *Stress, appraisal and coping.* New York: Academic Press.

McCarroll, J. E., Ursano, R. J., Fullerton, C. S., Liu, X., & Lundy, A. (2001). Effects of exposure to death in a war mortuary on posttraumatic stress disorder symptoms of intrusion and avoidance. *Journal of Nervous and Mental Disease, 189*(1), 44-48.

McCarroll, J. E., Ursano, R. J., & Fullerton, C. S. (1993). Symptoms of posttraumatic stress disorder following recovery of war dead. *American Journal of Psychiatry, 150*(12), 1875-1877.

McCarroll, J. E., Ursano, R. J., Wright, K. M., & Fullerton, C. S. (1993). Handling bodies after violent death: Strategies for coping. *American Journal of Orthopsychiatry, 63*, 209-214.

McIntosh, D. M., Silver, R. C., & Wortman, C. B. (1993). Religion's role in adjustment to negative life events: Coping with the loss of a child. *Journal of Personality and Social Psychology, 65*, 812-821.

Miles, M. S., Demi, A. S., & Mostyn-Aker, P. (1984). Rescue workers' reactions following the Hyatt Hotel disaster. *Death Education, 8*, 315-331.

Pargament, K. I. (1997). *The psychology of religion and coping: Theory, research and practice.* New York: Guilford Press.

Pargament, K. I., Smith, B. W., & Koenig, H. G. (1996, August). Religious coping with the Oklahoma City bombing: The brief RCOPE. Paper presented at the 104th Annual Convention of the American Psychological Association, Toronto, Canada.

Solomon, Z. & Prager, E. (1992). Elderly Israeli Holocaust survivors during the Persian Gulf War: A study of psychological distress. *American Journal of Psychiatry. 149*, 1707-1710.

Solomon, Z., Benbenishty, R., Neria, Y., Abramovitz, M., Ginzburg, K., & Ohry, A. (1993). Assessment of PTSD: Validation of the revised PTSD inventory. *Israel Journal of Psychiatry and Related Sciences, 30*, 110-115.

Solomon, Z., Ginzburg, K., Neria, Y., & Ohry, A. (1995). Coping with war captivity: The role of sensation seeking. *European Journal of Personality, 9*(1), 57-70.

Solomon, Z. (1995). *Coping with War Induced Stress: The Gulf War and the Israeli Response.* New York: Plenum Press.

Sutker, P. B., Uddo, M., Braisley, K., Vasterling, J. J., & Errera, P. (1994). Psychopathology in war-zone deployed and non-deployed Operation Desert Storm troops assigned graves registration duties. *Journal of Abnormal Psychology, 103,* 383-390.

Thoits, P. A., & Newitt, L. N. (2001). Volunteer work and well-being. *Journal of Health & Social Behavior, 42*(2), 115-131.

Tix, A. P., & Frazier, P. A. (1998). The use of religious coping during stressful life events: Main effects, moderation and mediation. *Journal of Consulting and Clinical Psychology, 66*(2), 411-422.

Tucker, P., Pfefferbaum, B., Nixon, S. J., & Foy, D. W. (1999). Trauma and recovery among adults highly exposed to a community disaster. *Psychiatric Annals, 29*(2), 78-83.

Ursano, R. J., & McCarroll, J. E. (1990). The nature of a traumatic stressor: Handling dead bodies. *Journal of Nervous and Mental Disease, 178,* 396-398.

Ursano, R. J., Fullerton, C. S., Kao, T. C., & Bhartiya, V. R. (1995). Longitudinal assessment of posttraumatic stress disorder and depression after exposure to traumatic death. *Journal of Nervous and Mental Disease, 183,* 36-42.

Wagner, D., Heinrichs, M., & Ehlert, U. (1998). Prevalence of symptoms of posttraumatic stress disorder in German professional firefighters. *American Journal of Psychiatry, 155*(12), 1727-1732.

Voice:
Ten Years Later?

Deena Yellin

This year marks the 10th year anniversary since I survived a suicide bombing in Israel. Miraculously, I emerged from the wreckage intact, but I want the ghastly memories to fade. Even after a decade, the gruesome scenes remain with me. I can still feel the blast, the power of its vibration was so strong I felt I had been thrown back 50 feet. I can still smell the smoke that spread the stench of explosives and filled my throat so I could barely breathe. I can still hear the young woman lying on the ground, her face covered in blood and crying harder than anyone I'd ever seen.

My husband and I were on our honeymoon in the Middle East and had spent three wondrous days exploring the Jordan Valley. We breathed in the scenery, remarked on its beauty, and took loads of pictures for our honeymoon album. On Friday, weary from touring an ancient Roman amphitheater, we sank into our seats on the 961 bus to Jerusalem. My nap was interrupted by the driver's announcement that we were stopping at a roadside café. I was too tired to move, but my husband urged me off. I approached the snack bar and asked a young Arab worker for an ice cream bar. He handed it over, and I pulled a 10-shekel bill from my wallet. Before I could pay, an earsplitting blast froze me in place. The earth vibrated and all around me I heard people screaming and running. My husband pulled me to the ground. I glanced at our bus, which

Address correspondence to: Deena Yellin (E-mail: dyellin@aol.com).

[Haworth co-indexing entry note]: "Voice: Ten Years Later?" Yellin, Deena. Co-published simultaneously in *Journal of Aggression, Maltreatment & Trauma* (The Haworth Maltreatment & Trauma Press, an imprint of The Haworth Press, Inc.) Vol. 10, No. 1/2, 2005; and: *The Trauma of Terrorism: Sharing Knowledge and Shared Care, An International Handbook* (ed: Yael Danieli, Danny Brom, and Joe Sills) The Haworth Maltreatment & Trauma Press, an imprint of The Haworth Press, Inc., 2005.

had been about 15 feet from where we were standing. In its place was a ball of fire spewing clouds of black smoke into the sky.

We learned later that Sahar Tamam Nabulsi, a 22-year-old Hamas member from the West Bank, had loaded his van with explosives and crashed it into our bus. The shrapnel that flew over the counter missed us but killed the worker who had handed me my ice cream. Had the bomb detonated moments earlier, when we were on the bus, or had it gone off after we re-boarded, the fatalities would have been numerous. Instead, only the café worker was killed and nine passengers were wounded. The bomber's sole casualty, Marwan Ibrahim Hajeb Abed Ghani, 25, an Arab, was from a nearby village. He was struck on the head by a fragment from the blast and died immediately. The Israeli cafe owner said that the worker, who had recently married, was like a "member of my family."

The passengers on 961 had been very lucky that day. My husband and I emerged from the attack unscathed for the most part, but the emotional scars were wrenching. Loud noises jar me. So do the images that invade my mind. Ours was the first suicide bus bombing in the history of the Palestinian-Israeli conflict. It was a new tactic by terrorists, who had previously done their work through ambushes, stabbings, and time bombs. Since our bombing, so many others have followed.

Feeling a kinship with the victims, I studied the news reports intently. Each time I saw footage of an explosion site, it brought back unwanted memories of my own experience. When I learned of other young American tourists who had been killed, I was sickened. I read their obituaries and marveled at their accomplishments. In many ways, their lives were more meaningful than my own. I buried my yellowed news clippings about my incident in a drawer and counted my blessings in silence.

A near-death experience should have inspired me, but the guilt of survival weighed me down. I wondered why I had survived while the others died, and a question lingered in my mind: What was I doing to own up to my second chance at life? As I approached the 10th anniversary of this milestone in April, I wondered how to mark it. Some suggested we celebrate our survival with a party, but with the escalating violence in the Middle East over the past decade, I felt a memorial service would have been more appropriate, for those who did not live to tell their stories.

I even mourned the bomber's life, which ended when he was 22. He had eight years of formal education, lived in an Arab village in the West Bank and made techina in his father's factory, a dish I am particularly fond of. I felt we shared common ground. Both of us came from small towns and tightly knit families. Both of us were young and passionate about our ideals. I too would give my life for some of my highest beliefs, although I would never harm others. I would like to think that, had our paths crossed in other circumstances, we might have become friends. Instead, he wasted his life attempting to kill strangers over a situation they did not create.

I mourn for others like Sahar who are indoctrinated to believe there is nobility in detonating oneself and others for a cause, when a resolution could be reached through compromise. Several weeks after the bombing, my husband and I returned to the scene. We were drawn there, hoping to find something that would help us make sense of the seemingly random act of violence. I wanted to look one more time at the ashes, the charred bus and the demolished kiosk to gain a sense of closure. Instead, we found the kiosk had been rebuilt into a sparkling, sleek roadside cafeteria. Smiling customers flanked the snack bar, going about their daily lives, seemingly indifferent to the bombing. I was disappointed, I had wanted the site to reflect what had happened, but this is the Israeli way. They cry, mourn, and clean up the mess quickly. Life goes on, albeit in some terribly altered way. Somehow the survivors brush themselves off and continue.

Now I am coming to see my experience as a sort of message of triumph over our current dark times. Just as America's troubles in Iraq will impact us in a myriad of ways, life will go on long after the hostilities are over. We can thwart our enemies just by going about our lives. I am also coming to see my close call as a message in my personal life.

Stephen Flatow, whose daughter Alissa was killed in a suicide bombing several years after my own brush with death, told me: "God could have easily let you be taken in the attack, so there must be a reason why you were spared. . . . Therefore, don't you have an obligation to become a better person?" My life was saved. Now I have to make sure it was worth saving.

Training and Mobilizing Volunteers for Emergency Response and Long-Term Support

Eleanor Pardess

SUMMARY. This article offers guidelines for the screening, assignment, and ongoing training of volunteers for active outreach, which are based on the experience of the Israel Crisis Management Center's countrywide volunteer network. Given ongoing support, volunteers can provide the vital immediate and long-term support that is particularly important to vulnerable populations. Issues in training include: (a) responding to loss and trauma, (b) collaboration, and (c) cultural sensitivity. Ways to minimize burnout through nurturing a sense of belonging, connectedness, and meaning are discussed. The unique contribution and need for special support of volunteer trauma survivors who are models of post-traumatic growth is described.

KEYWORDS. Volunteers, outreach, crisis intervention, immigrants, post-traumatic growth

Address correspondence to: Eleanor Pardess, MA, Selah-Israel Crisis Management Center, 15 Chevrat Shas, Tel-Aviv, Israel (E-mail: epardess@israsrv.net.il).

[Haworth co-indexing entry note]: "Training and Mobilizing Volunteers for Emergency Response and Long-Term Support." Pardess, Eleanor. Co-published simultaneously in *Journal of Aggression, Maltreatment & Trauma* (The Haworth Maltreatment & Trauma Press, an imprint of The Haworth Press, Inc.) Vol. 10, No. 1/2, 2005; and: *The Trauma of Terrorism: Sharing Knowledge and Shared Care, An International Handbook* (ed: Yael Danieli, Danny Brom, and Joe Sills) The Haworth Maltreatment & Trauma Press, an imprint of The Haworth Press, Inc., 2005.

Volunteers play a wide range of roles in the aftermath of trauma (i.e., as part of rescue teams, staffing crisis hotlines, at walk-in centers, in hospitals, and in outreach programs) providing crisis intervention and ongoing support. Despite the heavy reliance on volunteers by many organizations, there is a notable lack of literature on training volunteers who work with disaster victims and on ways of preventing volunteer burnout. This article describes ways in which organizations can mobilize and strengthen volunteer resources through appropriate screening, orientation, assignment, training, and ongoing support. The guidelines offered are based on the ten-year countrywide volunteer network experience of the Israel Crisis Management Center (Selah).

THE IMPORTANCE OF VOLUNTEERS IN THE AFTERMATH OF DISASTER

Volunteers are a valuable human resource that can help meet community needs which cannot be met by government agencies. They enable social agencies and human services to expand their services to vulnerable "high-risk" populations. Active outreach by volunteers has been described as one of the spontaneous community responses in the aftermath of disaster, where volunteers play a vital role in rescue, relief, and recovery efforts (Danieli, 2001; Drabek, 1986; Norris et al., 2002). However, these may be ineffective if not properly planned and organized, and the uncoordinated outpouring of volunteers may even interfere (Craig & Fuchs, 2002; Gillespie & Murty, 1994).

Volunteer resources during a time of disaster or other community-wide trauma may foster both individual and community resilience and post-traumatic recovery (Rosse, 1993). Volunteering is a form of collective action (Gidron, 1994; Wilson & Musick, 1997). Among the most important functions of volunteers in disaster work is the provision of social support, whether in the form of instrumental assistance, information, or direct emotional support.

Terrorism is an attack on the community to which volunteerism is a communal response. Trauma isolates, often threatening to destroy the bonds between the individual and the community. "The solidarity of the group provides the strongest protection against terror and despair, and the strongest antidote to traumatic experience" (Herman, 1992, p. 214). The social support that volunteers can provide is perhaps even more important in man-made disasters (i.e., terrorism) than in natural disasters (Danieli, 1996). Knowing that others are prepared to devote time and energy of their own free will can help restore the faith in humanity (Janoff-Bulman, 1985). The presence of volunteers conveys a message of caring and connectedness. The sense of belonging and being part of a community is most important in the process of reconstruction of meaning and resolution of trauma. Furthermore, in the aftermath of terrorism, anger at governmental authorities for having failed to provide protection may color relationships with official helping agencies (such as the National Insurance Institute). Under these circumstances volunteer help can be accepted more readily as it represents a sense of shared fate and public acknowledgment.

MOTIVATING VOLUNTEERS

Understanding volunteers' motivation is important in mobilizing them and reducing attrition rates (Davis et al., 2003; Lafer, 1991; Omoto & Snyder, 1990; Penner & Finkelstein, 1998). Volunteering in the aftermath of terrorism and other disasters is for many a way of coping and an avenue to self-growth. Instead of remaining passive spectators witnessing horrors on television, people choose to engage actively in reaching out to others and alleviating suffering. In the face of the ongoing threat of terror, the active nature of helping others can reduce the sense of helplessness and promote a feeling of connectedness. The worst of times can also bring out our best (Walsch, 2002) and enable us to discover inner strengths.

Along with the gratifying aspects of volunteering, it is important to recognize the risks of working with traumatized populations and to find ways to minimize burnout and secondary traumatization (Danieli, 1994; Figley, 1995). Support providers need to be supported. By providing adequate support, ongoing training, and guidance, agencies deploying volunteers can ensure an effective emergency and long-term support system while conserving and even enriching the volunteers' resources. The Selah volunteer network model illustrates these issues.

THE SELAH VOLUNTEER NETWORK: A MODEL OF OUTREACH

Selah carries out a wide range of support programs for new immigrants struck by crisis. Stepping into a vacuum ten years ago, it developed a comprehensive and culturally-sensitive program of outreach, crisis management, and long-term support tailored to meet the special needs of immigrant victims of terror attacks and other tragedies. Since its founding in 1993, it has helped over 10,000 distressed immigrants by providing both emergency and long-term essential emotional, material, and financial help.

The struggle that all people face following a tragedy is compounded for immigrants by language difficulties, the sense of uprootedness, and disorientation and, in many cases, the lack of a natural support system of extended family and friends. Selah operates through a mobile, nationwide support network of some 600 volunteers who come from a wide variety of professional backgrounds, including mental health professionals experienced in working in crisis intervention and trauma treatment. Volunteering brings together individuals from different age groups and countries, who speak different languages, native Israelis as well as veteran and new immigrants.

IMMEDIATE OUTREACH FOLLOWING A TERRORIST ATTACK

During the immediate emergency response to an attack, teams provide vital practical and emotional assistance, and serve as bridges to other resources. Volunteers visiting the hospitals or the homes of the families can assist in the complicated task of assessing the immediate needs and resources of the victims and their families. Volunteers can also stand by the bereaved families during the process of identifying bodies. They can provide essential information and solve problems regarding transportation, translation, and contact with family members in the country or abroad.

During the next stage of crisis support, volunteers may visit homes and help with developing needs, such as providing day-care for children of the injured or building a support system around a parent tending a hospitalized child. Other practical assistance at this stage may include finding shelter, household items, and medical equipment, thereby providing bridging support until government services take over.

LONG-TERM SUPPORT

Following a tragedy, there is usually an initial outpouring of help, which tends to subside within the first few weeks. Grief, trauma, and pain, however, do not go away quickly. Unfortunately, it is just when the reality of the loss begins to sink in that the victims are often the most alone. It is crucial, therefore, to channel as much of the initial volunteer resources as possible to the long term, when many vital needs begin to emerge that are not apparent in the first stage. In the long run, volunteers can help activate existing resources and strengthen the coping skills and social networks of bereaved parents, orphaned children, children who have lost siblings, and the physically injured or emotionally traumatized and their families.

The volunteers' support is most important during difficult times which trigger the most painful memories such as holidays or anniversaries when loneliness is heightened, security crises, terror alerts, or after major terror attacks. The importance of operating a "telephone chain" of volunteers reaching out to offer support cannot be overstated.

A person needs time and space to grieve (Volkan, 1981). However, often the bereaved are encouraged by others to "put the past behind them" and get on with their lives. The long-term presence of volunteers provides a protective shield and conveys society's acknowledgment of the pain and the message: We remember!

In addition to individual support, Selah provides group support programs that are primarily run by a multidisciplinary team. These programs bring people together, break through isolation, and create a protected space for working through trauma and sharing grief. Healing retreats for the injured and bereaved on weekends and vacation outings also include groups for mutual support that emphasize: (a) reconnecting through sharing grief; (b) rebuilding bridges (both personal and collective) between past, present, and future; and (c) restoring continuity in life. The presence of volunteers is central to this reconnection process.

ORIENTATION, SCREENING, ASSIGNMENT, AND TRAINING OF VOLUNTEERS

Orientation. Orientation for new volunteers is carried out in groups led by veteran volunteers. It usually covers: (a) the target community's needs and resources; (b) the volunteer organization's approach, activities, and programs; and (c) the various possibilities of volunteering in the organization (e.g., outreach, hotline, and mentoring). It is also important to discuss the commitment required as well as the stresses and challenges the volunteers are likely to encounter.

Screening. The overwhelming demands of crisis situations require highly motivated volunteers who possess self-confidence, initiative, problem-solving skills, sensitivity, and compassion. Screening for these qualities is one way to ensure that volunteers in emergency teams have the requisite emotional strength, commitment, and capacity. It also helps guard against burnout and attrition. Group screening, facilitated by experienced volunteers following an individual interview, has proven to be effective. The group screening involves three stages: (a) In-depth group discussion of motivations and expectations ("What has led you to consider volunteering?" or "What do you expect from the volunteering experience"); (b) Simulation of outreach and crisis intervention in an emergency situation; and (c) Space for sharing feelings and questions.

Training. The purpose of training is to empower volunteers to respond in a sensitive and responsible way by activating their natural listening skills, common sense, life experience, and inner strengths. Care should be taken not to discourage or overwhelm them with excessive amounts of information or theory that might erode their self-confidence and natural helping capacities.

The training process starts before deployment and continues well into the volunteering process. The main issues the training should address are communication skills, responding to loss and trauma, and cultural sensitivity.

Communication skills can be practiced in small groups through role-playing and sharing perceptions and feelings. The key skills are active listening, non-verbal communication, and reflecting feelings. Emphasis should be placed on setting aside preconceptions and judgments, and on tolerating individual differences in coping styles. Empathy is a major issue; stepping into another's shoes and stepping out of them should be modeled, and the difference between empathy and over-identification discussed.

Responding to Loss and Trauma. Grief and mourning processes should be discussed and volunteers encouraged to become aware of their feelings about bereavement and death. Crisis intervention skills should be covered, such as: (a) how to initiate contact with people in shock; (b) how to cope with their possible initial rejection or ambivalence; and (c) how to provide a quiet, responsive, responsible, and reassuring presence in the midst of chaos. The means of providing information, assisting in problem solving, and supporting family members of the wounded and bereaved should also be covered. Attention should be devoted to understanding the role that volunteers may play in the long run as outsider witnesses and facilitators of the telling and retelling of narrative (White & Epston, 1990) and reconstruction of meaning (Neinmeyer, 2000). Telling one's story to an understanding listener helps restore continuity, a sense of identity and connectedness.

Volunteers working with children require further specialized training in helping children of various age groups. Cultural sensitivity to differences in the ways people from different cultures cope with loss and trauma can be enhanced by narrative practices such as "reflecting" teams, and exploring one's "landscape of identity" (White & Epston, 1995), which can help promote self-awareness. The diversity of the volunteers themselves is an important resource in the training process.

The importance of collaboration with other agencies should be stressed so as to avoid uncoordinated, overlapping, or conflicting efforts. The training program should include information about the various community agencies involved in emergency response and the way they work, as well as to whom to report and how.

The Use of Language. Avoiding mental health terminology like "therapy," "patients," or "clients" is important in training volunteers as well as in helping them become more sensitive to the role language plays in shaping our views of others and ourselves. For example, individuals often do not want to be labeled as "victims" or to be objects of "pity" (which is different from compassion).

Guided visits to sites of the volunteer activity (e.g., hospital, forensic institute) enable the volunteers to learn how the agencies operate in times of emergency and give them the opportunity to share and process the strong feelings evoked by these encounters.

Mentoring is a crucial aspect of the early stages of volunteering. New volunteers should be sent out with experienced volunteers who serve as role models and sources of inspiration, and help them move on gradually from an observer role to active involvement in crisis intervention. Among other things, mentors model how to assess needs; check out availability of resources, prioritize, and make cool-headed judgments; and wait patiently through the confusion of disasters, as needs are revealed and information obtained bit by bit. The latter is important in light of the natural desire to "do something" in such situations. Mentors can model the value of just being there.

New volunteers often need help in establishing realistic expectations, accepting their limitations, and dealing with the sense of powerlessness engendered by disaster work. Past help recipients who are now volunteers themselves may be particularly helpful here. They can tell of the long and painful process of coming to terms with their loss, their initial ambivalence towards receiving help, and what the long-term meaning of that help was to them. This can help new volunteers avoid unrealistic expectations and "rescue fantasies" that may result in a sense of failure, guilt, frustration, or helplessness.

The training of volunteers may use a mixture of teaching methods ranging from theory and information to nonverbal expressive techniques that enhance self-awareness and facilitate the expression of experiences that are hard to put into words. Stress management techniques are also useful. Outdoor training can prepare helpers (especially professionals accustomed to indoor clinic settings) to apply their skills in a flexible manner in a variety of situations.

Assignment. The key in assignment, both for efficiency and for volunteer fulfillment, is to assign every volunteer to do whatever he or she is good at doing. In the aftermath of a terror attack, it is also important to strike a balance between under-recruitment and over-recruitment. Under-recruitment may result in a "hole" in the safety net provided by the volunteer network or in volunteers being overwhelmed with multiple tasks they cannot carry out. Over-recruitment may result in volunteers standing around with nothing to do, after they have left their own families and other pursuits. Both are potentially demoralizing. Given the unpredictability of emergency situations, it is desirable to maintain contact with volunteers waiting for assignments. Volunteers from "reserve" teams need to be kept updated and to feel they are part of the collective effort.

STRENGTHENING RESOURCES AND PREVENTING BURNOUT

Support providers working with disaster survivors are subject to risks ranging from emotional exhaustion and burnout, through heightened anxiety and nightmares, up to secondary traumatization marked by the full range of Post Traumatic Stress Disorder (PTSD) symptoms (Jenkins & Baird, 2002). The very characteristics that motivate volunteers and make their support so valuable (i.e., their empathy, sense of shared fate, authentic closeness, and lack of professional distance) often increase these risks.

Burnout among disaster volunteers stems primarily from the enormous stress of the work, with its many demands and the resulting sense that one can never do enough. Volunteers who do not receive adequate support may soon find their emotional resources depleted. Since stress occurs when demands exceed resources (Lazarus & Folkman, 1984), to reduce this risk of burnout we must provide ongoing support to conserve, strengthen, and build the volunteers' inner resources to meet the demands they face. Applying terminology of Conservation of Resources theory (Hobfoll, 1998), strengthening these resources through the support of an organization, peer support, and individual supervision may enable "a gain cycle" instead of a "loss" cycle to take place. A strength-based approach that acknowledges the difficulties as well as the rewards can promote volunteer motivation.

In group supervision, the most prevalent concerns can be addressed, including nightmares, survivor guilt, role ambiguity, and boundaries. It often reassures volunteers in this work to know how common nightmares are among them. Because of the salience of survivor guilt among disaster volunteers, with the attendant difficulties about enjoying themselves and even returning to their regular routine, it may be necessary to legitimize continuing life and living. To cope with the sense of powerlessness and helplessness they often feel, it is important to help volunteers come to terms with the impossibility of taking away pain. This is especially relevant since the desire to alleviate suffering is generally a major motive for their volunteering. Non-professional volunteers may need help in defining their roles, since they are not quite friends, yet do not act in a professional capacity. In general, support providers walk a tightrope between over-identification and protective distancing (Meichenbaum,

1997). Helping them to find an optimal interpersonal space reduces the risk of debilitating over-involvement.

Volunteers often ask, "Am I doing the right thing?" Meetings, workshops, and seminars can provide essential feedback, affirmation, and reassurance. The shocked, grieving, and traumatized people they work with cannot be expected to do this.

Group work can also help volunteers discover their strengths and maximize the gains from their participation in disaster relief work, such as increased understanding of self and others, improved ability to react logically in abnormal situations, and coping with pressure. It can help them gain perspective and learn to communicate with people from different backgrounds. The volunteer group validates the work that has been done and may help transform the potentially debilitating experience into a growth-promoting one.

Balancing the demands of family and volunteering (as well as work) is no simple matter. Volunteers may feel that their families and friends cannot understand what they go through. Indeed, after stressful encounters the transition to a regular home routine can be most difficult (Danieli, 2002). Having confronted so much pain, everyday matters can seem trivial and even irritating. Domestic issues may be dwarfed in comparison, and the volunteer may feel preoccupied with thoughts about the scenes s/he has witnessed and worry about those in distress. Family support can be mobilized by joint sessions or activities. Family members need to know about the challenges and stresses, as well as about the importance of the endeavor. This can help them achieve better understanding and acceptance of the volunteer's reactions upon returning home from difficult experiences.

Creating and maintaining a sense of belonging, meaning, and purpose is essential to preventing burnout. When volunteers feel part of a team, receive recognition for their efforts, and are involved in decision-making, their initial motivation is enhanced and the risk of burnout and secondary trauma is reduced.

VOLUNTEERS FROM AMONG TRAUMA SURVIVORS– MODELS OF POST-TRAUMATIC GROWTH

In addition to the support all volunteers need, special attention should be given to those who have coped with tragedy themselves and now reach out to help others. It is important to acknowledge their unique contribution and the ways they can help and be helped at the same time. Helping others is a survivor mission (Herman, 1992) which may serve as a way of reconstructing the personal world of meaning that has been challenged by their trauma and loss, reconnecting to the community, and restoring some sense of control.

Having experienced and navigated the painstaking course of working through their own trauma and loss, such volunteers have a special sensitivity, understanding, and perspective. Their contribution to the volunteer endeavor is immense. For the newly bereaved and injured, they often are able to offer a unique source of support that conveys a special understanding without their having to say a word. They act as role models of post-traumatic growth whose value has been demonstrated in clinical reports as well as research (Tedeschi, Park, & Calhoun, 1998).

As illustrated below, the most significant contribution of these volunteers is not necessarily at the first post-impact stage, but later. They can be excellent teachers for other volunteers by sharing their experiences of receiving support; what helped and what did not. They can also reassure volunteers who encounter initial rejection that they also rejected the volunteer who approached them in their grief, only to later appreciate the outreach as life-saving.

In addition to the ongoing support that all volunteers receive, these volunteers require space to share and work through their traumatic experiences and to address wounds reopened through helping others. Otherwise, they are prone to over-identification impeding their ability to provide support. They may need help in setting boundaries and differentiating between their own experience and coping strategies, and those of the people they help. Some of them must also be protected from taking too much on themselves too soon after their traumatic experience.

Volunteers who were themselves traumatized pass on what they have gained from the volunteers who reached out to them to the persons to whom they reach out. Tanya (names have been changed to protect identities) lost her son Vladik in a sniper attack some three years after her immigration from Belarus. At first she did not want to live. Luda, a volunteer whose son had been killed three years earlier, provided her with a role model for living. As Tanya told:

> "It was the first time I met a woman with the same fate. I saw a woman who was alive, who wants to continue living, working, eating; a woman with her two feet on the ground. At that moment I understood that I would actually live." When Tanya became an active Selah volunteer several years later, she visited other bereaved families. Telling of her first volunteering experience, she related: "I heard a bereaved mother saying, 'I don't want to live.' I clearly remembered how I felt exactly the same way. I spoke with her about how I had felt and how I continue to live. I believe it helped her, just like what I heard from Luda helped me."

Tanya also recounted the benefits of the processes she experienced in Selah seminars: "At home I cry alone, so that my husband won't see. And he does the same. In the seminar we cried and laughed together without being judged or criticized. The tools I received afterwards in the volunteer seminars helped me in dealing with my own grief. They are tools for life and not just for helping others in crisis: learning to listen, to reach out, and to share. When I give strength to others, I take strength from it. What I do as a volunteer is my own self-psychoanalysis. I never stop thinking of Vladik. When I share my experience, I keep his memory alive."

REFERENCES

Caplan, G. (1964). *Principles of preventive psychiatry*. New York: Basic Books.

Craig, S. J., & Fuchs, J. (2002). The heartland responds to terror: Volunteering after the bombing of the Murrah Federal Building. *Social Science Quarterly, 83*, 397-418.

Danieli, Y. (1994). Countertransference and trauma: Self-healing and training issues. In M. B. Williams & J. F. Sommer (Eds.), *Handbook of post-traumatic therapy* (pp. 540-550). Westport, CT: Greenwood Press.

Danieli, Y. (Ed.) (2001). *Sharing the front line and the back hills: International protectors and providers, peacekeepers, humanitarian aid workers and the media in the midst of crisis*. New York: Baywood Publishing.

Davis, M. H., Hall, J. A., & Meyer, M. (2003). The first year: Influences on the satisfaction, involvement, and persistence of new community volunteers. *Personality and Social Psychology Bulletin, 29*, 248-260.

Drabek, T. E. (1986). *Human system responses to disaster–An inventory of sociological findings*. New York: Springer-Verlag.

Figley, C. (1995). *Compassion fatigue: Coping with secondary traumatic stress disorder in those who treat the traumatized*. New York: Brunner/Mazel.

Gidron, B. (1984). Predictors of retention and turnover among service volunteer workers. *Journal of Social Service Research, 8*(1), 1-16.

Herman, J. L. (1992). *Trauma and recovery*. New York: Basic Books.

Hobfoll, S. E. (1998). *Stress, culture, and community: The psychology and philosophy of stress*. New York: Plenum.

Janoff-Bulman, R. (1985). The aftermath of victimization: Rebuilding shattered assumptions. In C. Figley (Ed.), *Trauma and its wake: Vol. 1. The study and treatment of posttraumatic stress disorder* (pp. 15-35). New York: Brunner/Mazel.

Jenkins, S. R., & Baird, S. (2002). Secondary traumatic stress and vicarious traumatization: A validational study. *International Society for Traumatic Stress Studies, 15*, 423-432.

Lafer, B. (1991). The attrition of hospice volunteers. *Omega, 23*, 161-168.

Lazarus, R. S., & Folkman, S. (1984). *Stress, appraisal and coping*. New York: Springer.

Meichenbaum, D. (1997). *Treating post-traumatic stress disorder: A handbook and practice manual for therapy*. John Wiley: Brisbane.

Neimeyer, R. A., Keesee, N. J., & Former, B. V. (2000). Loss and meaning reconstruction: Propositions and procedures. In R. Malkinson, S. Rubin, & E. Wiztum (Eds.), *Traumatic and non-traumatic loss and bereavement* (pp. 197-230). Madison, CT: Psychosocial Press.

Norris, F., Friedman, M., Watson, P., Byrne, C., Diaz, E., & Kaniasty, K. (2002). 60,000 disaster victims speak: Part I. An empirical review of the empirical literature, 1981-2001. *Psychiatry, 65*(3), 207-239.

Omoto, A. M., & Snyder, M. (1990). Basic research in action: Volunteerism and society's responses to AIDS. *Personality and Social Psychology Bulletin, 16*, 152-156.

Penner, L. A., & Finkelstein, M. A. (1998). Dispositional and structural determinants of volunteerism. *Journal of Personality and Social Psychology, 74*(2), 525-537.

Rosse, W. (1993). Volunteers and post-disaster recovery: A call for community self-sufficiency. *Journal of Social Behavior and Personality, 8*, 261-266.

Tedeschi, R., Park, C., & Calhoun, L. (Eds.) (1998). *Posttraumatic growth: Positive changes in the aftermath of crisis*. Mahwah, NJ: Lawrence Erlbaum.

Ursano, R. J., Fullerton, C. S., Vance, K., & Tzu-Cheg, K. (1999). Posttraumatic stress disorder and identification in disaster workers. *The American Journal of Psychiatry, 156*, 353-340.

Volkan, V. D. (1981). *Linking objects and linking phenomena*. New York: International University Press.

Walsh, F. (2002). Bouncing forward: Resilience in the aftermath of September 11. *Family Process, 41*(1), 34-36.

Weiss, T. (2002). Posttraumatic growth in women with breast cancer and their husbands: An intersubjective validation study. *Journal of Psychosocial Oncology, 20*(2), 65-80.

White, M., & Epston, D. (1990). *Narrative means to therapeutic ends*. New York: Norton.

Wilson, J., & Musick, M. (1997). Who cares: Toward an integrated theory of volunteer work. *American Sociological Review, 62*, 694-713.

Volunteers in Disaster Response: The American Red Cross

Susan E. Hamilton

SUMMARY. Terrorism directed against the United States abroad and at home during the 1990s, in conjunction with the ongoing terrorist threat and use of weapons of mass destruction, and mass casualty disasters demanded a reexamination of national security and disaster response. Strategies to confront current threats and meet population needs include increasing collaboration and cooperation among federal, state, and county agencies and voluntary organizations. The American Red Cross has implemented training to familiarize participants with terrorist threats and the characteristics of chemical, biological, radiological, nuclear, and explosive weapons and has introduced technological changes to speed up service delivery at disasters.

KEYWORDS. American Red Cross, disaster response, terrorism, volunteer

Address correspondence to: Susan E. Hamilton, PhD, American Red Cross National Headquarters, 2025 E Street NW, Washington, DC 20006 USA (E-mail: Hamiltons@usa.redcross.org).

[Haworth co-indexing entry note]: "Volunteers in Disaster Response: The American Red Cross." Hamilton, Susan E. Co-published simultaneously in *Journal of Aggression, Maltreatment & Trauma* (The Haworth Maltreatment & Trauma Press, an imprint of The Haworth Press, Inc.) Vol. 10, No. 1/2, 2005; and: *The Trauma of Terrorism: Sharing Knowledge and Shared Care, An International Handbook* (ed: Yael Danieli, Danny Brom, and Joe Sills) The Haworth Maltreatment & Trauma Press, an imprint of The Haworth Press, Inc., 2005.

After the bombing of the Alfred P. Murrah Federal Building in Oklahoma City in 1995, the model for disaster response in the United States changed. Prior to that day, government and volunteer agency response was geared toward hurricanes, tornadoes, floods, and earthquakes. During the 1970s the nature of disaster had subtly changed as manmade disasters increased to include oil spills, chemical plant accidents, and dam breaks. Following the 1979 nuclear power plant accident at Three Mile Island, Pennsylvania, the only request from the White House to the Red Cross was to plan for a potential mass evacuation. On April 15, 1995, when a bomb exploded in the truck parked outside the Murrah Building at 9:02 a.m., the sound was heard throughout the city, was felt 55 miles away, and measured 6.0 on the Richter scale (U.S. Department of Justice, 2000). The ensuing psychological impact reverberated throughout the country. Federal and state agencies responded with appropriate urgency. By 9:25 a.m., twenty-three minutes after the explosion, the State Emergency Operations Center was operational.

Joining the state agencies, the military, and the departments of health and education, was the American Red Cross (ARC), the only non-governmental agency of 27 that has responsibilities under the Federal Response Plan, presently undergoing revision to produce the National Response Plan. The Federal Response Plan, defined in the 1988 Robert T. Stafford Disaster Relief and Emergency Assistance Act, can be partially or fully activated upon a Presidential disaster declaration. Under 12 Emergency Support Functions (ESF), it groups the types of direct federal assistance that a state is most likely to need as well as the kinds of operational support required to sustain federal response actions such as communications and transportation. The Red Cross is the primary agency for ESF #6 (Mass Care), which includes providing emergency shelter for disaster victims, feeding victims and emergency workers, bulk distribution of emergency relief items, emergency first aid, and disaster welfare information regarding individuals residing within the affected area and their reunification. The Red Cross also serves as a support agency to ESF #5 (Information and Planning), ESF #8 (Health and Medical Services), and ESF #11 (Food).

When President Clinton declared Oklahoma City a federal disaster area, the Red Cross became the lead agency in providing mass care. The following day the Red Cross took charge of the management of The Compassion Center set up to serve victims and families. To support, the center's mental health professionals were mobilized from across the county along with local clergy, police, and military chaplains. Throughout the 16 days that the center remained open, approximately 400 mental health volunteers provided services daily.

Whenever a natural or manmade disaster occurs, a local chapter of the Red Cross immediately responds with, if the size warrants, support from the state.

As disasters reach a level when the need for resources is greater than the state can provide, the overall administration transfers to the national headquarters in Washington, D.C. Volunteers are recruited through a national database, the Disaster Services Human Resource (DSHR) system, and supplies are ordered and sent from regional warehouses. The goals are to provide an effective rapid response, empower the affected people and communities, and, as soon as reasonably possible, to return the responsibility for support to the local Red Cross chapter and the community.

VOLUNTEER RECRUITING AND TRAINING

Volunteers drawn from the general population become involved through their local Red Cross chapters. Many decide to become part of the DSHR system and are deployed to disasters throughout the continental United States and its territories. Young people who have not reached the age of majority in their state are not deployed across state lines. An August 2003 DSHR statistical analysis reported 22,641 volunteers, 86.9% of the total DSHR; 11% were chapter employees, 2.1% were national employees, totaling 26,048 (American Red Cross, 2003a). Their ages ranged from 10 to over 80. The largest age group consisted of people ages 50 to 59. Two hundred and ninety-nine volunteers were 80 years old or older, many of whom are retirees. The largest ethnic group is Caucasian and more women volunteer than men. New Red Cross strategic initiatives include engaging a more diverse volunteer population and increasing efforts to attract youth as well as strengthen relationships with the older generation.

After completing a basic training course which utilizes a video that depicts the upheaval and impact of a disaster and the responsibility for response that the Red Cross assumes, volunteers choose a specific function in which to be trained, one that employs or builds upon competencies they have developed previously or for which they have a special interest. A series of Red Cross procedural documents clarifies the responsibilities of each function.

Of the 23 functions in Disaster Services, five comprise the Direct Services and involve client contact. These include (a) Mass Care; (b) Family Services, which is the largest function; (c) Health Services (HS); (d) Mental Health Services (DMHS); and (e) Disaster Welfare Information (DWI). Mass Care volunteers work on the frontlines providing shelter, and fixed and mobile feeding to clients and workers. The Health Services function, responsible for the physical health of clients and workers, offers hands-on health care at shelters, service centers, feeding and reception sites and other service delivery sites, as well as making condolence calls and arranging for the replacement of medicines, eyeglasses, or other health-related items. Family Services volunteers are trained to interview individuals to determine their progress in recovery, to identify how the Red Cross can best meet their immediate needs, and give referrals if necessary. The DWI function receives and responds to inquiries from immediate family members through the local chapters about people within the affected area. Since the September 11 terrorist attacks in 2001, a reverse inquiry system has also operated, whereby people caught in disaster circumstances could phone the Red Cross information hotline and request the DWI function to inform their families that they are safe.

The health and mental health services functions require employees and volunteers to maintain current professional licenses or certification in the state where they live or, if they are retired, from the state in which they practiced before retirement. Internal Support Services functions interface between direct and indirect client services. An administrative team supervises the functions and the service delivery plan at a Disaster Relief Operation (DRO), while function officers can request technical guidance from their Function Leads, or designees, at Red Cross national headquarters.

Pre-screening occurs before anyone is deployed. Workdays on a disaster site can be long and the hardships of some relief operations are physically unsuitable for some volunteers. After arriving at the relief operation headquarters and before they are assigned to a job site, volunteers are interviewed by health services. They then attend an orientation to acclimate them to the environmental conditions and cultural aspects specific to the disaster. Additionally, they are given Red Cross vests and identification badges to wear. During the 9/11 operations at the Pentagon and in New York, the badges also signified zones where they were permitted to work.

DISASTER MENTAL HEALTH SERVICES

It became apparent during the 1989 operations in the Caribbean and the Carolinas after Hurricane Hugo and the Loma Prieta Earthquake in northern California that considerable emotional support was needed by workers and victims. A survey of disaster workers indicated that creating a separate mental health program was warranted. A year later, the DMHS function was established and by 1992 (revised 1995), a two-day training course was developed "to prepare participants to use their professional skills to provide the specific activities and interventions necessary to meet the immediate disaster-related mental health needs of Red Cross workers, their families, and people affected by disaster" (American Red Cross, 1998a, p. 1).

Experienced mental health volunteers familiar with current disaster regulations and procedures and agreements with other agencies providing disaster relief teach the course at Red Cross chapters. After completing the course, participants are able to: (a) identify the range of emotions experienced by clients, as well as Red Cross employees and volunteers, during disasters and Red Cross relief operations, (b) understand some of the factors that might influence the emotional impact on the community, (c) describe the role of Red Cross DMHS and how it supports Red Cross disaster relief operations on major relief operations as well as in local chapters, (d) describe the various setting in which DMHS operates, (e) demonstrate the mental health techniques used by DMHS, and (f) develop a plan of action for further involvement with the Red Cross (American Red Cross, 1998a, p. 1).

A disaster environment is a constantly changing milieu where flexibility and teamwork are imperative to success. The course is designed to build on existing skills and provide tools and techniques useful within Red Cross settings and does not teach clinical or crisis intervention skills. The competencies employed are those used in clinical practice. These include: (a) listening, (b) observing, and (c) reframing in order to monitor and reduce high levels of stress. Red Cross mental health workers do not provide psychotherapy. Experience has shown that 70% of the time they are engaged in education, problem solving, and advocacy, and during the remainder they provide interventions related to the crisis, stress factors, and coping strategies (American Red Cross, 1998a).

The Red Cross makes mental health brochures available for disaster victims of different age groups in English, Spanish, and several other languages, as well as brochures for volunteers and their families that explain stress management, the use of positive coping strategies, and how to monitor their own emotional well-being during their work and when they have returned home. In 2001, a three-hour DMHS Overview Course was developed to show the work of the mental health function to other volunteers, and when and how they could make referrals to mental health. Since its inception, the DMHS function has grown considerably, from less than a hundred people in August 1992 to 470 by mid-November 1993. Ten years later, in August 2003, it had grown to 3,464.

The mental health function works closely with the public affairs function, which is tasked with media dissemination, arranging radio, television and film interviews, as well as crafting messaging to the public at the local, state, and national level. At the Oklahoma City bombing the intense media intrusion had to be contained; mental health workers briefed and accompanied survivors and family members who were willing to speak with the press. However, not all clients wish to be shielded from the media. For cultural and/or political reasons families and survivors may seek media attention. In 1997, at the Korean Airlines disaster family assistance center in Guam, the media were highly visible, and the Korean family members wished very much to speak with them.

The advent of terrorist threat and from experience at two domestic and international exercises designed to produce a more effective, coordinated global response to Weapons of Mass Destruction/Terrorism (WMD/T), sensitized the Red Cross to the importance of risk communication. Immediately following a WMD/T event, multiple organizations release information to the public. Fear and confusion can increase and impinge upon people's ability to make life-saving decisions when information about the nature of the event is delayed. A Red Cross objective is to mount a post-event messaging strategy to reduce public fear through information and reassurance in the immediate aftermath of the event.

INTERAGENCY COOPERATION AND COLLABORATION

During the year following the events of September 11, 2001, the Red Cross conducted a survey to identify the lessons learned, key issues, and success factors that could be used in future disaster planning and preparedness. The impacted chapters and the operations voiced concern at the emotional toll on Red Cross responders. The survey findings indicated that rotating staff would be one way of lessening the emotional impact and the report emphasized the importance of continuing to increase mental health services capacity. Workers found that exit interviews during which they could discuss their experience were satisfying (American Red Cross, 2002). An emerging issue was that the staff was not fully prepared for the unique features of a terrorist attack and/or for an urban metropolitan disaster relief operation, nor had they been trained for a WMD/T response that involved high security. The survey showed that staff preparation and operational orientation is of paramount importance and that future planning must encompass both the need to respond quickly and the need for worker safety (American Red Cross, 2002). This requires coordination with local authorities and establishing safe zones for Red Cross and other responders.

If the Oklahoma bombing served to awaken agency cooperation and collaboration, six and a half years later the tragedies that resulted from the catastrophic terrorist attacks on September 11, 2001 accelerated government and volunteer agency action. The attacks exposed our vulnerability and the need for greater mitigation and interagency response planning. Both the bombing in Oklahoma City and those on 9/11 at the World Trade Center, the Pentagon, and in Shanksville, Pennsylvania occurred early in the day. On each occasion federal and state agencies, local emergency response departments and the numerous non-governmental volunteer agencies responded immediately. Mental Health All-Hazards Disaster Planning Guidance, published by the Center for Mental Health Services and the Substance Abuse and Mental Health Services Administration in 2003, details the planning necessary for coordinated State and local mental health agencies (www.samhsa.gov).

The National Voluntary Organizations Active in Disaster (NOVAD) is an umbrella organization that facilitates inter-agency cooperation and coordinates planning efforts, helping to avoid duplication by the 38 national member agencies. Besides the Red Cross, other prominent agencies include the Salvation Army, the National Organization of Victim Assistance, the Church of the Brethren, the Lutheran Disaster Response, Church World Services, the Adventist Community, Catholic Charities, and the International Critical Incident Stress Foundation. Non-governmental agencies can mutually support one another by cross-training and by engaging in ongoing dialogue. Since the events of 9/11, regular inter-agency meetings have been held to promote greater collaboration. The Red Cross DMHS function enjoys a strong relationship with the national mental health organizations and associations.

On September 11, 2001, as people began to understand the enormity of what had happened, a surge of spontaneous local volunteers, eager to help but with little or no previous disaster experience, arrived at the American Red Cross Greater New York chapter on Manhattan. This produced overwhelming difficulties for the recruitment system, as there were no systems in place to identify spontaneous volunteers with the needed special skills and then place them in appropriate roles. The systems to select, orient, train, and provide meaningful work were inadequate to meet the demands from the operations in New Jersey, New York City, and Washington, D.C. More than 51,000 people converged on the American Red Cross after September 11. They helped in any way they could, interpreting one or more of the 130 languages spoken by victims, making sandwiches for rescue workers, helping stranded passengers at airports where planes were grounded. Red Cross volunteers in Canada delighted stranded travelers with home-cooked meals, free taxi service, even new underwear for those separated from their luggage. Across the country people rallied.

It was quickly understood that service provision would be required beyond the usual time period; at four weeks the degree of activity was comparable to the second day at other large relief operations. It was crucial that the Red Cross institute ongoing volunteer training because the needs in New York and Washington far exceeded those normally occurring in a disaster.

At the New York Office of Emergency Management, Red Cross volunteers were among other volunteers who staffed the hotline used by families calling to learn whether and where their loved ones were hospitalized. The Red Cross hotline in Falls Church, Virginia, staffed by volunteers recruited from across the country had handled 43,000 calls by September 19, 2001. Callers phoned to express their grief, to find a way to assist those who were suffering, or to learn how to protect their families from another terrorist attack. Mental health volunteers handled phone calls to families whose loved ones had still not been found. Because of the disturbing nature of the calls received, the DWI function requested extra full-time support from mental health workers.

AVIATION INCIDENT AND MASS CASUALTY DISASTERS TRAINING

Fortuitously, between the time of the Oklahoma City bombing and the tragedies in 2001 the Red Cross had developed an Aviation Incident Response training and a Mass Casualty Disasters training. The Aviation Disaster Family Assistance Act of 1996 authorized the National Transportation Board (NTSB) to designate a not-for-profit organization to have primary responsibility for coordinating the emergency care and support of the families of passengers involved in aircraft accidents. NTSB chose the Red Cross to fulfill that responsibility, largely because of the Red Cross response in Oklahoma (American Red Cross, 1998b). The Aviation Incident Response (AIR) team was deployed for the first time at the Korean Airlines crash on Guam, and since then has been deployed at all major air crashes. The AIR team consisted of experienced volunteers from the functions who could support family care and mental health. These included: (a) Mass Care and Health Services; (b) Disaster Mental Health Services, to provide a supportive emotional presence at the Family Assistance Center; (c) Public Affairs, to circumnavigate the inexhaustible media inquiries; and (d) Administration, to give overall direction to the relief operation and submit daily reports to national headquarters. Other functions provided logistical and technological support. Volunteers were expected to have a thorough knowledge of all aspects related to aviation and transportation incidents.

CRITICAL RESPONSE TEAM TRAINING

During the summer of 2003 the AIR Team was expanded to a Critical Response Team (CRT), able to deploy within four hours for any mass casualty incident, and provided with additional training. The CRT provides services to aviation and other transportation disasters, events caused by weapons of mass destruction, and structural collapses resulting in large numbers of fatalities. The training given to the CRT includes issues that may arise during a critical incident including: (a) significant level of response at the scene of the incident; (b) survivors and victims triaged and treated at the scene and at hospitals or clinics; (c) need to recover the dead and initiate special morgue operations; (d) need for assistance to victims and/or survivors at the scene; (e) need for assistance to families of victims and/or survivors at the scene and, in transportation incidents, at points of origin or destination or at locations near families or communities affected by the disaster; (f) significant media attention; (g) major use of a wide range of health care providers; (h) hospitals and medical personnel may be overwhelmed; (i) involvement of governmental regulatory agencies; and (j) involvement of diplomatic agencies (American Red Cross, 2003b).

Immediate psychological effects may appear as physical complaints such as headaches or diarrhea, which can be confused as symptoms of exposure to an agent. As a result, many people may seek medical treatment even though the symptoms are caused by stress, not exposure. Materials on Mass Trauma Preparedness and Response from the Centers for Disease Control and Prevention web site (http://www.cdc.gov/masstrauma/default.htm) are discussed during the training program. An examination of past mass trauma events shows patterns of hospital use which indicate that within 90 minutes following an event, 50-80% of the acute casualties will likely arrive at the closest medical facilities via ground transportation or spontaneously while hospitals outside the area usually receive few or no casualties. One-third of acute casualties are critical while two-thirds are treated and released from the emergency department (American Red Cross, 2003b). It can be expected that a terrorist bombing would cause a similar casualty pattern.

Participants in the training are familiarized with the threats and characteristics of chemical, biological, radiological, nuclear, and explosive weapons (CBRNE). They are also trained to identify possible clients and their needs following a CBRNE incident and the safety and security concerns that follow a terrorist use of a CBRNE Weapon of Mass Destruction. The Red Cross holds the safety of its workers as the highest priority; before deployment, the CRT would conduct an initial threat assessment and gather essential information on the incident. There could be possible restrictions on normal service delivery methods. Among the first responders arriving at a WMD/T scene are Law Enforcement officials, the Fire Department and the Emergency Medical Service. It should be noted that the Red Cross is a second responder. When there is a concern over safety to unprotected individuals due to a hazard, Hazard Control Zones are established. The Red Cross works within the Incident Management System also known as Incident Command System and in WMD/T events takes direction from local/federal authorities regarding safety and hazardous conditions.

As well as understanding the threats, characteristics, and potential human impacts, Red Cross employees and volunteers need to understand what and how other government and other volunteer agencies become involved. Before the Department of Homeland Security was created, a variety of response plans governed response. In the future, the evolving National Incident Management System (NIMS) and the National Response Plan, a federal plan for an all-hazard response, will serve as the framework for response. Understanding the unification of plans and how the Red Cross relates to them is complex, not yet entirely clear, and an ongoing challenge.

NEW DEVELOPMENTS IN THE RED CROSS

Mainly in reaction to the 9/11 terrorist attacks, lessons learned, and consequent changes in Red Cross leadership and upper management, in 2002 the Board of Governors launched an organizational review. In 2003, the ARC announced a Strategic Plan for Fiscal Years 2004-2008 that describes a structure for planning across the organization. Among the contextual trends that influenced the plan were the enlarged population, increased diversity and age, the population shift to urban and coastal areas and toward more disaster prone areas, the increasing number and cost of disasters, and the pervasive reality of terrorism. The threat of terrorist activity meant that the Red Cross would have to strengthen its plan for Homeland Security to ensure an integrated response and preparedness effort across all its units and partner agencies. This translates into developing seamless, high quality client service, better partnering with other voluntary agencies, and inspiring a new and diverse generation of volunteers.

As part of the refocus on disaster, a task force examined the structure of Disaster Services and the Chapter Services Network to determine how most effectively to support the service delivery capacity of field units, and provide greater client satisfaction and swifter response. A Service Area system of operations will replace the current system of regions. Eight Service Area teams will be formed serving a defined area that is based on population density, geography and similarities in known potential hazards and threats, and similar population characteristics, such as demographics and culture. This will bring closer operational response.

The new Disaster Services Technology Integration Program (DSTIP) will bring challenges to Red Cross disaster workers. Larger relief operations will use high-tech tools that will be independent of local infrastructure. Employees and volunteers will use a new Client Relationship Management System to enter data and manage cases and those on-site will be able to share information with national headquarters. Already, many chapters are using the new Red Cross Client Assistance Card, a stored-value card activated through the Internet and used much like a bank debit card. The cards can be used to purchase emergency food and supplies. Volunteers wanting to work in this system will be required to develop or improve their computer skills.

A new volunteer management project will consolidate human resources data about paid staff, volunteers, and DSHR System members to match volunteer skills with function needs during a relief operation. Individual career development and training needs will be analyzed to improve capacity building. In a WMD/T response, this will speed the review of volunteer training and history, hastening their placement and speeding up service delivery.

The American Red Cross has embraced the challenges that arose in Oklahoma in 1995 and six years later in New York City and Washington. Today, the Red Cross is confronting the demands of relief operations in a dynamic and innovative way. What is emerging is a more efficient and more productive system that brings greater satisfaction to clients, employees, and volunteers. However, even though technology will enable the Red Cross to respond to disasters more promptly and efficiently, the foundation of Red Cross disaster relief remains, as it has always been, the compassionate volunteer.

REFERENCES

American Red Cross. (1998a). *Disaster mental health services 1* (ARC Publication No. 3077-1F). Washington, DC: Author.

American Red Cross. (1998b). *Statement of understanding between the American Red Cross and the National Transportation Safety Board.* Washington, DC: American Red Cross.

American Red Cross. (2001). *Disaster mental health services: An overview* (ARC Publication No. 3077-2). Washington, DC: American Red Cross.

American Red Cross. (2002). [American Red Cross Response to the events of September 11, 2002]. Unpublished raw data.

American Red Cross. (2003a). [American Red Cross DSHR analysis]. Unpublished raw data.

American Red Cross. (2003b). *Critical response team (CRT) course* (ARC No. 3079-4). Unpublished internal document.

Federal Emergency Management Agency. (1999). *Federal response plan* (FEMA Publication No. 9231.1-PL). Washington, DC: Federal Emergency Management Agency.

Public Law 104-264, title VII, Aviation Disaster Family Assistance Act of 1996, October 9, 1996.

U.S. Department of Health and Human Services. (2003). *Mental health all-hazard disaster planning guidance* (DHHS Pub. No. SMA 3829). Rockville, MD: Center for Mental Health Services, Substance Abuse and Mental Health Services Administration.

U.S. Department of Justice. (2000). *Responding to terrorism victims: Oklahoma City and beyond* (NCJ Publication No.183949). Washington, DC: U.S. Department of Justice.

Training Therapists to Treat the Psychological Consequences of Terrorism: Disseminating Psychotherapy Research and Researching Psychotherapy Dissemination

Lawrence V. Amsel
Yuval Neria
Randall D. Marshall
Eun Jung Suh

SUMMARY. In the wake of 9/11, the mental health community began to develop a model for recovery and preparedness. A public information campaign regarding the psychological consequences of terrorism was launched, and it succeeded in reducing the stigma of utilizing mental health services. However, as this campaign began to succeed, it became clear that most clinicians in the community had little training in evidence-based assessment and treatment procedures for the psychological sequelae of terrorism. This article describes the development, delivery, and initial assessment of one attempt to correct this problem by broadly disseminating an effective treatment for Post Traumatic Stress Disorder

Address correspondence to: Lawrence V. Amsel, MD, MPH, 245 West 107th Street, Suite # 14-F, New York, NY 10025-3064 USA (E-mail: LVA2@columbia. edu).

[Haworth co-indexing entry note]: "Training Therapists to Treat the Psychological Consequences of Terrorism: Disseminating Psychotherapy Research and Researching Psychotherapy Dissemination." Amsel, Lawrence V. et al. Co-published simultaneously in *Journal of Aggression, Maltreatment & Trauma* (The Haworth Maltreatment & Trauma Press, an imprint of The Haworth Press, Inc.) Vol. 10, No. 1/2, 2005; and: *The Trauma of Terrorism: Sharing Knowledge and Shared Care, An International Handbook* (ed: Yael Danieli, Danny Brom, and Joe Sills) The Haworth Maltreatment & Trauma Press, an imprint of The Haworth Press, Inc., 2005.

(PTSD). Using models of behavior change, we were able to study trainee attitudes and the training process in ways that will help improve training effectiveness beyond what traditional Continuing Professional Education (CPE) has been able to do.

KEYWORDS. Evidence-based medicine, mental health services, training evaluation

The psychological consequences of the 9/11 terrorist attacks were substantial and were not confined by time or space to those directly involved. Rather, these psychological effects were dispersed broadly throughout the larger community, and have persisted over an extended period of time. The psychological consequences of the 9/11 attacks thus constitute a significant mental health challenge to the broad population, and require a comprehensive public mental health response. In particular, a workforce of trauma-savvy mental health providers is needed to treat those who have developed serious psychiatric conditions such as PTSD and Major Depression in the wake of 9/11.

In its report on developing a public health strategy to prepare for the psychological consequences of terrorism, the Institute of Medicine (IOM) concluded that, as a workforce, mental health professionals are inadequately prepared to meet the needs generated by the events of 9/11 or any future mass trauma (Butler, Panzer, & Goldfrank, 2003). Most mental health professionals lack training in the appropriate treatments for the psychological effects of trauma. The IOM, therefore, stressed the need to ensure that mental health professionals rapidly obtain adequate training in the psychological aspects of trauma and disasters in general, and in the treatments of the serious psychological disorders that can result from such disasters in particular.

WHAT THERAPISTS DO NOT KNOW
ABOUT PSYCHOLOGICAL TRAUMA AND ITS TREATMENT

When it comes to the treatment of full syndromal Post Traumatic Stress Disorder (PTSD), there is a solid evidence base for effective psychotherapy treatment, as well as studies on the appropriate uses of medication (Davis, English, Ambrose, & Petty, 2001). In particular, a form of Cognitive Behavioral Therapy (CBT) that incorporates imaginal exposure exercises has been repeatedly shown to be the most effective psychotherapy treatment for PTSD (Taylor et al., 2003). Imaginal exposure is a therapeutic exercise in which an intense remembering of the trauma serves to desensitize and habituate the traumatic memories, and thus robs them of much of their toxic power. Because this is done repeatedly, it is referred to as prolonged exposure (PE), and the whole treatment is often abbreviated as CBT-PE.

Despite strong evidence for its efficacy, most clinicians are either unaware of CBT-PE or, if aware, do not practice it. A survey of psychologists conducted by Becker, Zayfert, and Anderson (in press) demonstrated that only 27% of the psychologists surveyed had been trained in the use of CBT-PE for PTSD, and only 9% reported that they use it with the majority of their PTSD patients. The most frequently cited reasons for not using CBT-PE with PTSD patients were either a lack of training (60%), resistance to manualized treatments (25%), or fears of re-traumatizing patients (22%).

Thus, while the public outreach and educational programs initiated after 9/11 seemed to be having the intended results of lowering stigma and bringing those in need to the clinic, the mental health professionals were poorly prepared to treat them, and were in sore need of training in treatments for the psychological sequelae of terrorism. In this context, the unit on Trauma Studies and Services (TSS) of the New York Psychiatric Institute/Columbia University, as part of establishing a mental health preparedness infrastructure, created and delivered a training program for the broad community of mental health clinicians practicing in New York. The size and scope of this dissemination project, as well as its potential consequences, were unprecedented. Our first goal was therefore to develop a training program based on the best available evidence of effective methods for disseminating psychotherapy. As this was going to be a very large dissemination effort, a second goal was to use the training program to answer questions about improving the effectiveness of large-scale psychotherapy training projects.

PRIOR EXPERIENCE WITH DISSEMINATING CBT-PE FOR PTSD

The last decade has seen a great effort to ground clinical practice in empirical evidence. This proved to be more difficult than anticipated (for a review see Beutler, Moleiro, & Talebi, 2002; Chambless & Ollendick, 2001). In particular, traditional Continuing Professional Education (CPE), which had been based on an information transmission model, has repeatedly been shown to be ineffective at producing the kind of change in clinicians' behavior that was required to achieve an evidence-based (EB) style of practice (Davis et al., 1999).

Nevertheless, there have been reports of successful psychotherapy dissemination projects, and, closer to our interests, programs focused specifically on CBT-PE (Cahill, Hembree, & Foa, in press). The first project described by Cahill et al. (in press) consisted of an intensive weeklong workshop followed by group weekly supervision, which continued for several years (see Foa, Hembree, Feeny, & Zoellner, 2002). Those patients who were treated by the trainees showed therapeutic outcomes comparable to those treated by the original research group, indicating a successful dissemination. These results were then replicated at several sites.

Another dissemination project more closely resembles our situation. Gillespie, Duffy, Hackmann, and Clark (2002) report on disseminating CBT-PE to community clinicians in the wake of the Omagh terrorist bombing in Northern Ireland in 1998 (see Campbell, Cairns, & Mallett, this volume). The dissemination model used was similar to the one described above. The training of five selected therapists began with intensive workshops lasting several days, and was followed by monthly group supervision based on videotaped therapy sessions. A total of 91 patients with PTSD directly related to the bombing completed the treatment. The patients showed significant improvement, and their outcomes were again comparable to that obtained with CBT-PE in research settings.

There are a number of difficulties with adopting the dissemination examples described above. First, they are focused on training a few select clinicians who intend to become experts in this treatment model. The huge investment of time and resources by trainees and trainers in intensive ongoing supervision was, therefore, both justified and feasible. However, the costs of intensive personal supervision for the hundreds of trainees involved in a community-wide dissemination project would be prohibitive and not clearly justified. In his review, Addis (2000) found these limitations to be a common problem for broad dissemination projects. A second difficulty is that the above-mentioned dissemination reports do not describe, in any specific fashion, the actual training process. Given that these research groups are highly experienced with describing therapeutic interventions in specific, measurable and reproducible fashion, it is surprising that their training methods are summed up by vaguely referring to an intense workshop and ongoing supervision.

The challenges for widespread dissemination projects that emerged from these considerations are, first, to find the most effective way to use the limited contact time with trainees in order to achieve maximum change in clinical behaviors and, second, to describe precisely a training process that can be empirically studied. Our work attempted to take some first steps in responding to these challenges.

METHODOLOGY: DESIGNING THE TRAINING PROGRAM AND EVALUATING TRAINEES' ATTITUDES

In designing our training program to reach as broad a group of clinicians as possible, we were faced with real world limitations relating to clinicians' time, clinics' abilities to release clinicians for continuing education, and available training funds. It thus became clear that, as a basic fixed parameter, the dissemination program would consist of workshops involving two full days of intensive training for groups of approximately 50 licensed mental health clinicians at a time. Within these limitations our challenge was to utilize behavior change theories and research to structure the trainings in a way that would maximize their impact on the factors that contribute to clinician behavior change. In particular we aimed, not at information exchange, but rather at impacting clinicians' attitudes towards CBT-PE, their perception of current therapeutic norms, their self-efficacy for specific therapy skills, and their intention to adopt these techniques.

The impact on clinical behavior of a dissemination or training intervention involves both the content of what is being disseminated and the training process. These two dimensions must be considered individually and interactively just as length and width are inseparable in the understanding of area. We begin with a discussion of aspects of the content.

First, the content of the training, which in our case is the treatment of PTSD by CBT-PE, needed to be decomposed into specifically defined and operationalized components. Only when these components are so identified can one begin to learn what therapists believe about these components, what their skill levels in executing these components are, and how likely they are to adopt these components into practice after a dissemination intervention. Of equal importance, one can then also identify the barriers to adoption for each of the specified components, and begin to address the identified barriers. Without this decomposition or dismantling, it is very difficult to understand how a complex, multi-part psychotherapy is being perceived and what helps or hurts its general adoption by front-line clinicians.

In identifying the individual components of CBT-PE we relied on work by Blagys and Hilsenroth (2002), which reviewed the psychotherapy process literature in order to identify elements of CBT that were distinctive from other forms of therapy. Using these findings as a starting point and reviewing Foa's treatment manual (Foa, Rothbaum, Riggs, & Murdock, 1991), we identified ten component recommendations for CBT-PE (see Table 1). We included psycho-education (which is not distinctive to CBT but rather applied very generally across many therapies) to serve as a control against which we could measure attitudes towards the other components.

TABLE 1. Component CBT for PTSD

1.	Diagnostic evaluation and patient selection.
2.	Prolonged exposure.
3.	Breathing retraining exercises.
4.	Psycho-education.
5.	In vivo exposure.
6.	Conduct the treatment according to the manual.
7.	The use of structured instruments or forms.
8.	Homework assignments and their documentation.
9.	Cognitive restructuring.
10.	The use of Subjective Units of Distress (SUDs).

Having decomposed CBT-PE into individual component recommendations, we measured trainees' attitudes toward these recommendations with questionnaires given at the start of the training. The Attitudes Towards CBT-PE Questionnaires asked participants to rate each recommendation on its favorability using a scale ranging from −5 (very unfavorable attitude) to +5 (very favorable attitude), as well as rating their ability, or self-efficacy, to carry out each recommendation, again rated on a scale from −5 (very hard to implement) to +5 (very easy to implement), as well as a number of other attitudes which we will not cover in this report. These questionnaires covered participants' responses to the content of the training.

As mentioned above, the second dimension of interest, which is often glossed over in the dissemination research, involved the specifics of the training process. The format of our training, which relied on the behavior change literature, involved the combined use of three educational modalities including: (a) Lectures were focused on addressing clinicians' beliefs regarding expected outcomes of the recommended interventions. This was done by presenting both a persuasive rationale for the treatment design, and convincing research evidence for the efficacy of the treatment. (b) Clinical demonstrations by faculty illustrated specific clinical techniques, such as the diagnostic interview. These demonstrations served to model clinical practice by an identified expert, and were expected to have their greatest impact on the perception of norms, and to impact skill acquisition. (c) Role-play by participant of specific therapeutic techniques involved trainees alternating in taking the part of the therapist and the patient. While lectures and clinical demonstration are passive teaching modalities, these role-play sessions were active. Research has shown that active practice is required to actually alter skill levels and self-efficacy, which is the perception of those skill levels (Smith, 2000). Questions and discussion were encouraged throughout all modalities of the program to address potential barriers to implementation for each technique being taught.

To evaluate participants' responses to the training process we developed the Teaching Modality Questionnaire, in which participants were asked to rate (on a scale from −5 to +5) how effective they believed each of the three modalities (i.e., lectures, demonstrations, and role-play) was at influencing each of seven educational factors: (a) conveying theoretical principles, (b) conveying methodological details of the therapy, (c) changing beliefs, (d) changing initial reservations or objections, (e) overcoming barriers to implementation, (f) promoting skill acquisition, and (g) motivating practice change.

RESULTS AND DISCUSSION I

Trainees' Attitudes Towards Workshop Content (CBT-PE)

The results reported here are based on an analysis of an initial group of 104 clinicians who participated in the training workshops and completed Questionnaires at the start of the training and at the close of the training. The group consisted of 81% female, with a mean age of 49. Demographically, the group was 81% white, 10% Hispanic, 6% Asian and 2% African American. The participants had a mean of 17 years in practice, and were in a variety of disciplines, with 57% in social work, 18% in psychology, 8% in psychiatry, 2% in nursing, and the rest in miscellaneous helping professions. In this section (see Table 2) we will present the results and discussion of the findings for the Attitudes Towards CBT-PE Questionnaire, and in the next section we will present results and discussion for the Teaching Modality Questionnaire.

As expected, subjects rated psycho-education differently than the other recommendations. The mean favorability rating for psycho-education was 4.6 (SD 0.7) out of a possible 5, while the mean rating for self-efficacy in performing psycho-education was 3.8 (SD 1.8). Clinicians' ratings on other recommendations were, in general, significantly lower both in terms of favorability and self-efficacy.

Second, for many recommendations there was a large difference between the favorability score and self-efficacy score. That is to say that there are recommendations that clinicians saw as somewhat favorable but, nevertheless, these same clinicians had low confidence in their ability to apply these recommendations successfully. We call this an "implementation gap," and it may represent the conflict that exists between a positive attitude toward a recom-

TABLE 2. Attitudes Towards CBT-PE Questionnaire

		Favorable Attitude (-5 to $+5$)	Self Efficacy Score (-5 to $+5$)	Implementation Gap (Favorability– Self-Efficacy)
Nonspecific Component	Psycho-education	4.6 (0.7)	3.8 (1.8)	0.8
CBT-Specific Components	Prolonged (imaginal) Exposure	2.5 (2.2)**	0.3 (2.8)**	2.2**
	In Vivo Exposure	2.6 (2.2)**	0.1 (3.0)**	2.4**
	Use of Manual	1.5 (2.6)**	0.3 (2.9)**	1.1
	Structured Instruments	2.9 (2.0)**	1.8 (2.7)**	1.1
	Homework	3.0 (2.1)**	0.7 (3.0)**	2.3**
	Cognitive Restructuring	3.0 (2.3)**	1.2 (2.9)**	1.8*
	Assessment	3.8 (1.9)	1.9 (2.8)**	1.9*
	SUDS Awareness	3.4 (1.7)	2.1 (2.6)**	1.3
	Breathing Training	4.1 (1.3)	3.2 (2.2)	0.9

** $p < 0.000$ two-tailed t-test in comparison with Psycho-education score
* $p < 0.01$ two-tailed t-test in comparison with Psycho-education score

mendation, on the one hand, and concerns about personal skills and abilities to apply the recommendation, on the other.

In theory we would, therefore, expect to see several patterns. At one extreme, clinicians both support a recommendation and are confident in their ability to implement it. For this pattern there is no implementation gap and there is a high likelihood of the recommendation being implemented. For these, there is also no need for an educational intervention in the first place. This is exactly the pattern seen in psycho-education, which proved to have the smallest gap of 0.8 (which we then used as the standard for further comparisons). The breathing retraining recommendation also received very high scores, with a favorability score of 4.1 (SD 1.3) and self-efficacy score of 3.2 (SD 2.2). Together, these ratings indicate that therapists were probably already incorporating breathing techniques into their therapies, even if they used few other CBT techniques. We confirmed this impression by informal polling of therapists, who overwhelmingly confirmed that they had already incorporated breathing techniques into their practice. To our knowledge, this constitutes the first empirical documentation of how widespread the use of breathing retraining has become for psychotherapists of all theoretical persuasions.

At the other extreme are recommendations with a low favorability rating and a low self-efficacy rating. We expect recommendations with this pattern to be the most difficult to change. The recommendation to use a manual to direct individual sessions was a prime example that fell into this category. It had the lowest favorability rating of 1.5 (SD 2.6), and the second lowest self-efficacy rating of 0.3 (SD 2.9). Note that the gap of 1.2 here is relatively small. Perhaps this means that therapists do not approve of the recommendation, have poor skills to apply it and are quite comfortable with this status quo. If this is the correct interpretation, this comfort level indicates a lack of motivation to change skills or practice regarding this particular recommendation. In other words, this is a stable clinical practice that is not likely to be affected by a simple training program, unless it were to fundamentally alter attitudes, skills, or both. This is confirmed by a number of previous findings of therapist objections to, and lack of comfort with, manualized psychotherapy procedures, as described below.

Interestingly, this finding is reflected in the psychotherapy research literature, where the role of manualization is being actively debated. Garfield (1998) has argued that under certain circumstances strict adherence to a manual might be detrimental to the efficacy of psychotherapy, as therapists would not be able to deviate constructively and respond to patients individual and unique needs. Castonguay (1996) found that, in treatment for depression, an overly rigid adherence to the CBT manual correlated negatively with treatment outcome. Gibbons (2003) takes an intermediate position. While she argues for the usefulness of manuals, she believes they need to be applied with flexibility. Her study demonstrated that highly trained therapists applied the manuals with considerable flexibility and sensitivity to patients' needs. What is certain is that manualization and standardization is a key issue in disseminating evidence-based psychotherapies, and in need of much more research.

Another pattern that emerged from the trainees' responses involved a high (or moderate) favorability rating but a low self-efficacy rating. Recommendations with these patterns should respond most robustly to skill-based trainings. Notably, both imaginal exposure and in vivo exposure fell into this category.

The favorability scores for recommendations regarding careful assessment, cognitive restructuring, assigning therapeutic homework, and use of structured assessment instruments were close to each other and higher than PE, thus falling somewhere in the middle of all recommendations. These recommendations were probably seen as the workhorse components of the treatment, not well known, but not particularly controversial. Again, skill-building training could be expected to have an important effect on the adoption rate of this group of recommendations.

In summary, at entry into our training, clinicians' attitudes divided the ten recommendations into five subgroups. (a) Manualization, representing the structured approach to psychotherapy, is in a class by itself both for the low favorability rating it received and for the low self-efficacy most clinicians have towards this approach to the interpersonal work of psychotherapy. (b) Exposure work, both in-session imaginal exposure and at-home in vivo exposure, raises concerns about harming the patient, and many clinicians feared that they lacked the skills to execute these techniques properly. At the same time, their potential benefit was acknowledged. (c) Cognitive restructuring, homework assignments, teaching patients to quantify their subjective units of distress, and using structured instruments, are seen as useful but unfamiliar techniques in need of more practice. (d) Initial assessment is seen as an essential skill important to proper delivery of therapy, and a skill that clinicians are mostly comfortable with, although its relatively lower self-efficacy score of 1.9 may represent an acknowledgment that this is a difficult task. (e) Psycho-education and use of breathing retraining are already adopted parts of everyday clinical practice, although when and how this occurred remains unclear.

Thus, starting with an evidence-based treatment for PTSD, we were able to break it down into ten specific recommendations. We were then able to assess trainees' baseline attitudes and self-perceived self-efficacy for each of these recommendations, thereby clarifying what educational deficits existed for each recommendation. Our next task was to assess which training modalities best addressed which educational needs on the part of trainees with the ultimate goal of designing an efficient workshop that used the appropriate modality to address the existing cognitive, skill, or motivational deficit that was preventing the given recommendations from being practiced.

RESULTS AND DISCUSSION II

Trainees' Attitudes Towards Workshop Process

While confirming some of our assumptions, in many areas the results were both surprising and illuminating (see Table 3). First, clinical demonstrations rated highest on every dimension, even where our theoretical assumptions would have predicted otherwise. Demonstration was rated superior to lectures in changing beliefs (2.8 vs. 1.5, $p < .005$), reversing reservations (3.0 vs. 1.4, $p < .005$), and most surprisingly, even in conveying the theoretical model (3.8 vs. 3.3, $p < .005$). These are functions that we usually attribute to the purely information-imparting aspects of lectures. Equally surprising, demonstration rated higher than role-play on skill acquisition (2.9 vs. 2.2, $p < .005$), even though role-play was designed specifically for that function. An important caveat here is that watching clinical demonstration of a PTSD treatment can be a highly dramatic and emotionally salient experience, and may unduly influence participants' assessment of which modality affected which training factor.

It is therefore also important to examine each modality by itself to determine its relative effect on each of the educational factors. For example, focusing on role-play alone, it had its greatest impact on skill acquisition (2.9), followed by methodological details (2.8), and motivation (2.7). Lectures do best in conveying theoretical principles (3.3), and conveying methodological details (3.0), and do poorly on skill acquisition (2.2), and overcoming barriers (1.3), all as we would expect. However, contrary to expectation, lectures have little effect on changing beliefs (1.5), or changing initial reservations (1.4). We also expected that the experience of role-play would have more impact on overcoming barriers, yet this was rated quite poorly (2.3).

While more definitive conclusions need to await further analysis, there are some lessons to glean that may be used to improve future training and education programs in evidence-based psychotherapy.

First, lectures should continue to carry the burden of conveying theory, which they do well, but be less focused on therapeutic details, which are best conveyed in other ways. The goal of lectures is to not to teach all the details but to motivate trainees to want to educate themselves further.

Second, role-play may not be the place to change belief systems or convey theory, but could be useful in skill acquisition, motivation and beginning to assimilate therapeutic details. Given the highly positive results for demonstrations, perhaps the role-play should be modified to a hybrid somewhere between the passive observation of an expert and the active try-out of role-play, for example, the so-called *fish bowl* in which a few trainees role play while the rest watch and critique. Interestingly, this resembles the training process involved in ongoing group supervision with videotaped therapy sessions.

Third, psychotherapy education often consists of theoretical lectures followed by a focus on trainees attempting the techniques and receiving supervision, often without having seen an expert perform these techniques. The very high rating that demonstrations received as a teaching tool may argue for more regular incorporation of clinical demonstrations by experts as a key component of training and dissemination. This also supports the idea that development of videotapes of clinical skills and techniques might be a very cost-effective way of enhancing dissemination. Moreover, by incorporating patient experience with

TABLE 3. Training Modality Questionnaire, Means (SD) and Comparisons

	Demonstration (D)	Role-Play (R)	Lecture (L)	Comparisons
Theory	3.8 (1.3)	2.5 (2.5)	3.3 (1.5)	D *> L*> R §
Details	3.8 (1.3)	2.8 (2.3)	3.0 (1.6)	D **>L > R §
Skills	3.5 (1.6)	2.9 (2.5)	2.2 (2.3)	D *> R > L $
Motivation	3.0 (1.9)	2.7 (2.7)	2.0 (2.3)	D > R > L $
Reservations	3.0 (1.9)	2.0 (2.5)	1.4 (2.3)	D **>R > L $
Beliefs	2.8 (1.9)	2.0 (2.5)	1.5 (2.3)	D **>R > L $
Barriers	2.8 (1.8)	2.3 (2.6)	1.3 (2.6)	D > R *>L $

KEY: (**>) Significantly greater at the p < .000 level.
    (*>) Significantly greater at the p < .005 level.
    (>) Greater than but not significant. To correct for multiple comparisons
    minimum significance set at p < .005
    § Demonstration significantly larger than Role Play (p < .000)
    $ Demonstration significantly larger than Lecture (p < .000)

expert therapist commentary, these videotapes can serve a powerful motivating function that lectures alone cannot achieve.

Finally, it should be noticed that all three modalities were relatively ineffective in overcoming barriers. Barriers may play a much larger role in preventing adoption of new therapies than was previously believed, and overcoming them may require an entirely new and dedicated training modality (see Gollwitzer, 2002).

DISCUSSION AND CONCLUSION

This study had a number of limitations, many of which resulted from the fact that the study was designed to take advantage of a training program with its own fixed parameters, rather than being designed de novo as a stand alone research project. First, the study participants were geographically limited to the metropolitan New York area and its surroundings. Mental health clinicians in other parts of the country may have different baseline attitudes towards CBT in general and CBT-PE in particular. Second, the participants within this geographic region were self-selected by their desire to participate in the training workshop. It is unclear how this self-selection biased their responses compared to what a random sampling of the region's mental health clinicians might have elicited. Third, the study was limited to self-report and thus cannot speak to actual clinical behavioral patterns or changes in those patterns. Fourth and closely related, the study did not follow up to see what effect the trainings might have had on actual clinical behavior in the months and years following the workshops. Finally, the study was observational rather than experimental, in that no element of the training was systematically altered to form an experimental comparison condition. In ongoing research our group is working to address a number of these limitations.

Nevertheless, there are some useful lessons that we can take from these findings regarding the steps that ought to be taken in designing a dissemination intervention. First, decompose the treatment or procedure into specifically defined and operationalized components, whose execution can be measured. Second, ascertain prior to training what trainees' attitudes, knowledge, self-efficacy, perceived norms, and barriers are for each of these components. Third, tailor the workshop to address specific gaps in knowledge, skills, and motivation. This differs from traditional needs-assessment, which focused only on gaps in knowledge and offered only information in return. Fourth, there is a need to evaluate effectiveness both via trainees' self-report and via actual measures of clinical behavior change if we are to understand how a dissemination project impacts on the actual clinical implementation of the relevant skills and techniques.

Future Directions

In the wake of the events of 9/11 we must adopt a community-oriented approach to mental health akin to the public health models that have effectively reduced communicable diseases and environmental hazards. This includes educating the public and the community of available clinicians about evidence-based prevention, assessment, and treatment for the serious psychological consequences of mass trauma. While evidence-based mental health, including practice guidelines, have been accepted as the ideal for nearly a decade, actually getting clinicians to practice this way has proven more challenging than anticipated (Poses, 1999). To conduct effectively such dissemination of empirically efficacious practices we must revamp the current system of developing CPE on the basis of perceived informational gaps alone. Instead, we must focus on creating trainings that are as efficacious in changing clinician behavior as our therapies are in changing patient behavior (Drake, 2001). To do this we must incorporate insights from the basic behavioral sciences of decision-making and motivation science (Fishbein, 1975), and we must research our training processes with the same rigor we use to research our therapeutic procedures (Waltz, Addis, Koerner, & Jacobson, 1993).

REFERENCES

Addis, M. E., & Krasnow, A. D (2000). A national survey of practicing psychologists' attitudes toward psychotherapy treatment manuals. *Journal of Consulting and Clinical Psychology*, 68(2), 331-339.

Becker, C. B., Zayfert, C., & Anderson, E. (in press). A survey of psychologists' attitudes towards and utilization of exposure therapy for PTSD. *Behaviour Research and Therapy*.

Beutler, L. E., Moleiro, C., & Talebi, H. (2002) How practitioners can systematically use empirical evidence in treatment selection. *Journal of Clinical Psychology*, 58(10), 1199-1212.

Blagys, M. D., & Hilsenroth, M. J. (2002). Distinctive activities of cognitive-behavioral therapy. A review of the comparative psychotherapy process literature. *Clinical Psychology Review*, 22(5), 671-706.

Butler, A. S., Panzer, A. M., & Goldfrank, L. R. (Eds.). (2003). *Preparing for the psychological consequences of terrorism: A public health strategy*. Washington, DC: National Academies Press.

Cahill, S. P., Hembree, E. A., & Foa, E. B. (in press). Dissemination of prolonged exposure therapy for posttraumatic stress disorder: Successes and challenges. In Y. Neria, R. Gross, R. D. Marshall, & E. Susser (Eds.), *September 11, 2001: Treatment, research and public mental health in the wake of a terrorist attack*. Cambridge: Cambridge University Press.

Campbell, A., Cairns, E., & Mallett, J. (2004). Northern Ireland: Impact of the Troubles. *Journal of Aggression, Maltreatment & Trauma*, 9(1/2/3/4), 175-184.

Castonguay, L. G., Goldfried, M. R., Wiser, S., Raue, P. J., & Hayes, A. M. (1996). Predicting the effect of cognitive therapy for depression: A study of unique and common factors. *Journal of Consulting and Clinical Psychology*, 64(3), 497-504.

Chambless, D. L., & Ollendick, T. H. (2001). Empirically supported psychological interventions: Controversies and evidence. *Annual Review of Psychology*, 52, 685-716.

Davis, D., O'Brien, M. A., Freemantle, N., Wolf, F. M., Mazmanian, P., & Taylor-Vaisey, A. (1999). Impact of formal continuing medical education: Do conferences, workshops, rounds, and other traditional continuing education activities change physician behavior or health care outcomes? *Journal of the American Medical Association*, 282(9), 867-874.

Davis, L. L., English, B. A., Ambrose, S. M., & Petty, F. (2001). Pharmacotherapy for post-traumatic stress disorder: A comprehensive review. *Expert Opinions in Pharmacotherapy*, 2(10), 1583-95.

Drake, R. E., Goldman, H. H., Leff, H. S., Lehman, A. F., Dixon, L., Mueser, K. T. et al. (2001). Implementing evidence-based practices in routine mental health service settings. *Psychiatric Services*, 52(2), 179-82.

Fishbein, M., & Ajzen, I. (1975). *Belief, attitude, intention and behavior: An introduction to theory and research*. Reading, MA: Addison-Wesley.

Foa, E. B., Hembree, E. A., Feeny, N. C., & Zoellner, L. A. (2002, March). *Posttraumatic stress disorder treatment for female assault victims*. In L. A. Zoellner (Chair), Recent Innovations in Posttraumatic Stress Disorder Treatment. Symposium presented at the annual convention of the Anxiety Disorders Association of America, Austin, TX.

Foa, E. B., Rothbaum, B. O., Riggs, D. S., & Murdock, T. B. (1991). Treatment of posttraumatic stress disorder in rape victims: A comparison between cognitive-behavioral procedures and counseling. *Journal of Consulting and Clinical Psychology, 59*(5), 715-723.

Garfield, S. L. (1998). Some comments on empirically supported treatments. *Journal of Consulting and Clinical Psychology, 66*(1), 121-125.

Gibbons, M. B., Crits-Christoph, P., Levinson, J., Gladis, M., Siqueland, L., Barber, J. P. et al. (2002). Therapist interventions in the interpersonal and cognitive therapy sessions of the Treatment of Depression Collaborative Research Program. *American Journal of Psychotherapy, 56*(1), 3-26.

Gillespie, K., Duffy, M., Hackmann, A., & Clark, D. M. (2002). Community based cognitive therapy in the treatment of posttraumatic stress disorder following the Omagh bomb. *Behaviour Research and Therapy, 40*(4), 345-357.

Gollwitzer, P. M. (1999). Implementation intentions: Strong effects of simple plans. *American Psychologist, 54*, 493-503.

Poses, R. M. (1999). One size does not fit all: Questions to answer before intervening to change physician behavior. *The Joint Commission Journal on Quality Improvement, 25*(9), 486-95.

Smith, W. R. (2000). Evidence for the effectiveness of techniques to change physician behavior. *Chest, 118*(2 Suppl.), 8S-17S.

Taylor, S., Thordarson, D. S., Maxfield, L., Fedoroff, I. C., Lovell, K., & Ogrodniczuk, J. (2003). Comparative efficacy, speed, and adverse effects of three PTSD treatments: Exposure therapy, EMDR, and relaxation training. *Journal of Consulting and Clinical Psychology, 71*(2), 330-338.

Waltz, J., Addis, M. E., Koerner, K., & Jacobson, N. S. (1993). Testing the integrity of a psychotherapy protocol: Assessment of adherence and competence. *Journal of Consulting and Clinical Psychology, 61*(4), 620-630.

Provider Perspectives on Disaster Mental Health Services in Oklahoma City

Fran H. Norris
Patricia J. Watson
Jessica L. Hamblen
Betty J. Pfefferbaum

SUMMARY. Seven years after the bombing of the Murrah Federal Building in Oklahoma City, 34 individuals affiliated with various organizations were interviewed about their experiences in providing disaster mental health services to victims and the community. Their perspectives elucidated the importance of preparedness, training and education, local control, interagency cooperation, and psychosocial support for providers. Significant conflicts emerged among providers about credentials,

Address correspondence to: Fran Norris, PhD, NCPTSD, VA Medical Center (MS 116D), 215 North Main Street, White River Junction, VT 05009 USA (E-mail: Fran.Norris@Dartmouth.edu).

Appreciation is extended to Josef Ruzek for assistance in conducting the interviews, Josef Ruzek and Bruce Young for assistance in developing the interview guide, and Dan Almeida for assistance in coding the data.

This work was funded by an interagency agreement between CMHS and NCPTSD, Matthew Friedman and Patricia Watson, Project Directors. Fran Norris' contributions were funded by NIMH Grant K02 MH63909.

This article provides a brief summary of results; a copy of the full report can be obtained from the authors.

[Haworth co-indexing entry note]: "Provider Perspectives on Disaster Mental Health Services in Oklahoma City." Norris, Fran H. et al. Co-published simultaneously in *Journal of Aggression, Maltreatment & Trauma* (The Haworth Maltreatment & Trauma Press, an imprint of The Haworth Press, Inc.) Vol. 10, No. 1/2, 2005; and: *The Trauma of Terrorism: Sharing Knowledge and Shared Care, An International Handbook* (ed: Yael Danieli, Danny Brom, and Joe Sills) The Haworth Maltreatment & Trauma Press, an imprint of The Haworth Press, Inc., 2005.

referrals, the quality of services provided, and the appropriateness, in this context, of basing services solely on a crisis counseling model. The lack of ongoing needs assessment or evaluation data further fueled the debates. On the basis of the findings, the authors outline several recommendations for planning mental health responses to future terrorist attacks.

KEYWORDS. Disaster, terrorism, mental health services, Oklahoma City bombing

On April 19, 1995, a truck bomb exploded in front of the Murrah Federal Building in Oklahoma City, Oklahoma (OKC), killing 168 people, including 19 children, and injuring another 500. The bombing generated immense concern among mental health professionals about how to meet the needs of direct victims, surviving family members, and the community as a whole. The primary response was Project Heartland, a crisis counseling program implemented by Oklahoma's Department of Mental Health and Substance Abuse Services (DMHSAS). Most of the funding for Project Heartland was provided by the Federal Emergency Management Agency (FEMA), as administered by the Center for Mental Health Services (CMHS). The Office of Victims of Crime, Red Cross, and various charities and grants also provided funding for mental health services.

Seven years after the bombing, our evaluation team visited OKC to document the perspectives of local people who had played important roles in developing, implementing, or providing disaster mental health services (DMHS). Our goal was to learn lessons from OKC's experience that could be useful to other communities that must respond to major disasters.

A systems perspective on service delivery (Figure 1) guided the study. DMHS systems are imposed upon host systems that have pre-existing missions. They are both assisted and constrained by the federal system of emergency management. Characteristics such as credibility and accessibility are criteria for evaluation of service delivery (Hodgkinson & Stewart, 1998). Forming the essential link between the DMHS system and the consumer, providers are influenced by (a) host system characteristics, especially preparedness; (b) fit between their own orientations and DMHS principles (Allen, 1993; Flynn, 1994; Jacobs & Kulkarni, 1999; Myers, 1994; Pfefferbaum,

North, Flynn, Norris, & DeMartino, 2002; Young, Ruzek, & Gusman, 1999); and (c) service coordination. Turf boundaries, poor interagency linkages, communication gaps, confusion, and ambivalence regarding outsiders have been identified as issues that interfere with service delivery and add to the stressfulness of disaster work (American Psychological Association [APA], 1997; Bowenkamp, 2000; Call & Pfefferbaum, 1999; Canterbury & Yule, 1999; Gillespie & Murty, 1994; Hodgkinson & Stewart, 1998; Lanou, 1993; Sitterle & Gurwich, 1998). A "culture of chaos" is endemic to disaster work, but coordinated networks provide workers with information, knowledge, and opportunities to support each other (Campbell & Ahrens, 1998). In summary, we began our work with the assumption that providers who function within *coherent and supportive* DMHS systems will deliver services that are perceived to be credible, acceptable, accessible, and proactive, thereby maximizing the reach of the program to those in need.

METHODS

In April 2002, four psychologists, working in pairs, interviewed 34 individuals affiliated with various organizations that provided a range of services after the bombing. Project Heartland (PH) was the federally funded crisis counseling program implemented by DMHSAS. Catholic Charities, Consumer Council, Community Counseling Center, and Latino Community Development Agency were PH subcontractors. The OKC Community Foundation administered funds received as charitable donations. First Christian Church was the site of the Compassion Center operated by the Red Cross in collaboration with the Oklahoma Psychological Association Disaster Response Network. The University of Oklahoma Health Sciences Center, Fire Department, Police Department, and VA Medical Center also played significant roles in the response.

None of the interviewers were from OKC or had provided services after the bombing. (Betty Pfefferbaum, one of the authors and planners of the study, did not conduct interviews or have access to the data.) The interview guide included broad questions about participants' roles, activities, training, interactions, stress management, service characteristics, and barriers. Interviews were audiotaped and transcribed.

Data were analyzed to identify key findings within six action-themes: (a) preparing for disaster, (b) training the workers, (c) negotiating insider-outsider dynamics, (d) implementing an interagency response, (e) caring for the workers, and (f) serving the consumer. *Data* refer to the verbatim transcriptions, *findings* to consensually agreed-upon paraphrases or summaries of the data, and *conclusions* to investigator interpretations of the findings.

FIGURE 1. Conceptual Framework: A Systems Perspective on Service Delivery

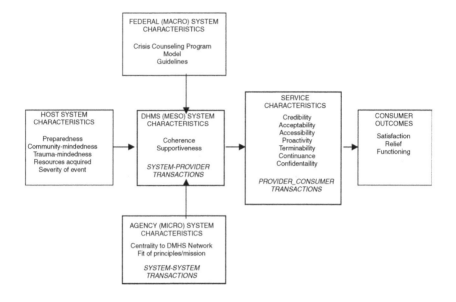

FINDINGS

Preparing for Disaster

Participants valued preparedness highly, often commenting on how their own preparedness or lack thereof influenced their ability to respond quickly, competently, and appropriately. Most participants did not perceive OKC to have been well prepared. Several findings emerged within this theme. First, participants noted that providers need to be prepared for their own anxiety and must understand how their own experiences will influence their ability to cope with their roles. Attention to providers' stress and health is crucial and should be part of the overall preparedness plan. Second, respondents emphasized the need to know how to create and manage an emergency mental health response. Developing networks, coalitions, and cooperative agreements ahead of time was seen as very important. The plan should indicate how key constituencies will be involved and how volunteers will be managed. Respondents also believed that advanced designation of responsibilities and chains of command would reduce confusion and conflict.

Participants identified many barriers to preparedness. Mental health professionals are often not interested in disaster response until a significant event occurs in their community. Necessary coalitions and networks may not exist ahead of time. Funding for training and planning is limited. Organizations that have played lead roles in one disaster may not want to take on this burden again.

Some data contradicted our finding that preparedness was viewed as critical. At the time of the interviews, the State still did not have a formal, written plan for conducting a disaster mental health response, expecting instead to draw on the rich experience gained in the aftermath of the bombing.

Training the Workers

Disaster mental health training (Red Cross and/or Critical Incident Stress Debriefing) was seen as very valuable. It was valued not only for the information it provided but also because of the access and credibility it afforded. Several nationally recognized experts came to OKC and provided training in specific topics such as PTSD and traumatic grief. With a few exceptions, comments about these trainings were positive. One participant noted that training served as a form of stress management by allowing her to take a break from direct service provision while thinking about the issues with more distance.

Limitations of training were also noted. Several participants were adamant that disaster mental health training alone was not adequate to prepare someone to work directly with trauma survivors and could not substitute for a professional education. Often, comments about the limitations of training co-occurred with strong criticisms of using paraprofessionals (e.g., persons with a Bachelor's degree or less) in disaster response.

According to participants, training should cover: (a) the range of mental health responses to trauma, including PTSD, acute stress, depression, suicidality, grief, and anger; (b) influences of pre-existing experiences and conditions; (c) family/marital issues; (d) psychological treatments; (e) workings/mandates of authorities; (f) skills for dealing with/using media; and (g) vicarious trauma and stress management. Participants recommended that trainings emphasize practical rather than theoretical issues. Case examples, mock scenarios, and drills were preferred modes. Trainings should be sensitive to perspectives of diverse cultures.

Negotiating Insider-Outsider Dynamics

Local professionals appeared to feel a strong sense of "ownership" of the disaster. Outsiders who implied that the local community was not capable of managing the situation were strongly resented. Because she asked the mayor what OKC was going to do until the "experts" arrived, newswoman Connie

Chung became a symbol of an arrogant outsider. She was mentioned in numerous interviews. Outsiders must be highly respectful of local people.

Unsolicited offers of help from self-identified experts were generally not received well. Having to deal with the volume of offers to help, letters, and donations placed a burden on gatekeepers in the community. However, individuals and organizations that were invited in because of their experience or expertise were seen as enormously helpful. The help was most appreciated when it played a supporting role to local leadership. Being invited to assist versus simply showing up was thus the most critical factor.

Implementing an Interagency Mental Health Response

The American Red Cross, First Christian Church, and local psychologists and clergy created a safe, protective environment for families of the bombing victims that came to be known as the Compassion Center. Local psychologists who played leadership roles at the Center were adamant about the necessity for minimal qualifications of those who worked with the families (masters degree) or served on death notification teams (doctorate degree). This structure did cause some conflicts. PH leaders who did not have Red Cross credentials were denied access to the Center and were very unhappy about this. Conversely, Compassion Center workers were "horrified" that PH staff had no prior training in disaster mental health.

Transitions from national to local leadership and from Red Cross to PH were not always accomplished smoothly. The sentiment was that local providers were able to coordinate and provide services more effectively once the national agencies left OKC. The Red Cross would not share its list of service recipients with state authorities, making it more difficult for the state to conduct its needs assessment. It was noted that other states have had the same problem. Implementation and management of PH posed numerous challenges. It was not initially clear who would serve as the lead agency for the FEMA-funded crisis counseling program. DMHSAS leadership struggled to keep up with meetings scheduled around OKC and plans made by various groups. A critical point was when the Governor's Office designated DMHSAS as the lead agency for the mental health response.

Both PH leadership and the subcontractors supported the idea, novel at the time, of using subcontractors to reach different segments of the population. The coordination of subcontractors was challenging at times. It was important to provide them oversight and technical assistance in creating materials for education and outreach. One subcontractor did not comply with the requirements of the subcontract, resulting in termination of the relationship. The subcontractors had a good sense of camaraderie, met often, and felt that management was highly supportive of their efforts. They believed they understood their specific responsibilities within the larger mission.

There were many examples of interagency cooperation. Participants who helped victims financially believed that PH had good relationships with other community-based agencies and that it was easy to make referrals to PH. The resource coordinating committee, which met on a regular basis to address the unmet needs of victims, aimed to provide "one-stop shopping" for the client and was well received.

However, considerable conflict emerged between PH and local psychologists and psychiatrists who often felt that PH staff were not equipped to deal with more severe problems and could not provide needed medication. Policies prohibiting record-keeping interfered with collaboration with medical professionals because of the latter's concerns about liability. Some participants believed that PH was closed to influence from professionals outside of the PH system. Some felt strongly that PH failed to refer their clients to other professionals as often as needed. This generally went hand in hand with the view that PH therapists were not particularly accomplished and "refused to let go of people" because of their own issues. PH staff believed they did make referrals when warranted and that more professionals should have been willing to offer their services for reduced fees. The sentiment was expressed, and told with salient examples, that private practitioners were "greedy" and "just after the money." Work styles (e.g., willingness to work within the school rather than in one's office) were identified as an additional barrier to working with private practitioners. According to PH, referral of rescue workers was particularly problematic; reluctance on the part of some rescue workers to have their care transferred to other providers after establishing a trusting relationship at PH complicated their treatment.

Caring for the Worker

Stories were relayed of providers who took years to recover and suffered serious consequences to their health (see also Wee & Myers, 2002). Stress and stress management were quite salient, and required that we spend more time discussing these issues with the participants than we had originally planned.

Features of disaster mental health work that make it extraordinarily stressful include its urgency and risk for emotional involvement with victims. "Self-imposed pressure" or an "internal need to hurry, hurry, hurry" led providers to put in long hours for an extended period. It was difficult for them to focus on and address their own needs. Normal activities were set aside or forgotten, creating problems at home that exacerbated the stressfulness of the work. Some participants noted the danger of getting too involved emotionally with victims. "If we can't separate ourselves from that, then we are going to be affected by it." As one participant noted, "It's hard to keep that distance, that professional distance, when you're seeing such intense pain. It was impossible for me." The extent of provider stress was not recognized until well after the event. Upper-level management said that they did not receive feedback until many of the problems were serious.

That stress can have consequences for the well-being of entire organizations, as well as individuals, was neither anticipated nor addressed by PH or other mental health programs. This fact was especially evident at the church that provided space for the Compassion Center. Church leaders became increasingly disenfranchised as the "bureaucracy" at the Center increased and their role diminished. They were scolded for inviting families to services, which seemed only hospitable to them, and criticized for using donations to repair the damage that had been done to the building by the thousands of adults, children, workers, journalists, and even animals that occupied it for weeks. Predictably, conflicts within the congregation emerged about what to do with the unsolicited financial donations the church received. As one lay leader summarized their experience, "No building can house that much pain without being affected by it."

Solutions often emphasized imposed, systemic constraints. Some participants believed it would be advisable to limit the hours worked per day (e.g., 6 hours) or the total amount of time devoted to this work (e.g., rotating off after one year). Adequate numbers of staff at all levels (administrative, counselors, support staff, media relations) must be hired to reduce the pressure on individuals. Weekly case supervision is essential, and individual therapy for workers should be made available as well.

Participants also provided advice about self-care, including being aware of one's own limits, knowing what jobs are a good match, and retaining social/recreational activities. Writing, whether academic or personal, was helpful for many, as were activities that foster relaxation, such as massage and deep breathing. Providers should avoid over-exposure to media coverage of the disaster.

Serving the Consumer

Participants were shown definitions of seven characteristics proposed to be important for DMHS (Hodgkinson & Stewart, 1998). With the exception of *terminability* (meaning that the service is seen as having an endpoint), participants agreed that the proposed characteristics served as valuable goals for service delivery in disaster-stricken settings. PH received high marks with regard to *accessibility* (service is provided in the heart of the affected community), *acceptability* (help does not demean the recipient), *confidentiality* (survivors believe that their privacy is assured), and *proactivity* (service reaches out to those most affected). *Credibility* (service is seen by survivors as offering something that will be of use) received the most discussion of the seven characteristics. Many participants disagreed with the definition provided, placing more emphasis on credentials and training as the central components of credibility. They also noted being trustworthy and knowing what one was doing, as reflected in the statement, "She gets us, she knows cops." *Continuance* (that the service must be present for a sufficient period to meet the need) was believed by many to have not been achieved because of the emphasis on short-term interventions. It was noted that PTSD and other responses to trauma persist and fluctuate in severity over time, making access to long-term care essential. Limits placed on the number of counseling sessions were perceived as very restrictive, especially for children, those who were grieving, and those from different cultures. Continuance may be even more important for rescue workers. Many of their problems were not acknowledged until years later. *Flexibility* was suggested as another important characteristic. Regulations that guide crisis counseling programs need to be flexible enough to allow for providing the most appropriate services for a particular event.

Several respondents noted the importance of meeting the needs of culturally diverse groups. The lack of fit between regular services grant requirements and culturally approved ways of helping may prevent some agencies from becoming involved in crisis counseling programs. Credibility is enhanced when consumers believe that providers understand their needs in the context of the culture with which they identify.

Several participants perceived discord between guidelines of the crisis counseling program and either their own orientations or the OKC context. Participants noted that the host system primarily serves the seriously mentally ill. Not all providers were comfortable with brief interventions and the emphasis on outreach as opposed to in-office activities. Many staff members were oriented toward case management, which was not allowed in crisis counseling guidelines. PH was not designed to serve those who needed more intensive treatment. Inherent conflicts between the goals of crisis counseling and those of long-term care were mentioned very frequently.

Many participants expressed concern, often quite strongly, about the use of paraprofessionals in outreach because they would not recognize PTSD and other serious conditions. They believed PH missed opportunities to serve people who may have needed their services the most. The alternative view was also expressed: paraprofessionals may be able to reach segments of the population that professionals ("the white coats") would not have access to, such as the homeless and the seriously mentally ill. According to one peer counselor,

"It doesn't take a rocket scientist to tell that someone is distressed." The use of paraprofessionals for running support groups in the schools was also challenged because these counselors were typically unlicensed and minimally trained. Some perceived as problematic that decisions about continued employment were based on number of client hours, a structure that discouraged referrals.

SUMMARY AND CONCLUSIONS

Participants recommended strongly that other communities not wait until after a disaster to plan a mental health response. Overall, it appeared that OKC was not and is not well prepared. Relying on prior experience is a questionable strategy, as the experience may rest in individuals who are not available in the advent of another major disaster. Programs, personnel, funding, and incentives are essential to assist state mental health authorities to become more prepared and better informed. Recent preparedness grants are now helping to make this possible.

Although it cannot substitute for professional education, training in disaster mental health was perceived as critical for service providers. Training imparts access and entry to systems as well as information and skills. There does not appear to be a training program focused on the longer-term mental health response, leaving communities to depend on non-standardized and unevaluated training programs provided by individual experts. A training program that provides credentialed, comprehensive, state-of-the-art and practical information and skills with regard to immediate, intermediate, and longer-term care would be an important addition to the field.

Although the emergence of insider-outsider dynamics was expected, we were surprised by the frequency with which the topic emerged in the interviews and the intensity of affect associated with it. Care is needed to avoid undermining the natural, appropriate, and empowering need for local control, yet it is unfortunate to deny communities access to information that could be helpful. Mechanisms for credentialing, managing, and coordinating national expertise would help communities find credible, knowledgeable, and respectful consultants. Outsiders who seek to do disaster work or consultation must foster pre-existing relationships with local professionals, mental health authorities, and/or national entities that provide entrée and credibility.

The response of local, state, and national organizations to the OKC bombing was swift and enduring. Providers' dedication and commitment to alleviating the pain of the victims shone through all their comments, even those describing conflicts regarding how best to accomplish shared goals. Further evaluation of the transition from the emergency period of disaster relief to the period of intermediate and long-term care is needed. Collaboration between the Red Cross, FEMA, and CMHS at the national level could facilitate transitions at the local level.

Project Heartland appears to have done many things well. The structure of using subcontractors to reach diverse segments of the population was novel at the time and largely successful. The subcontractors evaluated Project Heartland as coherent and supportive, which are essential characteristics in our framework. Private practitioners, however, were not well integrated into the long-term response. Relationships between the public and private sectors should be strengthened. CMHS should discuss issues regarding appropriate referrals, fees, and record-keeping with representatives of professional organizations. Professionals' concern about paraprofessionals may reflect some confusion between *outreach* and *triage*; these concepts need programmatic review. Programs need guidance regarding when and where these activities take place.

The stressfulness of providing services after a disaster of this magnitude was profound. A high level of affect was still observable seven years after the event. Systems of care need to be built into program structures, as all of the workers reported that most of their stress was self-imposed. A unilateral rule that creates a maximum term of service for all workers could interfere with program functioning and continuity. However, careful monitoring of provider stress levels is critical. Individual therapy should be made available to both line-workers and management in a process separate from case supervision. Program plans should be required to state explicitly how they will monitor and reduce provider stress. Danieli (2002) emphasized the importance of senior level support for providers, noting that it must be clear that no stigma follows from seeking psychological support. In accord with our observations, she also described trauma's capacity to create ruptures within entire organizations and encouraged "ongoing dynamic dialogues among all layers of involvement" (p. 388).

Findings on serving the consumer are complex and not easy to summarize. Services were evaluated as *accessible, acceptable, proactive*, and *confidential* but were not always perceived as having *credibility* and *continuance*. The criticisms of PH were, in general, criticisms of the FEMA crisis counseling model. It was not always clear how to conceptualize crisis counseling because the bombing had engendered unthinkable trauma. Many participants believed that consumers' problems were too severe to be treated by unlicensed mental health workers. FEMA and CMHS may need to review the adequacy of relying solely on a crisis counseling model. A more flexible structure, providing crisis counseling for most but true clinical care for a minority, may be required following major disasters.

The lack of assessment of community-level needs and status makes it impossible to say which side of this debate over treatment needs was accurate. It is quite possible that psychologists and psychiatrists in OKC overestimated the level of need for professional treatment in the community. Valid need assessments could resolve many of the controversies regarding the relative need for counseling versus professional treatment in the community.

Similarly, the lack of empirical evaluation data fueled debate over the quality of the work that was done. There are no data that can establish whether or not the services offered matched consumers' needs or helped them. Beliefs in the efficacy of crisis counseling approaches appeared to follow from perceivers' ideology rather than evidence. CMHS must continue to move in a direction that supports the inclusion of evaluation in program plans.

The limitations of our study should be acknowledged. We elicited only the perspectives of providers, and it will be critical for the voice of consumers to be heard before definitive recommendations can be made. Perspectives were embedded in one community's experience and may not generalize. Likewise, it would be premature to draw conclusions regarding the utility of our conceptual framework. Nonetheless, these findings do provide preliminary support for several of the framework's implications that: (a) host system preparedness facilitates postdisaster response; (b) the fit between providers' orientation and the system's orientation influences judgments regarding system coherence and service effectiveness; and (c) credibility, acceptability, accessibility, proactivity, continuance, and confidentiality compose a minimal set of criteria for postdisaster service delivery.

REFERENCES

Allen, R. (1993). Organizing mental health services following a disaster: A community systems perspective. *Journal of Social Behavior and Personality, 8,* 179-188.

American Psychological Association. (1997). *Task force on the mental health response to the Oklahoma City bombing.* Washington, DC: Author.

Bowenkamp, C. (2000). Coordination of mental health and community agencies in disaster *International Journal of Emergency Mental Health, 2,* 159-165.

Call, J., & Pfefferbaum, B. (1999). Lessons from the first two years of Project Heartland, Oklahoma's mental health response to the 1995 bombing. *Psychiatric Services, 50,* 953-955.

Campbell, R., & Ahrens, C. (1998). Innovative community services for rape victims: An application of multiple case study methodology. *American Journal of Community Psychology, 26,* 537-571.

Canterbury, R., & Yule, W. (1999). Planning a psychosocial response to a disaster. In W. Yule (Ed.), *Post-traumatic stress disorders: Concepts and therapy* (pp. 285-296). New York: Wiley & Sons.

Danieli, Y. (2002). Conclusion. In Y. Danieli (Ed.), *Sharing the front line and the back hills* (pp. 381-390). Amityville, NY: Baywood.

Flynn, B. (1994). Mental health services in large scale disasters: An overview of the Crisis Counseling Program. *NCP Clinical Quarterly, 4,* 1-4.

Gillespie, D., & Murty, S. (1994). Cracks in a postdisaster service delivery network. *American Journal of Community Psychology, 22,* 639-660.

Hodgkinson, P., & Stewart, M. (1998). *Coping with catastrophe: A handbook of post-disaster psychosocial aftercare* (2nd ed.). London: Routledge.

Jacobs, G., & Kulkarni, N. (1999). Mental health responses to terrorism. *Psychiatric Annals, 29,* 376-380.

Lanou, F. (1993). Coordinating private and public mental health resources in a disaster. *Journal of Social Behavior and Personality, 8,* 255-260.

Myers, D. G. (1994). Psychological recovery from disaster: Key concepts for delivery of mental health services. *NCP Clinical Quarterly, 4,* 1-3.

Pfefferbaum, B., North, C., Flynn, B., Norris, F., & DeMartino, R. (2002). Disaster mental health services following the 1995 Oklahoma City bombing: Modifying approaches to address terrorism. *CNS Spectrums, 7,* 575-579.

Sitterle, K., & Gurwich, R. (1998). The terrorist bombing in Oklahoma City. In E. Zinner & M. Williams (Eds.), *When a community weeps: Case studies in group survivorship* (pp. 161-189). Philadelphia, PA: Brunner/Mazel.

Wee, D., & Myers, D. (2002). Stress response of mental health workers following disaster: The Oklahoma City bombing. In C. Figley (Ed.), *Treating compassion fatigue* (pp. 57-83). New York: Brunner-Routledge.

Young, B., Ruzek, J., & Gusman, F. (1999). Disaster mental health: Current status and future directions. *New Directions for Mental Health Services, 82,* 53-64.

Guide:
Some Principles of Self Care

Yael Danieli

The following principles of self-healing were designed to help professionals recognize, contain, and heal their emotional and other reactions to trauma. They were originally conceptualized as event countertransferences (Danieli, 1988), namely, psychotherapists' reactions to the trauma event or the survivors' accounts rather than to the victims themselves. They have been recognized as ubiquitous, and are at the forefront of our concern in preparing and training professionals to work with victims and terrorized populations (see, for example, Danieli, 1994). Numerous protectors and providers worldwide have found them valuable (Danieli, 1996, 2002; Smith, Agger, Danieli, & Weisaeth, 1996). The main principles are as follows:

A. *To Recognize One's Reactions:*

1. Develop awareness of somatic signals of distress. One's chart of warning signs of potential countertransference reactions would include symptoms such as sleeplessness, headaches, and perspiration.
2. Try to find words to name accurately and articulate one's inner experiences and feelings. As Bettelheim (1984) commented, "what cannot

Address correspondence to: Yael Danieli, PhD, Group Project for Holocaust Survivors and Their Children, 345 East 80th Street (31-J), New York, NY 10021 USA (E-mail: yaeld@aol.com).

[Haworth co-indexing entry note]: "Guide: Some Principles of Self Care." Danieli, Yael. Co-published simultaneously in *Journal of Aggression, Maltreatment & Trauma* (The Haworth Maltreatment & Trauma Press, an imprint of The Haworth Press, Inc.) Vol. 10, No. 1/2, 2005; and: *The Trauma of Terrorism: Sharing Knowledge and Shared Care, An International Handbook* (ed: Yael Danieli, Danny Brom, and Joe Sills) The Haworth Maltreatment & Trauma Press, an imprint of The Haworth Press, Inc., 2005.

be talked about can also not be put to rest; and if it is not, the wounds continue to fester from generation to generation" (p. 166).

B. To Contain One's Reactions:

1. Identify one's personal level of comfort in order to build openness, tolerance, and readiness to hear anything.
2. Knowing that every emotion has a beginning, a middle, and an end, learn to attenuate one's fear of being overwhelmed by its intensity to try to feel its full life-cycle without resorting to defensive countertransference reactions.

C. To Heal and Grow:

1. Accept that nothing will ever be the same.
2. When one feels wounded, one should take time, accurately diagnose, soothe, and heal before being "emotionally fit" again to continue to work.
3. Seek consultation or further therapy for previously unexplored areas triggered by patients' stories.
4. Any one of the affective reactions (i.e., grief, mourning, rage) may interact with old, unworked through experiences of the therapists. They will thus be able to use their professional work purposefully for their own growth.
5. Establish a network of people to create a holding environment (Winnicott, 1965) within which one can share their trauma-related work.
6. Therapists should provide themselves with avocational avenues for creative and relaxing self-expression in order to regenerate energies.

Being kind to oneself and feeling free to have fun and joy is not a frivolity in this field, but a necessity without which one cannot fulfill one's professional obligations or professional contract.

REFERENCES

Bettelheim, B. (1984). Afterward to C. Vegh, *I didn't say goodbye* (R. Schwartz, Trans.). New York: E. P. Dutton.

Danieli, Y. (1988). Confronting the unimaginable: Psychotherapists' reactions to victims of the Nazi Holocaust. In J. P. Wilson, Z. Harel, & B. Kahana (Eds.), *Human adaptation to extreme stress* (pp. 219-238). New York: Plenum.

Danieli, Y. (1994). Countertransference, trauma and training. In J. P. Wilson and J. Lindy (Eds.), *Countertransference in the treatment of post-traumatic stress disorder* (pp. 368-388). New York: Guilford Press.

Danieli, Y. (1996). Who takes care of the caretakers? The emotional life of those working with children in situations of violence. In R. J. Appel & B. Simon (Eds.), *Minefields in their hearts: The mental health of children in war and communal violence* (pp. 189-205). New Haven, CT: Yale University Press.

Danieli, Y. (Ed.). (2002). Sharing the front line and the back hills: International protectors and providers, peacekeepers, humanitarian aid workers and the Media in the midst of crisis. Amityville, New York: Baywood Publishing Company, Inc.

Smith, B., Agger, I., Danieli, Y., & Weisaeth, L. (1996). Emotional responses of international humanitarian aid workers. In Y. Danieli, N. Rodley, & L. Weisaeth (Eds.), *International responses to traumatic stress: Humanitarian, human rights, justice, peace and development contributions, collaborative actions and future initiatives* (pp. 397-423). Amityville, NY: Baywood Publishing Company, Inc. Published for and on behalf of the United Nations.

Winnicott, D. W. (1965). *The maturational processes and the facilitating environment.* London: Hogarth Press.

Terrorism:
The Community Perspective

Mooli Lahad

SUMMARY. This article examines the effect of terrorism on communities. Its specific point of view is that of resiliency rather than psychopathology. To this end, both a review of the literature on the impact of terrorism on communities in general and the close to home experience of communities in the north of Israel comprise this study. The conclusions drawn lead to practical recommendations for preparing communities both on the national level and at the

Address correspondence to: Mooli Lahad, PhD, Director of the Community Stress Prevention Center, Kiryat Shmona, POB 797, Kiryat Shmona, 11012, Israel (E-mail: lahadm@netvision.net.il).

[Haworth co-indexing entry note]: "Terrorism: The Community Perspective." Lahad, Mooli. Co-published simultaneously in *Journal of Aggression, Maltreatment & Trauma* (The Haworth Maltreatment & Trauma Press, an imprint of The Haworth Press, Inc.) Vol. 10, No. 3/4, 2005; and: *The Trauma of Terrorism: Sharing Knowledge and Shared Care, An International Handbook* (ed: Yael Danieli, Danny Brom, and Joe Sills) The Haworth Maltreatment & Trauma Press, an imprint of The Haworth Press, Inc., 2005.

local authority level to deal with the long-term psychological results of terror.

KEYWORDS. Terrorism, resiliency, coping, uncertainty, psychopathology, community, preparedness, Israel

Although terrorism has a strong influence on individuals, its intended effect is to intimidate large groups, communities, and nations. The two major questions discussed in this article are, "Can we really assess the mental well-being of large communities?" and "What do we know about the ability of communities to live with terrorism and to build resiliency in the face of the uncertainty with which terrorism confronts us?"

In an Institute of Medicine (IOM) report, Stith-Butler (2003) states:

> Much of what is used to determine how individuals and communities may react to terrorism is derived from broader trauma literature, including that which examines disasters. Although there may be some similarities between other types of disasters and terrorism, the malicious intent and unpredictable nature of terrorism may carry a particularly devastating impact for those directly or indirectly affected. (p. 4)

In most cases of natural or industrial disasters, communities can predict the location, give some warning, and assess directives and routes to safety. More than anything, many of these catastrophes can be categorized under "acts of God" or unintended harm or neglect. None of the aforementioned is possible with acts of terrorism.

In a National Center for PTSD Fact Sheet, Norris, Byrne, and Kaniasty (2003a) scanned 177 articles that described results for 130 distinct samples comprising over 50,000 individuals who experienced 80 different disasters. These studies were coded for the presence of six sets of outcomes and rated for overall severity of impairment. Posttraumatic Stress Disorder (PTSD) was the most prevalent outcome (67%), followed by depression (37%) and anxiety (37%). Non-specific distress, social and interpersonal disruptions, and psychosocial resource losses each were found in 10% or less.

MAGNITUDE OF EFFECTS

To provide a rough estimate of the overall impact of the events studied, the results of each sample were classified on a four-point scale of severity (Norris, Byrne, & Kaniasty, 2003b):

1. Nine percent showed minimal impairment, meaning that the majority of the samples experienced only transient stress reactions.
2. Fifty-two percent showed moderate impairment, wherein prolonged but sub-clinical distress was the predominant result.
3. Twenty-three percent showed severe impairment, meaning that 25 to 49% of the samples suffered from criterion-level psychopathology.
4. Sixteen percent showed very severe impairment, meaning that 50% or more of the samples suffered from criterion-level psychopathology.

ASSESSING THE MENTAL WELL-BEING OF COMMUNITIES

The disruption and sometimes destruction of continuities manifest themselves in some communities by lowering the inhabitants' belief that anything will change, such as their self-perception as victims and their sense of "learned helplessness" (Kalish, 1999). The impact may be long lasting. Ayalon (1983a) described coping abilities of different communities when faced with terrorist invasions of their settlements. Her overall findings were that settlements that had pre-attack community organizational preparedness and support systems in place fared better than those with a loose community structure, where members felt less cohesion and did not have these systems. This study highlighted the benefits of a close-knit societal structure, such as the Kibbutz (an Israeli communal settlement based on socialist ideology of shared property and life style), that on calm days members may perceive as intrusive and domineering. The structure of these Kibbutzim enabled them to maintain four continuities:

1. Logical rules: There was a contingency plan in place.
2. Role: Each member knew his or her role, what was expected of him or her in that role, and who would replace him/her.
3. Social: The concerted way the Kibbutz was running enhanced the feeling of togetherness.
4. Historical: Continuity was reinforced by previous experiences of surviving hardship together and the ideology of shared fate and responsibility.

However, Niv (1994) showed that with the structural change of the Kibbutz movement towards more private life and privatization of services and property, the cohesion and emergency preparedness system collapsed. One example of this change became apparent after a massive attack in 1993 (10 days of shelling by terrorist organizations from southern Lebanon) on the same kibbutzim that functioned well in Ayalon's (1983b) study. They were unprepared, and the rate of unorganized, spontaneous evacuation of the Kibbutz was significant both socially and economically. Fewer people were available to take care of the children in the shelters, and some of the kibbutzim, for the first time in their history, were unable to work their dairy farms. Based on Niv's findings the regional council developed a new plan. The focus was on a coordinating body based on the existing manpower present in the Kibbutz at any given time, volunteering members to fill positions previously held by full-time workers, a psychosocial team, and an emergency plan for the education system based on volunteering parents (Lahad, 2000).

THE ABILITY OF COMMUNITIES TO LIVE WITH TERRORISM: LIFE ON THE BORDER 1974-2000

The northern town of Kiryat Shmona has seen multiple terrorist attacks for a period of almost 30 years, beginning with the 1970s Katyusha rocket attacks. However, it was not until the terrorists' infiltration in 1974 that the level of anxiety, helplessness, and hopelessness affected large parts of the population. Twenty-two inhabitants were killed in that attack, including mothers and children, and this seriously affected the routine of daily living in the town and in its inhabitants' basic sense of security.

Zuckerman-Bareli (1978) compared the abilities of villages to those of Kibbutzim in the inhabitants' perception of their ability to cope with the prolonged stress. She found the following factors to be responsible for villagers feeling much less secure than the kibbutzim: (a) low level of education, (b) dissatisfaction with the local leadership and with living conditions, (c) absence of organization for emergencies, (d) low income, and (e) personal anxiety not necessarily connected with a "real" attack. The kibbutzim fared better in local organization for meeting crises by having well defined roles for members, social support, and group cohesion.

Ahronstam and Wolf (1975) and Maoz, Weisenbeck, Rosenbaum, and Rabor (1975) conducted several studies on the impact of living under constant threat of terrorist attacks and described the impact on the young and the adult population. Their findings showed that fear, anxiety, and insecurity were prevalent across age groups. Adults showed somatic problems, including cardiac, insomnia, and respiratory difficulties, and children stuttered and suffered from enuresis. Military and civil defense operational planning were in place as the law required; however, the behavioral aspects, or the psychosocial elements of preparedness and response to crisis, were not developed and activities in this area were random, ad hoc, and uncoordinated.

Despite the known, detrimental consequences of the lack of preparation on the behavioral dimension, and despite the various recommendations of official reports, it took the local authorities in Kiryat Shmona 4 years until the first structured attempt to build a psychosocial response capability in the town began (Lahad, 1981). Based on Ayalon's study on the impact of face-to-face confrontation with terrorism and the conclusion of military surveys, the first psychosocial preparedness plan and training were conducted in two towns in the north of Israel, Nahariya on the eastern coast (Ayalon, 1993) and Kiryat Shmona (Ayalon & Lahad, 2000). The method adopted was a multi-agency simulation to reveal the behavioral, emotional, and social implications of exposure to terrorist attacks and the need for multi-agency preparedness and response capability.

THE COMMUNITY MODEL

The need for a coordinated psychosocial medical education and community-based intervention team was one of the foremost recommendations emanating from the 1980 10-day stay in shelters in the town of Kiryat Shmona. The comprehensive psychosocial plan drawn up at that time later developed into Tel Aviv's metropolitan preparedness program.

The community model was guided by the following assumptions:

1. There will never be enough professional workforces to respond to all needs.
2. There are areas where different professions overlap.
3. There are gaps in services that need to be detected.
4. There is a need to nominate a lead agency.
5. There is a need to coordinate interventions.
6. There is a need to agree on basic intervention protocols.
7. The aim should be as much as possible to help locals help themselves.
8. People are naturally resilient and most need only appropriate preparation and guidance to bring out the best in them under emergencies.

Based on these assumptions, a coordinating committee that consisted of the heads of social, education, mental health, school psychology, primary care, and community centers chaired by the social services was formed. Psychosocial intervention teams of mental health and social work professionals were formed and dispatched to assess the situation and intervene on the individual, family, or group level. A community outreach team comprised of welfare and community workers scanned the towns' shelters on a daily basis to identify needs, support those in need, and enhance self-care and leadership among the citizens. A third team of primary care nurses with a general practitioner and a psychologist was formed to be on call whenever any of the above two teams reported medical or emotional needs or when there were injuries as a result of the terrorist attack.

The education system and community center's staff developed informal education teams to support and activate children of all ages in the shelters or in the near vicinity. Last but not least, media and information dissemination services were developed. These were comprised of an information center, hotline telephone, local interactive TV broadcasting from the town to "meet your leadership," and a local radio station to give instructions and information. To shorten the distance and speed up the response to local needs, the community centers, schools, and kindergartens became neighborhood centers for locals to call in or ask for help. A major volunteer recruitment effort was launched to train in a variety of skills including medical first aid, emotional support, multi-lingual response at information centers, education, and practical skills.

ELEMENTS OF COMMUNITY PSYCHOSOCIAL PREPAREDNESS: RISK FACTORS IN A COMMUNITY

Just as there are risk factors that increase potential long-term negative effects of disasters on individuals, there are risk factors that affect a community's ability to respond to a disaster. Kulka et al. (1989) describe several.

Prolonged Exposure to Event. When there is prolonged exposure to a disaster, it is likely the community will experience a breakdown of significant portions of its infrastructure, making recovery much harder. As Williams, Zinner, and Ellis (1999) explain, "If the tragedy involved massive dislocation or relocation, long-term unemployment, and/or widespread property destruction, the catastrophe may challenge the identity and even the structure of that community" (p. 8).

Repetitive Events. Communities recover when there is a belief that things can return to "normal." This is not the case for communities that experience repetitive terrorist attacks. For them, there is a repeated risk and encounter with loss and damage.

Intentionality of Traumatic Events. Communities are at higher risk for intense grief or traumatic reactions when there is a sense that their trauma was brought specifically to them. This is very much the case with terrorist acts in which the terrorists specifically unleash destruction and fear on the population with the intention of inflicting horror and disrupting the routine of life.

Raphael's (1986) discussion of how a community's nature and culture influence its reactions to a natural disaster is applicable to communities struggling with terrorism. She notes that the most influential variables in determining how a community will respond to a natural disaster are its degrees of poverty, deprivation, underdevelopment, and socioeconomic vulnerability. She also states that a community's willingness or preparedness to cope with a disaster depends on its sense of vulnerability to the threats, the trust of its citizens in public authorities, its communication system, and the costs of preparedness and response.

One of the few organized attempts to address this issue was launched following the spontaneous evacuation of Kiryat Shmona by its residents in 1980, in reaction to a weeklong rocket attack resulting in two fatalities. The psychosocial and community center's recovery plan included home-based support groups led by community personnel, local officials, and military commanders. The main aim was to express the leadership's genuine interest in the public's opinions and feelings and to restore the citizens' trust in local government and the army's ability to protect them.

Other measures of the community recovery plan were: (a) training local women as civil defense officers and assigning them as "shelter commanders," (b) training parents as informal shelter education staff, (c) teaching them how to engage children through simple arts and crafts activities, and (d) training citizens in basic shelter maintenance skills. These measures ended their total dependence on the municipality for any and every service (Shapiro & Amit, 1982).

THE EMERGENCY BEHAVIOR OFFICER: A NEW PROFESSION

Decision-makers, be they mayors, chiefs of police, fire brigades, army officers, or ministers, typically are in charge of local emergency services, although often they lack training in understanding the needs of the public when responding to disasters. In some cases, because of their training, military or police officers confuse the public with the "enemy." A classic example of this was the Hillsborough football stadium disaster in Sheffield, England in April 1989, where 96 fans were crushed to death due to officials who were attempting to control the crowd and confusing fans trying to escape the crush with hooligans trying to invade the pitch (field). Very often, decision-makers and local councils hold myths about human behavior in emergency situations. In contrast to such myths, Dynes, Quarantelli, and Kreps (1972) described the following facts on the basis of 70 years of research:

1. Disaster victims cope very well. They help their families, neighbors, and co-workers.
2. Panic is so rare that it is not a problem.
3. Looting is rare. Crime rates fall after disasters.
4. People with emergency responsibilities do not leave their posts in a disaster. In more than 500 field studies, the Disaster Research Center at the University of Delaware did not discover a single example of role abandonment.

5. Organizations are at a disadvantage in disasters. Victims can look around them, see what has to be done, and then do it. Communication and transportation damage may make it impossible for organizations to do the same. They are ready and willing to help but may not have adequate access to information or equipment.

Myths become dangerous when organizations act on them. Fearing panic, radio stations hold back warnings. To prevent looting, police devote their resources to security. On the assumption that victims cannot cope, impact areas are evacuated. Imagining the victims to be helpless, outsiders rush to help, causing congestion.

The public may be viewed as helpless, resulting in a decision not to inform citizens about what is happening for fear they will panic. In other cases, the public may be viewed as unimportant, and thus public reactions are not considered as a factor in decision-making. People's natural resilience is not given its true weight. As a result of the establishment of the coordinating body of psychosocial medical and educational services, a new profession was designated–the Emergency Behavior Officer (EBO). The first body to adopt the concept and develop structure, organization, and method of operation was the Israeli Home Front. This role was further adopted by the Ministries of Education, Welfare, and Health.

During 1985-1986, the Community Stress Prevention Center (CSPC) trained the first group of EBOs in skills necessary to understand the human aspects of critical incidents and the many factors influencing public reactions. This training included disaster management, human reaction to disasters, organization and community reactions to disasters, and the difference between an individual-focused approach and an organization and community mental health focus. Some of the skills taught in this initial training were: (a) accumulation of data and information on mass behavior, (b) presentation of a central behavioral picture, (c) predicting public reaction using human sciences, anthropology, mass media, and social psychology, (d) offering suggestions and recommendations to decision-makers at the headquarters level, (e) supporting rescue operation teams, and (f) compiling recommendations based on alternative courses of action.

The overall frame of reference was of resiliency and coping based on the integrative model of resiliency BASIC Ph (Lahad, 1993) as a paradigm both for understanding how a community copes and as the basis for communicating with decision-makers and the public and using the media as a source of support (Lahad, Peled, & Cohen, 1995). To date, there are hundreds of trained EBOs in Israel and in other countries serving as consultants on human behavior and community stress prevention. The information in Table 1 was developed for the training of the EBOs in community stress prevention.

WHEN RESOURCES ARE SCARCE: REMOTE COMMUNITIES CARING FOR THEMSELVES

The capacity to provide the above services does not exist everywhere. Gilad and Cohen (1988) describe the attempts to establish a community self-help system where very little professional help is available, or where it would take time for it to arrive following a terrorist attack. This concept, later developed by many small communities in Israel, is based on three components:

1. Screening and mapping: Looking for professionals within the community.
2. Getting volunteers and training non-professionals: Using community outreach and empowering methods, locating volunteers to cover all aspects of community life: logistics, security, education, social, religion, medical, morale, emotional and information; training them in disaster management and community networking and support.
3. Self-management and information dissemination: Training volunteers (professionals and non-professionals) to operate the community as long as it takes and to be able to coordinate with outer bodies (e.g., government, army, hospitals, regional council) until the emergency is over.

Brender (2001) surveyed the operation of these community emergency teams for the Israeli Ministry of the Interior and found that overall satisfaction of the inhabitants with the teams' activity was very high (almost 94% of the interviewees). When he asked the teams what helped them to cope with the situation, they mentioned cooperation of citizens, volunteering of adults and youth, support from the community leadership and establishment, the team's training prior to the Intifada (the Palestinian uprising), simulations in the community, outside support, the welfare department of the regional council, and learning and rehearsing the procedures and contingency plans.

CONCLUSIONS AND RECOMMENDATIONS

Terrorism can be seen as the disease of the 21st century; its ability to influence masses will probably grow as a result of the availability of new technologies, weapons of mass destruction, and the construct of the "global village"

TABLE 1. The Public's Expectations from the Community Organization

Preparedness	Response	Recovery
(Primary prevention)	(Secondary prevention)	(Tertiary prevention)
* Contingency plans	* Quick response	* Resume control
* Prevention activities	* Save life & property	* Quick return to normal
* High competence of personnel	* Contain the risk	* Assistance in solving personal problems
* High readiness	* Control the damage	* Preserve victim's rights
* Keeping obligations	* Quick response to the victims	* Taking care of the public at risk
* Public preparedness	* Law enforcement	* Control the situation
* Information for public	* Provide clear instructions	* Long-term mental support (instructions, addresses)
	* Information dissemination	* Provide for victims' needs

that makes the impact of terrorism global. The psychosocial field is still very much behind other aspects of disaster planning and preparedness and will continue to be this way as long as decision-makers fail to understand the need to invest resources in this field comparable to those which are poured into the strategic and logistical ones. There is a clear paradox of investing billions of dollars in equipment and materials, whereas investment in social and emotional resiliency that pays off for years to come receives very little and in some cases next to no funding. The need for such investment is crucial for the sustainability of any nation's reactions to large-scale terrorist attacks and the concomitant mass disasters.

At the decision-making level, there is a need to see a raised public awareness of the impact of such incidents, bearing in mind that PTSD should not be the primary factor advocate but rather the immediate numbers of the public who are psychologically and behaviorally affected by the disaster. In a recent report of the Israeli Ministry of Health (Ben Gershon, 2003), the ratio is 1 physically injured to 13 people emotionally affected. This alerts us to the need to make plans to speed up the recovery and return to functioning of people who would otherwise be an enormous burden on the system, even for 3 to 6 weeks. The other side of this awareness is to instill the knowledge that the public will recover and that almost everyone will be able to function well if instructed beforehand and assisted, guided, and supported during and after the incident.

On a national level, a system focusing on the psychosocial aspects of disasters must be developed (the Emergency Behavior Consultancy System [EBCS]). The task of the EBCS should include (a) advising policy makers,

(b) building a database, (c) developing tools and methods to analyze information in "real time," and (d) coordinating agencies and services dealing with the public during normal times so that the response will be well organized and resources will be better utilized. The EBCS should function at all levels: (a) headquarters (decision-makers), (b) intervention teams, and (c) ground level (in the community). Additional factors would have to be taken into consideration with terrorist attacks, including the public's reaction to the perpetrators (such as the wish for revenge, not always directed at only the perpetrators) and the altered perception of what constitutes a safe activity (such as traveling on a bus and eating in a café).

Another aspect of psychosocial preparedness should be on the local authority level, building upon existing services and adopting the concept of "helping the public to help themselves," that is, enhancing "motivational resiliency." We recommend adapting the Israeli model of coordination teams of all the services and agencies dealing with the public, namely welfare, health, education, community services, non-governmental organizations (NGOs), clergy or other cultural services, information, public shelters, and mental health services. The community response teams model (Brender, 2001; Gilad & Cohen, 1988) is recommended for adoption by small, remote communities that may be subject to attacks and where distance or scarcity of professional help necessitate a locally-led response.

All plans and systems need to be culturally sensitive, utilizing local resources and communicating in a culturally accepted manner. As some research indicates that the source of support and information for many people lies in the neighborhoods, we suggest a neighborhood liaison system based on volunteers and existing services.

Finally, the family as a source of preparedness and support before, during and after the incident is another crucial element in the community's ability to face crisis. In the case of terrorist incidents, this crisis is generally longer term and much wider focused than after a natural disaster or accident. Parents and family need to be engaged in the process. Much has been written on this subject but very little done in this area, and even fewer studies were carried out to test what are the most important aspects of family preparedness (Rosenfeld, Caye, Ayalon, & Lahad, in press). The community provides its members with a context for coping with their daily life as well as for the meaning they attribute to disasters. It is, therefore, of major importance to study more carefully successful as well as unsuccessful attempts by communities to deal with the aftermath of disasters, and to develop tools to assess the capabilities or resilience of communities prior to catastrophes.

REFERENCES

Ahronstam, S., & Wolf, O. (1975). Kiryat Shmona project. *Journal of Psychology Counseling and Guidance in Education, 8,* 94-101. (Hebrew).

Ayalon, O. (1983a). Coping with terrorism: The Israeli case. In D. Meichenbaum & M. Jaremko (Eds.), *Stress reduction and prevention* (pp. 293-339). Cambridge, MA: Perseus Publishing.

Ayalon, O. (1983b). Face to face with terrorists. In A. Cohen (Ed.), *Education as encounter* (pp. 81-92). Haifa, Israel: Haifa University Press. (Hebrew).

Ayalon, O. (1993). Post traumatic stress recovery. In J. Wilson & B. Raphael (Eds.), *International handbook of traumatic stress syndromes* (pp. 855-866). New York: Plenum Press.

Ayalon, O., & Lahad, M. (1991). *Life on the edge: Coping with stress of war and peace.* Haifa, Israel: Nord Publications. (Hebrew).

Ayalon, O., & Lahad, M. (2000). Coping with uncertainty. In O. Ayalon & M. Lahad (Eds.), *Life on the edge: Coping with stress, war, security hazards, violence, 2000* (pp. 327-347). Haifa, Israel: Nord Publications. (Hebrew).

Ben Gershon, B. (2003, August). *The Israeli Ministry of Health preparedness plan for mass casualty incident.* Paper presented at the Cherish Conference, Cyprus, Nicosia. (Hebrew).

Brender, M. (2001, February). *Evaluation of the effectiveness of the Community Emergency Teams* (CET). Report presented to the Ministry of Interior, Jerusalem, Israel. (Hebrew).

Dynes, R., Quarantelli, E., & Kreps, G. (1972). *A perspective on disaster planning* (Report Series No.11). Newark, DE: Newark Disaster Research Center, University of Delaware.

Gilad, M., & Cohen, A. (1988). Preparing non-professional volunteers for crisis and Emergency. In M. Lahad & A. Cohen (Eds.), *Community stress prevention* (Vols. 1-2; pp. 154-159). Kiryat Shmona, Israel: Community Stress Prevention Center.

Kalish, N. (1999). *Youth in high school coping in an uncertain reality of life; The relationship between one's outlook on life, political awareness, declared level of religiosity and anxiety level.* Budapest, Hungary: Department of Education, Faculty of Arts at Eötvös Loránd University, Budapest.

Kulka, B. A., Schlenger, W. E., Fairbank, J. A., Hough, R. L., Jordan, B. K., Marmar, C. R., & Weiss, D. A. (1989). *Trauma and the Vietnam War generation: Reports of findings from the national Vietnam veterans adjustment study.* New York: Brunner/Mazel.

Lahad, M. (1981). *Preparation of children and teachers to cope with stress: An integrative approach.* Unpublished masters thesis, Hebrew University, Jerusalem, Israel. (Hebrew).

Lahad, M. (1993). BASIC Ph: The story of coping resources. In M. Lahad & A. Cohen (Eds.), *Community stress prevention* (Vols. 1-2; pp. 117-145). Kiryat Shmona, Israel: Community Stress Prevention Center.

Lahad, M., Peled, D., & Cohen, A. (1995). *Emergency behavior officer training manual.* Ramat Gan, Israel: DEMCO.

Lahad, M. (2000). *Kibbutz emergency contingency plan.* Kiryat Shmona, Israel: CSPC (Hebrew).

Maoz, B., Weisenbeck, H., Rosenbaum, M., & Rabor, M. (1975). *Community psychiatry in the Upper Galilee* (conference report) pp. 150-158. (Hebrew).

Niv, A. (1994). *Communities under fire–The Kibbutzim of the Upper Galilee.* Report to the United Kibbutzim Movement, Ruppin Institute, Working paper. (Hebrew).

Norris, F. H., Byrne, C. M., & Kaniasty, K. (2003a). *Risk factors for adverse outcomes in natural and human-caused disasters: A review of the empirical literature. A national center for PTSD fact sheet.* Retrieved from, *http://www.ncptsd.org/facts/ disasters/fs_riskfactors.html*

Norris, F. H., Byrne, C. M., & Kaniasty, K. (2003b). *The range, magnitude, and duration of effects of natural and human-caused disasters: A review of the empirical literature: A national center for PTSD fact sheet.* Retrieved from, *http://www.ncptsd. org/facts/disasters/fs_range.html*

Raphael, B. (1986). *When disaster strikes: A handbook for the caring professions.* London: Hutchinson.

Rosenfeld, L. B., Caye, J., Ayalon, O., & Lahad, M. (in press). *When their world comes apart: Helping families and children manage the effects of disasters.* Washington, DC: NASW Press.

Shapiro, D., & Amit, M. (1982, September). *Survey of tendencies to stay or leave Kiryat Shmona following a terrorist attack.* A survey for the Kiryat Shmona Municipality. Kiryat Shmona, Israel: Kiryat Shmona Municipality publication. (Hebrew).

Stith Butler, A., Panzer, A. M., & Goldfrank, L. R. (Eds.) (2003). *Preparing for the psychological consequences of terrorism: A public health strategy.* Washington DC: National Academies Press.

Williams, M. B., Zinner, E. S., & Ellis, R. R. (1999). The connection between grief and trauma: An overview. In E. S. Zinner & M. B. Williams (Eds.), *When a community weeps: Case studies in group survivorship* (pp. 3-16). Philadelphia: Brunner/Mazel.

Zuckerman-Bareli, C. (1978). The effect of border tension on the adjustment of kibbutzim and moshavim on the northern border of Israel: A path analysis. In C. D. Spielberger & I. G. Sarason (Eds.), *Stress and anxiety* (pp. 81-91). New York: McGrew-Hill International Book Company.

Community Mental Health
in Emergencies and Mass Disasters:
The Tel-Aviv Model

Nathaniel Laor
Zeev Wiener
Smadar Spirman
Leo Wolmer

SUMMARY. Mass disasters are widespread and intensive, affecting individuals, families, communities, society, and culture. Mental health services must play a crucial role in order to meet non-routine challenges that put basic professional issues to the test both in theory and in practice. In the Tel Aviv Model, responsible planning is based on a broad system of mediators and activities during normal times, supplemented by intervention personnel and techniques set in motion during emergencies. This operation is coordinated with municipal and governmental support systems, which must be aware of the importance of comprehensive and flexible emergency systems for treating the population.

Address correspondence to: Nathaniel Laor, MD, PhD, Tel-Aviv Community Mental Health Center, 9 Hatzvi Street, Tel-Aviv 67197, Israel (E-mail: nlaor@netvision.net.il).

[Haworth co-indexing entry note]: "Community Mental Health in Emergencies and Mass Disasters: The Tel-Aviv Model." Laor, Nathaniel et al. Co-published simultaneously in *Journal of Aggression, Maltreatment & Trauma* (The Haworth Maltreatment & Trauma Press, an imprint of The Haworth Press, Inc.) Vol. 10, No. 3/4, 2005; and: *The Trauma of Terrorism: Sharing Knowledge and Shared Care, An International Handbook* (ed: Yael Danieli, Danny Brom, and Joe Sills) The Haworth Maltreatment & Trauma Press, an imprint of The Haworth Press, Inc., 2005.

KEYWORDS. Disaster, emergency, municipal, mental health

Israel is continually threatened by terrorism and the ever-present possibility of an all-out war. Border incidents, the 1991 Iraqi missile attacks, unrelenting terrorism, and the second Gulf War presented government authorities with the challenge of coping with a distinctive new reality, which necessitates a rapid and ongoing response to a wide range of problems deriving from the emergency situation and from fundamental changes to the everyday routine.

No existing system can provide an adequate response to these challenges. Until now, preparations for emergencies were made without enlisting the proper organizational and professional frameworks for dealing with the changed reality and without legislation to allocate the necessary resources. No clear definition of potential disaster scenarios exists, either on the national or on the local level, and the boundaries of responsibility for disaster management are blurred in both realms. Furthermore, essential coordination is lacking among all organizations involved in coping with emergencies. Health organizations, particularly those providing mental health services, operate within the local government authorities through autonomous frameworks with diverse organizational and professional languages, non-uniform levels of proficiency, and poorly defined public obligations. Because emergency hospitalization procedures are not coordinated with community procedures, the continuity crucial to proper treatment is lacking.

This article addresses the shortcomings outlined above and provides a working model: the Tel Aviv Model. It first discusses basic theoretical terminology, namely, disaster, disaster syndrome, and system disassociation. Second, it presents the professional preparation theory with its operational principles for mental health teams, including central, theoretical, and practical recommendations for enhancing the resilience of the population. Finally, it describes the Tel Aviv Model as an example of theory implementation and the actual operation of emergency mental health procedures. This model served as a blueprint for the Israel Ministry of Health guidelines for disaster preparedness and intervention in the area of community mental health.

WHAT IS A DISASTER?

A disaster is a radical, sudden, and surprising occurrence that causes extensive damage and shakes the physical and social foundations of life. It may occur as a result of intentional human actions (terrorism), human negligence (an explosion in a chemical plant), or the forces of nature (earthquake). The damage can be immediate, ongoing, or delayed, disrupting the routine of individuals and the community for days, weeks, or even years afterwards. The stages of a disaster may be based upon the intervening systems (army, local government authority, health services), according to the population's responses at various times (Danieli, 1998; Laor, 2001; World Health Organization, 1991), or both.

Clinical Stages of Disaster

Pre-Disaster/Preparation. This stage is characterized by warning signs and a sense of insecurity. Since not every disaster has warning signs, and ignoring such signs even if they are present is common, this stage is usually defined retrospectively.

The Event and Its Immediate Aftermath. A relatively short stage characterized by destruction, chaos, confusion, heightened emotions, and helplessness.

Initial Response. This stage is characterized by extensive and regressive structural and functional changes on the individual, organizational, and community levels. After the initial optimism caused by resource allocation at the disaster site and media attention, disillusionment sets in, accompanied by feelings of helplessness and isolation when victims deal with the bureaucratic systems designated to take care of them.

Stabilization. In this stage, survivors cope with physical, psychological, and ideological losses, which may have ramifications for collective ideology and identity.

Massive damage to the physical, socio-psychological, and cultural foundations of society may also be the result of sub-acute processes of rolling disasters, such as civil war, continuous terrorism, drought, and famine. In these cases, the initial erosion of infrastructure may allow for adaptive and normal life. With time, however, deep chinks may appear, soon becoming prominent cracks that impinge on what was thought to be normal and organized life, heralding a total systemic collapse.

In the case of terrorism, this continuous attack on public-civil space sets more significant changes in motion: the social fabric (ethnic, political, religious) begins to unravel; a blow is dealt to ethical foundations (killing of innocent people, use of ambulances for terrorist purposes, attacks on places of worship, hospitals and schools, the trampling of civil rights); political and ideological symbols are undermined; economic infrastructure is sabotaged (money laundering, smuggling, counterfeiting currency, bribery, organized crime); and the rule of law is weakened (violence, governmental corruption). As a result, a serious economic decline sets in (unemployment, poverty, diluted social services) and presents an existential threat to a large part of society.

MASS DISASTER SYNDROME

The mass disaster syndrome is comprised of a combination of post-traumatic and dissociative symptoms that appear while coming to terms with, and mourning, diverse losses on the individual and community levels. The phases of this syndrome's development are similar to the clinical stages of a disaster. First comes the shock induced by exposure to the massive destruction. Next is an intense emotional and cognitive response to different types of losses: loss of people, support systems, routine, and basic assumptions regarding security and order. Dissociative symptoms then begin to appear in the hours and days following the event. These are caused by a surreal experience of the self or the environment and reflect a reaction to experiential inundation. Psychological symptoms (anger, anxiety, sadness) and behavioral symptoms (sleep disturbances, violence) later complete the clinical picture (Norwood, Ursano & Fullerton, 2000; Vogel & Vernberg, 1993). If the traumatic response to the disaster is limited and controlled, most symptoms will disappear within the first year (Shalev, 2000). In more difficult cases, primarily those characterized by the collapse of social functions and support systems (the fourth stage), the symptoms will remain active for years and may become chronic (Laor, Wolmer, Mayes, Gershon, Weizman, & Cohen, 1997; Pynoos et al., 1993).

SYSTEMIC DISSOCIATION

Systemic dissociation is a process in which the system loses control of its parts during a disaster. For example, during a mass population evacuation, tent cities are set up detached from ordinary life and run according to different and autonomous rules. Often, the overall system retains some element of control and functioning while implementing goals determined by sub-systems (Laor & Wolmer, 2002). Thus, for example, at times of military takeovers, the military sub-system utilizes the economy and the health services to maintain governmental stability. In such situations, individuals, communities, and systems can remain detached from governmental bodies for quite a long time, as well as from their values and major objectives. The educational system, for example, will continue with the old curriculum, ignoring that changing needs and the emergency situation dictate a change in organization, educational content, and values. Thus, although dissociation appears in the name of maintaining routine and a sense of normality, it ultimately serves to cut off individuals and systems from reality and damages their ability to cope.

The following examples demonstrate the detrimental consequences of systemic dissociation. Mutual responsibility gives way to tribal convergence and withdrawal to sectorial and family groups; language becomes interwoven with traumatic words and images that differ completely from their original meanings; technologies change their purposes, serving the primary sub-system rather than the good of all; organizations become alienated and passive; cultural pride and a defined sense of identity lose their historical, cultural, and geographical context; and loyalty to one's people and nation is eroded by feelings of alienation, shame, disappointment, and betrayal.

PROFESSIONAL PREPARATION

In mass disasters, mental health services must play a crucial role to meet non-routine challenges that put basic professional issues to the test both in theory and in practice (Laor, Wolmer, Spirman & Wiener, 2003). The traumatized public, in confusion, disappointment, and anger, may need some source of stability within the chaotic conditions induced by the disaster. Mental health teams may be called upon to serve as anchor for community well-being and thus find themselves stretched beyond their designated roles and professional capabilities (Danieli, 2002).

The emergency operation of mental health teams is based on the following principles:

1. A comprehensive preparedness plan intended to provide solutions for various disaster scenarios, routinely implemented during emergencies that occur during normal times.
2. An ecological work plan based on the principles of preventive medicine, public health, community action, education, and urban planning (Laor & Wolmer, 2002).
3. A systemic social and community-oriented approach that copes with the impact of disaster on individuals, families, communities, society, and culture, integrated with the local government leadership, with special emphasis on populations at risk (e.g., children, elderly, minorities) and sensitivity to cultural diversity.
4. Wide-ranging multi-systemic coordination, laying a common operational foundation for the medical, mental health, educational, and welfare systems.
5. Empowerment of mediating agencies and professionals, such as the educational system, welfare services, primary medical care, volunteers, and community leadership.
6. Two-stage operation, beginning with a lack of differentiation among the intervention teams (everyone does everything), followed by functional differentiation according to profession and level of training.

7. Multidisciplinary operation integrating medical, mental health, welfare, educational, and community/urban leadership.
8. Continuity of care and services for those directly harmed by the emergency situation and those indirectly affected.
9. A professional infrastructure, characterized by expertise in allocating resources according to needs that can change unexpectedly, including the ability to work under constant pressure and to function within a variety of systems (primary and secondary medicine, mental health, public health, welfare, education, and government agencies) and at diverse locations (individual and community, education and culture, within the establishment and with non-government agencies).
10. Operational infrastructure for the mental health teams to enjoy both mobility and communication to improve command and control.

THE MENTAL HEALTH SYSTEM IN A DISASTER

The local government authority is responsible for operating the emergency services network in a disaster. Therefore, the urban mental health services must come under the auspices of the local government authority rather than remain subject to the routine command of the regular health systems (HMOs, Ministry of Health). This systemic change is essential to enable integration of the municipal systems of engineering, security, and welfare with professionals such as psychologists, social workers, primary care physicians, and psychiatrists in the community to create a comprehensive and coordinated system.

In a disaster, the mental health system alone cannot meet all needs. Responsible planning for mental health services during a disaster must be based on a broader system of mediating agencies (e.g., teachers, nurses) and of activities implemented during normal times, with the help of municipal and governmental support systems (Goenjian, 1993; Pynoos, Goenjian, & Steinberg, 1998).

Most of the position papers on how mental health services should cope with disasters focus on interventions after the event (DeWolfe, 2000; Young, Ford, Ruzek, Friedman, & Gusman, 1998), concentrating on the biological and psychological implications of alleviating pain and suffering. Almost no reference is made to advance preparation or fostering personal and community resilience along the lines of preventive medicine and urban/community planning. Coping with disaster necessitates intensive, ongoing preparations, starting at the governmental level and including all those involved in the local sub-systems, to create procedures for feedback from top to bottom, and vice versa.

Traditionally, the community mental health system consists of clinics and centers that treat patients referred by their family physicians, emergency rooms, as well as walk-ins. In some Western societies (such as the US), the delivery of mental healthcare services is largely privatized. As a result, community mental health systems tend to be smaller in size and geared primarily to the care of the chronically mentally ill. Furthermore, both the private and public mental health systems lack integration with social and educational services. The forecasting of disaster scenarios behooves decision makers of all systems involved to work collaboratively and create a coherent preparedness and resilience program for the community.

During a disaster, community mental health centers and clinics can serve as specialized trauma centers. Trained personnel of these institutions can be integrated into immediate intervention teams to assess, diagnose, and offer initial treatment. Likewise, they may serve as backups and supervisors for empowered clinical mediators from existing institutions, such as welfare services, family health clinics, schools, and community centers (Wolmer, Laor & Yazgan, 2003).

The responsible role of mental health specialists is to lead the multidisciplinary and inter-institutional teams by providing training and support for the mediators and treatment for victims in need of further specialized help. The merit of clinical mediators is in their being part of the natural communal environment and, as such, their activity is characterized by immediacy, familiarity, and lack of stigmatization. Hence, social workers in the municipal welfare system, educational counselors in the educational system, or nurses in the primary care clinics, could screen, identify, and provide initial treatment, maintaining ongoing contact with patients.

The principles of intervention can be summarized as follows (Laor & Wolmer, 2002):

Anticipation and Planning. Building an integrative forecast for functioning during disasters; predicting a variety of scenarios and developing appropriate programs; training skilled personnel; diverting material and human resources according to plan and need; constructing therapeutic protocols; developing local, national, and international networks; encouraging cooperation among systems; obtaining public funding and recognition.

Re-Differentiation. Evaluating the social losses of individuals and systems and their derivative functional failures; planning the functional classification stage in each system and between systems; building multidisciplinary teams.

Empowerment. Assimilating the know-how and training of those professionals and key organizations that come in direct contact with the victims; defining precisely the role of these organizations during a disaster; delegating authority to these bodies regarding assessment and initial treatment (Rappaport, 1987).

Supervision and Assessment. Setting functional boundaries; delegating know-how, expertise, and support among the therapeutic organizations; evaluating and developing plans in accordance with changing needs identified by feedback.

Treatment, Follow-Up, and Rehabilitation. Focusing on rehabilitating individuals and families while anticipating delayed reactions; coping with systemic and socio-cultural ramifications.

THE EMERGENCY MENTAL HEALTH SYSTEM–TEL AVIV MODEL

The Population Command

The operational coordination of the emergency system (including the mental health) headquarters comes under the Population Command in the local government, which is responsible for the management of evacuation, assistance, and casualties. The mental health headquarters is coordinated with the district emergency headquarters of the Ministry of Health, to which it reports (Spirman, Friedman, & Buchner, 2001).

The Population Command is responsible for preparedness and intervention strategies on both organizational and professional levels. This command consists of representatives from the various services of the local government (welfare and education, educational psychology, public health, tourism, communication, security, and emergency). The Population Command also includes representatives of other vital urban services and governmental bodies (HMOs, the army's Home Front Command, the regional offices of the Ministries of Health, Social Welfare, and Education; the National Insurance Institute, and the Religious Council).

The Population Command is comprised of five headquarters: (a) Welfare (provides immediate and ongoing psychosocial assistance; ensures that life goes on as normal and enhances community as well as individual resilience; (b) Education (activates formal and informal educational frameworks in accordance with the Ministry of Education and municipal policy); (c) Health (coordinates community medical services [HMO clinics], in accordance with instructions from the Ministry of Health); (d) Evacuation and Absorption (runs municipal evacuation and absorption centers for displaced populations); (e) Tourism (coordinates assistance to foreign visitors and workers, in coordination with the Ministries of Tourism and of Foreign Affairs).

The Mental Health Headquarters

The Donald J. Cohen and Irving B. Harris Center for Trauma and Disaster Intervention was established to alleviate the institutional and professional fragmentation in the community. It has a three-prong structure that brings together the municipal emergency system, the community primary care and mental health services, and the army's counterparts.

In calm times, among its other activities, the Center is involved in developing and implementing resilience and preparedness programs. In emergencies, the Center's professional leadership forms the Mental Health Headquarters for the metropolitan area, which is part of the Welfare Headquarters.

The Mental Health Headquarters is made up of five units, which are integrated with local government emergency teams (see Figure 1). The mental health emergency staff is regionally deployed in three trauma centers (a community mental health center can be designated as a regional trauma center within each local government or regional council).

Centers for Trauma and Disaster Intervention

Each Trauma Center specializes in: Screening and Evaluation (intake, screening prior to treatment, and evaluation of causation and disability), Treatment (individual, group, and family interventions for people of all ages), and Community Intervention (multidisciplinary teams, also posted in evacuation centers in coordination with the Home Front Command).

Training

Provides training and continuing education for professional and para-professional staff, and support through the "Who will Help the Helper?" unit.

Information and Evaluation

Gathers data about the population in all groups affected by the disaster; develops tools for evaluating individual, group, and community interventions.

Communications and Population Behavior

Offers information to the public via written and electronic media, including a "hotline" that provides emotional first aid over the phone.

Community Preparedness and Intervention

Plans and implements preparedness as well as community intervention and rehabilitation programs, consistent with the needs of special groups: preschoolers, children, and adolescents; elderly, disabled, and sick population groups; special populations (new immigrants, foreigners, minorities). This complex operation is carried out through the regional trauma centers as well as through teams of the municipal welfare headquarters:

FIGURE 1. The Municpial Mental Health Headquarters

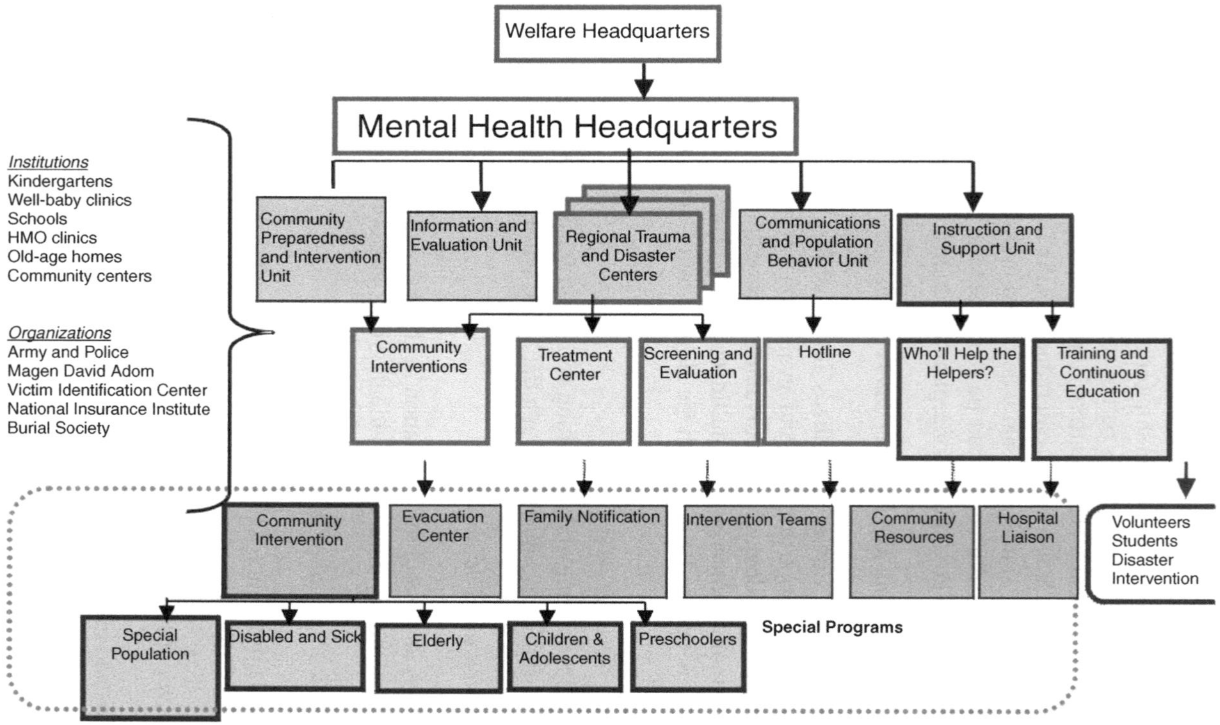

Intervention Teams. Provide immediate physical and mental assistance at the disaster site, at the National Institute for Forensic Medicine (victim identification center) or at evacuation centers. These multidisciplinary teams consist of social workers, psychologists, educators, physicians, nurses, and professional support staff.

Community Intervention. Plans and implements steps toward rehabilitating and treating individuals, families, communities, and institutions. These teams are involved in program development, outreach and treatment of special populations, and clinical and community intervention. These programs are implemented in community institutions, schools, kindergartens, well baby clinics, primary care medical clinics, mental health clinics, nursing homes, and community centers.

Hospital Liaison. Coordinates between the medical and mental health systems in the hospitals and the emergency headquarters.

Family Notification. Notifies the families of the deceased and assists in funeral arrangements. Each team has six members: a member of the city council, a clergyman, a physician/paramedic, two social workers, and a police officer.

Evacuation Center. Provides ongoing medical and mental health screening and treatment for displaced victims as well as coordinates the safe return to the community. Each team is made up of social workers, psychologists, a nurse, a professional support worker, and a social coordinator, backed up by community primary care clinics.

Community Resources. Supports the mental health system by means of planned and organized use of trained volunteers and activists to empower and rehabilitate the community.

THE EMERGENCY MENTAL HEALTH SYSTEM IN ACTION

Thus far, we have described the structure of the emergency system. The following describes dynamically the system as it responds to an emergency. Municipal multidisciplinary intervention teams consisting of social workers, psychologists, educators, physicians, and nurses arrive on the scene immediately after emergency rescue teams have completed their tasks. These teams conduct screening in the vicinity, refer identified victims to Regional Trauma Centers, and provide immediate physical and mental assistance at the disaster site and/or at the evacuation centers, should evacuation be deemed necessary. At the Regional Trauma Center, multidisciplinary teams (psychologists, psychiatrists, and social workers) are responsible for assessing and treating individuals, families, and entire communities. Hospitalized victims are followed up by members of the Liaison Unit, who visit them at their homes upon discharge. If needed, members of the Liaison Unit refer victims to Regional Trauma Centers.

During emergencies, the information offered to families of the dead and of the wounded needs to be managed with sensitivity. Information about casualties is transferred from the hospital and from the victim identification center to the Family Notification Unit. The latter notifies the families and assists in every detail of the funeral arrangements. The Victim Identification Center also provides liaison representation to intervention teams working with families waiting for information, because many of these families may need to participate in the daunting process of identifying the remains of their loved ones. Furthermore, special mental health teams work closely with the pathologist and the families during and after the identification process.

In case of emergencies affecting civilians and soldiers as well as army reserve units, this operation is run in collaboration with the army's Home Front Command and with the Department of Mental Health (Medical Corps). Of particular interest is the model developed for reserve units returning from combat with high casualty rates. In these cases, professionals from the army and from the Cohen-Harris Center team up to intervene with the goal of revitalizing and reactivating whole units to facilitate their return in due course to active duty.

In cases of mass disasters, the emergency system also takes responsibility for the process of evacuation; early evaluation and assessment of risk as guide for interventions; the construction and revitalization of newly created artificial communities; the implementation of protocols dealing with the disaster syndrome (e.g., posttrauma, grief, dissociation) for individuals, families, and the community; and lastly, occupational rehabilitation to create the suitable conditions for the reintegration of disaster survivors in their original community (Laor & Wolmer, 2002).

Finally, the Cohen-Harris Center established the School for the Study of Trauma, Preparedness, and Community Resilience. The school offers a two-year program for leaders of the various disciplines coming from different institutions in the community who are involved with disaster management and intervention. It intends to introduce state-of-the-art knowledge, common protocols of assessment, intervention, and information management, all serving to create integrated disaster preparedness and intervention programs for the metropolitan area of Tel-Aviv.

CONCLUSION

The overwhelming nature of a disaster and its concomitant massive losses generate a complex clinical and social picture whose impact is physical, psychological, social, and communal. In order to prepare adequately for the potential damage, to run a comprehensive intervention program geared to the changing needs of the victims, and to preserve the social and emotional functioning of individuals and the community as a whole, professionals must adopt an ecological and systemic approach for coping with disaster. Such an approach is based upon integrating multi-systemic and multidisciplinary teams while using mediating agents trained for the task by mental health specialists. The training process is ongoing and cyclical; it takes place during ordinary times and not only in preparation for emergencies.

All this, however, is not sufficient; peripheral and complementary organizations and institutions in the mental health field must also be prepared to act as mediators and helpers for specialized professionals. This way, systemic mediation is both along vertical (top-down) and horizontal (cross-sectional) lines. Even in societies where mental healthcare services are largely privatized, local governments as well as national institutions must be aware of the importance of comprehensive and flexible emergency systems for treating the population. It is their responsibility to invest continually and proactively in disaster preparation rather than to react after such events occur.

In our era, environmental risks ought to be taken seriously lest we jeopardize human existence. Most societies find it extremely hard to invest resources based on long-term considerations, and decide to spend resources only when faced with concrete challenges. Surprised by disaster, these societies may find themselves all-too-vulnerable. In today's global village, under the constant threat of terrorism, no community is free from commitment to preparedness. Yet, no community must cope with disaster on its own, nor is it capable of doing so. Working together can save lives, reduce the damage, alleviate pain, and maintain hope for a better world.

REFERENCES

Danieli, Y. (1998). Conclusions and future directions. In Y. Danieli (Ed.), *International Handbook of Multigenerational Legacies of Trauma* (pp. 669-689). New York: Plenum Press.

DeWolfe, D. J. (2000). Field manual for mental health and human service workers in major disasters. *Center for Mental Health Services*. Retrieved November 10, 2002 from http://www.mentalhealth.org

Goenjian, A. (1993). A mental health relief programme in Armenia after the 1988 earthquake: Implementation and clinical observations. *British Journal of Psychiatry, 163*, 230-239.

Laor, N. (2001, April). *The role of mental health professionals after mass disasters.* Paper presented at the Promised Childhood Congress, Tel Aviv, Israel.

Laor, N., & Wolmer, L. (2002). Children exposed to disaster: The role of the mental health professional. In M. Lewis (Ed.), *Textbook of Child and Adolescent Psychiatry* (3rd ed., pp. 925-937). Baltimore, MD: Williams and Wilkins.

Laor, N., Wolmer, L., Mayes, L. C., Gershon, A., Weizman, R., & Cohen, D. J. (1997). Israeli preschoolers under Scuds: A thirty-month follow-up. *Journal of the American Academy of Child and Adolescent Psychiatry, 36,* 349-356.

Laor, N., Wolmer, L., Spirman, S., & Wiener, Z. (2003). Facing war, terrorism, and disaster: toward a child-oriented comprehensive emergency care system. *Child and Adolescent Psychiatric Clinics of North America, 12*(2), 343-361.

Norwood, A. E., Ursano, R. J., & Fullerton, C. S. (2000). Disaster psychiatry: Principles and practice. *Psychiatry Quarterly, 71,* 207-266.

Pynoos, R. S., Goenjian, A., Tashjian, M., Karakashian, M., Manjikian, R., Manoukian, G. et al. (1993). Post-traumatic stress reactions in children after the 1988 Armenian earthquake. *British Journal of Psychiatry, 163,* 239-247.

Pynoos, R. S., Goenjian, A. K., & Steinberg, A. M. (1998). A public mental health approach to the postdisaster treatment of children and adolescents. *Child and Adolescent Psychiatric Clinics of North America, 7*(1), 195-210.

Rappaport, J. (1987). Terms of empowerment/exemplars of prevention. Towards a theory for community psychology. *American Journal of Community Psychology, 15,* 121-145.

Shalev, A. Y. (2000). Post-traumatic stress disorder: Diagnosis, history and life course. In D. Nutt, J. R. T. Davidson, & J. Zohar, (Eds.), *Post-traumatic stress disorder: Diagnosis, management and treatment* (pp. 1-15). London: Martin Dunitz.

Spirman, S., Friedman, Z., & Buchner, N. (2001). *Mass emergency treatment system.* Tel-Aviv, Israel: Tel Aviv-Jaffa Municipality.

Vogel, J. M., & Vernberg, E. M. (1993). Children's psychological responses to disasters. *Journal of Clinical Child Psychology, 22,* 464-484.

Wolmer, L., Laor, N., & Yazgan, Y. (2003). Implementing relief programs in schools after disasters: The teacher as clinical resource. *Child and Adolescent Psychiatry Clinics of North America, 12*(2), 343-361.

World Health Organization. (1991). *Psychosocial guidelines for preparedness and intervention in disaster.* Geneva, Switzerland: WHO, MNH/PSF/91.3.

Young, B. H., Ford, J. D., Ruzek, J. I., Friedman, M. J., & Gusman, F. D. (1998). *Disaster mental health services: A guidebook for clinicians and administrators.* Department of Veterans Affairs. The National Center for Post-Traumatic Stress Disorder. Retrieved October 12, 2002 from http://www.ncptsd.org

Challenges of Urban
Mental Health Disaster Planning

Lloyd I. Sederer
Kelly L. Ryan
Kimberly B. Gill
Joshua F. Rubin

SUMMARY. Establishing disaster preparedness is an urgent matter, particularly with regard to mental health. This article examines the challenges of mental health disaster planning in the context of an urban setting, which may differ from those pertaining to rural areas. The need to better integrate public health disaster planning and mental health disaster planning is critical. This document particularly focuses on the challenges involved in leading, coordinating, and convening an urban mental health disaster response. With time, dedication, resources, and creation of effective policy, successful mental health response capability will evolve and endure.

Address correspondence to: Lloyd I. Sederer, MD, Department of Health and Mental Hygiene, 93 Worth Street, Room 410, New York, NY 10013 USA (E-mail: lsederer@health.nyc.gov).

[Haworth co-indexing entry note]: "Challenges of Urban Mental Health Disaster Planning." Sederer, Loyd I. et al. Co-published simultaneously in *Journal of Aggression, Maltreatment & Trauma* (The Haworth Maltreatment & Trauma Press, an imprint of The Haworth Press, Inc.) Vol. 10, No. 3/4, 2005; and: *The Trauma of Terrorism: Sharing Knowledge and Shared Care, An International Handbook* (ed: Yael Danieli, Danny Brom, and Joe Sills) The Haworth Maltreatment & Trauma Press, an imprint of The Haworth Press, Inc., 2005.

KEYWORDS. Disaster mental health, terrorism, urban planning, disasters, community, resilience

Disasters and terrorist attacks have become an inevitable reality. The question is not if they will happen, but when and of what kind, natural or person-made, accidental or intentional. Most cities have well-developed protocols in place to respond to fires, floods, tornadoes, earthquakes, and other such incidents. However, the terrorist attacks of September 11, 2001 and the ongoing threat of future terrorist attacks beg for a better understanding of what it means to be prepared for a "disaster." Disaster preparedness, as discussed in this article, pays special attention to acts of terrorism.

A particular challenge to successful disaster planning is the need to depend on hypotheticals. It is simply not possible to anticipate every scenario that could occur. Furthermore, disaster responses are typically enacted after a disaster has occurred and only for a specified period of time, which might suffice for a flood, but would be less effective in responding to a terrorist attack. A mental health disaster response to terrorism must prepare for phases of response before and after an event occurs. The mere threat of harm for a prolonged period of time, as many have experienced since September 11, 2001, in conjunction with a limited sense of what one can do to protect oneself, is akin to a prolonged, chronic disaster, which necessitates a similarly protracted mental health response. This is a much different model than issued for other areas of disaster preparedness and response.

Consequently, mental health disaster planning must be both flexible and comprehensive. Any response will depend heavily upon the context of the disaster. A terrorist attack is likely to elicit psychological reactions that differ from those resulting from a natural disaster, such as a hurricane. Feelings of having been intentionally wronged contribute to the complexity of reaction in the case of terrorist attack (Stern, 1999). Furthermore, the response to a biological, chemical or radiological terrorist attack will differ significantly from the response to a "traditional" terrorist attack, such as a bombing. Many biological, chemical, and radiological agents are difficult to identify, spread rapidly, and raise the question of contamination, making the 'event' difficult to recognize. In contrast, a bombing tends to be contained in one defined area, even a large area like the Alfred P. Murrah Federal Building in Oklahoma City, and is typically at a specific point in time in terms of the active attack (Stern, 1999).

While establishing disaster preparedness is an urgent matter, there are obstacles, particularly with regard to mental health. This article will examine the challenges of mental health disaster planning in the context of an urban setting, which may differ from those pertaining to rural areas. We will discuss the need to better integrate public health disaster planning and mental health disaster planning; review the challenges involved in mental health disaster preparedness within an urban setting; consider the challenges involved in leading, coordinating and convening an urban mental health disaster response; and emphasize the difficulty of ensuring the quality of a mental health disaster response.

DISASTER PLANNING, PUBLIC HEALTH, AND MENTAL HEALTH

Before one can begin to discuss the specifics of mental health disaster preparedness, it is essential to address the role of disaster planning in relation to public health and mental health, respectively. It is also important to consider mental health with respect to its role as an essential component of both public health and disaster preparedness. The interdependency of mental health, public health, and disaster planning is inescapable.

The public health consequences of the September 11, 2001 attacks, such as air pollution, water contamination, dangerous working conditions, and injuries, make it difficult to ignore the importance of disaster preparedness within the field of public health (Klitzman & Freudenberg, 2003). In response to a biological, chemical, or radiological attack, the role of public health workers is particularly critical. Minimizing the damage of an attack requires a swift and effective response from the many specialty areas of public health. While most understand that mental health is a specialty component of public health, confusion and ambivalence remain as to how it should be incorporated into public health initiatives and planning.

Articles by Bleich, Gelkopf and Solomon (2003), Butler, Panzer, and Goldfrank (2003), Cardenas, Williams, Wilson, Fanouraki, and Singh (2003), Danieli, Engdahl, and Schlenger (2003), Klitzman and Freudenberg (2003), Linley, Joseph, Cooper, Harris, and Meyer (2003), North and Pfefferbaum (2002), Schlenger et al. (2002), Silver, Holman, McIntosh, Poulin, and Gil-Rivas (2002), and Simeon, Greenberg, Knutelska, Schmeidler and Hollander (2003) document in detail the direct and indirect, immediate and long-term mental health effects of terrorist attacks, such as 9/11. The mere anticipation of another terrorist act, consistent warnings and threats, combined with the lack of information on when, where, or how a future event might occur, and therefore how to protect oneself, is likely to produce additional psychological effects (Karon, 2002). In fact, one of the essential aims of terrorism is this intentional intimidation of a population (Butler et al., 2003; Stern, 1999).

The fields of "health" and "mental health" are distinct in various ways, but the two domains should not be considered separate when considering overall well-being. To paraphrase former Surgeon General David Satcher, there is no health without mental health. Moreover, physical illness likewise affects mental health. Further, integrating mental health concerns into public health activities will help to create a more comprehensive definition of "public health" and enable comprehensive public health disaster preparedness.

Advancing mental health disaster planning as an essential function in any public health agenda cannot be done without the support of leaders, administrators, and policymakers. The first of many struggles in achieving such integration exists within the field of mental health. Many in the mental health community do not yet understand the critical responsibility that mental health administrators and practitioners have in disaster preparedness (Butler et al., 2003). Considering the psychological consequences that result from a disaster, or simply the threat thereof, mental health leaders must acknowledge and meet their responsibility in achieving disaster preparedness. They must do so by obtaining and dedicating resources, developing policy, educating constituents, and, of course, accepting responsibility for a significant portion of the public's overall health. In essence, the role of mental health administrators is to prepare an effective response to the mental health consequences of terrorism while continuing to develop policies and allotting funds that will enable such a response to be fully realized and maintained.

SPECIAL CHALLENGES OF AN URBAN SETTING

Based on factors such as population density, infrastructure, and previous attacks, urban areas are generally considered vulnerable to possible terrorist attacks (Perlman, 2003; U.S. Department of Homeland Security, 2003). Urban areas have unique transportation characteristics including bottlenecking entryways, such as bridges and tunnels, as well as substantial mass transportation infrastructures such as subways and buses. Cities are easily accessible and often densely populated, making it difficult to locate particular individuals, assess need, and control the spread of various chemical, biological, and radiological agents. Preparedness activities that are effective in less dense areas are often impractical for an urban setting. Storage of large emergency response kits and extra sets of car keys may be useful for a family living in a suburban or rural area, but may be less germane to many residents in urban areas who often live in small apartments and rely on public transportation.

The distinctive characteristics of a city must be considered when approaching mental health disaster preparedness. One of the greatest assets of many cities, varied demography, can represent a challenge for mental health disaster planning. New York City is an excellent example with eight million residents, representing a tremendous diversity in ethnicity, nationality, religion, socioeconomic status, language, and culture. Over one million New Yorkers are not proficient in the English language; thus, language is a particular consideration for any and all planning activities (New York City Department of City Planning, 2001). Additionally, mental health disaster preparedness must also take into account specific and vulnerable populations that have particular needs, for example, refugees, children, older adults, and individuals with mental retardation, developmental disabilities, chemical dependencies, or mental illnesses. Urban areas also have more homeless individuals, many of whom have mental health needs, and are likely to be without health insurance (National Coalition for the Homeless, 1999).

Further, these challenges make it more difficult to gain access to communities and to conduct needs assessments. Identifying where needs exist and the most appropriate way to address them is confounded by culture and belief systems, making it also more challenging to conduct quality outreach in an attempt to increase awareness of the availability of services and understand the depth of need. Within many cultures, the formal mental health system is not the preferred arena to seek or obtain help. This must, too, be respected and accommodated in planning and outreach efforts.

IMPORTANT CONSIDERATIONS IN MENTAL HEALTH DISASTER PLANNING

Community Resilience

Building community resilience, or building a community's ability to withstand past and future adversity and reinforcing belief in this ability, is a crucial, but not an easy, element of mental health disaster planning. By some counts, there are over 400 communities in New York City (Citizen's Committee for NYC, 2003). Furthermore, there are significant and complex questions about how to define a community. One must also learn the community's values and identify its official and unofficial leaders before resilience work is undertaken.

Once the foundation is established, alliances can be formed with de facto and non-traditional mental health providers in communities. Social networks can then be identified or built, or repaired and strengthened, and then connected to other networks, including government and other mental health disaster planners. Support must be developed and offered in ways that are acceptable and relevant to particular communities and involve their members. True community resilience cannot be implanted from without. There may be a role for government to initiate a process of building community resilience (e.g., by fostering linkages within and among communities), but the approach is best when it enables community members on all levels to lead and own it from the start (Sederer, Ryan, & Rubin, 2003).

Any one community's process of building its points of cohesion will look different from another's, as the local values and systems will determine what is needed and how it will be provided. However, while each process will be unique, each should celebrate people's strengths and promote positive individual and community self-images. Building community resilience is not only an important aspect of mental health disaster preparedness; it is the very context in which such preparedness should occur. Examples of models of such community-building initiatives can be reviewed in Bell (2001), Boss, Beaulieu, Weiling, Turner, and LaCruz (2003), Everly (2003), and Ottenstein (2003).

Continual Stress

Throughout all communities in the United States, people have been experiencing a consistently increased level of terror alert for over two years (Danieli et al., 2003). Many people do not acknowledge the continued impact of threats of terrorism, and symptoms of chronic stress and fear are not always obvious, may be misunderstood, or simply ignored, and therefore go unaddressed (Project Liberty/New York City Department of Health, 2001). Chronic stress can also impact physical health. Some people abuse or increase their abuse of alcohol and other drugs, including tobacco. Many individuals coping with chronic stress experience elevated blood pressure, decreased energy and efficiency, lower motivation to exercise, and are more distracted, jeopardizing safety and increasing risk of accidents (Butler et al., 2003; Project Liberty/New York City Department of Health, 2001; Vlahov et al., 2002).

People often become desensitized and inured to such warnings and are therefore less likely to take precautions, remain vigilant, or report suspicious activity. In addition, while successful adaptation to a new reality of continual threat might involve a certain level of routinization or normalization, there is a fine balance between protecting oneself from perpetual stimulation and not attending to the psychological reactions to persistent threat (Kron & Mendlovic, 2002).

It is, however, important to distinguish between the use of these defense mechanisms and the concept of resilience. Defense mechanisms may be adaptive when there is an actual threat and there are limited protective actions available, but they are not adaptive when it is in fact possible to do something or when they persist when threat no longer exists (Kron & Mendlovic, 2002). Ideally, resilient communities cease to employ defense mechanisms when a threat no longer exists.

THE ROLE OF GOVERNMENT

The number and diversity of services and resources available in New York City is an invaluable asset in the planning process. Professionals working throughout the City are often trusted by, and familiar to, people in the community. Many have established relationships with the public and therefore have a good sense of its needs. New York City is fortunate to have the benefit of an extensive mental health network, as well as a remarkable system of over 75 hospitals and half a dozen academic medical centers.

However, challenges abound. Government must harness and organize a vast array of resources, and this new set of organizational hurdles can delay the development of a comprehensive mental health disaster plan. When organizing a plan in a resource-rich urban environment, it is necessary first to identify the functions where assistance is necessary, such as assessment of needs, deployment of responders, communication with responders and the public, credentialing of those who will assist in a response, and outreach to ensure that communities access the assistance available to them. One must then identify which individuals, organizations, agencies, or institutions will be most useful, based on their core competencies. This will help avoid confusion, duplication of services, exhaustion of personnel, depletion of resources, and revictimization (Pfefferbaum, 1996; Tucker, Pfefferbaum, Vincent, Boehler, & Nixon, 1998).

Disaster resources are found within the de facto, or natural, provider communities as well. People often turn to clergy and other key community members such as teachers, nurses, or salon workers to obtain informal support. It is necessary to involve these indigenous providers in the planning process, as they are sometimes closest to those community members who are hardest to reach. They should also be involved in the formal planning process so that they can be supported, trained, evaluated, and integrated, both into the government response plan and among themselves.

Furthermore, it is helpful to organize the relevant functions for each phase of a disaster: pre-event, acute, post-acute, and long-term. This is quite challenging, however, given that defining the specific, predetermined timeframes of these phases can be arbitrary. Depending on the event, the acute phase of a disaster could be three days or three months. Furthermore, one cannot be sure that the impact of an event will not intensify, rather than deescalate, as time passes.

The need to draw heavily upon, and extensively coordinate, hospitals and mental health agencies in order to develop high levels of preparedness places an unprecedented demand upon planners. Coordinating a comprehensive mental health disaster plan raises questions about prioritizing functions, defining jurisdiction, and reexamining role definition and hierarchy. Some agencies and hospitals may have collaborated or partnered in the past and have extensive histories, good and bad, with one another. Intervening in these long-term relationships is thus a delicate process. When depending upon external responders, there is also the potential for overlap in resources.

It is especially critical that safety net providers are functioning in the aftermath of a disaster. Considerations include relief systems for responders, command structures when community leaders are unavailable, contingency plans for programs, and policies on temporary relocation, emergency communications plans, and computer backup. These can be developed in governmental contracts or memoranda of understanding.

BEST PRACTICES: MENTAL HEALTH DISASTER RESPONSE

One of the most critical, and least developed, components of a mental health disaster response is *quality*. The effectiveness of any particular response intervention, how interventions are taught, and the credentials of those who respond to disasters are all important factors in developing best practices for mental health disaster response. However, empirical information and professional consensus to support decisions in this area are limited at best (National Institute of Mental Health [NIMH], 2002).

There are numerous methods of intervention and treatment for addressing the mental health consequences of terrorism. More detailed information on such treatment interventions following incidents of terrorism and traumatic experiences can be found in Danieli et al. (2003), Marshall and Suh (2003), and Miller (2003). Consequently, there is variation in mental health disaster response and treatment, yet not all traditional trauma interventions will be of value in response to a community-wide disaster (Hiley-Young & Gerrity, 1994). It is therefore necessary to advance particular curricula to ensure that the training of mental health disaster responders is constructive. This is not to say that there is one single training method that is of the most value; there are likely several. However, there is a need for some uniformity in response (Butler et al., 2003; NIMH, 2002). To date, neither the United States federal government nor professional organizations have provided such guidance. A report by the Institute of Medicine, *Preparing for the Psychological Consequences of Terrorism* (Butler et al., 2003), acknowledges the same lack of consensus.

In fact, in the immediate days following a disaster, basic needs such as food, water, shelter, and locating loved ones are generally of much greater importance to an affected individual than talking about their emotions, which is an important point for any clinician or responder to bear in mind. This too further points to the need for a common understanding among responders, and for uniform training in disaster mental health response, bearing in mind that the effects of trauma differ based on how it is inflicted on the victim, so responses to trauma must follow suit (North & Pfefferbaum, 2002).

Moreover, many individuals impacted by a disaster may be unaware of, or unconcerned about, their own need for self-care, particularly in an acute phase. Others hesitate to seek mental health treatment, in part because of the stigma associated with mental illness (U.S. Department of Health and Human Services, 1999). This presents another challenge in organizing a mental health response. To reach individuals in order to provide them with information on accessing mental health services, it is important to integrate mental health services throughout an overall disaster response system in both subtle and direct ways. For example, direct mental health service in the immediate aftermath of a disaster might include administering medication, triage, and referral. However, individuals who are ambivalent about acknowledging mental health concerns in an acute phase of a disaster may benefit from the distribution of mental health information pamphlets, along with other social service information, that they may refer to at another time. An understanding of psychological reactions to a disaster should be integrated in all medical, public health, and human service responses to a disaster.

Training and credentials of disaster mental health responders are essential to the quality of response. The qualifications, education, and experience of mental health clinicians vary and, as a result, it is not always clear what it means to be a trauma, grief, or crisis "expert." Standardized training should be developed and added to accredited programs through which responders obtain their degrees.

Finally, in the wake of a disaster, people are eager to provide assistance. Many spontaneous volunteers come forward to offer mental health aid. While it is comforting to see a community unite, it can be problematic to involve volunteers in a mental health disaster response when they are not connected to a trusted institution or their credentials are not easily verified. This underscores the need for uniformity in disaster mental health training, consensus on best clinical practices, and reliable credentialing.

FUTURE DIRECTIONS

In this document, we have attempted to outline a few of the many challenges in developing and leading an urban mental health disaster response.

While identifying responders, harnessing resources, and creating communications plans are some of the greatest challenges, urban areas present a rich array of resources that can be mobilized. With time, determination, and some limited resources, a plan to coordinate and convene a response can be achieved. To the extent that preparedness is built into permanent infrastructures, over time effective response capability will endure.

As we work to further integrate mental health into public health, we urge that mental health screening be better integrated into general medical practice and pediatric care. Undetected mental health disorders such as depression, anxiety, and PTSD have profound ramifications on individuals, communities, and the economy. Mental healthcare coverage, or lack thereof, greatly impacts access to services.

Comprehensive mental health disaster preparedness will require developing best clinical practices. Research and guidance is needed in the areas of needs assessment, clinical intervention, triage, training, credentialing, and resource allocation (NIMH, 2002). Such guidance will enable policymakers and leaders to provide sound recommendations for mental health disaster planning.

REFERENCES

Bell, C. (2001). Cultivating resiliency in youth. *Journal of Adolescent Health, 29*, 375-381.

Bleich, A., Gelkopf, M., & Solomon, Z. (2003). Exposure to terrorism, stress-related mental health symptoms, and coping behaviors among a nationally representative sample in Israel. *Journal of the American Medical Association, 290*, 612-620.

Boss, P., Beaulieu, L., Weiling, E., Turner, W., & LaCruz, S. (2003). Healing loss, ambiguity, and trauma: A community-based intervention with families of union workers missing after the 9/11 attack in New York City. *Journal of Marital and Family Therapy, 29*, 455-467.

Butler, A. S., Panzer, A. M., & Goldfrank, L. R. (Eds.). (2003). *Preparing for the psychological consequences of terrorism: A public health strategy.* (Committee on Responding to the Psychological Consequences of Terrorism, Board on Neuroscience and Behavioral Health). Washington, DC: Institute of Medicine of The National Academy of Sciences, The National Academies Press.

Cardenas, J., Williams, K., Wilson, J. P., Fanouraki, G., & Singh, A. (2003). PTSD, major depressive symptoms, and substance abuse following September 11, 2001, in a midwestern university population. *International Journal of Emergency Mental Health, 5*, 15-28.

Citizen's Committee for NYC. (2003). *Neighborhood link.* Retrieved June 3, 2003 from http://ccnyc.neighborhoodlink.com/ccnyc

Danieli, Y., Engdahl, B., & Schlenger, W. E. (2003). The psychological aftermath of terrorism. In F. Moghaddam, A. J. Marsella, & A. Bandura (Eds.), *International ter-*

rorism and terrorists: Psychosocial perspectives (pp. 223-246). Washington, DC: American Psychological Association.

Everly, G. S. (2003). Pastoral crisis intervention in response to terrorism. *International Journal of Emergency Mental Health, 5*, 1-2.

Hiley-Young, B., & Gerrity, E. T. (1994). Critical incident stress debriefing (CISD): Value and limitations in disaster response. *NCP Clinical Quarterly, 4*. Retrieved June 17, 2003 from http://www.ncptsd.org/publications/cq/v4/n2/hiley-yo.html

Karon, T. (2002). Terrorizing ourselves. *Time*. Retrieved June 17, 2003 from http://www.time.com/time/nation/article/0,8599,241309,00.html

Klitzman, S., & Freudenberg, N. (2003). Implications of the world trade center attack for the public health and health care infrastructures. *American Journal of Public Health, 93*, 400-406.

Kron, S., & Mendlovic, S. (2002). Mental health consequences of bioterrorism. *The Israeli Medical Association Journal, 4*, 524-527.

Linley, P. A., Joseph, S., Cooper, R. Harris, S., & Meyer, C. (2003). Positive and negative changes following vicarious exposure to the September 11 terrorist attacks. *Journal of Traumatic Stress, 16*, 481-485.

Marshall, R. D., & Suh, E. J. (2003). Contextualizing trauma: Using evidence-based treatments in a multicultural community after 9/11. *Psychiatric Quarterly, 74*, 401-420.

Miller, L. (2003). Family therapy of terroristic trauma: Psychological syndromes and treatment strategies. *Psychotherapy: Theory, Research, Practice Training, 39*, 283-296.

National Coalition for the Homeless. (1999). *Health care and homelessness: NCH fact sheet #8*. Retrieved May 29, 2003 from http://www.nationalhomeless.org/health.html

National Institute of Mental Health. (2002). *Mental health and mass violence: Evidence-based early psychological intervention for victims/survivors of mass violence*. A workshop to reach consensus on best practices. NIH Publication No. 02-5138, Washington, DC: U.S. Government Printing Office. Retrieved February 24, 2003 from http://www.nimh.gov/research/massviolence.pdf

New York City Department of City Planning, Population Division. (2001). *NYC 2000, results from the 2000 consensus, socioeconomic characteristics*. Retrieved June 26, 2003 from http://www.ci.nyc.ny.us/html/dcp/pdf/census/sociopp.pdf

North, C. S., & Pfefferbaum, B. (2002). Research on the mental health effects of terrorism. *Journal of the American Medical Association, 288*, 633-636.

Ottenstein, R. J. (2003). Coping with threats of terrorism: A protocol for group intervention. *International Journal of Emergency Mental Health, 5*, 39-42.

Perlman, E. (2003, May). Can we talk? *Governing*. Retrieved May 30, 2003 from http://www.governing.com/archive/2003/may/interop.txt

Pfefferbaum, B. (1996). *The Oklahoma City bombing: Organizing the mental health response*. Retrieved May 22, 2003 from http://www.aaets.org/arts/art5.htm.

Project Liberty/New York City Department of Health. (2001). *New York needs us strong; Coping after Sept. 11*. Retrieved May 22, 2003 from http://www.nyc.gov/html/doh/html/liberty/english.html

Schlenger, W. E., Caddell, J. M., Ebert, L., Jordan, B. K., Rourke, K. M., Wilson, D. et al. (2002). Psychological reactions to terrorist attacks. *Journal of the American Medical Association, 288*(5), 581-588.

Sederer, L. I., Ryan, K. L., & Rubin, J. F. (2003) The psychological impact of terrorism: Policy implications. *International Journal of Mental Health, 32*, 7-19.

Silver, R. C., Holman, A. E., McIntosh, D. N., Poulin, M., & Gil-Rivas, V. (2002). Nationwide longitudinal study of psychological responses to September 11. *Journal of the American Medical Association, 288*, 1235-1244.

Simeon, D., Greenberg, J., Knutelska, M., Schmeidler, J., & Hollander, E. (2003). Peritraumatic reactions associated with the world trade center disaster. *American Journal of Psychiatry, 160*, 1702-1705.

Stern, J. (1999). *The ultimate terrorists*. Cambridge, MA: Harvard University Press.

Tucker, P., Pfefferbaum, B., Vincent, R., Boehler, S. D., & Nixon, S. J. (1998). Oklahoma City: Disaster challenges mental health and medical administrators. *Journal of Behavioral Health Services and Research, 25*, 93-99.

U.S. Department of Health and Human Services. (1999). *Mental health: A report of the Surgeon General*. Rockville, MD: U.S. Department of Health and Human Services, Substance Abuse and Mental Health Services Administration.

U.S. Department of Homeland Security. (2003). *Securing the homeland: Protecting our states and cities*. Retrieved June 4, 2003 from http://www.whitehouse.gov/news/releases/2003/04/20030408-5.html

Vlahov, D., Galea, S., Resnick, H., Ahern, J., Boscarino, J., Bucuvalas, M. et al. (2002). Increased use of cigarettes, alcohol, and marijuana among Manhattan, New York, residents after the September 11th terrorist attacks. *American Journal of Epidemiology, 155*, 988-996.

Integrating Behavioral Aspects into Community Preparedness and Response Systems

Dori B. Reissman
Shauna Spencer
Terri L. Tanielian
Bradley D. Stein

SUMMARY. This article examines the role of psychosocial and behavioral dimensions of terrorism that influence community preparedness and homeland defense efforts. Public health interventions will fail if people do not follow the recommendations. A broader public health model is applied to help identify the interactions between risk and safety appraisals, social factors, and behavioral response to uncertain and stressful situations. Community preparedness would benefit by linking disparate programmatic and advocacy initiatives that already exist. It stands to reason that improving the cohesiveness of existing systems of

---

Address correspondence to: Dori B. Reissman, MD, MPH, Commander, U.S. Public Health Service, Senior Advisor for Disaster, Terrorism, and Mental Health, Office of the Director, Division of Violence Prevention, National Center for Injury Prevention and Control, Centers for Disease Control and Prevention (CDC), 4770 Buford Highway, NE, Mailstop K-68, Atlanta, GA 30341-3742 USA (E-mail: dreissman@cdc.gov).

[Haworth co-indexing entry note]: "Integrating Behavioral Aspects into Community Preparedness and Response Systems." Reissman, Dori B. et al. Co-published simultaneously in *Journal of Aggression, Maltreatment & Trauma* (The Haworth Maltreatment & Trauma Press, an imprint of The Haworth Press, Inc.) Vol. 10, No. 3/4, 2005; and: *The Trauma of Terrorism: Sharing Knowledge and Shared Care, An International Handbook* (ed: Yaël Danieli, Danny Brom, and Joe Sills) The Haworth Maltreatment & Trauma Press, an imprint of The Haworth Press, Inc., 2005.

social organization would strengthen community resilience and serve as effective countermeasures for terrorism.

KEYWORDS. Psychosocial, mental health, public health, emergency response, community resilience, terrorism, psychological consequences, social consequences, community violence

Terrorist activities in 2001 challenged the United States of America to learn new ways of preparing and responding that would provide a sense of safety and security to the public (Hyams, Murphy, & Wessely, 2003). Increased information has been provided to improve community preparedness, such as encouraging families and schools to have plans for an emergency that include food and water supplies, activities for children, medications, flashlights and batteries, contact information, and reunification plans if children and parents are not co-located. The "new normal" has required extensive collaborations across culturally and organizationally disparate systems such as law enforcement, emergency management, public health, clinical laboratory, mass media, education agencies, and medical response systems from all levels of public enterprise. Priority in health planning has focused initially on the acute investigational challenges and medical treatment or prophylaxis, and secondly on the surge capacity to provide scalable medical and public health responses. However, the events of September 11, 2001 (hereinafter referred to as 9/11) highlighted the need for a well-coordinated public mental health response system (Hyams et al., 2003; Institute of Medicine [IOM], 2003).

Response system coordination requires that public and private mental and behavioral health networks participate in joint planning and community-based or regional exercises with other response system components; namely, public health, emergency management, law enforcement, business communities, civic and faith-based organizations, schools, special needs facilities, and medical care systems. Currently, planning for "mental health" needs after large-scale public health emergencies is commonly limited to providing clinical service or psychological first aid designed to mitigate directly or lessen the severity of the psychological impact on victims, responders, and nearby community members (Centers of Disease Control [CDC], 2003a). Yet, little attention has been paid to preparedness involving the broader psychological, social, functional, and behavioral issues that influence recovery efforts at the community level.

The term "community" can be applied in many ways that influence strategic public health intervention efforts. A community can be defined by geographic proximity, common governance, or a variety of social, cultural, religious, and economic parameters. The notion of community may be defined in terms of social networks arising from common experiences, such as childcare, occupation, workplace, school, hobby, or through exposure to disastrous events. Since emergency response is coordinated at a local jurisdictional level, community preparedness is a key ingredient for homeland security. Response readiness needs to consider both individual and collective behavior and function within the social and cultural contexts of impacted communities (Kaniasty & Norris, 1999).

LIFECYCLE OF PUBLIC HEALTH EMERGENCIES

Phases of Disaster from a Community Perspective

Four common collective psychosocial and behavioral response phases occur during the lifecycle of a disaster (Myers & Zunin, 2000). A heroic period has been noted in the early aftermath of disasters requiring intense search and rescue efforts. The community then experiences a honeymoon phase where survivors and less impacted others are more likely to exhibit altruistic behaviors, including donating money, clothing, food, medicine, blood, and volunteering for service with civic and faith-based organizations. This is a time where the desire to help others overcomes the usual communication barriers due to social hierarchy and infrastructure. Disillusionment, resentment, and group fragmentation often appear as reimbursement plans and disbursements of donated goods and services fail to meet expectations to reconstruct social position and infrastructure. During this time, there may be intensifying frustration and emotional pain associated with multiple losses, such as (a) real or perceived social support (either through death, relocation, or compassion fatigue); (b) physical vitality or integrity (due to injury, disability, or disfigurement); (c) social infrastructure (due to loss of job, home, or neighborhood connections); and (d) other concurrent life event stressors unassociated with the disaster (Kaniasty & Norris, 1999). At the same time, stigma and retaliatory acts (e.g., hate crimes) may emerge due to blame and disparities involving reimbursement and available services that exacerbate underlying tensions within community-based social hierarchies (Taintor, 2003). In the recovery phase, a community attempts to rebuild while the membership continues to process the event and all of its ramifications. This may take years, and residual tensions or traumatic bereavement may be rekindled by reminders of the traumatic events (e.g., anniversaries; Myers & Zunin, 2000).

While this model illustrates how communities often respond after a disaster, not all communities will proceed in the same fashion. Some communities may skip phases, or become entrenched in one phase for prolonged periods, or revisit prior phases. The speed with which communities recover may be influenced by the implementation and organization of the response components (Hyams et al., 2003). For example, movement into the recovery phase can be facilitated by communities who feel well-informed and reassured. On the other hand, disillusionment can be exacerbated and prolonged if fragmented groups believe they are being misled, ignored, or treated unfairly (Kaniasty & Norris, 1999). This could instigate behavioral responses with significant political and economic consequences. For example, if individuals lose faith or trust in some institutions, they may withdraw membership or support or change their purchasing behavior. Thus, information sharing, communication, and social cohesion become important factors in predicting the economic and political consequences of traumatic events.

Utilizing a Broader Public Health Approach

Other articles in this volume address the range of psychological sequelae. However, after 9/11 more prolonged and complex concerns about maladaptive behavior and impaired function at both the individual and the community level arose. The IOM (2003) has proposed a broader public health model, built upon the classic epidemiologic triad to represent the transmission of infectious disease (see Figure 1). In the traditional model, the term "agent" refers to a microbe or toxin that causes disease or illness. The "host" refers to a person that is susceptible to infection by virtue of intrinsic factors (e.g., genetics, behavior, gender). The "environment" refers to the physical setting or extrinsic exposure factors (e.g., climate, ventilation system) that bring the host and the agent together, resulting in disease. Sometimes a "vector" or "vehicle" is needed to bring the agent in contact with the host, such as the mosquito, whose bite can inject the West Nile virus into a susceptible host and cause viral encephalitis. In the adapted model (see Figure 2), the agent is defined as a terrorist act or threat (resulting in fear and dread of future attacks). The environment is defined by the social or community context in addition to physical exposure parameters. The vector is determined by the hazards and exposure pathways selected to propagate terror, such as the deliberate contamination of mail, food, air, or potable water with infectious pathogens, or the destruction of symbolic structures by bombs or collisions with hijacked airplanes. The host is defined by those individuals or populations affected by the terrorist action. The model considers phases and factors before, during, and after terrorist events to conceptualize issues pertinent to preparedness, response, and recovery, respec-

FIGURE 1. Epidemiologic Approach to Explain Disease Transmission

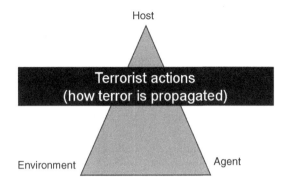

FIGURE 2. Psychological Consequences of Terrorism.

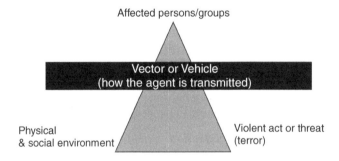

tively. The model is fluid and adaptable because of its ability to vary the focus (transmission or prevention), complexity, and scale of any of its dimensions for preparedness, mitigation, response, or recovery considerations.

The severity and duration of psychological and behavioral sequelae may vary due to the event characteristics and the societal context that surrounds terrorist action. Event characteristics include consideration of the following: (a) the number of affected sites (single or multiple); (b) the proximity of affected sites (clustered or widely dispersed); (c) the relationship of affected sites (random or targeted); (d) the timing of the attack (significant dates or important events); (e) the temporal sequence of events (singular, repeated, or propagating); (f) the immediacy, severity, and emotional impact of adverse health effects; and (g) the disruption of community services and support (Hall, Norwood, Ursano, & Fullerton, 2003; Hyams et al., 2003).

READINESS IN TERMS OF PERCEPTION AND BEHAVIOR

Destruction of symbols of financial and military strength (e.g., World Trade Towers; Pentagon) and perceptions about hazardous exposures or health effects may fundamentally alter perceptions of safety and threat (Grieger, Fullerton, Ursano, & Reeves, 2003; Hyams et al., 2003; Kaniasty & Norris, 1999). Changes in frequency, destination, or mode of travel (e.g., flying, use of mass transit) provide behavioral signals about altered perceptions of safety or threat by individuals, or within communities or businesses (IOM, 2003). Air travel dropped remarkably after the aircraft-related terrorist attacks of 2001 and during the 2003 severe acute respiratory syndrome (SARS) epidemic. Six to nine months after 9/11, 25% of New York City's adult residents were still drinking and smoking more than they had prior to the attacks (Vlahov et al., 2002).

Medical science seeks to find new drugs and vaccines to counter illness due to emerging disease threats. Many of the measures we employ for infection control practices are, in essence, behavioral countermeasures; they rely upon people to take some action to mitigate the risk or impact. The transmission of SARS, for example, was halted via prudent social and behavioral practices, such as increased social or contact distance (e.g., quarantine and isolation of exposed or infected persons), use of barriers (e.g., wearing facemasks, gowns, gloves, goggles), and hand-washing (Twu et al., 2003).

Critical Issues in Workforce Retention

One year after the terrorist attacks of 2001 (Pentagon, anthrax), a series of sniper attacks randomly killed 10 and wounded 2 (including a teenage boy) in the Washington, DC, Maryland, and Virginia area. The randomness of these shootings increased uncertainty and fear in the community as residents had little information to use in assessing their own risk, and resulted in marked behavioral changes in the surrounding communities (Grieger et al., 2003). A study of highly educated hospital employees in the Washington, DC area was conducted one week after the two suspects were arrested for the serial sniper attacks. Thirty-eight percent ($n = 382$) reported lower perceived safety, 40% reported higher perceived threat, and 3% increased their alcohol use. Health care workers reported fewer than usual routine activities either for themselves or their family outside the home (e.g., being in public places, buying gas, sending children to school or extracurricular activities, attending large public gatherings, traveling by public transportation, traveling by car, and attending faith-based activities). The psychological and behavioral impact of emerging and continuing threats raises important questions about our ability to retain adequate health care staffing and surge capacity during times of uncertainty. The inability to retain appropriately functioning health care workforces during an epidemic or exposure period can erode the public's sense of safety and impair regional mutual aid for medical response capacity.

In a similar vein, if absenteeism causes closure of child-serving institutions (e.g., child care, schools), then working parents with children may be forced to stay home. This can diminish the ability of critical organizations to implement their response plans or to maintain economic viability. Preparedness needs to address the psychosocial aspects of critical workforce retention during periods of high stress, fear, and uncertainty.

INCORPORATING BEHAVIORAL HEALTH INTO PUBLIC HEALTH PREPAREDNESS

Social Networks Influence the Effectiveness of Public Health Interventions

Terrorism is a form of psychological warfare, whose intent is to frighten and demoralize people, induce chaos, and disrupt the fabric of society (Hall et al., 2003; Hyams et al., 2003). Activities that promote a sense of community well-being and social cohesion would thus be effective countermeasures to this disruption. Current response plans incorporate extensive knowledge about epidemiological and laboratory investigations to identify risk and protective factors and disease or injury transmission pathways (CDC, 2003a). These investigations inform the design of public health interventions and recommendations that will "contain and control" the spread of injury, illness, or disease and disability. Most of the recommendations made by public health authorities involve behaviors designed to reduce exposure, seek help, comply with recommended treatment, or change the nature of social contact. The best scientifically-based advice can be rendered, but the success of a public health intervention depends on public compliance or adherence to recommended actions. However, recent experience tell us that adherence cannot be taken for granted, particularly when there is marked uncertainty about exposure and health consequences, as well as the risks involved with following the recommended protective measures (e.g., prolonged prophylactic use of antibiotics; Shepherd et al., 2002).

Knowledge Impacts the Risk Appraisal Process

Recently, there has been increased attention paid to issues related to education and communication, such as target audiences and delivery vehicles (e.g., toll free information line, Internet, public service announcements, workplace or civic literature; CDC, 2003b; Hall et al., 2003; Hyams et al., 2003). Emergency risk and crisis communication training programs have emerged due to the expanded role of public health in national security, as highlighted in the anthrax bioterrorist events of 2001. Extensive outreach efforts were conducted in New York City, the Washington, DC area, and New Jersey after the terrorist actions of 9/11 and the anthrax bioterrorism. Creativity, passion, and persistence enabled these outreach programs to function successfully. Various strategies were attempted to capitalize on established messaging channels, emphasizing risk reduction and health promotion, to offer opportunities to communicate with community-based or workplace populations and provide information aimed at reducing anxiety, improving positive coping, and promoting early intervention screening. Further research is needed to evaluate the efficacy of these outreach interventions and to create a matrix of interventions that consider the event characteristics.

Appraisals Influence Behavior

Public health preparedness guidance has often been behaviorally naïve, that is, not incorporating all that we know about the complexity of decision-making at the individual level under situations of great stress and uncertainty (Tversky & Kahneman, 1974). Compliance or adherence to recommended public health action is a complex subject that has psychological, sociocultural, anthropological, and political underpinnings. Adherence behavior is determined, in part, by individual appraisal of the risks and benefits derived by either following recommended actions or not. Individual risk appraisals are derived from past experiences, biases, beliefs, knowledge, and social influences.

Effective terrorism response strategies need data about collective behavior, psychological reaction, and the heuristics people apply to situations involving greater levels of uncertainty about the potential for exposure, health effects, and availability and efficacy of treatment and protective measures. More input is needed to assess the functionality of social networks that influence and support decision-making and coping in such events (Kaniasty & Norris, 1999). Without such information, critical components needed for successful education, communication, and preparedness may be overlooked, thereby undermining attempts to respond effectively.

Recent Attention to Behavioral Preparedness
Through Federal Grant Language

For the first time, federal funding for terrorism and public health emergency preparedness and response incorporated language (CDC, 2003c) to address "issues of psychological health and their behavioral manifestations. This represents a strongly recognized need that the Nation prepares to protect both the physical and psychological health of those potentially victimized by terrorism" (p. 4). This language was included in grant programs administered by both the CDC and the Health Resources Service Administration (HRSA) of the U.S. Department of Health and Human Services (DHHS). Resource planning and attention to special subpopulations (e.g., physically or mentally disabled, senior citizens, children) are to be coordinated across public health, mental health, and medical response systems. Grant language included the formation of cross-disciplinary planning teams, service provider networks, and attention to short-term and long-term psychosocial service delivery. However, it is difficult for state mental health authorities to broaden their mission to include the welfare of the public at-large with current funding and staffing levels. The Substance Abuse and Mental Health Services Administration (SAMHSA, part of DHHS) and the National Association of State Mental Health Program Directors (NASMHPD) jointly discovered that few states had a state-level disaster mental health plan. Subsequently, SAMHSA and NASMHPD published guidance to help states develop appropriate disaster mental health plans that would be integrated into state emergency management operations (SAMHSA, 2003).

FURTHER RESEARCH NEEDED ON BEHAVIORAL HEALTH

Longitudinal Needs and Functioning of a Community Recovering from Terrorism

More research is needed on the longitudinal needs and functioning of a community recovering from terrorism or other forms of community violence. Longitudinal needs assessments must address the adequacy of information, clinical services (medical and psychiatric), social services, community services, financial resources, and supportive social networks to buffer distress and foster recovery. Empirically, we might assume that the honeymoon phase of the disaster lifecycle presents an opportunity to engage disparate or fragmented groups in collaborative efforts that will facilitate the speed and extent of community recovery. Engaging the community during this period might help to inoculate residents against the disillusionment and splintering that often follows. However, successful engagement requires pre-disaster planning and outreach. Other inoculation strategies have been suggested during the pre-disaster phase, like public education campaigns (Glass & Schoch-Spana, 2002) about the lifecycle of disasters, uncertainties in scientific endeavors to identify hazardous exposures, and why a range of protective actions (e.g., pro-phylactic medicine or vaccine, personal protective equipment, sheltering, etc.) might be recommended. Further research is needed to define the boundaries of communication and education that successfully alert and motivate healthy adaptive individual and collective behavior, without raising undue anxiety and distress.

Problems in this arena were evident with the postal workers in the Wash-ington, DC area. They had to deal with the emotional impact of displacement from their worksite, stigma related to their potential exposure, the illness and death of coworkers, inconsistent practices of nasal swabbing for anthrax spore exposure, different antibiotic prophylaxis than those exposed on Capitol Hill, and referral to their personal medical provider. There was an implicit assump-tion that existing health care relationships would be sufficient to manage on-going questions and issues as they arose. Opportunity was not available to assess the postal workers' perception about the trustworthiness of information sources, nor was there an understanding by providers of how the flow of infor-mation was managed throughout the organization.

On a different note, our globally mobile society and "just-in-time" hospital and food supply practices have wrought new challenges for community disas-ter preparedness. Additional guidance needs to be developed to support the implementation of exposure protection practices like sheltering in place or various levels of quarantine. Credentialing the workforce that will provide critical services (e.g., food, medicine and medical attention, water, sanitation) and those who might intervene to diffuse escalating tensions within house-holds or congregate settings or provide social contact for those in isolation should be considered.

To bolster a sense of community resilience, psychosocial preparedness might also include creative linkages between local business, civic and faith-based organi-zations, and informal community or opinion leaders. Resilience refers to the ability of a community to withstand adversity and maintain cohesion and healthy function-ing. Regional capacity and programmatic efficiency might be achieved by linking disparate initiatives that already exist. For example, relationships could be devel-oped among existing injury prevention and violence prevention programs, pro-grams to help victims of assault (sexual or physical; adult or child), and community enhancement programs stemming from urban renewal initiatives. There are numer-ous questions about what constitutes healthy community functioning, which needs to be examined across different disciplines: sociology, anthropology, community psychology and psychiatry, urban planning, and grass-roots efforts. It stands to rea-son that improving the cohesiveness of existing systems of social organization would strengthen community resilience and serve as effective countermeasures for terrorism.

Searching for Indicators of Community Resilience

How might we apply standard assessments of community function (or adaptation) to evaluate interventions? There are a multitude of questions about "resilience" and whether it can be used to describe a community that can withstand adversity and successfully recover or adapt to new circumstances. Can we identify factors that promote or impede community resilience? Is it feasible to measure such items?

Can we study collective behavior within communities and determine the psychological and behavioral impact of events that breed uncertainty about personal or community risk? Collective behaviors might be assessed by estimating the frequency or rate of many different behavioral domains or indicators of psychological impact within communities. Such domains and indicators may include a sampling of the following: (a) the use and the type of social support (e.g., religious, family, friends, workplace, etc.); (b) spending patterns; (c) attendance at large public gatherings; (d) use of public transportation; (e) altered patterns of substance use (e.g., tobacco, illicit drugs, alcohol); (f) patterns of healthcare utilization (e.g., specific injuries, sexually transmitted infections, teen pregnancy, diagnoses or syndromes consistent with co-morbid anxiety or depression); (g) indicators of risky behaviors (e.g., speeding, unprotected sex with multiple partners); (h) records of violent crimes (e.g., sexual or physical assault, hate crimes); (i) records of work or school absenteeism or performance measures; (j) unemployment rate; (k) stigmatizing behavior; and (l) selection of and adherence to recommended protective actions or other actions perceived to lower risk of harm to loved ones (e.g., social distancing, use of masks, hand-washing, medication use). All of these should include comparative data for the various cultural groups within the community. Evaluation studies would be needed to assess the predictive efficiency of selected domains and indicators.

Stigma raises a number of concerns at the community level. Despite the small number of SARS-infected persons in the U.S., stigma was a huge problem as the SARS epidemic progressed, mostly targeted at persons of Asian descent (CDC, 2003d). Fear of disease transmission led to avoidance of restaurants and markets in American "Chinatowns," creating economic hardships for business owners. Institutions of higher education were trying to prevent persons from SARS-infected countries from matriculating or attending graduation ceremonies. Hate crimes against Muslims increased after 9/11 (Taintor, 2003). Postal workers revealed anecdotes about their children being stigmatized in school because of the parent's workplace and fear that the children were going to spread the anthrax.

Healthcare utilization increases in the aftermath of disasters, which may reflect distress responses, including exacerbations of underlying medical conditions (Engel, in press; Hyams et al., 2003). Somatically-based health complaints can be complex and confusing in the aftermath of terrorist events, and might be confounded by other concurrent life event stressors. However, acute presentations of somatically-based distress could overwhelm healthcare systems as individuals seek out formal medical evaluations due to concerns and uncertainties about terrorist events and hazardous exposure, or in mass casualty situations (Hall et al., 2003). Engel (in press) proposes a four-part model to suggest "that physical factors (e.g., coexisting disease or injury), cognitive factors (e.g., community or individual beliefs regarding a trauma), behavioral factors (e.g., patterns of health care use), and health service experience (e.g., iatrogenic harm, satisfaction with care, and differing provider and patient explanations for symptoms) may impact the onset, course, and duration of multiple idiopathic physical symptoms (MIPS) and related distress and disability" (p. 5). Patient-provider relationships can be torn apart by differences in appraisals after extensive evaluations fail to provide medical evidence to explain persisting health complaints after terrorist events.

Community-based settings, particularly those experienced in the health care of special populations, may be better positioned to link victims with family and community networks and resources, especially to reach populations that would not otherwise seek and accept support. Community-based needs assessment instruments and population-based screening tools for psychiatric referral should be designed to inform each other and reduce survey burdens on the affected population. Using community-based health settings to supplement screening initiatives may offer the opportunity for cultural competence and facilitate the recovery cycle. Unless we can greatly improve the sensitivity and specificity of the potential screening instruments that currently exist, screening may be of limited use. Psychosocial interventions should focus on optimizing recovery, rather than treat disease (Shalev et al., 2003).

Given the growing recognition of the power of terrorism to target its goal of weakening social capital, public health strategies must not only recognize its effects on social connectedness, but adopt broad interventions that recognize the interdependence of community health and social connections.

REFERENCES

Centers for Disease Control and Prevention. (2003a). *Crisis and emergency risk communication: CDCynergy training tools.* Retrieved November 05, 2003, from http://www.cdc.gov/communication/emergency/erc_overview.htm

Centers for Disease Control and Prevention. (2003b). *Emergency preparedness and Response: Preparation and planning.* Retrieved October 30, 2003, from http://www.bt.cdc.gov/planning/index.asp

Centers for Disease Control and Prevention. (2003c). *Continuation guidance for cooperative agreement on public health preparedness and response for bioterrorism–budget year four. Program announcement 99051.* Retrieved November 05, 2003, from http://www.bt.cdc.gov/planning/continuationguidance/index.asp

Centers for Disease Control and Prevention. (2003d). *Interim guidance for institutions or organizations hosting persons arriving in the United States from areas with Severe Acute Respiratory syndrome (SARS).* Retrieved November 05, 2003, from http://www.cdc.gov/ncidod/sars/hostingarrivals.htm

Engel, C. C. (in press). Somatization and multiple idiopathic physical symptoms: Relationship to traumatic events and posttraumatic stress disorder. In P. P. Schnurr & B. L. Green (Eds.), *Trauma and health: Physical health consequences of exposure to extreme stress.* Washington, DC: American Psychological Association.

Glass, T. A., & Schoch-Spana, M. (2002). Bioterrorism and the people: How to vaccinate a city against panic. *Clinical Infectous* Diseases, 34:2, 217-23.

Grieger, T. A., Fullerton, C. S., Ursano, R. J., & Reeves, J. J. (2003). Acute stress disorder, alcohol use, and perception of safety among hospital staff after the sniper attacks. *Psychiatric Services, 54*(10), 1383-1387.

Hall, M., Norwood, A., Ursano, R., & Fullerton, C. (2003). The psychological impacts of bioterrorism. *Biosecurity and Bioterrorism, 1,* 139-44.

Hyams, K. C., Murphy, F. M., & Wessely, S. (2003). Responding to chemical, biological, or nuclear terrorism: The indirect and long-term health effects may present the greatest challenge. In P. R. Lee & C. L. Estes (Eds.), *The nation's health* (7th ed., pp. 289-304). Boston, MA: Jones and Bartlett Publishers.

Institute of Medicine. (2003). *Preparing for the psychological consequences of terrorism: A public health strategy.* Washington DC: The National Academies Press.

Kaniasty, K., & Norris, F. (1999). The experience of disaster: Individuals and communities sharing trauma. In R. Gist & B. Lubin (Eds.), *Response to disaster: Psychosocial, community, and ecological approaches* (pp. 25-62). Philadelphia, PA: Brunner/Mazel.

Myers, D., & Zunin, L. (2000). Phases of disaster. In D. DeWolfe (Ed.) (2nd ed.), *Training manual for mental health and human service workers in major disasters.* (DHHS Publication No. ADM 90-538). Washington, DC: U.S. Government Printing Office. Retrieved February 4, 2002, from http://www.mentalhealth.org/publications/allpubs/ADM90-538/index.htm

Shalev, A. Y., Adessky, R., Boker, R., Bargai, N., Cooper, R., Friedman, S., et al. (2003). Clinical intervention of survivors of prolonged adversities. In R. Ursano, C. Fullerton, & A. Norwood (Eds.), *Terrorism and disaster: Individual and community mental health interventions* (pp. 162-88). Cambridge UK: Cambridge University Press.

Shepard, C. W., Soriano-Gabarro, M., Zell, E. R., Hayslett, J., Lukacs, S., Goldstein, S., et al. (2002). Antimicrobial postexposure prophylaxis for anthrax: Adverse events and adherence. [Electronic version]. *Emerging Infectious Diseases, 18*(10). Retrieved November 05, 2003, from http://www.cdc.gov/ncidod/EID/ vol8no10/02-0349.htm

Substance Abuse and Mental Health Services Administration. (2003). *Mental health all-hazards disaster planning guidance.* (DHHS Publication No. SMA 3829). Washington, DC: U.S. Government Printing Office.

Taintor, Z. (2003). Addressing mental health needs. In B. S. Levy & V. W. Sidel (Eds.), *Terrorism and public health: A balanced approach to strengthening systems and protecting people* (pp. 49-69). New York: Oxford University Press and American Public Health Association.

Tversky, A., & Kahneman, D. (1974). Judgment under uncertainty: Heuristics and biases. *Science, 185*, 1124-1130.

Twu, S-J., Chen, T-J., Chen, C-J., Olsen, S. J., Lee, L-T., Fisk, T. et al. (2003). Control measures for severe acute respiratory syndrome (SARS) in Taiwan. [Electronic version]. *Emerging Infectious Diseases, 19*(6). Retrieved June 05, 2003, from http://www.cdc.gov/ncidod/EID/vol9no6/03-0283.htm

Vlahov, D., Galea, S., Resnick, H., Ahern, J., Boscarino, J. A., Bucualas, M. et al. (2002). Increased use of cigarettes, alcohol, and marijuana among Manhattan, New York, residents after the September 11th terrorist attacks. *American Journal of Epidemiolgy, 155*, 988-96.

Finding the Gift in the Horror: Toward Developing a National Psychosocial Security Policy

Claude M. Chemtob

SUMMARY. This brief article proposes an analysis of the risks society faces in coping with terrorism, and suggests broad outlines of a plan to increase national resilience through creating a national strategy for enhancing psychosocial security. The analysis is based on survival mode theory, which posits two survival sub-systems in human beings: the threat detection system and the human bonding and attachment system. It proposes to redefine the concept of national security policy to go beyond the traditional military aspects of defense to include establishing psychological countermeasures that define maintaining psychological safety as a key marker of the defense against terrorism.

Address correspondence to: Claude M. Chemtob, PhD, Department of Psychiatry and Pediatrics, Mt. Sinai School of Medicine, One Gustave L. Levy Place, New York, NY 10029 USA (E-mail: claude.chemtob@mssm.edu).

[Haworth co-indexing entry note]: "Finding the Gift in the Horror: Toward Developing a National Psychosocial Security Policy." Chemtob, Claude M. Co-published simultaneously in *Journal of Aggression, Maltreatment & Trauma* (The Haworth Maltreatment & Trauma Press, an imprint of The Haworth Press, Inc.) Vol. 10, No. 3/4, 2005; and: *The Trauma of Terrorism: Sharing Knowledge and Shared Care, An International Handbook* (ed: Yael Danieli, Danny Brom, and Joe Sills) The Haworth Maltreatment & Trauma Press, an imprint of The Haworth Press, Inc., 2005.

KEYWORDS. Psychosocial security, terrorism, survival mode, resilience

Terrorism is a psychological weapon. Its success is measured by the perceptible and social harm it creates in the people targeted. Engendering fear triggers a cascade of consequences usually culminating in economic and social harm. The long-term effects of terrorism include increased social fragmentation that weakens the resolve of a nation by reducing its ability to maintain a sense of common purpose in the face of an enemy. More subtly, the recurrent threat posed by terrorism can cause a hardening of attitudes that undermines the ideals and creativity of a society. Ultimately, the challenge posed by terrorism to a nation is whether the nation will become more rigid in its pursuit of safety or respond to the challenge by refining its values to increase its capacity for creativity in the face of adversity. The choice a nation faces is whether to become more resilient or merely more vigilant. The risk of hyper-vigilance is that it may lead to sacrificing cherished values.

This brief article proposes an analysis of this risk, and suggests the broad outlines of a plan to increase national resilience through creating a national strategy for increasing psychosocial security. In short, terrorism gives us the opportunity to redefine the concept of national security policy to go beyond the traditional military aspects of defense to include establishing psychological countermeasures that define maintaining psychological safety as a key marker of the defense against terrorism. This re-definition posits that national security is defined not only by marshalling protection against external enemies, but also by investing the resources needed to establish an expectation of mutual cooperation in the face of risk that assures *psychosocial security* as a human right, a government obligation, and a basic duty of competent citizens. This redefinition may transform the threat of terrorism into an opportunity for social and cultural growth rather than an occasion for increased rigidity.

Historically, states have invested in developing and fielding technology and personnel to protect national resources, the security of citizens, and the stability of the government. Traditional security policy might be likened to an immune system that directs itself to the repelling of external invaders. The social body (group/organization/community/nation) identifies the external stressor (enemy) and mobilizes the resources needed to block or destroy the attackers effectively. National security provides for defense and maintains an effective organization of resources to sustain mobilization in the face of threat. This approach to defense relies on natural processes of social mobilization that have evolved to regulate fear and anxiety in times of danger.

This structured process of responding to threat represents a set of adaptations that have evolved over time. My colleagues and I (Chemtob, Roitblat, Hamada, Carlson, & Twentyman, 1988; Chemtob & Taylor, 2002) have described these adaptations to threat as a "survival mode" of functioning. We have proposed that when people are faced with threat, specialized cognitive information processing mechanisms are activated in threatening contexts. These cognitive structures are activated automatically and are characterized by peremptoriness, suppression of normal modes of cognition, and a loss of self-monitoring. People in survival mode usually are not aware that they are responding differently.

We have proposed that there are two survival sub-systems in human beings. These are the threat detection system and the human bonding and attachment system. The threat detection system, when activated, is characterized by (a) a shift to gestalt processing, (b) a confirmation bias for threat (that translates into more generalized negative expectations), and (c) a lowered threshold for action (whether it be flight or aggression). We posit that the human bonding survival subsystem reflects the fact that human beings depend for survival on social inclusion in a group. Exclusion from the group can be as dangerous as facing a tiger. Social threats are consequential because exclusion from the group reduces fitness dramatically. In the context of the bonding system, activation of survival mode is associated with (a) significantly increased intra-group solidarity; (b) increased identification with one's identity as part of a collective; (c) reduced self-differentiation from the group; and (d) increased primacy of non-verbal social information.

Importantly, this theory applies equally to individuals and groups. Thus, similar to the shifts in information processing at the individual level, when groups are faced with significant threats, they mobilize their defense capacity by rallying around a leader more cohesively and suppressing intra-group differences in the service of increased cooperation and the greater good. These dynamics are largely automatic and increase the fitness of a group. They have been used by leaders throughout history to marshal enhanced internal cohesion through invoking a common external enemy. In short, survival mode when mobilized in the context of a threat supports adaptive fitness. However, when survival mode is activated in a non-threatening context by virtue of its automaticity it undermines effective response.

Terrorism, whether consciously or merely through sophisticated intuition, takes advantage of these adaptive evolutionary structures to undermine the adaptive fitness of a group. In the context of the metaphor of the immune system we proposed earlier, terrorism seeks to take advantage of the fact that when people mobilize to face a threat they automatically, peremptorily, and without self-monitoring, turn their attention and aggression to face an external enemy. In a sense, they mobilize to identify and repel or destroy an external organism, akin to the immune system's mobilization to identify and destroy a noxious bacterial invader. The defense system depends for its effective operation on a relatively simple differentiation between the external attacker (enemy) and the repelling insider (self and community). In contrast, viral infections are characterized by taking over the host cell's machinery to accomplish the invading organism's aims. The challenge in that circumstance is to avoid treating the self as if it were an enemy. Similarly, in an autoimmune reaction the disorder arises because normally adaptive systems are too reactive and attack the self rather than legitimately defined external enemies.

Terrorism, by definition and by procedure, seeks to break down the barrier between what is safe (i.e., what is inside the group) and what is dangerous because it comes from the enemy outside. It seeks to create sufficient confusion about where the enemy is located that intra-group aggression causes internal damage leading in the long term to a breakdown in the ability to mount an effective response to threat. In the metaphorical sense, terrorism seeks to provoke an autoimmune response by creating social confusion in defining who is friend and who is foe.

The events of September 11, 2001, as well as the terrorist strategies that have been used in Israel, are highly illustrative. Very much like in the case in viral attacks that commandeer the host's own cells to carry out the purpose of the invading virus, the 9/11 terrorists commandeered the nation's own planes. They turned an otherwise benign system that had earned over decades the status of being a safe means of transportation into a symbol of unconstrained threat and danger. Because flying in airplanes was no longer perceived as "safe" by a significant number of people, the air transportation system was economically damaged and productive social interaction and cooperation were undercut.

The high saliency of the use of aircraft to attack highly symbolic targets commandeered media attention. In turn, the mass media served the terrorist's purpose by dramatizing and publicizing the attacks, thereby magnifying their impact. In Israel, to give but one example, terrorists have capitalized on blurring the distinction between in-group and enemy by dressing like orthodox Jews who wear distinctive garb, using fashion and style to suggest Israeli identity. These ploys had the advantage not only of foiling internal defenses but also of increasing intra-group mutual suspiciousness, thus undercutting social support and rendering vigilance less effective.

These terrorist strategies take advantage of evolutionarily structured biases in responding to external and social threats to undermine psychosocial security. Traditionally, security policy has depended on the ready discrimination of friend as internal (within a defined border boundary) and external (outside that same boundary). To enforce this clarity, treason and spying have been treated as extremely serious, usually capital, offenses. Historically, the discrimination of friend and foe was abetted by relatively homogeneous populations within nations. However, in the context of terrorism, we are faced with a new challenge for which we have not been well prepared by evolutionary history, the discrimination of foe from friend in the context of multi-ethnic societies characterized by considerable cross-border traffic. Moreover, in the case of the United States, there has been little experience with respect to managing threats from enemies on domestic soil.

Much of the reaction following 9/11 is consistent with this analysis, namely, the increased consciousness of collective identity represented by widespread wearing of flag lapel pins, rallying to the President, the salient definition of a homeland security agenda, and increased preoccupation with defining foe and friend at the border. However, while that reaction represents increased vigilance in discriminating friend from foe, it has not included a focus on managing the increased fearfulness of the population. Nor has it addressed the dynamics of fear contagion that, while not panic-like, nevertheless sufficiently influence behaviors to have a significant impact on social and economic life.

Nor has there been recognition that in times of emergency, traditional first-responders represent only the most visible aspect of internal national defense and recovery. Interestingly, little has been made of the fact that the one plane that did not reach its intended target was stopped by civilians. Nor has enough attention been paid to the fact that the "shoe bomber" was stopped by vigilant passengers seated next to him. The difficulties faced by non-traditional first responders such as teachers, who are asked to become de facto first-responders in times of crisis despite a lack of training and preparation, have also not been systematically addressed.

In short, if terrorism is a psychological weapon, we must develop psychological countermeasures as part of our defense posture. These must increase the nation's capacity to resist the contagious fear effects triggered by terrorism and significantly increase the nation's skill to recover from crisis. To accomplish this, we must define and promulgate protective attitudes related to the impact and anticipation of terrorism, systematically disseminate knowledge regarding fear and its secondary impacts, and increase skills to contain and recover from terrorist attacks. In addition, we must systematically increase coordination among key stakeholders in each of our neighborhoods in order to establish a significant reserve of social capital that can be drawn on in times of need both for social support and for concrete competence in effectively marshalling resources for recovery. Finally, recognizing that many professions will be called upon to be first-responders that are not traditionally recognized as such, we should develop role-specific emergency response competencies. These role-specific competencies must include expertise in establishing coordinated action with other stakeholders. We have developed a model to guide the development of these competencies. This model is the ASK and C model. It refers to the need to identify and promulgate the Attitudes, Skills, and Knowledge that together with social Connections support resilience and recovery. Systematic enhancement of social competencies in managing emergencies has not been included in the current strategy of the U.S. and many other nations for combating terrorism. Indeed, while this article has put its emphasis on the need to address preparing non-traditional responders, the same problem of supporting collaboration and coordination is bedeviling preparation and response efforts of traditional uniformed responders.

The chief dangers to the success of this preparedness strategy is that people grow disinterested as the threat fades and policy makers are far more supportive of investment in tangible goods such as gas masks and medication stockpiles. These necessary investments are well defined and do not put policy makers in the politically risky posture of drawing attention to fearfulness. Remarkably, therein the bridge to the development of national psychosocial security policy may be forged. Defining psychosocial safety as part of defense policy means that one must articulate clear expectations of protecting citizens both physically, through the maintenance of armed forces, and psychologically, through the definition of competencies to manage emergencies and threats to the psychological safety of people. This renewed expectation will require that we counter the attempt at confusing friend and foe by increasing the competency of caring for each other. We should counter increased ability to undermine our sense of community by learning to define and protect community better than ever before.

Doing so for purposes of national defense against terrorism requires establishing preparedness in such a way that it is practiced on a daily basis. The protection of children from threat, establishing mechanisms to detect children whose safety has been compromised, and disseminating recovery procedures for these children, may be the way to begin establishing psychosocial security as part of national security policy. It is natural to begin with children because they are the Achilles' heel of a society and a critical rallying point for a community. To that end, establishing clear expectations and competencies regarding protecting the most vulnerable among us, children, from threat and the consequent fear begins to define a dual-use civilian and military investment. The same role-specific competencies to maintain and restore the psychological safety of a child that we disseminate among policemen, pediatricians, clergy, and teachers (in short, all who come into contact with children) are ultimately the skills needed to protect children in emergencies. Most critically, integration of these new skills into a circle of care around each child serves to reduce fear of terror by activating consciously and intentionally the protective power of cooperation and community that children naturally engender. This approach counters the corrosive effects of terrorism that are mediated through the activation of survival mode in the absence of a defined threat by activating the equally powerful and protective human capacity for bonding in the face of danger.

REFERENCES

Chemtob, C. M., Roitblat, H., Hamada, R., Carlson, J., & Twentyman, C. (1988). A cognitive action theory of post-traumatic stress disorder. *Journal of Anxiety Disorders, 2*, 253-275.

Chemtob, C. M., & Taylor, T. L. (2002). The treatment of traumatized children. In R. Yehuda (Ed.), *Trauma survivors: Bridging the gap between intervention research and practice* (pp. 75-126). Washington DC: American Psychiatric Press.

The Need for a Continuum
of Trauma Services:
Who Feeds the Birds?

Talia Levanon
Elisheva Flamm-Oren
Gilah Kahn-Hoffmann

SUMMARY. Since September 2000, residents of Israel have experienced a prolonged period of terrorist attacks that shows no sign of abating. The ramifications of the ongoing trauma permeate every facet of life. Since existing services provided by government and Non-Governmental Organizations (NGOs) are unable to meet the needs that have emerged, the Continuum of Trauma Services (CTS) was developed for victims of terrorist attacks, their families, friends, emergency and mental health professionals and the community at large. This article also describes the Israel Trauma Coalition and its interest groups, which may be seen as the embodiment of an evolving CTS.

Address correspondence to: Talia Levanson, MSW (E-mail: TLevanon@herzog hospital.org).

[Haworth co-indexing entry note]: "The Need for a Continuum of Trauma Services: Who Feeds the Birds?" Levanon, Talia, Elisheva Flamm-Oren, and Gilah Kahn-Hoffmann. Co-published simultaneously in *Journal of Aggression, Maltreatment & Trauma* (The Haworth Maltreatment & Trauma Press, an imprint of The Haworth Press, Inc.) Vol. 10, No. 3/4, 2005; and: *The Trauma of Terrorism: Sharing Knowledge and Shared Care, An International Handbook* (ed: Yael Danieli, Danny Brom, and Joe Sills) The Haworth Maltreatment & Trauma Press, an imprint of The Haworth Press, Inc., 2005.

KEYWORDS. Trauma, terrorism, service delivery, continuum of services, NGO

Six-year-old Sasha[1] was badly hurt in a terror attack outside a shopping mall in Netanya in May, 2001. His father was killed and his mother Olessia was seriously injured. His uncle's fiancée was also killed. Sasha's uncle Germann, Olessia's 20-year-old brother, a soldier in the Israel Defence Forces, was the family's only relative in the country.

Immediately after the attack, the National Insurance Institute (NII) provided services mandated by law, and volunteers from Israel Crisis Management Center (SELAH) were at the family's side. A volunteer from SELAH provided Germann with a bed in her home, so that he could be close to the hospital. SELAH volunteers accompanied him as he buried his fiancee and his brother-in-law. They sat next to little Sasha in the hospital, and watched over Olessia in the Intensive Care Unit as she struggled back to consciousness and the realization of her terrible loss. SELAH brought Germann and Olessia's mother to Israel so she could help care for her wounded daughter and grandson, and a volunteer was at the airport to greet her when she arrived. When Sasha had to leave his bed for an X-ray, it was suddenly discovered that he had no slippers–a SELAH volunteer ran out and bought them for him. And it was a SELAH volunteer who took Sasha's precious pet lovebirds into her own home, to care for them until he recovered and could resume taking care of them himself. Sasha survived, and on his first day out of the hospital he was taken to visit his lovebirds.[2]

TWO SAFETY NETS

Despite the prevalence of terror attacks in Israel since the founding of the state, during the past three years of the armed Palestinian uprising, or Intifada, inhabitants of the country have been facing a national situation unlike any that they have previously experienced. With its human bombs and its attacks on men, women and children, the Intifada has fundamentally affected every person in Israel. The population is living in a state of ongoing trauma, which may be visualized as a "stream" of traumatic events, which may also be described as an inter-traumatic (Onno Van der Hart, personal communication, October 29, 2003) or peri-traumatic phase. It is as if they are trapped in this phase, as the conflict shows no sign of coming to an end. All inhabitants of the country, from infants to the elderly, native-born to newly-arrived, are potential targets of terrorism. Every city, town, and suburb in Israel is a possible site of attack.

There are no safe places and no safe times. Day or night, awake or asleep, no one is immune. First and foremost, the terror touches its victims, but also their families, close friends, surrounding communities and the population at large, as well as helpers such as emergency teams and mental health care workers, who play multiple roles since they are simultaneously members of the groups listed above.

When the Intifada began, two safety nets were already in place. The first, provided by the state, attempts, through the Benefits to Victims of Hostile Acts Law of 1970, to meet the needs of direct victims of terrorist attacks. This law embodies the obligation and ideological commitment of the state to provide assistance to terror victims with medical, financial, psychological and rehabilitation needs (see Baca Baldomero, Baca-García, Pérez-Rodríguez, & Cabanas, this volume). Immediately following a small or medium scale traumatic incident, specially trained trauma response teams are made available on the scene and in hospital emergency rooms for approximately six hours (see Ben-Gershon, Grinshpoon, & Ponizovsky, this volume). Following a large-scale traumatic incident, municipal welfare personnel are also available for 48 hours. After this 48-hour period, the NII provides services, but only for those who meet their criteria for direct victims of terrorism. After every terrorist attack, an authorized committee is convened to determine whether the event is recognized as a terrorist attack and then, which of its victims are recognized as victims of terrorism and would be eligible for government assistance.

The second safety net is provided by Non-Governmental Organizations (NGOs). The story of Sasha and his family, recounted above, illustrates the need for the type of intervention that these organizations provide. Despite the fact that Sasha was a recognized direct victim, the young boy had needs that the law does not meet. The seemingly trivial issue of his pet birds, who needed a caretaker while Sasha and his mother were recovering in the hospital, appeared to be an insurmountable problem for Sasha. For a native-born Israeli or veteran immigrant with lifelong friends, neighbors and extended family this would not have been a problem, but without the NGO this tiny immigrant family would have been lost. Here, the intervention of an NGO was the only possible solution.

SELAH's work, like that of other NGOs, extends far beyond the feeding of pets to include such support as financial assistance, ongoing emotional support and healing retreats for victims and their families. These NGOs that have either been expanded or created to fill gaps assist those who do not qualify for government aid or whose needs are not provided for within the framework of the law. NGOs tend to be more flexible than government agencies as well as more linguistically and culturally attuned. They have the ability to respond rapidly to newly emerging needs with an array of responses (Schmidt, 1998; Schmidt & Sabbagh, 1991).

And yet, despite the existence of both these safety nets, the government and the NGOs that may complement each other (Katan, 1988; Salamon 1995), as attacks continued, it became apparent that numerous victims and individual needs are still overlooked.

THE CONCEPT OF A CONTINUUM OF TRAUMA SERVICES

The trauma-related needs of the population in Israel have increased greatly over the past three years (Bleich, Gelkopf, & Solomon, 2003) and many of those who previously functioned normally have suddenly found themselves in need of help. Emerging needs are more complex and diverse, extending further and reaching deeper into peoples' lives. The security situation is wearing down individuals and systems, eroding their basic sense of security and well-being. The consequences of trauma extend like ripples in a pond, affecting victims according to their degree of exposure to the traumatic event (Ayalon & Lahad, 1991). The hardest hit are direct victims. This is especially true because the trauma extends to relatives, close friends, first responders, second responders, witnesses, near misses and the community at large.

During the initial stages of the Intifada, the responses from government and NGOs may be described as scattered or isolated. To cope with the plethora of needs that is constantly being uncovered, it is critical to develop new, complementary services and to connect them with the isolated services. The integration of these services into a more holistic and comprehensive unit, rather than merely a reactive model, was the first step toward a Continuum of Trauma Services (CTS).

The Continuum both broadens and strengthens existing services. It also supplies additional safety nets stretched below the existing two to ensure that a response is available for those still in "free fall," who are not supported by either of the two nets already in place.

The responsibility for a CTS should be shared by government and NGOs. Its creation reflects a strengthened commitment both to assume responsibility for the needs of trauma victims and to provide additional safety nets of trauma-related services in response to the gaps in existing services. A CTS is also responsible for enhancing resilience in the community at large, which contributes to the ability to cope better with normal, or developmental, trauma as well.

The ability of tiers of safety nets to self-regulate (i.e., to upgrade their services or extend them as necessary or to direct an individual to the most appropriate net) is built in. The previous response to the need for trauma services was a linear model, while the ideal model is spiral. At its most effective level of performance, a CTS functions as a self-regulating spiral, ceaselessly monitoring needs and developing and improving the means and ability to respond to those needs, as well as providing new solutions where necessary. These solutions are also constantly evaluated, enabling further enhancement of the network. The identification of needs can be facilitated by connecting those affected by trauma to a number of continuums.

THE LEVELS OF EXPOSURE CONTINUUM

The scope of each traumatic event (i.e., the number of casualties and the size of the area impacted, as well as the fact that the trauma is not one specific event but one event in a chain of many), may influence the reactions to the incident and should be reflected in the crafting of appropriate responses. It has been shown that there is a relation between level of exposure and coping with the traumatic events (Kleber & Brom, 1992; Vogel & Verenberg, 1993).

Direct Victims. Direct victims are those who are present at a terror attack and directly affected physically and/or emotionally. This group is recognized by law and eligible for benefits (see also Baca Baldomero et al., this volume).

Relatives (and Close Friends). Relatives and close friends include parents, grandparents, spouses, siblings and children whose lives are drastically changed by the event. Some members of this group are recognized by law and eligible for benefits, as determined by the law. Some relatives and all close friends are not eligible for benefits. Nearly all are in need of various kinds of support (Ayalon & Lahad, 1991; Kfir, 1998; Rosenfeld, Caye, Ayalon, & Lahad, in press; see also Baca Baldomero et al., this volume).

Others. None of the following are recognized by law as victims and therefore none are eligible for benefits from the state:

First Responders. First responders include police, firefighters, body identification units, Magen David Adom (the Israeli Red Cross), mental health care professionals and volunteers. Members of this group are first on the scene, providing first aid, evacuating victims and working on-site (see also Baca Baldomero et al., this volume).

Second Responders. Second responders include emergency room personnel, hospital personnel, social workers who accompany relatives of terror victims to the morgue, and social workers who work for the Ministry of Defense or the National Insurance Institute, who treat survivors of attacks. Members of these groups also require assistance in processing their experiences, training and upgrading their skills, as well as support designed specifically to prevent burnout (see also Baca Baldomero et al., this volume).

Eyewitnesses. Eyewitnesses include individuals who are also in need of support to help them process events they have witnessed or described in detail as part of their job. This group also includes members of the media who cover terror attacks.

Near Misses. Near misses include individuals that may also be traumatized by knowing that they had intended, were supposed to be, or had just left the site of an attack but for some reason were not there when it took place.

Community. The community parallels the group which includes those exposed to various media reports describing terror incidents as well as exposure to the experiences of school mates, neighbors, and colleagues.

The subdivision of the population into an age or time continuum, like the model of an exposure continuum previously described, facilitates mapping of needs and enables clear identification of services required for the widest possible spectrum of the population. Naturally, most people belong simultaneously to a number of categories. Two of these additional examples of continuums follow:

Age Continuum. The age continuum includes toddlers, children, adolescents, adults, and the elderly. Each developmental stage has its own unique characteristics which dictate the particular needs to be addressed when developing age-appropriate responses to trauma. An individual's reaction to trauma is determined by his or her level of cognitive, emotional, linguistic, moral and social development (Lonigman, 1991).

Time Continuum. This extends from the event to immediate intervention, to post-event intervention, then to long-term intervention. Reactions of individuals differ in nature and intensity at each point on the time continuum and each requires the appropriate interventions (Danieli, Engdahl, & Schlenger, 2003). The type of assistance indicated immediately following a traumatic event would not be sufficient at a later stage.

SIX LEVELS OF CTS INTERVENTION

The six levels of intervention that a CTS ideally provides for first responders to terrorist attacks are:

Training. As those first on the scene, first responders provide direct, immediate aid to victims and others in the area and, to a great extent, shape their experience. To handle the interpersonal aspect of their job while simultaneously functioning at the highest possible professional level, they require upgrading of their interpersonal and communication skills.

Primary Prevention. Due to the gruesome and profound nature of their jobs, first responders require ongoing support as well as training and upgrading of their coping skills, to strengthen their resilience and prevent the development of post traumatic symptoms.

Post-Event Intervention. Immediately following an event, first responders are also in need of specific interventions designed to limit the impact of vicarious traumatization and to prevent burnout.

Screening. Screening programs are needed to identify professionals who have developed post traumatic symptoms and require clinical interventions.

Clinical Interventions. Clinical interventions, such as individual and group therapy, should be provided when indicated (Lahad & Cohen, 2003; see also Kutz & Bleich, this volume).

Support for Families. The families of first responders, who absorb much of their relatives' distress, need support and acknowledgement of the important role they play in supporting their loved ones as they work in horrific situations.

THE NEED FOR A COMPREHENSIVE RESPONSE

The Continuum of Trauma Services is a comprehensive response to trauma that encompasses the entire population. It ensures widespread availability of trauma services to the diverse geographic, ethnic, linguistic and professional communities represented in Israel's cultural mosaic. It includes coordination among service providers, mapping of existing services and their efficacy, identifying unmet needs and crafting solutions; evaluating interventions, the development of a body of knowledge based on evaluation and documentation, development of best practice models and standardized protocols; training agencies in service delivery, and education of the public as to the availability of services. It encompasses preventive, re-silience-building efforts and immediate, post-event, and long-term interventions.

While maintaining an inventory of resources, it also ensures that successful programs can be replicated nationwide while preventing duplication of effort. It assumes responsibility for educating professionals and upgrading their skills by providing basic and advanced training to non-professional providers of services to trauma victims and providing support for these "helpers" to prevent burnout. The services provided are developed by both lay leaders and professionals from NGOs, enabling them to benefit from each organization's ideology, resources and experience.

RESTORING CONNECTIONS

Trauma is a brutal disruption (Danieli et al., 2003). The world view of trauma victims is often reduced to a clean split, as most tend to perceive their lives as divided into two periods: the time before the traumatic event and the period since the event. Victims of trauma tend to flounder in the present, in the vortex of their suffering. The establishment of a continuum of services would help to re-establish connections on both the micro and the macro levels.

The word "continuum" reflects healthy functioning while the word "trauma" implies fragmentation. A parallel may be drawn between the individual's experience of trauma and the system's response to it. The essence of trauma therapy is to help the victim to regain a sense of control. The processing and healing that should be part of the therapeutic experience restore a person's sense of continuity, which is the entry point to living a normal life.

THE ISRAEL TRAUMA COALITION

As trauma fragments lives and isolates people from one another, so the creation of a CTS reintegrates shattered parts of a system struggling to meet critical needs. The CTS brings a healing approach to the organizational sphere, where the embodiment of the continuum is the Israel Trauma Coalition (ITC).

It is beyond the scope of any one organization or system, each of necessity occupied with its own survival and its own particular niche, to be aware of all existing trauma needs, resources and possible responses. This is why a coalition of key service providers, with combined, intimate knowledge of needs and services in the field, is the optimal mechanism of response.

The ITC is a national network of organizations that seeks to ensure that effective trauma-related services are available to all people living in Israel. It was founded in January 2002 as part of the initiative of the United Jewish Appeal (UJA)-Federation of New York, in response to the escalating and pervasive acts of terrorism in Israel. The idea was to seat members of different NGOs providing trauma-related services together around the table so that they could pool knowledge and resources.

Together, the members of the Coalition bring a wider perspective to the entire field of trauma services. In their roles as Coalition members they can step back from their individual concerns and the taxing work of managing a trauma services organization to consider the national situation. The peer group of experts, who sit on the Coalition's Coordinating Board, examines the macro issues of mapping and service availability and processes the information with respect to different sectors of the population. They decide how best to utilize existing services to fill gaps, whether this means matching resources to needs, replicating successful programs or creating what is lacking.

The firm and broad base upon which the Coalition must rest is provided by the interest groups that have been formed. The government is mandated by law and limited in its ability to provide services by availability of funds and political concerns. In the absence of interest groups, NGOs work in isolation, and there is often duplication of effort and an unequal distribution of services. The ITC strives to remedy this situation, through the four active interest groups that it has founded.

School-Based Interest Group

This interest group coordinates the implementation of screening projects and interventions from pre-school through high school, with programs for both teachers and students. The activities of this interest group also include the development and production of manuals and the development of treatment protocols.

Hospital Interest Group

This interest group is developing an Acute Stress Reaction (ASR) assessment tool to be used in hospital Emergency Rooms as well as an ASR best practices protocol. The protocol will be taught to staff at ten at risk hospitals and the training will be followed with evaluation.

In addition, the group is developing a nationwide training program in the treatment of Acute Stress Disorder (ASD) for mental health experts in general hospitals so that 1-3 mental health professionals in each general hospital will be equipped to provide ASD treatment for clients diagnosed with the disorder.

The Child and Adolescent Treatment Interest Group

All meetings of this interest group include lectures and are followed by discussion and peer group consultations. Evaluation and assessment tools are pooled and discussed and participants collaborate on research questions.

The Community Interest Group

A wide array of programs is being developed and implemented by members of this interest group. They include Helping the Helpers workshops, provided for "helpers" who are prone to burnout in various organizations and services, from volunteers to the first responders previously described.

The first walk-in crisis center providing short-term crisis intervention, free of charge, is the result of the work of this group. Other services provided by members of the Community Interest Group include 24-hour, emotional first aid hotlines; a hotline for victims of terror and war; direct trauma therapy; long-term trauma care; an array of post-event community interventions; training of therapists in trauma treatment; volunteer support in the form of seminars and retreats; parenting workshops to improve coping and emotional resilience; work with new immigrant trauma victims; work with Holocaust survivors for whom the current trauma triggers past traumas; and work with the Druze community, who experience the trauma in their unique way.

The work of the Coalition transforms the ideology of the CTS into a practical reality by continuously bringing more agencies into the fold through the interest groups and creating new interest groups as needed. Members of the interest groups identify, prevent and treat various forms of trauma and expand cadres of professionals who have training and knowledge and identify themselves as care providers who dispense trauma information, tools and supports.

The desired outcome is that, over time, government agencies will adopt the models that lend themselves to state-supported, nationwide replication. The ministries of health and education are already involved through the ITC interest groups, and hopefully their involvement will deepen as the CTS continues to develop. At the same time, it is clear that there will always be a need for the complementary services provided by NGOs.

The ITC was designed to meet needs engendered by terror-related emotional trauma. And yet, through the continuum of trauma services that it provides to direct victims, children, family members, witnesses, first responders, helping professionals and the community-at-large, it has transformed a response to a tragic situation into an uplifting experience, as it improves coping, builds emotional resilience and provides professional services.

Despite the context in which it was forged, the ITC has empowered and enriched tens of thousands of residents of Israel, impacting the country as a whole. Individuals profit from improved coping skills and strengthened emotional resilience, while professional organizations reap the benefits of collaboration, immeasurably exceeding the sum of their parts.

As the Coalition develops, the reality of a CTS, a continually evolving process, moves closer to its goal of supporting different circles of trauma victims and combating the scourge of terrorism as it attempts to rob the population of its right to live a terror-free life.

In line with the vision of the CTS, the Coalition has moved from emergency reactive response to a model that is much more comprehensive, involving almost all trauma-related service providers in Israel. It has moved from providing direct services to developing services, fostering collaboration, mapping, evaluation and research and developing a body of knowledge.

NOTES

1. All names were changed to protect the identity of participants in this study.
2. A story provided by SELAH, the non-profit organization providing emergency aid and long-term support to new immigrants who have experienced terror, tragedy and trauma.

REFERENCES

Ayalon, O. & Lahad, M. (1991). *Living on the edge*. Haifa, Israel: Nord.

Baca, E., Baca-García, E., Pérez-Rodríguez, M. M., & Cabanas, M. L. (2004). Short- and long-term effects of the terrorist attacks in Spain. *Journal of Aggression, Maltreatment, & Trauma*, 9(1/2/3/4), 157-170.

Ben-Gershon, B., Grinshpoon, A., & Ponizovsky, A. (2004). Mental health services preparing for the psychological consequences of terrorism. *Journal of Aggression, Maltreatment, & Trauma*, 10(1/2/3/4), 743-753.

Bleich, A., Gelkopf, M., & Solomon, Z. (2003). Exposure to terrorism, stress-related mental health symptoms, and coping behaviors among a nationally representative sample in Israel. *Journal of the American Medical Association, 290*, 612-620.

Danieli, Y., Engdahl, B. & Schlenger, W. E. (2003). The psychological aftermath of terrorism. In F. Moghaddam, & A. J. Marsella (Eds.), *Understanding terrorism: Psychosocial roots, consequences, and interventions* (pp. 223-246). Washington, DC: American Psychological Association.

Katan, J. (1988) Voluntary organizations–A substitute for or a partner to state activity in the social arena. *Social Security–Journal of Welfare and Social Security Studies, 32*, 57-73.

Kfir, N. (1998). *Crisis intervention verbatim*. Philadelphia, PA: Hemisphere Publishing.

Kleber, R. J., & Brom, D. (1992). *Coping with trauma: Consequences, prevention and treatment*. Lisse, The Netherlands: Swets.

Kutz, I., & Bleich, A. (2004). Mental health interventions in a general hospital following terrorist attacks: the Israeli experience. *Journal of Aggression, Maltreatment & Trauma*, 9(1/2/3/4), 425-437.

Lahad, M., & Cohen, A. (2003). The development of debriefing in Israel. In O. Ayalon, M. Lahad, & A. Cohen (Eds.), *Community stress prevention* (Vol. 5, pp. 117-126). Kiryat Shmona, Israel: Community Stress Prevention Center.

Lonigman, C. T. (1991). Children's reactions to natural disaster: Symptom severity, and degree of exposure. *Advanced Behavior Research Treatment, 13*, 135-153.

Rosenfeld, L. B., Caye, J., Ayalon, O., & Lahad, M. (in press). *When their world comes apart: Helping Families and children manage the effects of disasters*. Washington, DC: National Association of Social Workers Press.

Salamon, L. (1995). *Partners in public service*. Baltimore: The Johns Hopkins University Press.

Schmid, H. (1998). For-profit and nonprofit human services: A comparative analysis. *Social Security–Journal of Welfare and Social Security Studies, 51*, 29-42.

Schmid, H., & Sabbagh, C. (1991). Organizational and structural aspects of public and private organizations delivering services to the frail elderly–A comparative analysis. *Social Security–Journal of Welfare and Social Security Studies, 36*, 49-67.

Vogel, M., & Vernberg, E. (1993). Children's psychological responses to disaster (Task Force Report). *Journal of Clinical Child Psychology, 22*(4), 464-484.

Voice:
Right After the Bomb Went Off

Danny Brom

The bomb went off at 8:45 am in the bus in Jerusalem. A suicide bomber exploded himself in the middle of a bus full of people going to work and children on their way to school. Seven people died immediately, another four later in the hospital. The news of the bomb spread rapidly throughout the city. Cell phones rang everywhere: "Did you hear? Where are you? Did you speak to all the children?"

The social service machinery went into action immediately. Municipal social workers rushed to the scene of the bombing. An emergency center was set up in the municipality to coordinate everything. The hospitals prepared places in their emergency rooms. The social workers in the hospitals got ready to receive the wounded and people in shock. Specially trained psychiatrists, psychologists and social workers from mental health institutions hurried to the hospitals to back up and assist the hospital teams. Everyone knows his/her task and where to go; it's a known scenario. The crisis walk-in center gets organized: send information to the media, call more personnel as backup. Most wounded and people in shock are in the hospital by 9:30 a.m.

The fire fighters and police are the first on the scene and they work until they give the green light to the other emergency teams. The 25 or so ambulances that have arrived drive to and fro with the wounded, having selected who goes first, who can wait.

Address correspondence to: Danny Brom, PhD, Director, Temmy and Albert Latner Israel Center for the Treatment of Psychotrauma, Herzog Hospital, P.O.B. 3900, Jerusalem Israel, 91035.

[Haworth co-indexing entry note]: "Voice: Right After the Bomb Went Off." Brom, Danny. Co-published simultaneously in *Journal of Aggression, Maltreatment & Trauma* (The Haworth Maltreatment & Trauma Press, an imprint of The Haworth Press, Inc.) Vol. 10, No. 3/4, 2005; and: *The Trauma of Terrorism: Sharing Knowledge and Shared Care, An International Handbook* (ed: Yael Danieli, Danny Brom, and Joe Sills) The Haworth Maltreatment & Trauma Press, an imprint of The Haworth Press, Inc., 2005.

The trauma center is in contact with the headquarters of the fire fighters, with the ambulance services, and with the municipality. The ZAKA-unit that collects body parts (Solomon & Berger, this volume) calls: can someone come to talk to the team? The fire fighters would like someone to come at 12:00. The ambulance service would like to have someone at 12:30. The municipal social workers go around the scene and the surroundings, asking who was there and offering their help. The municipal emergency coordinator calls: is there a team that can work with a group of very distressed people from a social work agency in town who lost a colleague? Totally booked, the trauma center calls a colleague from the Israel Trauma Coalition. The Tel Aviv group readily agrees to take this upon themselves.

Families come to the hospitals looking for their loved ones. Social workers receive them. For some there is information, for some there is not. The hospitals share their information with each other, so that family members don't have to search for their loved ones. For some the horrible news is broken; someone needs to go to the body identification unit in Tel Aviv. The municipal social worker will accompany the family. Volunteers flow to the hospital to take care of the needs of the families, giving out drinks, being there, and providing transportation.

The schools make a list of who did not come to school and contact the families. Rumors start quickly: ten kids from one school were in the bus, 6 kids from another. The schools notify their psychological services. Three people come to the crisis walk-in center the same day, another 24 in the 20 days after that, some referred by other services, others self-referred.

After the first day, the social workers of the Social Insurance Institute take over. They get the lists from the hospitals of all hospitalized patients, visit all the wounded, and the families of those who died.

The next day the school psychological service calls the trauma center: two schools have lost children. They want an evening for parents; can you do it? The other school would like someone to talk to the seventh graders; can someone do that?

In the first week a tremendous amount of services are delivered by the municipality, the Social Insurance Institute, the trauma/crisis center, hospitals, and mental health providers. All are in contact with each other, referring, asking questions, offering help. A known and well-trained scene.

REFERENCE

Solomon, Z., & Berger, R. (2004). Coping with the aftermath of terror–Resilience of ZAKA body handlers. *Journal of Aggression, Maltreatment & Trauma, 9*(1/2/3/4), 353-364.

Mental Health Services Preparing for the Psychological Consequences of Terrorism

Bella Ben-Gershon
Alexander Grinshpoon
Alexander Ponizovsky

SUMMARY. The Israeli population has been subjected to the stresses of war and terrorist attacks since long before the state was founded. Confronting this extensive experience of terrorism-related psychological trauma, the Mental Health Services of the Ministry of Health designed and implemented a comprehensive emergency response system that operates in general hospitals and community settings to meet the psychological needs resulting from terrorism at both the individual and the population levels. This article describes general premises, basic elements, administrative structure and functioning of this system, as well as training programs for various service providers working with the victims.

Address correspondence to: Bella Ben-Gershon, MSW, National Coordinator for Emergency Preparedness and Trauma Treatment, Mental Health Services, Ministry of Health, 2 Ben Tabai Street, Jerusalem 93461, Israel (E-mail: bella.ben-gershon@ moh.health.gov.il).

[Haworth co-indexing entry note]: "Mental Health Services Preparing for the Psychological Consequences of Terrorism." Ben-Gershon, Bella, Alexander Grinshpoon, and Alexander Ponizovsky. Co-published simultaneously in *Journal of Aggression, Maltreatment & Trauma* (The Haworth Maltreatment & Trauma Press, an imprint of The Haworth Press, Inc.) Vol. 10, No. 3/4, 2005; and: *The Trauma of Terrorism: Sharing Knowledge and Shared Care, An International Handbook* (ed: Yael Danieli, Danny Brom, and Joe Sills) The Haworth Maltreatment & Trauma Press, an imprint of The Haworth Press, Inc., 2005.

743

KEYWORDS. Terrorism, mental health services, emergency situation, policy

The Israeli population has been subjected to the stresses of war since long before the state was founded in 1948. In addition to multiple terror attacks, its history has been punctuated by numerous wars with its neighbors. Its small size and close-knit social structure mean that all Israelis experience a feeling of deep involvement whenever a terrorist attack occurs (Bleich, Gelkopf, & Solomon, 2003). More recently, chemical, biological, radiological, and nuclear terrorism have become an immediate threat for the world community and Israel as well (DiGiovanni, 2001; Gardemann, 2002; Shalev, 2001; Weinberger, Meisel & David, 1996; Yitzhaki, Solomon & Kotler, 1991). The main significance of all of these threats is the psychological damage and demoralization they intend to cause rather than their potential for mass destruction (DiGiovanni, 2001; Kutz & Bleich, 2003; Moscrop, 2001). The broad nature of the psychological consequences demands a full public health response (Breslau et al., 1996).

BASIC PREMISES

The following assumptions form the basis of the disaster preparedness system of the Ministry of Health:

- One of the responsibilities of the mental health care system is responding to emergency situations that have the potential of causing severe psychological damage (Gardemann, 2002).
- Most disasters and terrorism casualties are those caused by stress (North & Pfefferbaum, 2002; Silver, Holman, McIntosh, Poulin & Gil-Rivas, 2002).
- Anxiety, fear, and demoralization impair individual well-being and can even result in mental disability. It can also affect people *en masse*, placing huge pressure on the health care system (Schlenger et al., 2003; Somasundaram & Sivayokan, 1994).
- To cope adequately with disasters of varying scale, the health care system should be able to care for stress casualties at both general hospital and community levels.
- Early intervention reduces stress and improves the chances of recovery (Caplan, 1963).
- The number of stress casualties is steadily increasing, which means there is a necessity to further develop community-based services, train more

mental health professionals, and improve the coordination of services and care agencies.

HISTORICAL REVIEW

Mental Health Services of the Israel Ministry of Health provide a professional response and care to a wide range of mental disorders. For many decades mental health care staff provided traditional forms of treatment in psychiatric hospitals and attached outpatient clinics. This care was mainly psychopharmacological treatment or long-term psychodynamic/psychoanalytically oriented therapy.

Psychological trauma has been seen more frequently by the Israel Defense Forces' mental health professionals (Neria, Solomon & Dekel, 1998; Yitzhaki, Solomon, & Kotler, 1991) and by a few experts in the private sector (Solomon, 2001; Solomon et al., 1993). During the first Intifada (1987-1993), a mass Palestinian terrorist activity, the media paid no attention to psychological casualties, nor were governmental services established to care for this client group. Since the Gulf War in 1991, however, when a whole civilian population found itself on the firing line and threatened with total destruction by chemical and biological warfare, unprecedented attention has been given to mental health issues, among them psychological resilience and trauma prevention and care (Bleich, Dycian, Koslovski, Solomon, & Weiner, 1992; Sokolone, Baras, Plati, & Epstein, 1996; Solomon et al., 1993; Weinberger et al., 1996). At the same time, the related activities of the Mental Health Services, Welfare and other agencies, which faced psychological trauma, have been unsystematic and uncoordinated. These uncoordinated efforts have resulted in agencies being overwhelmed by floods of clients, in duplication of treatment, and even in inadequate treatment.

The current Intifada began, and in addition to the multiplication and density of terrorist attacks, it has also brought the threat of a large-scale war. Once the Intifada started, the numbers of psychologically traumatized terror victims climbed steadily; during this time, the ratio of patients admitted to emergency rooms who are psychologically traumatized to those physically traumatized by suicide bombings has increased from 4:1 to 20:1. These developments have exposed severe inadequacies in the professional response to psychological trauma and traumatized population behavior. As a result, the Mental Health Services decided to set up the Population Behavior and Psychological Trauma Prevention and Care Unit. The Unit quickly became an integral and vital component of both general and emergency mental health care. The Unit aims to strengthen psychological resilience and the ability to cope with traumatic events at national, community and individual levels. The Unit acts in an advisory capacity to the Director of the Mental Health Services, the Ministry of Health's senior management, the Emergency Period Services Division, and the Supreme Hospitalization Authority. Its specific roles include helping to compile theory and contingency planning on coping and population management during emergency. The Unit also accomplishes public communication and dissemination of information in these two subject areas as well as provides advice and guidance to health care professionals. Since the Unit operates in the two large arenas, general hospitals and community settings, we will describe the two separately.

REINFORCEMENT OF GENERAL HOSPITALS

To assist general hospitals and to prevent the development of psychiatric disability, a unique mental health support system was developed that includes training of special teams. The typical team consists of a senior psychiatrist (team leader) and eight mental health professionals: two psychiatrists, two clinical psychologists, two clinical social workers, and two psychiatric nurses (half of the team specialize in children and the other in adults). Immediately following an attack/disaster, they are required to arrive at the Emergency Department (ED) of the relevant hospital to examine all injured persons, including those suffering from psychological traumatic shock. After receiving first aid, the patients are brought to a special area of the hospital, the Stress Unit (SU), which is located at some distance from the ED to prevent secondary traumatizing caused by seeing severely injured victims. All individual and group interventions have been performed in the SU. No patient is discharged without being examined by a mental health professional. Figure 1 shows the schema of trauma intervention in a general hospital.

The interventions include: (a) psycho-educational explanations about the nature and course of psychological trauma, (b) emotional support, and (c) information about ongoing psychological and social security assistance. In addition, each person is provided with written information available in various languages (Hebrew, English, Russian, Arabic, and Amharic) about the nature of traumatic symptoms, recommended ways of coping and ways to reach mental health regional coordinators for further assistance. An additional function of the team is emotional support provision to the doctors and personnel involved in treatment of the most severe victims (e.g., younger victims, patients with severe burns and missing body parts), which is drastically different from their usual experience.

FIGURE 1. Trauma intervention in general hospitals.

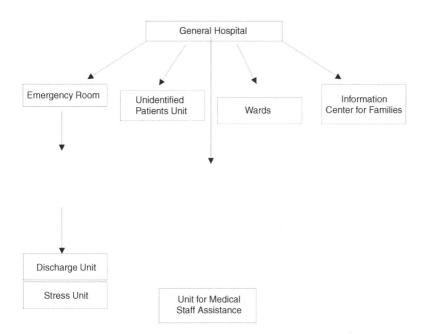

The hospital social workers provide contact between a victim and his/her family members and friends, helping them to cope with stress and to deal with grief manifestations. They also accompany family members to the hospital morgue when the identification of loved ones is required. When team members encounter patients at high risk for the development of Acute Stress Disorder (ASD; Shalev, 2002; Solomon et al., 1993), they refer those in need to outpatient mental health clinics for continuing treatment. Follow-up procedures have been put in place for patients discharged to the community.

Though no systematic data on the effectiveness of interventions have been collected, we receive consistent reports from ED professionals about an obvious improvement in the emotional status of victims. There is also some evidence for improving clinical diagnosis and prognosis with regard to ASD and post-traumatic stress disorder (PTSD; Campfield & Hills, 2001; Everly, 2000; Shalev, 2001).

REINFORCEMENT OF COMMUNITY SETTINGS

In times of both normalcy and emergency, the Unit is one of the agencies consulting the Supreme Hospitalization Authority (SHA). Under SHA auspices, the Mental Health Services Director and the Unit Head serve as national coordinators of the response to psychological trauma. The administration of a district's community-based mental health services is the direct responsibility of the District Psychiatrist. Together with the District Physician, they head the local District Health Bureau. The powers of District Psychiatrists with respect to emergency arrangements and the care of psychological trauma allow them to activate and administer all professional mental health care resources (Ministry of Health, Mental Health Services, 2003a). Figure 2 shows the schema of trauma intervention in the community settings.

These resources are divided into a number of areas:

1. The District Psychiatrist has overall charge of the specialist teams set up to respond to a range of planned scenarios of similar community events. Depending on a scenario, five categories of reinforcement teams have been established to manage the psychological consequences of terrorism:

    a. In mega-terrorist attacks (Ministry of Health, Mental Health Services, 2003b).
    b. To clinics conducting mass inoculations (Ministry of Health, Mental Health Services, 2003c).
    c. To evacuation (Ministry of Health, Mental Health Services, 2003d).
    d. For antibiotic distribution (Ministry of Health, Mental Health Services, 2003e).
    e. To general hospitals (Ministry of Health, Mental Health Services, 2003f).

2. The District Psychiatrist has under his direct administration Emergency Period Coordinators. These are senior staffers in 90 mental health outpatient clinics across Israel, all of whom have received a six-month training in psychological trauma care and disaster management. The Coordinators are responsible for training the staff of their clinics and for organizing immediate case management for trauma survivors discharged from general hospitals and for others who turn up or are referred to the clinic for outpatient care. Through the Coordinators, the District Psychiatrist operates all mental health clinics as trauma centers, providing a 24-hour coverage service with 12-hour shifts of working staff.
3. The psychiatric hospitals and various rehabilitation centers also come under the oversight of the District Psychiatrist, who will also take over their operation in times of emergency when they are called upon to put

their training into practice. Specially trained mental health professionals are in charge of other models of trauma care in a number of settlements in the Administered Territories (the West Bank and the Gaza Strip).

The professional care system clearly could not answer all needs, especially to provide the general population mental first aid and referrals to further sources of treatment and support. Therefore, the core needs of the general population must be fulfilled in the first turn, such as first psychological aid and referrals to further sources of treatment and support. For this purpose, ERAN, the Association's telephone crisis assistance network, was recruited to handle calls from members of the public suffering from fears, anxiety and uncertainty. The volunteer-staffed hotline with 24-hour coverage in five languages has activated immediately after every terrorist attack or disaster; the volunteers are working under the supervision of psychological trauma experts from the mental health services.

The family doctor is naturally the general population's first port of call for both mental and physical injury (Ponizovsky, Grinshpoon, Yagur, & Ben-Gershon, 2003). A special effort was thus made to develop family doctors' skills for identifying psychological trauma and referring sufferers to appropriate agencies. These doctors were provided with special training and information sheets (Ministry of Health, Mental Health Services, 2003g). Another domain now under development is the coordination between governmental mental health services and other relevant agencies for establishing a care succession between them. Figure 3 shows the scheme of the interrelations between government and community agencies.

FIGURE 2. Trauma intervention in the community.

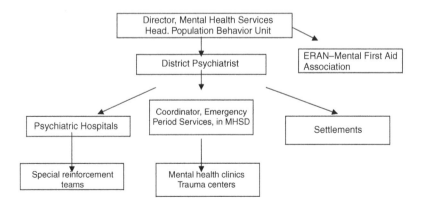

FIGURE 3. The interrelations between government and community agencies.

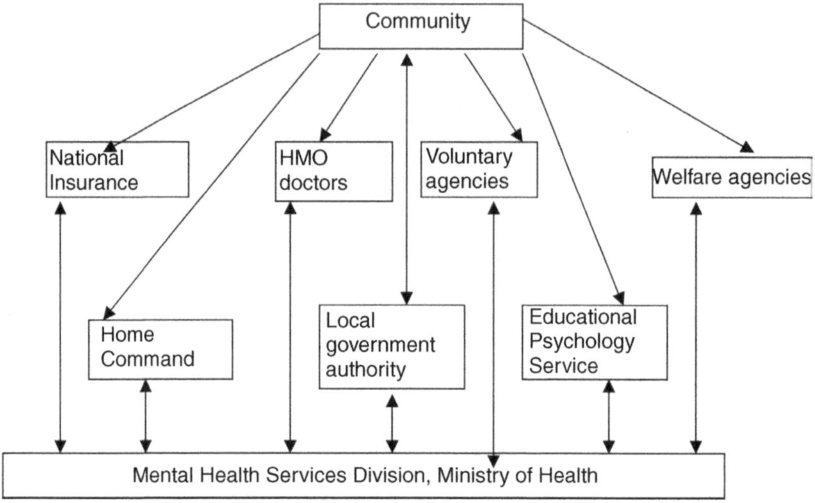

CONCLUSIONS

Preliminary data from the governmental mental health clinics indicate that few citizens seek care in the aftermath of terrorist attacks (Schuster et al., 2001). This suggests that the majority of sufferers prefer seeking help from private sector therapists or community trauma centers. Alternatively, most trauma-exposed persons may consider their suffering as a normal psychological reaction and do not believe that mental health services are the adequate address to obtain relief from their suffering. In addition, the stigma of "mental illness" still can prevent people from seeking help for their trauma from mental health services. The solution might be developing community trauma centers away from the existing clinics. The Israel Center for the Treatment of Psychotrauma in Jerusalem (http://www.traumaweb.org/) offers a successful model for replication, especially in the cities with the most frequent and intense terrorist attacks (e.g., Jerusalem, Haifa, Hadera, Kfar Saba, and Shderot).

The mental health professionals sent out to reinforce general hospital staffs after terrorist events are suffering from workplace burnout. Team members are quitting, for example, because of the emotional overloading in ED. We suggest that this phenomenon will be worsened over time. Relief teams need to be recruited and trained; for every team member massive support must be provided, including additional rest days, financial reward, advice and guidance as well as the organizing of supportive groups.

The mental health care network in the community maintains direct contact with a number of government agencies. However, professional leadership and collaborative relations with the local authorities have not been provided. Operational integration of other public agencies, such as the Educational Psychology Service, the welfare services, and the National Insurance Institute, are required in most areas of the country. In order to improve collaboration and integration, professional trauma care leadership in the local authorities should be established, joint operational guidelines developed and joint training carried out.

An important point requiring attention is the capacity of the mental health services to deal with psychological trauma and reinforce psychological resilience of residents of settlements in the Administered Territories. The personal insecurity makes it hard to find mental health professionals willing to work in the field. To solve this problem, we suggest utilizing novel medicine technology, such as telemedia networks, linking clinics inside Israel proper with the Territories' clinics for guidance, consulting and treatment.

Finally, we conclude that the Mental Health Services at the Ministry of Health have created a unique model for protecting the public and developing the population's psychological resilience to psychological effects of terrorism. Implementation of this model involving the cooperation of additional community agencies should be extended.

REFERENCES

Bleich, A., Dycian, A., Koslovski, M., Solomon, Z., & Weiner, M. (1992). Psychiatric implication of missile attacks on a civilian population: Israeli lessons from the Gulf War. *Journal of the American Medical Association, 268*, 613-615.

Bleich, A., Gelkopf, M., & Solomon, Z. (2003). Exposure to terrorism, stress-related mental health symptoms, and coping behaviors among a nationally representative sample in Israel. *Journal of the American Medical Association, 290*, 612-620.

Breslau, N., Kessler, R. C., Chilcoat, H. D., Schultz, L. R., Davis, G. C., & Andreski, P. (1998). Trauma and posttraumatic stress disorder in the community: The 1996 Detroit Area Survey of Trauma. *Archives of General Psychiatry, 55*, 626-632.

Campfield, K. M., & Hills, A. M. (2001). Effects of timing of critical incident stress debriefing (CISD) on posttraumatic symptoms. *Journal of Traumatic Stress, 4*(2), 327-340.

Caplan, G. (1963). *Principles of preventive psychiatry*. New York: Basic Books.

DiGiovanni, C. (2001). Pertinent psychological issues in immediate management of weapons of mass destruction event. *Military Medicine, 166*, 2, 59-60.

Everly, G. S. (2000). Crisis management briefings (CMB): Large group crisis intervention in response to terrorism, disasters, and violence. *International Journal of Emergency Mental Health, 2*(1), 53-57.

Gardemann, J. (2002). Primary health care in complex humanitarian emergencies: Rwanda and Kosovo experiences and their implication for public health training. *Croatian Medical Journal, 43*, 55-148.

Kutz, I., & Bleich, A. (2003). Conventional, chemical and biological terror of mass destruction: Psychological aspects and psychiatric guidelines. In J. Shemer & Y. Schoenfeld (Eds.), *Terror and medicine* (pp. 533-544). Lengeirich, Germany: Science Publishers.

Ministry of Health, Mental Health Services. (2003a). *Nohal hafalat briut hanefesh bakehila besheat herum* [Guidelines for the operation of mental health services in emergency]. Jerusalem: Ministry of Health.

Ministry of Health, Mental Health Services. (2003b). *Nohal tigbur bemega irua al yedei briut hanefesh* [Mega-terrorism operational guideline]. Jerusalem: Ministry of Health.

Ministry of Health, Mental Health Services. (2003c). *Nohal hafalat briut hanefesh betarhish ababuot shgorot* [Smallpox vaccination operational guideline]. Jerusalem: Ministry of Health.

Ministry of Health, Mental Health Services. (2003d). *Nohal tigbur merkazei pinui al yedei briut hanefesh* [Evacuation centers operational guideline]. Jerusalem: Ministry of Health.

Ministry of Health, Mental Health Services. (2003e). *Nohal hitargenut sherutei briut hanefesh betarhish antrax* [Anthrax scenario operational guideline]. Jerusalem: Ministry of Health.

Ministry of Health, Mental Health Services. (2003f). *Nohal petihat atarei dahak bevatei holim klaliim* [Opening stress-treatment stations in general hospitals guideline]. Jerusalem: Ministry of Health.

Ministry of Health, Mental Health Services. (2003g). *Nohal tigbur mirpaot rishoniot* [Primary care clinic intervention guideline]. Jerusalem: Ministry of Health.

Moscrop, A. (2001). Mass hysteria is seen as main threat from bio-weapons. *British Medical Journal, 323*, 1023.

Neria, K., Solomon, Z., & Dekel, R. (1998). An eighteen-year follow up study of Israeli prisoner of war and combat veterans. *Journal of Nervous and Mental Disease, 186*, 174-182.

North, C. S., & Pfefferbaum, B. (2002). Research on the mental health effects of terrorism. *Journal of the American Medical Association, 288*, 633-636.

Ponizovsky, A, Grinshpoon, A., Yagur, A., & Ben Gershon, B. (2003). War stress in primary care clinic in Gilo, a neighborhood of Jerusalem. In J. Shemer & Y. Schoenfeld (Eds.), *Terror and medicine.* Lengeirich, Germany: Pabst Science Publishers.

Schlenger, W. E., Caddell, J. M., Ebert, L., Jordan, B. K., Rourke, K. M., Wilson, D. et al. (2003). Psychological reaction to terrorist attacks: Findings from the National Study of Americans' Reaction to September 11. *Journal of the American Medical Association, 288*, 581-588.

Schuster, M. A., Stein, B. D., Jaycox, L. H., Collins, R. L., Marshall, G. N., Elliott, M. et al. (2001). A national survey of stress reactions after the September 11, 2001, terrorist attacks. *New England Journal of Medicine, 345*, 1507-1512.

Shalev, A. Y. (2002). Acute stress reaction in adults. *Biological Psychiatry, 51*, 532-543.

Shalev, A. Y. (2001). What is posttraumatic stress disorder? *Journal of Clinical Psychiatry, 62*, 4-10.

Silver, R. C., Holman, E. A., McIntosh, D. N., Poulin, M., & Gil-Rivas, V. (2002). Nationwide longitudinal study of psychological responses to September 11. *Journal of the American Medical Association, 288*, 1235-1244.

Sokolone, V., Baras, M., Plati, H., & Epstein, L. (1996). Exposure to missile attacks: The impact of the Persian Gulf War on physical health behaviors and psychological distress in high and low risk areas in Israel. *Social Science and Medicine, 42*, 1039-1047.

Solomon, Z., Laor, N., Weiler, D., Muller, U. F., Hadar, O., Waysman, M. et al. (1993). The psychological impact of the Gulf War: A study of acute stress in Israeli evacuees. *Archives of General Psychiatry, 50*, 320-321.

Solomon, Z. (2001). The impact of posttraumatic stress disorder in military situations. *Journal of Clinical Psychiatry, 62*(17), 5-11.

Somasundaram, D. J., & Sivayokan, S. (1994). War trauma in civilian population. *British Journal of Psychiatry, 165*, 524-527.

Weinberger, D., Meisel, S. R., & David, D. (1996). Sudden death among the Israeli population during the Gulf War–incidents and mechanisms. *Israel Journal of Medical Science, 32*, 95-99.

Yitzhaki, T., Solomon, Z., & Kotler, M. (1991). The clinical picture of acute combat stress reaction among Israeli soldiers in the 1982 Lebanon War. *Military Medicine, 156*, 193-197.

Mental Health Response to Terrorism in the United States: An Adolescent Field in an Adolescent Nation

Brian W. Flynn

SUMMARY. This article discusses the organization and delivery of psychosocial response to terrorism within the United States. The context is the state of a relatively young science and practice evolving in a relatively young nation. Specifically, the article describes the structure of preparedness and response at various levels of government and among groups and organizations with differing responsibilities. Sources of more detailed descriptions of program and practices are provided. The article describes the assets intrinsic in the organization and delivery of services within the United States as well as the considerable challenges faced by the field and country.

KEYWORDS. mental health, terrorism, government, disaster, emergency, psychological

Address correspondence to; Brian W. Flynn, EdD, P.O. Box 1205, Severna Park, MD 21146 USA (E-mail: Brianwflynn@aol.com).

[Haworth co-indexing entry note]: "Mental Health Response to Terrorism in the United States: An Adolescent Field in an Adolescent Nation." Flynn, Brian W. Co-published simultaneously in *Journal of Aggression, Maltreatment & Trauma* (The Haworth Maltreatment & Trauma Press, an imprint of The Haworth Press, Inc.) Vol. 10, No. 3/4, 2005; and: *The Trauma of Terrorism: Sharing Knowledge and Shared Care, An International Handbook* (ed: Yael Danieli, Danny Brom, and Joe Sills) The Haworth Maltreatment & Trauma Press, an imprint of The Haworth Press, Inc., 2005.

The mental health response to terrorism in the United States is emerging in a unique mixed context of long standing government support for disaster and emergency services and adaptation to the "new normal" as a nation that is the target of terrorism. The nation enjoys relatively abundant human and financial resources, yet a constricting mental health and increasingly difficult to access service system. Perhaps the greatest challenge lies in a public policy inability or unwillingness to understand that psychosocial factors are central to the very purpose of terrorism. This article will describe the structure of mental health response in the United States, the focus of those interventions, current controversies, and challenges that lay ahead.

The politics and practice of disaster mental health are emerging in a manner that reflects both the country and the culture. The "can do" creative problem solving approach in a nation relatively rich in mental health resources and expertise is moving the field ahead in an extremely robust manner. At the same time, the cultural imperative that seeks the "quick fix," "anybody can do anything," "we know best," a historic perspective complicates the picture (Danieli, Engdahl, & Schlenger, 2003). Paradoxically, a nation that treasures individuality as a cornerstone of its culture seems driven to one size fits all solutions to complex challenges. Mental health response to disaster is no exception. The current status of the United States approach to the mental health aspects of terrorism reflects its most significant assets as well as its challenges.

STRUCTURE

The organization and implementation of general response to disaster is a function of magnitude, scope, intensity, and type. Response to terrorist events, while sharing some models of intervention as well as system responsibilities, differs as a result of these events being intentional, potentially ongoing, and, in addition, criminal acts. As a result, the requirement that underpins governmental response to disaster (e.g., that needs exceed resources thereby activating resources at higher levels of government) is less critical than the ability of public and private resources to come together and provide adequate and integrated response that meets the wide variety of needs of directly and indirectly impacted populations. Terrorism requires tuning of existing plans, procedures, and relationships as well as developing new ones. The goal is a structure of preparedness, response, and recovery that builds upon existing infrastructure yet incorporates the challenges of terrorism that are so new to the United States.

FEDERAL AGENCIES

Several segments of the federal government are involved with disaster mental health matters while actual response following a terrorist incident is governed by the Federal Response Plan (FRP; available at www.fema.gov/rrr/frp). The federal agency with primary responsibility for leading the federal mental health service response is the Substance Abuse and Mental Health Services Administration (SAMHSA; www.samhsa.gov), within the Department of Health And Human Services (DHHS). Within SAMHSA, the most significant program for all types of disasters, including terrorism, is the Crisis Counseling and Training program funded by the Federal Emergency Management Agency (now part of the Department of Homeland Security; www.fema.gov). That program is described in more detail later in this article.

Parts of the federal government that are involved in disaster mental health activities, but are not assigned primary mental health response functions include: (a) the National Institute of Mental Health (NIMH; www.nih.gov), a part of the National Institutes of Health (NIH), (b) the Department of Health And Human Services (DHHS), and (c) NIMH, the federal government's lead agency for research in disaster and emergency mental health activities.

Centers for Disease Control and Prevention (CDC; www.cdc.gov). This DHHS component is playing an increasing role in integrating mental health into public health surveillance and monitoring, especially in events that result in large scale health impact.

Health Resources and Services Administration (HRSA; www.hrsa.gov). This DHHS Agency includes mental health concerns in its responsibilities for supporting health care programs (both hospital and community based) and in preparing health professionals to appropriately respond to terrorist events.

Office for Victims of Crime (OVC; www.ojp.usdoj.gov/ovc). This component of the Justice Department provides a wide variety of support (including mental health) services to crime victims. While not a major supporter in most natural disasters, this Office provides significant service to victims of terror both at home and abroad.

Department of Veterans Affairs (www.va.gov). This department has long provided mental health services to traumatized veterans and is now bringing its considerable experience and human resources base, to the aftermath of terrorist events. The National Center for Post Traumatic Stress Disorder (NCPTSD; www.ncptsd.org) is taking on a rapidly expanding role in bringing research to practice and in assisting SAMHSA in preparation of training and technical assistance materials.

Safe and Drug Free Schools Program (www.ed.gov/index.jsp). This Department of Education component makes funding, consultation, and technical assistance available to school systems to prepare for, and respond to, emergencies of all types including disasters and terrorism.

Department of Defense (DOD). While primarily serving the mental health needs of uniformed services members and their families, because of a long history of dealing with psychological trauma, DOD components have played an invaluable role in bringing that history to bear not only for DOD personal but by sharing expertise and exploring its application to broader populations. The Center for the Study of Traumatic Stress (www.usuhs.mil/psy/traumaticstress/center) in the Department of Psychiatry at the Uniformed Services University of the Health Sciences plays a central role in this regard.

THE FEDERAL RESPONSE PLAN

Overall federal disaster and terror mental health response is organized through the FRP, which provides the comprehensive guide to the response of the federal government and governs relationships with states, and states' various components. In the FRP, various federal departments and agencies are assigned primary, and sometimes secondary, responsibilities. Central to the FRP are a number of Emergency Support Functions (ESF). Mental health service issues are found primarily within ESF-8 (Health and Medical). As noted above, SAMHSA is the lead federal agency with primary responsibility for mental health service response when the FRP is activated.

FEDERAL DISASTER MENTAL HEALTH LEGISLATION

The United States is the only nation known to this writer that has standing federal legislation providing for mental health services following major disasters and emergencies. The most significant advantage of this legislation is its capacity to provide services and establish the legitimacy of meeting the mental health needs of victims and survivors without having to debate its relevance in every new event. The enabling legislation is the Robert T. Stafford Disaster Relief and Emergency Assistance Act (1999) administered by the Federal Emergency Management Agency (FEMA) currently located in the Department of Homeland Security (DHS) and its provisions for crisis counseling, education, and training services following disaster that receive a Presidential Declaration. In the more than three decades since its inception, the Crisis Counseling Program has become one of the federal government's largest programs serving disaster victims and survivors. It provides short-term informal crisis counseling services, as well as general targeted information and education outreach to individuals and communities, and referral for those who may need formal treatment for a mental disorder. More detailed information about this program can be obtained from The Center for Mental Health Services within SAMHSA (http://samhsa.gov/centers/cmhs/cmhs.html). The program provides federal funds, through the states, to local service providers.

While most agree that it is a sound (if not well researched) approach, many feel that when implemented in terrorist incidents the program has several shortcomings. These include its typical reliance on trained nonprofessionals for many services, relatively short duration (almost always perceived as shorter than needed), and its inability to provide services directly to those in need of ongoing formal mental health services for diagnosed disorders, who are referred to existing mental health services.

Beyond this FEMA legislated program, in terrorist events, significant services are provided by the Office for Victims of Crime (OVC) in the Justice Department, the Red Cross (see Hamilton, this volume), and other national organizations (e.g., National Organization of Voluntary Agencies Active in Disasters [NOVAAD]).

All programs are searching for ways to be more responsive to the needs of victim/survivors of terrorism and assure that services are coordinated and integrated. Results are often mixed.

STATE AND LOCAL STRUCTURE

Most states and territories have an emergency response structure that basically reflects the federal structure. Overall disaster and emergency preparedness and response authority and responsibility rests with the state Emergency Management Authority (EMA). Each state also has a Mental Health Authority (MHA) that has primary responsibility for implementing mental health preparedness and response functions. Each MHA has an Emergency Coordinator. Unfortunately, in most cases, because of budget and human resource constraints, emergency responsibilities are only a small portion of that person's larger responsibilities and, as a result, attention to comprehensive preparedness is often compromised. Only a handful of states have a full time person responsible for emergency preparedness and response. States then rely upon local structure such as counties, or increasingly, specific contract organizations, for actual mental health program implementation.

THE DECLARATION PROCESS

Historically, disasters followed a long standing of successive governmental "declarations" involving scope of, impact of, and resources available for response to, extraordinary events. Most natural disasters are first declared disasters or emergencies at the local level and, when local resources are overwhelmed, a disaster declaration is proclaimed by the governor making available broader state resources. When state resources are overwhelmed, the Governor requests a declaration from the President (through FEMA). A Presidential declaration activates eligibility for a wide variety of special funding and programs for both physical and human recovery. The Crisis Counseling Program requires a Presidential Disaster Declaration to be implemented.

The governmental leadership, structure, and process is somewhat different in cases of terrorism where the Federal Bureau of Investigation is the initial lead governmental agency. FEMA then assumes the lead for recovery activities.

FOCUS

While there is not a single mandated/authorized mental health program for terrorism in the United States, most government supported efforts incorporate the following as foundations of their approaches to preparedness, response, and recovery: (a) preparedness, (b) response, and (c) recovery.

Preparedness. In the wake of recent terrorism visited upon the United States, nearly all institutions, agencies, and government departments, including those with special standing (e.g., tribes, pacific island jurisdictions, and foreign and domestic military bases) place renewed focus on preparedness. Within federal, state, and local governments a consistent format for *all-hazards* preparedness has been adopted. This planning model does away with older, hazard specific focus and approaches planning from the standpoint of common elements and processes in all types of extraordinary events and then identifies the special factors, requirements, and relationships necessary to respond to specific event types. While not required by law, most state MHAs are developing and revising their disaster plans using the all-hazards model (DHHS, 2003).

Nearly all health care organizations (e.g., clinics and hospitals) are revising their disaster and mass casually plans. Extreme variation exists in the extent to which they incorporate planning for the psychosocial needs of both their patients and staff members.

Response. Variability and controversy exist regarding nearly all aspects of delivering a mental health response to terrorism. However, several beliefs and principles, discussed throughout this volume, underlie nearly all early mental health response:

- While exposure may vary, no one who experiences a terrorist incident is unaffected by it.
- While many, if not most, people will experience psychological distress a far fewer number will develop a psychiatric disorder.
- Most psychological response is a normal response to a very abnormal event.
- Provision of information, education and anticipatory guidance are considered universal interventions.
- Many types of providers (including mental health professionals, trained nonprofessionals, clergy, community leaders) can play important roles in reducing distress. Of particular note is how leaders communicate in a crisis in ways to reassure the public, reduce distress, and optimize positive behavior (USDHHS, 2002).
- Responses and reactions vary over time, resulting in different psychosocial needs over the response and recovery period.
- Outreach to victims/survivors is a central component of all post-event interventions.
- There is always both individual and collective effect and programs should address the needs of, and interaction between, both.
- The special characteristics, risk, and protective factors of various population subgroups should be taken into account in preparedness, response, and recovery. These include, but are not limited to, racial and ethnic minorities, refugees, children, the frail elderly, people with serious and persistent mental illness, those with learning disabilities and cognitive impairment, those who are injured, and families of dead and injured (for detailed guidance, see USDHHS, 2003).

Recovery. In meeting the mental health needs of victims/survivors of terrorism, the distinction between response to and recovery from the terrorist event often seems artificial. However, it becomes important because of the nature of resources available.

As previously described, in the aftermath of a terrorist event, for about a year, there are often government and other resources available to a broad population of those exposed. As those resources decline and eventually vanish, while the needs of many have been met, many needs typically remain. In the United States, the system providing for the more long-term needs is far less comprehensive and well developed than in the response and early recovery phase. The challenges of access to care are described below.

ASSETS AND ADVANTAGES

The United States has many significant assets that have resulted in, or have the potential to, formulate and deliver significant mental health programs to address mental health needs resulting from terrorism. Ironically, many of these assets also present challenges, described in the following section. Among these assets and advantages are:

- A relatively well developed (if differently focused) mental health service system.
- A relatively high number of mental health professionals.
- National legislation that has existed for more than thirty years that enables the provision of some types of mental health services (Robert T. Stafford Disaster Relief and Emergency Assistance Act, 1999).
- An experience base developed during and following natural disasters.
- An emerging (if too slowly for many) societal recognition of the importance and pervasiveness of psychosocial response to extreme events (including terrorism).

CHALLENGES AND CONTROVERSIES

The existence of an evidence-based comprehensive and coordinated approach to the mental health aspects of terrorism remains an unfulfilled goal. While the trend is positive, there is significant work ahead in many arenas.

FEDERAL LEADERSHIP

Perhaps the greatest challenge is the acute and continuing need for policy makers, at the highest levels, to embrace the notion that the mental health consequences of terrorism are critical issues of homeland/national security. Since the infliction of psychological distress (i.e., terror) is the very purpose of these acts, federal leadership, in the form of terrorism legislation, funding, policy, and cognitive frame, has been slow to embrace what many see as obvious.

HORIZONTAL INTEGRATION

Preparedness and response to terrorism in the post 9/11/01 era has produced both positive and negative results impacting on mental health considerations. Positive developments include a focus on preparedness and response at every level of government and within nearly all systems (e.g., education, health care, public health, law enforcement, etc.). At the same time, very little horizontal integration is taking place resulting in disconnected and uncoordinated preparedness. This "stove piping" will need to be significantly reduced if the goal of integrated response is to be realized.

This lack of horizontal integration is most dramatic with bioterrorism, where optimal behavioral health response requires the seamless integration of the mental health, public health, and medical care systems. Historically and currently, these systems are separate, largely independent, and typically unco-ordinated.

MENTAL HEALTH SYSTEM ISSUES

A credible system of preparedness, response, and recovery from terrorist incidents requires a *population based* approach that anticipates a wide range of individual and collective reactions ranging from emotional distress, to changes in behavior, to emerging psychiatric illness. A model for such a system is articulated in the Institute of Medicine (IOM) study (IOM, 2003). That goal exists within the context of a long standing mental health system in the United States that has significant strengths and weaknesses (DHHS, 1999).

A community mental health system that could easily accommodate such an approach was prevalent in the United States prior to 1980 but, except in some rural areas, has all but disappeared from the landscape. Instead, the current public mental health system in the United States is based on services largely to those who live with serious and persistent mental illness. As a result, it is often politically, legislatively, fiscally, and conceptually difficult for these systems to embrace the notion of comprehensive preparedness and response to the mental health sequelae of terrorism.

The private mental health sector is fundamentally driven by payment for services based upon a diagnosed mental disorder, making preventive and community-based services rare. Worse, in many managed systems, patients may face considerable temporal and procedural barriers to care from a mental health professional.

INTERVENTION ISSUES

While the field of disaster mental health is rapidly growing, fundamental questions remain unanswered. The core question is what interventions, provided to/for whom, delivered by whom, at what time before, during, and after an event, and tailored to what type of events, to provide the most efficacious results? While some evidence-based answers have emerged to a few of these questions, our interventions continue to be conceptually divergent, inconsistent, and often driven more by belief and marketing than evidence.

Influencing provider and consumer behavior in ways that assure the delivery of the appropriate level of intervention to a population with diverse needs in the aftermath of a terrorist event is a fundamental challenge. In events involving weapons of mass destruction (especially biological agents), the situation is even more complex because of anticipated surges on health care organizations based on both actual and psychogenic symptoms. In natural disasters, there is seldom if ever this surge of requests for health services and the acute need to both simultaneously triage levels of psychological need and differentiate between the effects of actual and perceived/believed exposure.

Unfortunately, few good tools and models currently exist to perform these simultaneous tasks. Military models of integrating psychiatrists, psychologists, and social workers in medical units may provide some leads in civilian situations. It is clear, however, that the following elements are important components of meeting this need: (a) Pre-event education of the public regarding behavioral and other health effects of various types of terrorist events; (b) Clear, believable, and direct instruction to those exposed or potentially exposed; (c) Integration of behavioral health professionals into the health care system to assist with assessment, triage, and referral; and (d) Health care plans and assessment/treatment approaches that recognize the centrality and importance of dealing with those who might be exhibiting psychogenic symptoms (and not derisively labeling them as the "worried well" and viewing them as annoyances in dealing with the "really" ill and injured). These *are* the behavioral health effects of terrorism.

HUMAN RESOURCES ISSUES

While a human resource rich country compared to many, issues of availability, accessibility, and appropriate training of mental health professionals are inconsistent and sometimes problematic. In rural areas, there simply may not be enough mental health professionals to provide adequate services at any time, let alone in a response to a terrorist event. In addition, as noted earlier, the nature of financing of health and mental health services in the United States often results in financial, procedural, and temporal barriers to treatment and intervention.

Moreover, there is controversy regarding *who* is qualified to provide *what* types of services to victims and survivors following disasters and terrorist events. While there is consensus that many can and should assist in recovery, little consensus exists regarding the appropriate nature and limits of services provided by trained nonprofessionals and other professionals, such as clergy and school personnel.

Appropriate and adequate training is a continuing challenge. Very few academic programs include training consistent with the foci described above to prepare mental health professionals to function optimally following a terrorist incident. While many may be qualified to provide treatment of psychiatric disorders such as PTSD, clinical depression, and acute stress disorder, few are prepared to function in the diverse roles and environments following large scale traumatic events. (See further, National Institute of Mental Health, 2002; USDHHS, 2000; Ursano, Fullerton, & Norwood, 1995, 2003.)

DIVERSE POPULATIONS

Developing and implementing a national program to provide comprehensive mental health intervention following terrorist incidents is extraordinarily difficult given the diversity of the United States population. The population differs on such demographic variables as race and ethnicity, socioeconomic status, age, prior life experience (including trauma history), urbanicity, family and community support, community intactness, and health status.

STIGMA

Virtually all documentation of the status of mental health in the United States describes the continued presences and impact of stigma against those who live with mental illness. In spite of its pervasiveness following disasters and terrorism, psychological distress, not surprisingly, also carries stigma. Ironically, the field of disaster mental health has probably helped destigmatize mental health problems because these difficulties are so pervasive and visible following large scale traumatic events. At the same time, one cannot help but speculate that stigma is a significant part of the failure to recognize that the intent of terrorism is to psychologically destabilize individuals and communities.

THE WORKPLACE

In the United States, public and private health and mental health systems, education, and employment have very distinct characteristics. Government approaches to mental health issues in terrorism, while nominally intended to serve all people, are primarily implemented through public systems. Most individuals employed in private sector business and industry, if they receive support for mental health related problems, typically receive it through Employment Assistance Programs and/or employer subsidized or supported health care.

The attack on the World Trade Center in New York on 9/11/01 dramatically demonstrated the artificiality of these boundaries when the vast majority of fatalities (and their surviving families) were privately employed, yet the psychological damage went well beyond those most immediately impacted. Provision of mental health response taxed the capacity of both public and private resources.

Workplace issues that go beyond direct health and mental health services, including policies and practices, are a largely unexplored and undeveloped area. Recognizing that traumatic events may affect families, productivity and workplace cohesion, cause concentration difficulties and resulting accidents and absenteeism, thereby impacting on business recovery.

TITRATION OF RESOURCES

Like many countries, the United State typically experiences an outpouring of both goodwill and resources of all types following extraordinary events. The appropriate titration of qualified resources in a significant challenge. With respect to mental health resources, there is often an outpouring that exceeds the ability of the impacted service system to absorb and utilize meaningfully. It is also extremely difficult to assure quality and appropriateness of volunteer services in the midst of a response. In fact, the management of volunteer mental health resources is a significant clinical, managerial, and systems problem.

Unfortunately, the willingness and interest of those who immediately and spontaneously volunteer do not last much beyond the initial phase. When these additional resources may be most needed, months later, they are usually difficult to find and utilize (see Hamilton, this volume, and Pardess, this volume).

Events involving bioterrorism present additional significant problems. If the event involves a contagious agent (or one feared to be contagious), the initial outpouring described above may well not occur. In fact, it may be difficult to get scheduled workers to perform their duties, presenting new types of titration challenges.

CONCLUSION

In describing the United States' preparedness for, response to, and recovery from, the mental health sequelae of terrorist events, it is hard to make an overall assessment. In some ways, the old cigarette advertisement that proclaimed,

"You've come a long way, baby" applies. At the same time, Robert Frost's (1923) verse, "I've miles to go and promises to keep before I sleep," seems most accurate. In the domain of mental health, the state of preparedness and response is actively and rapidly growing with much yet to be done. Compared to some other nations, the United States is less experienced in many arenas and has only recently had to come to grips with large-scale terrorism. We must apply our best talent, learn form other nations, and integrate the resources that are emerging. The nation, and the field of disaster mental health, both remain relatively young, enjoying great energy, vitality, and potential. At the same time, there is much knowledge, wisdom and maturity yet to be gained.

REFERENCES

Danieli, Y., Engdahl, B., & Schlenger, W. E. (2003). The psychological aftermath of terrorism. In F. Moghaddam, A. J. Marsella, & A. Bandura (Eds.) *International terrorism and terrorists: Psychosocial perspectives* (pp. 223-246). Washington, DC: American Psychological Association.

Department of Veterans Affairs. Retrieved April 5, 2004, from www.va.gov

Frost, R. (1923). Stopping by woods on a snowy evening. In *New Hampshire*. New York: Holt.

Hamilton, S. E. (2004). Volunteers in disaster response: The American Red Cross. *Journal of Aggression, Maltreatment, & Trauma, 10*(1/2/3/4), 621-632.

Institute of Medicine. (2003). *Preparing for the psychological consequences of terrorism: A public health strategy*. Washington, DC: The National Academies Press.

National Institute of Mental Health. (2002). *Mental health and mass violence: Evidence based early intervention for victims of mass violence. A workshop to reach consensus on best practices*. (NIH Publication No. 02-5138). Washington, DC: U.S. Government Printing Office.

Pardess, E. (2004). Training and mobilizing volunteers for emergency response and long-term support. *Journal of Aggression, Maltreatment & Trauma, 9*(1/2/3/4), 609-620.

Robert T. Stafford Disaster Relief and Emergency Assistance Act, 42 U.S.C. §§5121-5204c (updated, 1999).

U.S. Department of Health and Human Services. (1999). *Mental health: A report of the surgeon general*. Rockville, MD: U.S Department of Health and Human Services, Substance Abuse and Mental Health Services Administration, Center for Mental Health Services, National Institutes of Health, National Institute of Mental Health.

U.S. Department of Health and Human Services. (2000). *Training manual for mental health and human service workers* (2nd Ed.). (DHHS Pub. No. ADM 90-5383641). Rockville, MD: Center of Mental Health Services, Substance Abuse and Mental Health Services Administration.

U.S. Department of Health and Human Services. (2003). *Mental health all-hazards disaster planning guidance*. (DHHS Pub. No. SMA 3829). Rockville, MD: Center of

Mental Health Services, Substance Abuse and Mental Health Services Administration.

U.S. Department of Health and Human Services. (2003). *Designing culturally competent disaster mental health programs.* (DHHS Pub. No. SMA 3828). Rockville, MD: Center of Mental Health Services, Substance Abuse and Mental Health Services Administration.

U.S. Department of Health and Human Services. (2003). *Communicating in a crisis: Risk communication guidelines for public officials.* (DHHS Pub. No. SMA 3641). Rockville, MD. Center of Mental Health Services, Substance Abuse and Mental Health Services Administration.

Ursano, R. J., Fullerton, C. S., & Norwood, A. E. (1995). Psychiatric dimensions of disaster: Patient care, community consultation, and preventive medicine. *Harvard Review of Psychiatry*, *3*, 196-209.

Ursano, R. J., Fullerton, C. S., & Norwood, A. E. (2003) *Terrorism and disaster: Individual and community mental health interventions.* Cambridge, UK: Cambridge University Press.

Guide:
Building Bi-National Collaboration
in the Face of Terrorism

Shelley Horwitz
Roberta Leiner
Danny Brom
Claude M. Chemtob

In the face of public emergencies, philanthropic organizations can assume a leadership role beyond fundraising and traditional grant-making by developing and supporting transformative approaches to humanitarian crisis. We describe a specific response by a philanthropic organization, UJA-Federation of New York, to terrorism in the United States and Israel to illustrate opportunities to define innovation in catastrophes.

UJA-Federation of NY is the world's largest local philanthropy. It is a non-political, non-sectarian, human-service organization that helps 1.4 million people in New York, 3 million in Israel, and sustains activities in 60 other countries. UJA-Federation, representing the philanthropic commitment of New York Jews to Israel, brings to bear a unique bond, encapsulated by a shared heritage and identification that exceeds the typical funder/grantee relationship. Following the outbreak of the Al Aksa Intifada, UJA-Federation

Address correspondence to: Shelley Horwitz, MSW, UJA-Federation, 130 East 59th Street, New York, NY 10022 USA (E-mail: horwitzs@ujafedny.org).

[Haworth co-indexing entry note]: "Guide: Building Bi-National Collaboration in the Face of Terrorism." Horwitz, Shelley et al. Co-published simultaneously in *Journal of Aggression, Maltreatment & Trauma* (The Haworth Maltreatment & Trauma Press, an imprint of The Haworth Press, Inc.) Vol. 10, No. 3/4, 2005; and: *The Trauma of Terrorism: Sharing Knowledge and Shared Care, An International Handbook* (ed: Yael Danieli, Danny Brom, and Joe Sills) The Haworth Maltreatment & Trauma Press, an imprint of The Haworth Press, Inc., 2005.

made a strategic decision to establish and fund a coalition of trauma-related service providers in Israel to strengthen the trauma response capacity of the Israeli mental health system, bringing together Israeli experts and organizations with the goal of creating a continuum of trauma care in Israel.

September 11th prompted expansion of the concept of cooperative trauma service coordination to include New York City agencies involved in providing trauma recovery services. Bi-national collaboration was developed between trauma professionals and organizations through deployment of community organization principles to create a community of interests between experts and agencies in each of the countries.

A shared long-term strategic vision was developed through a series of forums, bi-national conferences, and videoconferences. The vision elements are: (a) decreasing fragmentation in trauma services, (b) collaborating to increase knowledge, skills, and services, (c) developing a comprehensive model of trauma services based on the application of a model for trauma response (preparedness, mitigation, intervention, and recovery), and (d) maintaining a vision of recovery that recognizes the opportunity for growth even under the worst circumstances. As a result, pre-existing collaborative projects were reorganized and became more bilateral as the shared experience of terrorism and trauma led to an increased identification and understanding, a deepening of connections and increased sharing of expertise, and ultimately, to the establishment of joint projects.

True partnership requires that partners derive essential benefits that may be practical, financial, intellectual, emotional, ethical, or religious. It is important to identify mutual benefits as well as divergent or sometimes conflicting interests. For example, among the benefits for American professionals: (a) deriving satisfaction from contributing expertise, (b) expanding knowledge by learning from a country living with ongoing terrorism, (c) field-testing concepts with the potential to advance the field of trauma services, and (d) strengthening the feeling of community. Among the benefits for Israelis: (a) financial resources, (b) additive perspective of 'outside eyes,' particularly helpful in mitigating the frequent tendency of trauma and crisis professionals to become over-involved, (c) connection and psychological support that helps counteract the isolation associated with coping with life-threatening circumstances, (d) professional development, and (e) upgrading of existing services.

A cornerstone of the bi-national collaboration has been shared learning and technology transfer. A sense of mutuality and respect rather than a paternalistic approach contributed toward building an effective bi-national team with different functions, from resource development and allocation to organizing and planning services, designing methods, and delivering direct services.

Engaging and mobilizing various constituencies (donor and professional) is an important element in successful collaboration. Funders may have competing emergencies, limited resources, compassion fatigue, policies or guidelines dictating time-limited projects, and interest in model development or seeding new projects. To the grantee, these may appear to reflect short attention spans, lack of commitment, or preferences for " boutique funding." Recruiting and building organizational support in both countries based on a strategic goal is a critical factor.

Creating a strategic vision is a crucial element in local empowerment and garnering support. It maximizes the potential for structural change and leveraging existing resources. The inherent challenge of assessing and responding to emergency needs while concurrently engaging in strategic short- and long-term planning is continuous.

Maintaining cross-cultural sensitivity is important, as cultural differences in collaborative style impact assumptions of shared understandings. The current situation intensifies the Israeli proclivity to adapt, assimilate, and integrate new ideas, models, and strategies, into a panoply of practice options (e.g., 'coping by doing'). Thus, circumstances and style do not leave sufficient time for reflection or deliberation. Americans tend to plan less incrementally, and the luxury of reflective space enables a broader perspective with time for method development, designing tools, and enhancing research and evaluation capacities. The need for explication, flexibility, and honesty is of the utmost importance in building true collaboration while acknowledging limitations and differences in approaches in order to minimize disappointments.

Establishing trust is an important element. The time-intensive work of building trusting relationships while operating in different time zones is an additional challenge that led, at times, to a bi-furcated planning process. Time differences can occasionally be used to an advantage, but impose long, stressful hours. Like the ebb and flow of any relationship, collaborations go through stages of mistrust, suspicion, ambivalence, disappointment, anger, rifts, and reconciliation along with idealization, intense bonding, dependency, hopefulness, and excitement, as well as passionate connection engendered by a shared vision and partnership.

There may be additional layers of complexities, since small and medium non-government organizations (NGOs) have individual interests in survival and accessing financial resources. Survival thus takes on additional dimensions: individual, organizational, and existential. The importance of continuous, honest, and transparent communication, as well as the acknowledgement of organizational differences, vested interests, divergent individual and/or organizational perspectives, even when sharing an overall vision and goal of changing a societal condition, is of critical necessity.

Sustainability is an important focus in establishing lasting change. Building a bi-national team and sharing a collective vision designed to capitalize on various strengths, assets, expertise, organizational capacities, and resources is key in fostering a successful international collaboration. Although philanthropy may initiate projects, ultimately linkages with government or creative public/private partnerships are an essential element for sustainable services.

Voice:
Assault on the United Nations:
Baghdad, 19 August 2003

Martin Barber

The Press Conference was drawing to a close. I had followed Sergio's[1] advice and expressed heartfelt sympathy to the people of Iraq for the pollution of their country by explosives of all kinds. Sergio was convinced that, given the chance, Iraqis could clean up the mess with some help from friends in the international community. A French journalist had asked a question. It was 4:30 p.m.

When the bomb went off, three things happened simultaneously: a deafening explosion, pitch darkness, and dust everywhere. I didn't move. I didn't feel surprise. I remember thinking, "Oh, so that's when it happens."

Those first three hours until we were taken back to the hotel passed in a blur, time seemingly suspended, but with many powerful images that would remain etched in my memory. I remember dead and dying colleagues covered in blood being brought out on the grass in front of the building. I remember a young black American soldier sitting disconsolately on the ground alone (he had been on guard duty at the front of the building). I remember Alan Johnson shouting "stay calm!" in the first seconds after the blast, and returning several times from his

Address correspondence to: Martin Barber, Director, United Nations Mine Action Service, 2 United Nations Plaza, Room 610, New York, NY 10017 USA (E-mail: barberm@un.org).

[Haworth co-indexing entry note]: "Voice: Assault on the United Nations: Baghdad, 19 August 2003." Barber, Martin. Co-published simultaneously in *Journal of Aggression, Maltreatment & Trauma* (The Haworth Maltreatment & Trauma Press, an imprint of The Haworth Press, Inc.) Vol. 10, No. 3/4, 2005; and: *The Trauma of Terrorism: Sharing Knowledge and Shared Care, An International Handbook* (ed: Yael Danieli, Danny Brom, and Joe Sills) The Haworth Maltreatment & Trauma Press, an imprint of The Haworth Press, Inc., 2005.

efforts to rescue Sergio from the rubble with increasingly desperate reports of his chances of survival. I remember the sudden outburst of grief from women who had worked in the cafeteria, when they were told that one of their co-workers had died. I remember holding a phone to Todd's ear as he told his wife in New Zealand that he loved her, and I remember the young Polish colleague who gave me his Australian bush hat as we sat in the open under the sun, because it was feared the fire from the blast would reach the fuel tanks.

What I am left with now is a terrible sadness for the loss of brilliant young people at the dawn of their lives and careers, gratitude for the spirit and bravery of those who risked their lives to rescue their colleagues from the building, compassion for the loved ones of those who died, who have to live the rest of their lives with that aching hole of loss in their hearts, and a sense that the time I am enjoying now is a bonus, extra innings, in which I must exceed my own expectations of myself.

Someone asked me if I felt unlucky to have been there. Even though I was a visitor to Baghdad, scheduled to spend only a few hours in the building, I have felt rather lucky that I was not in Sergio's office, as Arthur Helton was, when the bomb went off. I have not felt angry, perhaps that's my Buddhist training, but I feel terribly sorry for those suffering the guilt of feeling that they might have done more to prevent the disaster.

In 1997, I had been working in the UN Mission in Sarajevo, when word came that a helicopter carrying 12 of our colleagues had gone down in central Bosnia. All were killed. I became instantly absorbed in the arrangements for the memorial service and return of the bodies to families; this time, as a survivor, more of a numbing shock, a sense that violent emotions have been drummed out of me. This time, the messages from friends and colleagues have been hugely comforting. I consider myself a rather private person, who does not express emotions often or easily, but the experience of reading some of those messages presses home the importance of communicating with people who have suffered or lost. It may seem ridiculous to say this, but I have felt the impact of these messages almost literally like the effect of a healing ointment on a gaping wound. There is a feeling of relief, of being able to breathe more easily, of relaxing taut muscles, after sensing the compassion behind the words on the page.

NOTE

1. Sergio Vieira de Mello was the Special Representative of the United Nations Secretary-General in Iraq when the UN Headquarters at the Canal Hotel was hit by a terrorist bomb on 19 August 2003. He died in the rubble of the building about 90 minutes after the blast.

CONCLUSION

Sharing Knowledge and Shared Care

Yael Danieli
Danny Brom
Joe Sills

SUMMARY. This concluding article presents the main themes that emerged from this volume within a multidimensional, multidisciplinary integrative framework conceptualizing the consequences of the trauma of terrorism and informing optimal prevention and intervention methods. It reviews short- and long-term findings of the effects of terrorism on adults, children, families, communities, and societies and makes numerous research recommendations. Viewing terrorism as psychological warfare against the community, it advances community-based, culturally congruent interventions, with a public mental health approach, in an ongoing, integrated network of services promoting community and indi-

Address correspondence to: Yael Danieli, PhD, Group Project for Holocaust Survivors and their Children, 345 East 80th Street (31-J) New York, NY 10021 USA (E-mail: YAELD@aol.com).

[Haworth co-indexing entry note]: "Sharing Knowledge and Shared Care." Danieli, Yael, Danny Brom, and Joe Sills. Co-published simultaneously in *Journal of Aggression, Maltreatment & Trauma* (The Haworth Maltreatment & Trauma Press, an imprint of The Haworth Press, Inc.) Vol. 10, No. 3/4, 2005; and: *The Trauma of Terrorism: Sharing Knowledge and Shared Care, An International Handbook* (ed: Yael Danieli, Danny Brom, and Joe Sills) The Haworth Maltreatment & Trauma Press, an imprint of The Haworth Press, Inc., 2005.

vidual resilience, specialized training, international collaboration, and continued dialogue concerning the role of the media.

KEYWORDS. Trauma models, consequences of terrorism, community-based interventions, public mental health, integration of services, resilience, training, international collaboration, the role of the media

The preceding articles and voices capture some of the origins, nature, methods, and effects of terrorism, one of humanity's most tragic scourges. They also present some of today's most innovative and advanced, worldwide, comprehensive, compassionate, and effective responses to it.

This rich variety of approaches reflects the many challenges of the field, including: the difficulty in developing a comprehensive yet adequately parsimonious definition of terrorism; documenting the responses of individuals, families, and societies, and local, national, and international communities to specific acts of terrorism; and the development of a systematic and integrated network of services to counteract the devastating effects of terrorism. The three models proposed in this volume (Danieli's framework in the Introduction; Ayalon's in Berger; and the inverted psychosocial pyramid in Friedman) also attest to the complexity of the phenomena in that they all recognize the necessity for a multidimensional, multidisciplinary (e.g., psychological, educational, social, economic, legal, political), integrative framework for conceptualizing, analyzing, and designing optimal interventions. These models hold promise for the next generation of services.

Terrorism today is a force that influences the world in ways we would not have expected even a few years ago. The use of violence to instill fear as a means to political change is not new. The use of extreme showcase attacks such as 9/11, however, is unprecedented in both its enormity and its influence throughout the world. It also challenged all of us to create a "new normality" whose central question is: *How do we live with growing levels of threat, anxiety, fear, uncertainty, and loss?* If terrorism cannot be stopped by military or police action, individuals and societies must learn to live with this new sense of vulnerability. How does it affect us? How then do we protect ourselves?

Many authors point out that psychological responses to terrorism are neither simple nor easily predicted. Silver, Poulin, Holman, McIntosh, Gil-Rivas, and Pizarro's work on adults' responses to September 11 in the United States concludes that the "traditional" assumptions that only direct exposure to attacks matters are not valid. While post-9/11 surveys suggest that direct exposure to an attack is closely related to PTSD symptoms in adults, it is not related to non-specific distress, most of which is transient and self-limiting. These early studies indicate that adults who reported higher exposure to other traumatic events prior to 9/11 were significantly more likely to report higher levels of symptoms of depression, anxiety, and PTSD. Clearer definitions of the nature and effects of "exposure" are needed.

Future research should address the relation of television watching and prior traumatic events, among others. General population studies of the relationship between television watching and probable PTSD may help us understand those with prior traumatic experiences who were exposed to the current event only through television.

Reviewing empirical post-9/11 studies in adults, Schlenger concludes that the population- and community-based epidemiological studies should be considered preliminary. He calls for future studies to consider using well-validated measures of clinically significant symptoms, and to assess retrospective recall bias, probability samples, and the strong need for longitudinal design. More systematic study of the sequelae of terrorism, designed to support more definitive causal inferences, is needed. This research should: (a) clarify the full range of psychological responses to terrorism; (b) identify the most malignant aspects of terrorism and their specific pathogenic mechanisms, either of which may refine existing diagnostic constructs and/or lead to the development of new ones; and (c) identify effective early interventions and treatment interventions that combine to improve comprehensively victims' functioning.

Indeed, "a new normality" is the most productive concept for making sense of adaptations previously considered pathological. Hypervigilance, which can be highly functional and reframed as watchfulness in a society such as Israel, which is under constant threat of terrorist attacks, is an example (Solomon & Laufer, this volume). There is agreement that, for both analytical and operational purposes, a broader framework is essential. "A multidimensional, multidisciplinary framework provides the perspective to move beyond the starting points provided by symptom checklists and psychiatric diagnoses" (Engdahl, this volume).

Work on the impact of terrorism on children and adolescents is only now emerging. To date, no single pattern of post-attack outcomes has been identified and no studies so far have used a longitudinal design to assess the long-term impact of 9/11 on children. Further work on the impact of terrorism on developmental trajectories is thus necessary. Pfefferbaum, DeVoe, Stuber, Schiff,

Klein, and Fairbrother's review shows that children who are directly exposed to a terrorist attack are particularly vulnerable to adverse outcomes, but children with indirect exposures are also at risk. The authors suggest further investigation into age-specific vulnerabilities and competencies, including the capacity to assess danger and to make sense of a terrorist event, the significance of caregivers in shaping children's post-event adaptation, and a host of cultural factors.

Recognizing the need to address the full post-terrorism experience, this volume also focuses on grief and bereavement. In addition to Pivar and Prigerson's conclusion that researchers have been slow to recognize the necessity of measuring grief in the context of terrorism, Malkinson, Rubin, and Witztum emphasize the importance of a multi-dimensional assessment in cases of traumatic grief following terrorism in order to determine intervention strategies suited for the individual case.

Extending the findings to the family, community, and societal dimensions, Campbell, Cairns, and Mallett state that the 30 years "troubles" in Northern Ireland have touched most families and communities. An unanticipated finding was the major impact on the social fabric, as indicated by increased residential and educational segregation. Somasundaram highlights the "subtle but pernicious development of pathology in social structures and functioning that will need to be addressed if [Sri Lankan] society is to recover." Some of the collective, cumulative effects of terror there are deep suspicion and mistrust, passiveness and submissiveness, and social deterioration and brutalization, indexed by declines in sexual mores and social ethics and increased child abuse and suicide rates.

Consistent with many international findings, Khaled states: "Terrorism is not a temporary, time-limited phenomenon. Its effects extend–like an epidemic–in time and scope. The after effects are expected to last for many years to come and to extend to generations that have not been directly exposed to the crisis." Tracing a history of multiple traumata along the time dimension at different stages of development reveals that while for many people time heals ills, for *traumatized* people time may not heal, but may magnify and extend their response to further trauma and may carry intergenerational implications (Danieli, 1998). Norris, Watson, Hamblem, and Pfefferbaum noted the high level of affect still observable seven years after the Oklahoma City attack. Nonetheless, there seems to be little planning for the long-term effects of terrorism. Policies, plans, and projects are necessary internationally to address these needs. Additional systematic research is needed to document in detail the long-term course of the aftermath of repeated exposure to human-made traumata, including terrorism. Even though current findings on the effects of trauma on babies, toddlers, and children indicate that a main factor in the response in early childhood is determined by the state of the parent (see Danieli, 1998), the multigenerational effects of terrorism have not yet been sufficiently studied.

TERRORISM AND THE COMMUNITY: THE NEED FOR COMMUNITY-BASED MENTAL HEALTH PROGRAMS

The psychological and societal mechanisms to counteract threat have a common base, the need for human connection. When people are together and can share their experiences and concerns, fear diminishes. This may also mitigate at least some of the potential detriment of the *conspiracy of silence* (Danieli, 1985, 1993). Many of the programs described in this volume create frameworks for human connection in the aftermath of terrorist violence. To serve mental health and welfare needs, and thereby increase the ability of the population to withstand the stress of our times, existing institutions should be utilized, such as schools, workplaces, places of worship, community centers, and primary health care centers. Terrorism, by definition, is directed at the community, even when individuals are attacked. Its apparent randomness amplifies the entire community's fears. The community is targeted and responds as a community. However, much of the psychological trauma literature, certainly the research literature, focuses on the consequences for the individual. The more that wars and terrorists target civilian populations, the more important it becomes to develop approaches that conceptualize the community as their focus. Such approaches do not neglect individuals in need, but view the coherence and well-functioning of the community not only as contributing to successful coping with trauma at the individual and societal levels, but also as a defense against terrorism (Chemtob, this volume).

When communities feel threatened, a heightened bonding, coined the "honeymoon response" in the disaster literature, occurs. After terrorist attacks, people are also highly motivated to help others. These enhanced attachment responses and motivation to help can have strong societal benefits and should be harnessed and utilized for community health in general and in the planning for response to terrorism. In most instances, leaders spontaneously step forward to help. They should be informed about the need for and encouraged to promote psychosocial recovery efforts.

A community-based public health approach is "new territory for traditional clinicians, but one that addresses the needs of the population-at-large rather than self-selected individuals in distress who seek conventional, office-based treatment" (Friedman, this volume). In peacetime, the general attitude of service providers is passive, namely, needs express themselves through clients who seek services. In response to terrorist attacks, because of the potential number of people in need where waiting might create additional problems, there has been a shift to active outreach to victims. This integration of clinical and public health models demands a more active approach on the part of service providers and necessitates major training/inoculation efforts. This preparedness training is one of the core challenges for post-terrorism mental health care. While complex, the ongoing training including self-care and productive, yet responsible, use of non-professionals, paraprofessionals, and volunteers (see Pardess, this volume) are critical elements in strengthening support networks and preparing a community-based mental health response to terrorism.

"Cultural, religious, and ethnic differences are important elements in the prevention, assessment, and treatment of post-terrorism psychological sequelae" (Nader & Danieli, this volume). Culturally congruent intervention approaches that rely on the full range of indigenous resources and that the victims find acceptable and meaningful should be used (Danieli, Engdahl, & Schlenger, 2003). In Operation Recovery, initiated following the bombing of the U.S. embassy in Kenya in 1998, Kenyan mental health care providers adapted the western PTSD framework and counseling approaches as a starting point to local cultural and economic realities (Thielman, this volume). Project Liberty, created by the Federal Emergency Management Agency and the Community Mental Health Service in the New York City area in October 2001 after the attack on the World Trade Center, is "the largest disaster counseling effort ever" (Waizer, Dorin, Stoller, & Laird, this volume). It established the value of using culturally appropriate therapies as well as therapies that incorporated religious and spiritual beliefs into the healing process. A central element was the recruitment of a culturally, ethnically, and linguistically diverse staff that could reach out to New York City's large, foreign-born, and often previously traumatized community. Well-respected community members, rather than clinicians, were trained to use some basic counseling techniques based on the approach that the problem is a normal, expectable reaction to overwhelming stress. The critical role of spiritual caregivers became apparent as places of worship dramatically overflowed. The need to train and integrate disaster spiritual caregivers into disaster mental health care also became clear. Following 9/11, leaders in the field of disaster spiritual care have been determining "best practices" and developing standards for certification and training modules to assure appropriate care giving (Davidowitz-Farkas & Hutchinson-Hall, this volume). Incorporating volunteers into services after terrorist attacks can augment the community's capacity to respond. However, this should be done with caution to prevent relegating professional work to non-professional and insufficiently trained volunteers.

An interesting yet formidable challenge is to explore in-depth the meaning of community in different regions of the world, with differing levels of development, different cultures, in homogeneous and heterogeneous societies, in rural and urban settings. Most current worldwide research flows from a western academic framework and cultural background, and relies primarily on clinical reports. Indigenous community orientations and practices in developing countries may help and inform western cultures' newly appreciated focus on the community.

THE PUBLIC MENTAL HEALTH APPROACH

There is broad agreement among the contributors to this volume that the community-oriented and preparedness approach to post-disaster mental health should be akin to a public health model whose canon is the emphasis on wellness rather than illness, and is collaborative, multi-agency, and multidisciplinary. The fact that in a natural recovery process most somatic and psychological symptoms experienced after terrorist attacks are self-limiting makes it essential to differentiate nonspecific psychological distress from psychiatric illness. What may be required following major disasters then is "A more flexible structure, providing crisis counseling for most but true clinical care for a minority" (Norris, Watson, Hamblen, & Pfefferbaum, this volume).

Vardi calls for developing simple, innovative, and inexpensive methods to screen children for PTSD in primary health settings to bring those reluctant to seek treatment to professional caregivers. Pat-Horenczyk advocates a school-based screening method for detection of PTSD in youngsters and suggests that it be provided in a non-stigmatizing and non-clinical manner. Baum's program aims at empowering teachers and making them partners of mental health professionals.

Despite the finding that the majority of the people exposed who develop clinically significant psychological symptoms recover without formal intervention, the services available to individuals exposed to terrorism have developed from the clinical perspective, where the emphasis is on the psychopathological consequences and their treatment. Historically, the public mental health perspective has occupied a more meaningful place in the literature on natural rather than human-made disaster. This volume presents a compilation of conceptual and operational recommendations for closing this gap. In its strong emphasis on the community perspective, it underlines the need to integrate mental and public health.

If successful, one of the legacies of September 11 as well as of this volume would be a renewed and improved model for the delivery of mental health care that may reduce the prevailing stigmas associated with seeking and receiving mental health services. These stigmas are frequently culturally-based (i.e., there is a taboò against expressing mental health problems; Nader & Danieli, this volume). In the field of post-terrorism intervention, as in the trauma field in general, there is a fierce debate over the need for immediate intervention and how it should be delivered. Can we prevent ASD? Treat it? There is too little known about ways to prevent post-traumatic distress by immediate intervention. We know what does not work, but we have not actually seen validated methods for initial intervention. A systematic, worldwide comprehensive, comparative, cross-cultural study on the impact of interventions will provide invaluable data. "We must test the hypotheses spawned by a public mental health approach with the same scientific rigor we have utilized to evaluate psychosocial and pharmacological treatments developed for DSM-IV psychiatric disorders" (Friedman, this volume).

The threat of *bio*terrorism raises additional complications since bioterrorism is likely to create casualties presenting a mix of symptoms related both to the biologic agent itself and the terror experienced. Thus, the broader health care system must be prepared to recognize and serve individuals with this mixed symptomatology. In particular, the system must avoid dismissing the distress associated with the attack and be as forthcoming as possible about its known and unknown effects. Engel (2001) noted that "Polarized public discussion over science, policy, and media evidence following such incidents may reinforce the notion of cover-ups, create mutual doctor-patient mistrust, amplify symptom-related psychosocial distress and disability, and lead to unnecessary use of services. Under these circumstances, the clinician must always show respect, empathy and validation for a patient's concerns" (p. 48).

The Development of Integrated Services. Many articles in this volume indeed emphasize the organizational aspects of service delivery in the aftermath of terrorism. Focusing on citywide organization of services at the operational level, Laor, Wiener, and Wolmer call for integrating "multi-systemic and multidisciplinary teams while using mediating agents trained for the task by mental health specialists" (see also Jehel & Brunet, this volume). Levanon, Flamm-Oren, and Kahn-Hoffman, as well as Brom, outline a continuum of trauma services. These concepts, developed in response to war and terrorism, represent a new generation of approaches and attest to the validity of the need for a multidimensional, multidisciplinary integrative framework. Prevention, treatment, and welfare are no longer viewed as separate, but as interrelated elements of an integrative, seamless service framework. From the perspective of the time dimension, there is a need to build ongoing sustainable programs that ensure responsiveness and response-ability from a solid foundation. The timeline is to solidify *before*, keep flexible enough to respond to various forms *during* incidents of terrorism, and (re)adjust the programs and the responders *after*.

It is understandable, though disturbing, that collaboration among care agencies at all levels develops largely in response to threats to safety and mainly after actual disasters. Authors agree that waiting until after a disaster to plan a response is a recipe for failure as is a "one size fits all" approach. A major challenge for policymakers is to design and put into place realizable and sustainable response mechanisms in advance of the need for them. Alas, summarizing their interviews in Oklahoma City seven years after the bombing of the Murrah Building, Norris, Watson, Hamblen, and Pfefferbaum stated, "it appeared that Oklahoma City was not and is not well prepared." The state still had no formal, written plan for a future disaster mental health response.

Integration entails ongoing communication, collaboration, coordination, and cooperation. Elsewhere, Danieli, Rodley, and Weisaeth (1996) noted the risks of using these concepts uncritically. In addition, they emphasized that it is essential for agencies and programs to further define and develop complementary roles in their responses. Complementarity involves the tolerance of, respect for, and capitalizing on the differing strengths of the various partners: governments, NGOs, and the communities they serve. Sederer, Ryan, Gill, and Rubin emphasize prioritizing functions, defining jurisdiction, and reexamining role definition and hierarchy, and consider critical that safety net providers be included in the system's response. However, the principle remains that the interventions should address the broad set of dimensions that may be affected. Local involvement in its full contextual complexity is crucial to the success of any integrative attempt, particularly when outside assistance is involved; so is the reliance on existing infrastructures and long-term relationships.

RESILIENCE

Many of the articles consider individual and community resilience an important psychosocial protective factor in the struggle against the consequences of terrorism in particular and trauma exposure in general. Reissman, Spencer, Tanielian, and Stein define community resilience as "the ability of a community to withstand adversity and maintain cohesion and healthy functioning." Similarly, individual resilience can be defined as the ability of the individual to withstand adversity and maintain a sense of identity and a good level of functioning. Pre-disaster planning and outreach, in conjunction with public education campaigns, are needed in communities in order to bolster a sense of community resilience.

Resilience is a complex concept that unites multiple factors that determine the adequacy of the coping process. A person can be resilient in the face of one kind of traumatic event, while rendered helpless and symptomatic in another; s/he can maintain a good self-image in the face of horrific experiences, but at the same time adopt a cynical attitude toward the world. Cohen, Brom, and Dasberg (2001) have shown that high levels of posttraumatic symptoms in child survivors of the Holocaust do not necessarily mean that they suffer from general symptoms of psychosocial distress. People exhibit a mixture of symptoms and resilience. In time, they may congeal to adaptational styles (Danieli, 1985, and Introduction to this volume). The findings that survivors have areas of vulnerability as well as resilience is no longer paradoxical when viewed within a multidimensional framework for multiple levels of post-traumatic adaptation. Research still needs to explore questions such as: Does increasing resilience decrease/prevent psychopathology? What is the interplay over time of resilience and symptomatology? The answers should guide program development and prevention efforts.

Many projects described in this volume claim to increase resilience in different populations: Baum in teachers and school-age children; Waizer, Dorin, Stoller, and Laird, as well as Berger, within a wide range of community settings. Part VII addresses the resilience of the care system under the threat of terrorism. These efforts form the basis of the protection of the population against terrorism. However, there is an urgent need to develop valid measures of the multidimensional communal strengths and resources, community-level measures of traumatization, resilience, and recovery. Only when such measures exist will we be able to evaluate the efficacy of these efforts and intervene effectively to foster and promote resilience and recovery. The development of community assessment and intervention tools is an essential component of the future of the field of care. While a few tools are available to assess damage to, and resilience of, the community, their paucity presents a major challenge for service providers and researchers alike. "There are a lot of questions about what constitutes healthy community functioning. There is a need to examine this question across different disciplines: sociology, anthropology, community psychology and psychiatry, urban planning and grass-roots efforts" (Reissman, Spencer, Tanielian, & Stein, this volume).

SOME ISSUES IN TRAINING

A critical challenge in designing training is to tailor it to professionals and others who are at differing levels of knowledge and experience in trauma work. Training, credentialing, supervising, and monitoring of responders, including para-professionals and laypeople, are essential to ensure quality. Surprisingly little evidence has been gathered on the effectiveness of training (Amsel, Neria, Marshall, & Suh, this volume). Exposure to trauma has been shown to affect the interveners in multiple ways, both directly (sharing the same environment with the victims) and indirectly (listening to, or even reading, victims' accounts of their experiences in the context of attempting to help them or taking their testimonies). Those who help victims on the front lines are thus at high risk for double exposure. Danieli (2002) has addressed the costs they pay and their organizations' responsibility to train and support them before, during, and after their missions. The ubiquity of countertransference reactions has moved to the forefront of concern in the preparation and training of all professionals and others who work with victims and trauma survivors. Processing and working through *event countertransference* (Danieli, 1994), variously referred to as *vicarious traumatization* (Pearlman & Saakvitne, 1995), *secondary traumatic stress* (Hudnall Stamm, 1995), *burnout* (Maslach, 1982) or *compassion fatigue* (Figley, 1995), in the context of self-care (Danieli, this volume) are essential elements in training as well as during trauma work.

INTERNATIONAL COLLABORATION

An important element in the F.E.G.S. Project Liberty effort to define its approach to behavioral and infrastructure service was the contribution of Israeli colleagues who "taught . . . new approaches to staff training and a more flexible mix of mental health practice and public health outreach" (Waizer, Dorin, Stoller, & Laird, this volume). Horowitz, Leiner, Brom, and Chemtob prescribe bi-national cooperation "through deploying community organizing principles to create a community of interests between experts and agencies in each of [the] countries." International collaboration has the advantage of providing "an outside view" that allows people to see themselves through the eyes of the other when designing systems of self-care, evaluation, and service improvement. Continuing investigation of the causes of terrorism, as complex as they may be, is essential to informing policy choices aimed at controlling them.

As noted in the Foreword and the Introduction to this volume, the immediate response by the United Nations Security Council and General Assembly to the events of 9/11 included the creation of the Counter-Terrorism Committee (CTC), the goal of which is to aid member states in developing the legal, political, and operational capacity to carry out their responsibilities under Security Council Resolution 1373 to take specific actions to combat terrorism. Especially important is the continuous monitoring by the CTC of steps taken by member states to implement the provisions of Resolution 1373. The CTC needs also, with the support of donor nations, to supply technical and financial assistance to those countries lacking the capacity to implement these provisions. This volume, with its foci on the victims' experiences and combating and preventing the effects of terrorism, should supplement the work of the CTC.

The unanimous adoption in April 2004 by the Security Council of a resolution aimed at keeping chemical, biological, and nuclear weapons out of the hands of terrorists is a further step forward. It requires all UN member states to take legal steps to block the flow of these weapons, and establishes monitoring for a two-year period.

Another major policy issue is that of resources. The need for a greatly expanded system of mental health response to terrorism has been overwhelmingly established by this volume. If this need is to be met, research, preparation, and evaluation of mental health responses to terrorist attacks must be given higher priority and the necessary financial resources provided. The sheer organizational and financial resources required for prevention of terrorist risks and impacts and early detection of those at risk are daunting. As Laor, Wiener, and Wolmer note: "Most societies find it extremely hard to invest resources based on long-term considerations, and decide to spend resources only when faced with concrete challenges." This notwithstanding, major donor nations (e.g., the United States, the nations of Europe, Japan, and others) and the World Bank should incorporate funding for these needs into their development programs. Without such external support, there is little prospect that countries such as Sri Lanka or Algeria can implement the programs that are required.

This book should lead to greater bi-national and multinational cooperation in fighting terrorism and its malignant consequences. As difficult as it may be to accomplish, international collaboration will enhance intervention, research, and policy development.

Perhaps the most difficult policy issue raised in this volume is "terrorism's toll on civil liberties" (Strossen, this volume). It would be difficult enough to embrace many of the reductions in civil liberties that accompany the "war on terrorism" in the United States even had they been shown to be effective in reducing the threat of terrorism. However, there is little evidence that they are doing so. This central concern must be raised in countries whose regimes, historically repressive, are using the battle against terrorism as a cover for persecuting those who oppose them. It must remain at the forefront of formulating policies for meeting the threat of terrorism and mitigating its effects.

THE ROLE OF THE MEDIA

Terrorists view the media as a powerful tool in their psychological warfare. Television and the Internet are increasingly used to cover terrorists' attacks, their demands, and the retributions inflicted when these demands are not met.

A fundamental question concerning issues of policy, press freedom, and journalistic ethics arises: Should the media provide full and immediate coverage of terrorist attacks, interview their leaders, and publicize their threats and demands, basing decisions solely on judgments of newsworthiness, knowing fully that they are doing exactly what the terrorists want? Or can they be expected to exercise limits on their coverage in order to avoid being used by terrorists? Weimann calls for "reducing and censoring news coverage of terrorists acts" thus "minimizing the terrorists' capacity for manipulating the media." He and others feel, however, that self- rather than externally-imposed restrictions and guidelines should be used.

A second question related to the media involves the effects of coverage. Several authors note the strong association of PTSD symptom levels with extensive watching of television coverage of the September 11 attacks. Some, however, recognize the power of the media to generate positive effects and their responsibility, as members of society, to the victims and to society. Gina Ross views the media as an asset in helping the public cope with fear and terror. It is reasonable to expect the media to regularly print and broadcast information and warnings regarding terrorism as they do with natural disasters. In addition, in consultation with the relevant authorities and substantive experts, the media could voluntarily assist in frustrating the goals of terrorists as well as in aiding in the healing of the population following terrorist attacks (see also Thielman, this volume). Compassionate articulation (Spratt, 2002) is a feature shared by good leaders and good reporters.

The Media section in Danieli (2002) discussed the costs paid by journalists exposed to trauma and destruction, and the impact on their reporting and their lives (see also G. Ross, this volume). It also emphasized the obligation of news organizations to train and support them before, during, and after these assignments.

There is an ongoing discussion among governments, non-governmental organizations, and the media about these questions in the context of responsible journalism. The editors applaud this debate and call for its continuation and expansion in full recognition of the paramount issues involved.

Ruzek (2002) notes that the use of the Internet as venue for delivery of a broad range of psychosocial interventions will likely increase in importance given relatively low development costs, its ability to reach large numbers of people, the potential to "customize" content to particular disasters and audiences, and the ability to exert quality control over content. Groups of survivors can also use the Internet to access virtual support facilitated by discussion forums that may provide them with a tool to articulate their collective concerns and needs.

AS WE GO TO PRESS

As we go to press, this seemingly never-ending scourge continues. On the morning of March 11, 2004, in Madrid, Spain, a series of coordinated terrorist bombings against the commuter train system killed 191 people and wounded more than 1,800, shocking both the nation and the international community. We are outraged and haunted by this attack and the horrific terrorist attack on the Beslan school in Russia on September 1, 2004, the first day of the term. While proud parents were escorting their children to their classes, the school was seized by heavily-armed terrorists who took over 1,300 hostages. During the three-day siege, they were threatened with improvised explosive devices, and with execution. According to government figures, some 340 innocent people–half of them children–were killed.

Those who survived–especially the children, bereaved parents, grandparents, but also their community as a whole–will bear the mental scars from these atrocities. Their psychological wounds cannot simply be put behind them; they cannot be expected to "get on with their lives" lest they create a pathogenic *conspiracy of silence*. Their healing will be a difficult, complex, long process. They must be given the right kind of therapeutic care throughout the years ahead. Otherwise, their suffering would continue unabated not only for their own lifetimes but multigenerationally.

These tragedies still await serious systematic research. Answers need to be found to help prevent the wounds from festering, perhaps even to avert future cycles of violence.

CAN THERE BE A DIALOGUE?

Terrorists see themselves as fighters for a worthy cause, even though others may argue that some terrorists are seeking destruction only. Narratives of terrorists and their victims differ vastly. While terrorists often see themselves as freedom fighters, others view them as evil criminals. While survivors see themselves mostly as innocent victims of violence, the terrorists see them as symbols of oppressive and evil regimes. These counterposing perceptions are key obstacles to a dialogue that may lead to peace and cessation of terror rather than to the continued inflaming cycles of violence around the world.

We do find hope for healing and reconciliation in initiatives such as the Parents Circle-Families Forum of Israeli and Palestinian bereaved families (www.theparentscircle.org). Since its foundation in 1995 by family members who have lost a close relative due to the ongoing violence in the Middle East, the Families Forum has promoted reconciliation as an alternative to the prevailing cycle of hatred and revenge. Some 500 Forum members have chosen to play a unique role of showing by example that even those who have suffered the most can, through dialogue and mutual understanding, acknowledge and share the other side's pain and develop tolerance and trust rather than seek revenge for their loss.

Since the Intifada, direct dialogue has been extremely difficult. As a partial solution, the organization has set up a free telephone line (Hello Peace) to enable Palestinians and Israelis to share their experiences, important or mundane. There is only one rule: that the person on the other side must listen. Since its inception in October 2002, some 800,000 people have spoken to one another through this telephone line.

As part of an ongoing educational effort embodying the very essence of the Forum, personal contact among people on opposite sides of the conflict that allows meeting actual people behind the stigmas and the stereotypes, bereaved families share their stories and their pain in lectures to high school students, adult audiences, and policy makers (1,600 over the past year). Without this process of humanization of both societies, they believe that peace agreements signed by leaders will never lead to a lasting peace.

This universal message by those who share some of humanity's most intense and lasting pain is the seed of hope that trauma need not necessarily lead to further violence. This is the hope that motivated the editors and authors of this book.

REFERENCES

Cohen, M., Brom, D., & Dasberg, H. (2001). Child survivors of the Holocaust: Symptoms and coping after 50 years. *Israel Journal of Psychiatry, 38*(1), 3-12.

Danieli, Y. (1985). The treatment and prevention of long-term effects and intergenerational transmission of victimization: A lesson from Holocaust survivors and their children. In C. R. Figley (Ed.), *Trauma and its wake* (pp. 295-313). New York: Brunner/Mazel.

Danieli, Y. (1993). The diagnostic and therapeutic use of the multi-generational family tree in working with survivors and children of survivors of the Nazi Holocaust. In

D. Meichenbaum (Series Ed.) & J. P. Wilson & B. Raphael (Vol. Eds.), *Stress and coping series: International handbook of traumatic stress syndromes* (pp. 889-898). New York: Plenum Publishing.

Danieli, Y. (1994). Countertransference, trauma and training. In J. P. Wilson & J. Lindy (Eds.). *Countertransference in the treatment of post-traumatic stress disorder* (pp. 368-388). New York: Guilford Press.

Danieli, Y. (Ed.). (1998). *International handbook of multigenerational legacies of trauma.* New York: Kluwer Academic/Plenum Publishing Corporation.

Danieli, Y. (Ed.). (2002). *Sharing the front line and the back hills: International protectors and providers, peacekeepers, humanitarian aid workers and the media in the midst of crisis.* Amityville, NY: Baywood Publishing Company, Inc.

Danieli, Y., Engdahl, B., & Schlenger, W. E. (2003). The psychological aftermath of terrorism. In F. M. Moghaddam & A. J. Marsella (Eds.), *Understanding terrorism: Psychological roots, consequences, and interventions* (pp. 223-246) Washington, DC: American Psychological Association.

Danieli, Y., Rodley, N. S., & Weisaeth, L. (Eds.) (1996). *International responses to traumatic stress: Humanitarian, human Rights, justice, peace and development contributions, collaborative actions and future initiatives.* Published for and on behalf of the United Nations by Baywood Publishing Company, Inc., Amityville, NY.

Engel, C. (2001). Outbreaks of medically unexplained physical symptoms after military action, terrorist threat, or technological disaster. *Military Medicine, 166*(Suppl. 2), 47-48.

Figley, C. R. (Ed.). (1995). *Compassion fatigue: Coping with secondary traumatic stress disorder in those who treat the traumatized.* New York: Brunner/Mazel.

Hudnall Stamm, B. (Ed.). (1995). *Secondary traumatic stress: Self-care issues for clinicians, researchers, & educators.* Lutherville, MD: Sidran Press.

Maslach, C. (1982). *Burnout: The cost of caring.* Englewood Cliffs, NJ: Prentice-Hall.

Pearlman, L. A., & Saakvitne, K. W. (1995). *Trauma and the therapist: Countertransference and vicarious traumatization and psychotherapy with incest survivors.* New York: W. W. Norton & Company.

Ruzek, J. (2002). Dissemination of information and early intervention practices in the context of mass violence or large-scale disaster. *The Behavior Therapist, 25,* 32–36.

Spratt, M. (2002, August 28). *9/11 Media may comfort, terrify.* Retrieved on August 29, 2002 from: http://www.dartcenter.org

Epilogue

Sir Jeremy Greenstock

I am sitting in the protected Green Zone of the Coalition Provisional Authority Headquarters in Baghdad and wondering how my diplomatic career, its retirement clock stopped to allow a final contribution to the rebuilding of Iraq, has left me in this cage of concrete walls, Marine guards, and Close Protection teams. The world of democracy, choice, economic opportunity, and tolerance, which I imagined I was here to promote, has to be built by communication and the release of the human spirit. How can the hatred, resentment, and bloodthirstiness of a tiny minority of twisted souls have so constrained the instincts and wishes of the vast majority?

At the time of writing, it is two years and five months (is that all?) since that strange news flash, as I drove to a United Nations (UN) meeting in East Manhattan, about someone hitting the World Trade Center with an aircraft. An accident waiting to happen? There were two aircraft. Was it a deliberate act? They were airliners. It has to be terrorism. Other planes have crashed into the Pentagon and into the ground in Pennsylvania. It must, I said to myself and then to my European Union colleagues, be Bin Laden.

It would prove to be weeks, months, and then years before we could calculate the full breadth of the implications of that morning: not just the number of people killed and the much greater number of lives overturned and disrupted by their loss, but also the need to nurse a shocked society back into normal, if

---

Address correspondence to: Sir Jeremy Greenstock, GCMG (E-mail: AandJlondon@aol.com).

[Haworth co-indexing entry note]: "Epilogue." Greenstock, Sir Jeremy. Co-published simultaneously in *Journal of Aggression, Maltreatment & Trauma* (The Haworth Maltreatment & Trauma Press, an imprint of The Haworth Press, Inc.) Vol. 10, No. 3/4, 2005; and: *The Trauma of Terrorism: Sharing Knowledge and Shared Care, An International Handbook* (ed: Yael Danieli, Danny Brom, and Joe Sills) The Haworth Maltreatment & Trauma Press, an imprint of The Haworth Press, Inc., 2005.

changed, ways of living. The recognition of the psychological impact of terrorism on individuals, communities, societies, and nations, and of the need to strengthen our capacity to aid its victims and limit its reverberating effects, is what this volume has all been about. This expression of collective concern must parallel our efforts both to stop in their tracks those who plan and perpetrate terrorism and to understand and address its underlying causes.

On that horrifying Tuesday, we had to evacuate the UN Headquarters building soon afterwards because the UN itself had come up on the screen as a potential target. But then the UN took up with a will the task of constructing its own substantive response. Within 24 hours, the Security Council had met and unanimously adopted, without argument, Resolution 1368 condemning the attack as a terrorist act and opening the way to legitimate action by the United States to defend itself militarily. The General Assembly, with no opposing vote, followed suit the next day. Cultural, political, and diplomatic differences in that great boiling-pot of subjective argument were stilled in overwhelming sympathy for the victim of an act of world-perturbing brutality.

Sixteen days after SCR 1368, the Security Council passed SCR 1373 (September 28, 2001) by fifteen votes to nil. The draft, an American proposal, was the most severe collection of measures ever put forward in the UN to require every Member State to take specific action against offenders of the UN Charter. There was virtually no argument about the draft. The most awkward questioning of its precise terms came in fact from the United Kingdom, which had specific concerns over the operative sub-paragraph on asylum.

By 4 October 2001, the Committee established under SCR 1373 to monitor implementation was up and running under my Chairmanship, itself an unusual step as Chairs of Committees are the provenance of Non-Permanent Members of the Council. For the next 18 months, we met every week, sometimes every day of the working week, to bring the whole membership of the UN to take the requirements of 1373 seriously. It is unheard of to find 100% of the UN's 191 members fulfilling their obligations under a particular resolution. Fifty percent is enough of a miracle. By the time I handed over the chair to my Spanish colleague on 4 April 2003, all but seven states had taken up the task.

That in itself was of course not going to bring terrorism to its knees. We all knew that. The phenomenon of the use of shocking violence to deter resistance or break down normal defences has a long history. But 9-11 indicated a change of scale and reach. Governments everywhere immediately looked less capable of defending the peace on their territory. The costs of law and order had risen because free societies could no longer take goodwill and respect for freedom for granted, and because the power of modern weapons exploited by tiny numbers in an open world had been demonstrated. But something more had to be done than action by the United States and its Allies to seek out and deal with those who were guilty of actual terrorist murder. Terrorism had to be starved of room to grow and oxygen to breathe across the planet; and this could not be left only to those states with power to reach beyond their own borders. The United States subscribed to that proposition just as strongly as anyone else. All Governments had to act. We all knew, too, that we were setting in hand an exercise which would take many years, perhaps decades, of hard work to bring to effective results. That spirit of universal shock and disgust at the perpetration of 9-11 had to be distilled into a global determination to brand terrorism an enemy of the new Millennium. So far, these aims have only begun to be realised. Going global in this way has become part of the psychological remedy for the collective trauma of 9-11: we have all been affected and must all respond.

Modern life with its short-term focus is, alas, hard on ideals that take time and care to fructify. The whole world came out in sympathy with the US over 9-11. But hardly any other country was prepared to write a blank cheque for the United States on its own to compose the comprehensive follow-up required. The questions soon started coming in. How can we define terrorism to everyone's satisfaction? What are the root causes of terrorism and do they not include world poverty and deprivation? How far can the right to use force in self-defence be taken? Is there a basis for pre-empting the use of violence against an individual or a state? The doubts sown and the political subjectivism released threatened to overwhelm the collective will to deal with the mindless use of force. They still do.

This is why settling the new Iraq matters for the sanity of the modern world, beyond all the controversy about the reasons for military action and the legitimacy of the current phase. There are two conflicts active on Iraqi soil. One is a despairing attempt by the leftovers of Saddam's regime to prove anything but despotism a forlorn hope for the ruling of the country. The weight of Iraqi opinion against that view will tell. The other is an effort by the most dangerous of the organised global terrorists to take on the champions of the Western vision of an ordered world, on what they see as their ground politically and geographically.

We do not yet know for sure how it will turn out. The American-led alliance cannot be defeated in strategic terms. But the avoidance of civil strife between the communities of an Iraq awash with weapons and historical resentments, the guarantee that a bomb will not go off somewhere, against whatever undeserving and indiscriminately chosen target to prove the elusiveness of the rule of law, the granting of the wish of the vast majority of Iraqis for a peaceful life under a government they have chosen, all these are hard prospects when life and C4 explosive have become so cheap. Once again, Iraqis (not foreigners on their soil) will be the arbiters of that. Non-Iraqi groups of killers are no more wanted in their midst than foreign governors.

The roots back to 9-11 will be clear when the full history of these times is written. The destruction of the Twin Towers signaled a deviation from the positive and upward march of globalisation that we should have predicted, because freedom nearly always profits the criminal before the law-abiding. It takes time for people of goodwill to mobilise. The comparative advantage of using indiscriminate violence in an otherwise peaceful environment is a danger that the modern world has not yet learned to counter. Using powerful weapons in large-scale response is not the solution, or not the solution on its own. Ending Saddam Hussein's rule is only one element of a broader strategy. There has to be cultural and political understanding to match the global spread of communication, travel, and trade; or these three make a lack of understanding all the more explosive.

Plenty of wise voices have said as much at the UN and elsewhere, though almost always they have said it to make a political or a cultural point. That is not good enough. There has to be an absolute commitment by a very large number to address comprehensively the implications of global interchange. And that requires people and governments to put the global before the national priority. I do not see this being a practical concept except through the workings of the United Nations, our only global institution, whose potential strengths have not yet been fully realised. If the UN can find a fresh courage, the courage of a De Mello writ large, in this next phase in Iraq, it may be able to demonstrate a new capacity for leadership, in the most complex of international circumstances and in the face of the most unpleasant form of terrorism. Then there is a chance that the right lessons will have been learned from the trauma of 9-11 and its aftermath, and that the care and sympathy generated to restore the spirits of those most affected by terrorist violence will spread through the international community as a whole.

Index

The *Journal of Aggression, Maltreatment & Trauma* Monographic "Separates"

Robert Geffner, PhD, ABPN, Senior Editor

Below is a list of "separates," which in serials librarianship means a special issue simultaneously published as a special journal issue or double-issue *and* as a "separate" hardbound monograph. (This is a format which we also call a "DocuSerial.")

"Separates" are published because specialized libraries or professionals may wish to purchase a specific thematic issue by itself in a format which can be separately cataloged and shelved, as opposed to purchas-ing the journal on an on-going basis. Faculty members may also more easily consider a "separate" for classroom adoption.

"Separates" are carefully classified separately with the major book jobbers so that the journal tie-in can be noted on new book order slips to avoid duplicate purchasing.

The Trauma of Terrorism: Sharing Knowledge and Shared Care, An International Handbook, ed-ited by Yael Danieli, PhD, Danny Brom, PhD, and Joe Sills, MA, (Vol. 9, No. 1/2 and 3/4, 2004 and Vol. 10, No. 1/2 and 3/4, 2005. *"This book pulls together key programs that enable society to cope with ongoing terrorism, and is thus a rich resource for both policymakers and those who aid terrorism's victims directly. It demonstrates the invaluable collaboration between govern-ment and private initiative in the development of a resilient society." (Danny Naveh, Minister of Health, Government of Israel)*

The Victimization of Children: Emerging Issues, edited by Janet L. Mullings, PhD, James W. Marquart, PhD, and Deborah J. Hartley, MS (Vol. 8, No. 1/2 [#15/16] and 3 [#17], 2003). *"A fascinating, illuminating, and often troubling collection of research on child victimization, abuse, and neglect. This book . . . is timely, thought-provoking, and an important contribution to the literature. No other book on the market today provides such an authoritative overview of the complex issues involved in child victimization." (Craig Hemmens, JD, PhD, Chair and Associate Professor, Department of Criminal Justice Administration, Boise State University)*

Intimate Violence: Contemporary Treatment Innovations, edited by Donald Dutton, PhD, and Dan-iel J. Sonkin, PhD (Vol. 7, No. 1/2 [#13/14], 2003). *"Excellent. . . . Represents 'outside the box' thinking. I highly recommend this book for everyone working in the field of domestic violence who wants to stay fresh. Readers will be stimulated and in most cases very valuably informed." (David B. Wexter, PhD, Executive Director, Relationship Training Institute, San Diego, CA)*

Trauma and Juvenile Delinquency: Theory, Research, and Interventions, edited by Ricky Greenwald, PsyD (Vol. 6, No. 1 [#11], 2002). *"Timely, concise, compassionate, and stimulating. . . . An impressive array of authors deals with various aspects of the problem in depth. This book will be of considerable interest to clinicians, teachers, and researchers in the mental health field, as well as administrators and juvenile justice personnel handling juvenile delinquents. I highly commend Dr. Greenwald on a job well done." (Hans Steiner, MD, Professor of Psychiatry and Behavioral Sciences, Stanford University School of Medicine)*

Domestic Violence Offenders: Current Interventions, Research, and Implications for Policies and Standards, edited by Robert Geffner, PhD, and Alan Rosenbaum, PhD (Vol. 5, No. 2 [#10], 2001).

The Shaken Baby Syndrome: A Multidisciplinary Approach, edited by Stephen Lazoritz, MD, and Vincent J. Palusci, MD (Vol. 5, No. 1 [#9], 2001). *The first book to cover the full spectrum of Shaken Baby Syndrome (SBS). Offers expert information and advice on every aspect of prevention, diagnosis, treatment, and follow-up.*

Trauma and Cognitive Science: A Meeting of Minds, Science, and Human Experience, edited by Jennifer J. Freyd, PhD, and Anne P. DePrince, MS (Vol. 4, No. 2 [#8] 2001). *"A fine collection of scholarly works that address key questions about memory for childhood and adult traumas from a variety of disciplines and empirical approaches. A must-read volume for anyone wishing to understand traumatic memory." (Kathryn Quina, PhD, Professor of Psychology & Women's Studies, University of Rhode Island)*

Program Evaluation and Family Violence Research, edited by Sally K. Ward, PhD, and David Finkelhor, PhD (Vol. 4, No. 1 [#7], 2000). *"Offers wise advice to evaluators and others interested in understanding the impact of their work. I learned a lot from reading this book." (Jeffrey L. Edleson, PhD, Professor, University of Minnesota, St. Paul)*

Sexual Abuse Litigation: A Practical Resource for Attorneys, Clinicians, and Advocates, edited by Rebecca Rix, MALS (Vol. 3, No. 2 [#6], 2000). *"An interesting and well developed treatment of the complex subject of child sexual abuse trauma. The merger of the legal, psychological, scientific and historical expertise of the authors provides a unique, in-depth analysis of delayed discovery in CSA litigation. This book, including the extremely useful appendices, is a must for the attorney or expert witness who is involved in the representation of survivors of sexual abuse." (Leonard Karp, JD, and Cheryl L. Karp, PhD, co-authors, Domestic Torts: Family Violence, Conflict and Sexual Abuse)*

Children Exposed to Domestic Violence: Current Issues in Research, Intervention, Prevention, and Policy Development, edited by Robert A. Geffner, PhD, Peter G. Jaffe, PhD, and Marlies Sudermann, PhD (Vol. 3, No. 1 [#5], 2000). *"A welcome addition to the resource library of every professional whose career encompasses issues of children's mental health, well-being, and best interest . . . I strongly recommend this helpful and stimulating text." (The Honorable Justice Grant A. Campbell, Justice of the Ontario Superior Court of Justice, Family Court, London, Canada)*

Maltreatment in Early Childhood: Tools for Research-Based Intervention, edited by Kathleen Coulborn Faller, PhD (Vol. 2, No. 2 [#4], 1999). *"This important book takes an international and cross-cultural look at child abuse and maltreatment. Discussing the history of abuse in the United States, exploring psychological trauma, and containing interviews with sexual abuse victims,* Maltreatment in Early Childhood *provides counselors and mental health practitioners with research that may help prevent child abuse or reveal the mistreatment some children endure."*

Multiple Victimization of Children: Conceptual, Developmental, Research, and Treatment Issues, edited by B. B. Robbie Rossman, PhD, and Mindy S. Rosenberg, PhD (Vol. 2, No. 1 [#3], 1998). *"This book takes on a large challenge and meets it with stunning success. It fills a glaring gap in the literature . . . " (Edward P. Mulvey, PhD, Associate Professor of Child Psychiatry, Western Psychiatric Institute and Clinic, University of Pittsburgh School of Medicine)*

Violence Issues for Health Care Educators and Providers, edited by L. Kevin Hamberger, PhD, Sandra K. Burge, PhD, Antonnette V. Graham, PhD, and Anthony J. Costa, MD (Vol. 1, No. 2 [#2], 1997). *"A superb book that contains invaluable hands-on advice for medical educators and health care professionals alike . . . " (Richard L. Holloways, PhD, Professor and Vice Chair, Department of Family and Community Medicine, and Associate Dean for Student Affairs, Medical College of Wisconsin)*

Violence and Sexual Abuse at Home: Current Issues in Spousal Battering and Child Maltreatment, edited by Robert Geffner, PhD, Susan B. Sorenson, PhD, and Paula K. Lundberg-Love, PhD (Vol. 1, No. 1 [#1], 1997). *"The Editors have distilled the important questions at the cutting edge of the field of violence studies, and have brought rigor, balance and moral fortitude to the search for answers." (Virginia Goldner, PhD, Co-Director, Gender and Violence Project, Senior Faculty, Ackerman Institute for Family Therapy)*

T - #0442 - 101024 - C0 - 212/152/50 - PB - 9780789027733 - Gloss Lamination